Concepts in Pharmacogenomics

Martin M. Zdanowicz, Ph.D., MA
Professor of Pharmaceutical Sciences
South University School of Pharmacy
Savannah, GA

American Society of Health–System Pharmacists®
Bethesda, MD

Any correspondence regarding this publication should be sent to the publisher, American Society of Health-System Pharmacists, 7272 Wisconsin Avenue, Bethesda, MD 20814, attention: Special Publishing.

The information presented herein reflects the opinions of the contributors and advisors. It should not be interpreted as an official policy of ASHP or as an endorsement of any product.

Because of ongoing research and improvements in technology, the information and its applications contained in this text are constantly evolving and are subject to the professional judgment and interpretation of the practitioner due to the uniqueness of a clinical situation. The editors, contributors, and ASHP have made reasonable efforts to ensure the accuracy and appropriateness of the information presented in this document. However, any user of this information is advised that the editors, contributors, advisors, and ASHP are not responsible for the continued currency of the information, for any errors or omissions, and/or for any consequences arising from the use of the information in the document in any and all practice settings. Any reader of this document is cautioned that ASHP makes no representation, guarantee, or warranty, express or implied, as to the accuracy and appropriateness of the information contained in this document and specifically disclaims any liability to any party for the accuracy and/or completeness of the material or for any damages arising out of the use or non-use of any of the information contained in this document.

Director, Special Publishing: Jack Bruggeman
Acquisitions Editor: Rebecca Olson
Senior Editorial Project Manager: Dana Battaglia
Production Editors: Kristin Eckles and Bill Fogle
Composition: Yvonne Yirka
Cover and page design: Carol Barrer

Library of Congress Cataloging-in-Publication Data

Concepts in pharmacogenomics / [edited by] Martin M. Zdanowicz.
     p. ; cm.
  Includes bibliographical references.
  ISBN 978-1-58528-234-0
  1. Pharmacogenomics. I. Zdanowicz, Martin M. II. American Society of Health-System Pharmacists.
  [DNLM: 1. Pharmacogenetics. QV 38 C7445 2010]
  RM301.3.G45C665 2010
  615'.7--dc22
                              2010002089
ASHP is a service mark of the American Society of Health-System Pharmacists, Inc.; registered in the U.S. Patent and Trademark Office.
ISBN 978-1-58528-234-0

Dedication

I would like to dedicate this textbook to my wife Christine and to my children Alex and Olivia. You are the source of all the joy, love, and inspiration that fills my life.

Preface

Before I began to outline potential chapters for this text, I sat for a long while in my office just pondering how I could tell the story of pharmacogenomics in a way that would be practical and interesting to pharmacists, pharmacy students, and healthcare providers in general. I thought back to my own graduate training in pharmacology during the 80s and 90s. It was an exciting time in the field of pharmacology, because molecular biology was really taking hold and the technology was becoming available for the first time to investigate how drugs could affect cells and organisms at the actual molecular level. As wonderful and amazing as many of these advances in molecular pharmacology were to us pharmacologists, it was a science that remained principally one discussed and applied in research laboratories and pharmaceutical company drug development and discovery divisions.

While the science behind molecular pharmacology gradually found its way into pharmacy school curriculums, it had little direct impact on the day-to-day practice from the pharmacist's perspective. This is not the case with pharmacogenomics. Although classic drug training for pharmacists focused (and still does) on medicinal chemistry, pharmacology, pharmacokinetics, and therapeutics, students of pharmacy are taught that patients are individuals and that drug responses from person to person can vary. The potential for pharmacokinetic and pharmacodynamic variability is emphasized. Discussion often focuses on how aging or the presence of various disease states can alter a patient's pharmacokinetic response to drugs. Drug-food and drug-drug interactions are likewise highlighted as potential factors that can lead to variability in drug response. Practitioners have long been aware that even perfectly healthy patients given the same dose of the same drug can have different responses. Some patients are recognized as just being "fast" or "slow" metabolizers of certain drugs.

In short, pharmacists are used to treating patients as individuals who oftentimes require customized drug regimens. In recent years, a new factor has emerged, which clearly and unequivocally can alter individuals' response to drugs, their genetic makeup. Genetics is just one more factor along with age, body mass, liver and kidney function, etc., that pharmacists must now consider when choosing the best drug regimen for their patients. Reviewing key features of a patient's genetic makeup should, therefore, not seem foreign to pharmacists who already consider a number of factors in their individual patients when choosing the correct drug and dose.

In the past few years, several colleagues and I have been interested in looking at the current state of pharmacogenomics education and application in both the didactic and experiential portion of the curriculum in schools of pharmacy. One of the findings of our studies was that textbooks and various other resources that pharmacists could use to further their own education regarding pharmacogenomics were lacking. That finding, coupled with our own interest in offering a solid elective course in pharmacogenomics, was a main driving force behind this text. When compiling a list of topics for inclusion, there were several key elements I felt that needed to be emphasized if this book was going to be successful. First, the chapters needed to be written in a manner that was simple, clear, and organized. I stressed to the individual chapter authors that their material needed to be written in a way that facilitated clear understanding and direct application. It was written at a level that would have broad usefulness to pharmacists practicing in all areas as well as to fellows, residents, and students at various points in their training and with varying knowledge of pharmacogenomics. Second, I felt it was vital that chapters be written by individuals who used, taught, or had a thorough understanding of pharmacogenomics and the impact it could have in their particular area of expertise. Third, it needed to be fully up to date when published. Because the field of pharmacogenomics is so rapidly evolving, a companion website is envisioned on which authors can post regular updates and other supplemental materials for their chapters. Lastly, the text was organized in such a manner that would facilitate its use as a primary resource for both required and elective courses in pharmacogenomics. From an organizational standpoint, the presentation is divided into three distinct sections. The first focuses on the basic science involved in pharmacogenomics with emphasis on current methodology, pharmacodynamics, and pharmacokinetics. The second section presents a system-based approach to therapeutic applications of pharmacogenomics, while the third section focuses on related topics (bioethical considerations, educational issues, PG testing, pharmacists role, etc.) that are essential for a thorough understanding and appreciation of pharmacogenomics.

This textbook incorporates a number of features that are designed to enhance its usefulness and practicality. Key definitions are included at the front of each chapter so readers can be clear on the meaning of certain important words before they delve into the chapter. Case studies are also embedded within each chapter in order to stimulate critical thinking and clinical application by the reader. Clinical pearls are sprinkled throughout the chapters at select points to emphasize important concepts and highlight clinical applications. Numerous summary tables and figures are also included within the text to enhance and supplement each author's presentation.

It is my hope that after completing this text, readers will have a new appreciation and understanding of the potential impact of pharmacogenomics, regardless of whether they are a new student of pharmacy or a seasoned practitioner. I particularly hope that pharmacists who read this text will come to appreciate how their unique qualifications and training make them ideally suited for playing a leading role in bringing this important new discipline into the mainstream of clinical practice.

Martin M. Zdanowicz
November 2009

Contributors

Miriam A. Ansong, Pharm.D.
Director, Drug Information Center
Department of Clinical & Administrative Sciences
Sullivan University College of Pharmacy
Louisville, Kentucky

Christina L. Aquilante, Pharm.D.
Assistant Professor
University of Colorado Denver School of Pharmacy
Aurora, Colorado

John D. Cleary, Pharm.D., FCCP
Professor & Vice-Chairman of Research
Department of Pharmacy Practice
Schools of Pharmacy & Medicine
Antimycotic Program Director
Mycotic Research Center
Department of Medicine, Division of Infectious Diseases
University of Mississippi Medical Center
Jackson, Mississippi

Arthur G. Cox, Ph.D.
Assistant Professor
Department of Pharmaceutical Science
South University School of Pharmacy
Savannah, Georgia

Michael A. Crouch, Pharm.D., FASHP, BCPS
Professor and Chair
Department of Pharmacy Practice
South University School of Pharmacy
Savannah, Georgia

Megan Jo Ehret, Pharm.D., BCPP
Assistant Professor
University of Connecticut
Storrs, Connecticut

Jeffery D. Evans, Pharm.D.
Assistant Professor of Pharmacy Practice
University of Louisiana College of Pharmacy
Clinical Assistant Professor
Family Medicine and Comprehensive Care
Louisiana State University Health Science Center
Shreveport, Louisiana

James W. Fetterman, Jr., Pharm.D.
Associate Professor
Department of Pharmacy Practice
Experiential Education Coordinator
South University School of Pharmacy
Savannah, Georgia

Tawanda Gumbo, MD
Associate Professor of Medicine
Department of Medicine
Division of Infectious Diseases
University of Texas Southwestern Medical Center
Dallas, Texas

Pamela F. Hite, Pharm.D.
Assistant Professor (Critical Care)
Department of Pharmacy Practice
South University School of Pharmacy
Savannah, Georgia

Sally A. Huston, Ph.D.
Assistant Professor
University of Georgia College of Pharmacy
Athens, Georgia

Ajoy Koomer, Ph.D., MS, E.M.B.A.
Assistant Professor of Pharmaceutical Sciences
Director, Office of Program Assessment
Sullivan University College of Pharmacy
Louisville, Kentucky

Taimour Y. Langaee, MSPH, Ph.D.
Research Associate Professor
Department of Pharmacotherapy and Translational Research
Director, Center for Pharmacogenomics Genotyping Core Lab
University of Florida College of Pharmacy
Gainesville, Florida

W. Greg Leader, Pharm.D.
Interim Dean
Professor, Clinical Pharmacy Practice
University of Louisiana Monroe College of Pharmacy
Monroe, Louisiana

Kathryn M. Momary, Pharm.D., BCPS
Assistant Professor
Department of Pharmacy Practice
Mercer University College of Pharmacy and
   Health Sciences
Atlanta, Georgia

Jaekyu Shin, Pharm.D., MS, BCPS
Assistant Professor of Clinical Pharmacy
Department of Clinical Pharmacy
University of California School of Pharmacy
San Francisco, California

Helen E. Smith, MS, Ph.D., R.Ph.
Assistant Professor
Department of Pharmaceutical Sciences
Feik School of Pharmacy
University of the Incarnate Word
San Antonio, Texas

Todd A. Thompson, Ph.D.
Assistant Professor
Department of Pharmaceutical Sciences
University of New Mexico College of Pharmacy
Albuquerque, New Mexico

Kathy D. Webster, Pharm.D., Ph.D.
Associate Dean of Academic Affairs and Professor
University of Maryland Eastern Shore School of
   Pharmacy
Princess Anne, Maryland

Emily Weidman-Evans, Pharm.D., AE-C, CPE
Associate Professor, Department of Clinical and
   Administrative Sciences
University of Louisiana College of Pharmacy
Clinical Pharmacist, Department of Family Medi-
   cine
Louisiana State University Health Sciences Center
Shreveport, Louisiana

G. Scott Weston, R.Ph., Ph.D.
Associate Professor of Medicinal Chemistry
Director of Curricular Development
Department of Pharmaceutical Sciences
Harding University College of Pharmacy
Searcy, Arkansas

Martin M. Zdanowicz, Ph.D., MA
Professor of Pharmaceutical Sciences
South University School of Pharmacy
Savannah, Georgia

Reviewers

David W. Dyer, Ph.D.
Professor
Department of Microbiology and Immunology
Oklahoma University Health Sciences Center
Oklahoma City, Oklahoma

Y. W. Francis Lam, Pharm.D., FCCP
Associate Professor of Pharmacology and Medicine
University of Texas Health Science Center at San
   Antonio
San Antonio, Texas
Clinical Associate Professor of Pharmacy and
James O. Burke Endowed Fellow in Pharmacy
University of Texas at Austin
Austin, Texas

Daryl Jay Murry, Pharm.D.
Associate Professor
University of Iowa College of Pharmacy
Iowa City, Iowa

Amal Al Omari, Ph.D.
Assistant Professor
Al Isra University College of Pharmacy
Amman, Jordan

Contents

Part 1

Fundamentals of Pharmacogenomics

Chapter 1

Pharmacogenomics: Past, Present, and Future

Martin M. Zdanowicz, Ph.D., MA

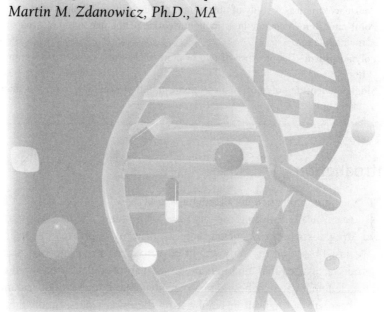

Learning Objectives

After completing this chapter, the reader should be able to
- Explain the meaning of key terms used in pharmacogenomics.
- Describe the effects of genetic polymorphisms on drug pharmacokinetic and pharmacodynamics.
- Discuss the potential benefits of pharmacogenomics on healthcare and the various roles pharmacists might play in its application.
- Summarize some of the major obstacles to the expansion of pharmacogenomics in clinical practice.
- Specify ways in which pharmacists might take the lead in utilizing the discipline of pharmacogenomics to enhance their practice.

Key Definitions

Allele—One of a pair of genes on a specific location of a chromosome that control the same trait.

Pharmacodynamics—The study of how a drug exerts its effects in the body.

Pharmacogenetics—The study of inherited differences or variations in drug metabolism and response.

Pharmacogenomics—The study of the role of inheritance in individual variation in drug response. It refers to the general study of all of the many different genes that determine drug behavior.

Pharmacokinetics—A study of absorption, distribution, metabolism, and excretion of drugs.

Point mutation—A change in a single nucleotide of the genome that occurs in 1% or less of the population.

Polymorphism—The presence of two or more alleles for a gene or DNA sequence in a population.

Single nucleotide polymorphism—A point mutation occurring in greater than 1% of the population.

Introduction

The phrase "one size fits all" might work for socks but certainly not for drugs. For many years, healthcare professionals have been taught the classic approach to determining drug doses in their patients. The vast majority of pharmacologic agents used today are simply dosed based on the body weight of the patient. Even in pediatric patients where it has long been recognized that "children are not miniature adults," specialized dosage formulations and detailed pharmacokinetic and pharmacodynamic studies are still lacking. Pharmacists have always been at the forefront in emphasizing the importance of individualizing drug therapy. In pharmacokinetics they are taught the many factors that can influence drug disposition in their patients including, organ function, blood flow, age, body fat, etc.[1] However, a key component of what makes a patient an individual, namely their unique genetic make-up, is often overlooked. The science of pharmacogenomics is a dynamic and developing field of study whose goal is to understand how the unique genetic composition of an individual can alter the pharmacokinetic and pharmacodynamic responses of that patient to a specific drug or class of drugs. The majority of drugs administered today are still administered based on a population average dose. Beyond tailoring a drug to an individual based on their size or weight or age, the science of pharmacogenomics strives to tailor drug therapy to individual patients based on their own unique molecular characteristics such as individual differences in drug metabolizing enzymes, drug transporter activity, receptor sensitivity, etc. Ultimately, it is hoped that such an approach can augment our current knowledge of pharmacotherapy to further improve the efficacy of drugs we use while reducing their unwanted side effects and potential toxicities.

The earliest clinical observations related to the impact of genetics on drug disposition and effects were made in the 1950s. Kalow published a landmark paper in 1956 in which he described several patients who did not exhibit a typical response to succinylcholine due to a genetic "variation" in the activity of their plasma cholinesterase enzymes.[2] That same year another study by Carson reported that a genetic deficiency in glucose-6 phosphate dehydrogenase enzyme was responsible for the excess hemolysis observed in primaquine-sensitive individuals.[3] Several years later, Evans detailed how genetic difference in metabolizing enzymes gave rise to patients who were "slow inactivators" or "rapid inactivators" of the antituberculosis drug isoniazid.[4] The actual term *pharmacogenetics* was first used by Fredrich Vogel in 1959.[5]

While studies in the new discipline of pharmacogenomics continued to expand throughout the 1960s, it was in the early 1970s that the next major expansion of this field occurred with the documentation of several genetic variations in key drug metabolizing enzymes of the liver. Mahgoub published a study in 1977 that quantitated measurable differences in elimination of the antihypertensive drug debrisoquine in 94 volunteers.[6] Variability in drug disposition in these individuals was due to genetic variation in the debrisoquine hydroxylase, an enzyme later identified as cytochrome p450, 2D6 (CYP2D6). Since this initial finding, numerous other drugs have also been shown to be substrates for CYP2D6 and thus potentially affected by genetic variation in this enzyme.

In the 1980s, genetic variability in other drug metabolizing enzymes such as thiopurine methyltransferase (involved in 6-mercaptopurine methylation) and CYP2C19 were also identified.[7,8] As the emerging science of pharmacogenetics continued to evolve, it eventually made its way into mainstream clinical pharmacy journals in 1992.[9,10] At this same time there was an explosion in molecular biology and a widespread availability of new genetic biotechnology that would directly impact the pace at which pharmacogenetics progressed in the next decade. In 1988, Congress commissioned formation of the Human Genome Project. Jointly run by the National Institutes of Health (NIH) and the Department of Energy, the goal of the Human Genome Project was to sequence the entire human genome. Information obtained from this project was to be made freely available to all interested parties via a database set up by the National Center for Biotechnology Information. The final results of the human genome project were presented in 2003—a full 2 years ahead of the anticipated finish date.[11] In 1999, 10 large pharmaceutical companies and the U.K. Wellcome Trust philanthropy joined together to form the SNP Consortium. The purpose of this collaboration was to find and map 300,000 common single nucleotide polymorphisms (SNPs). The ultimate goal of the consortium was to generate a widely accepted, high-quality, extensive, publicly available map using SNPs as markers evenly distributed throughout the human genome. When this group completed its initial work a total of 1.8 million SNPs were actually identified.

In 2000 the NIH established the Pharmacogenetics Research Network (PGRN). This nationwide collaboration of scientists was formed with three main goals: 1) to examine the relationship between genetic variation and drug response; 2) to become a resource through which researchers in the field of pharmacogenomics could interact and share knowledge, tools, and data; and 3) to create a publicly available data base thorough which researchers and other professional could freely access information regarding the link between various phenotypes and genotypes (pharmgkb.org). In an article published in 1990, Speedie predicted that the newly emerging biotechnology related to pharmacogenomics would have great impact on both pharmacy education and practice in the coming years, an opinion we hope to validate within this text.[12]

Case Study—Warfarin

Warfarin is a highly effective and widely used oral anticoagulant. The response of an individual patient to warfarin is highly variable and the dose of warfarin from patient to patient can vary significantly.

Questions:

1. What patient parameters are most commonly considered when determining a drug dose for an individual?
2. What specific parameters are used to guide the dose of warfarin administered to a patient?
3. Discuss specific genetic variants that might be responsible for the variability that might be observed in patients' responsiveness to warfarin.
4. How can knowledge of pharmacogenetics improve the safety profile of a potentially dangerous drug like warfarin?

Sources of Genetic Variability in Drug Response

At present it is estimated that the human genome contains between 30,000 and 40,000 distinct genes. When one factors in alternative splicing and posttranslational modifications, the human genome may code for in excess of 100,000 individual proteins. While genetic variation may arise due to a rare mutation, it most commonly occurs as random *variation* between the nucleotide sequences of different individuals. It is estimated that the genomes of any two given individuals differ by approximately one nucleotide in every thousand, or a difference of approximately 3 million base pairs in total. Single base-pair substitutions that occur with a frequency of ≥1% in a population are referred to as *single nucleotide polymorphisms (SNPs)*. SNPs are the most common type of variation found in human DNA. These substitutions can occur anywhere in the DNA. To date, over 1.4 million SNPs have been identified with more than 60,000 occurring in the coding regions for proteins. The genes that code for the CYP enzymes 2A6, 2C9, 2C19, 2D6, and 3A4 for example have been shown to be polymorphic with functional variations in a significant percentage of certain ethnic groups. A second, less common form of genetic variation stems from insertion, deletion, or duplication of bases. These types of mutation rarely occur within the coding regions of genes.

The most common and best studied genetic polymorphisms to date are those that affect drug pharmacokinetics; however, an increasing number of polymorphism are being identified that can affect drug pharmacodynamics as well. Since the overall effect of a drug in the body is based on both pharmacokinetic and pharmacodynamic interactions, pharmacogenomics will need to expand its future focus to include polygenic variations that can affect both facets of a drugs action.

Genetic Variability and Drug Pharmacokinetics

The pharmacokinetic profile of a particular drug may be determined by four main factors: 1) the extent to which a drug is absorbed from its site of administration; 2) how the drug is distributed in various body compartments once absorbed; 3) the extent and means by which a drug is metabolized within the body; and 4) how a drug is excreted from the body (e.g., kidney, liver, GI, etc.). The single greatest source of pharmacogenetic variability identified to date is those that occur in drug metabolizing enzymes. Phase I metabolism generally involves oxidation and reduction reactions carried out by the CYP450 system of the liver. Phase II reactions are conjugation reactions designed to made the product of the reaction more polar and water soluble in order to facilitate its elimination by the kidneys. Clinically important polymorphisms have been identified in most of the major enzymes involved in both phase I and phase II drug metabolism (Table 1-1).[13] The majority of the genetic variations in CYP450 genes are due to single amino acid substitutions. While a number of the genetic variants have not been reported to significantly alter activity of the enzyme they code for in vivo, several have clearly been associated with altered activity of the enzyme to the point where it impacts drug disposition. The CYP2D6 family of enzymes, for example, exhibits a number of polymorphisms that results in diminished activity of numerous enzymes within this family (e.g., CYP2D6*4, CYP2D6*5), while other polymorphisms (mainly duplicated or amplified alleles) result in enzymes that metabolize their substrates more rapidly or extensively (e.g., CYP2D6*2).

Table 1-1

Examples of the Impact of Pharmacogenomics on Drug Pharmacokinetics

Gene Product	Affected Drug	Clinical Impact
CYP2C9	Warfarin	Altered anticoagulant effect
CYP2C19	Omeprazole	Altered efficacy in treating H. pylori
CYP2D6	Anti-psychotics	Increased incidence of serious side effects (tardive dyskinesia)
CYP3A4	Tacrolimus	Altered efficacy & toxicity of immunosuppressants
N-acetyltransferase (NAT)	Isoniazid	Altered drug efficacy & toxicity
Thiopurine methyltransferase (TPMT)	Mercaptopurine	Life-threatening myelosuppression
Angiotensin Converting Enzyme (ACE)	ACE Inhibitors	Altered efficacy and toxicity of ACE inhibitors
P-glycoprotein	Digoxin	Altered plasma concentrations of digoxin

Enzymes from the CYP2D6 family are involved in the metabolism of many important and widely utilized drugs such as codeine, fluoxetine, haloperidol, and propranolol. Approximately 5% to 10% of the Caucasian population may be classified as "poor metabolizers" of agents metabolized by CYP2D6 due to the presence of a polymorphism in genes for this particular CYP family. In patients of Asian and African heritage, a higher prevalence of certain CYP subtypes (CYP2D6*10, and CYP2D6*17, respectively) have been identified that are associated with reduced rates of drug metabolism for certain substrates. Other polymorphisms in CYP2D6 can lead to the phenotypic presentation of patients that are rapid or ultra-rapid metabolizers (UM). In some populations (e.g., Ethiopian) the prevalence of the UM phenotype can be as high as 29%.[14]

The actual clinical effect of CYP2D6 polymorphism will depend on the specific drug being metabolized. In cases where the drug being acted on by CYP2D6 enzymes is a prodrug or less potent compound (e.g., the conversion of codeine to more potent morphine), poor metabolizers might require higher doses of drug to obtain the required therapeutic effect. If the drug is inactivated by CYP2D6 enzymes, then individuals who are poor metabolizers would require lower doses to yield the desired clinical effect. Clinical effects that might be in part attributable to CYP2D6 polymorphisms include altered codeine efficacy, the risk of tardive dyskinesia from antipsychotics, and the overall efficacy of certain beta blockers.

The CYP2C9 and CYP2C19 families of liver enzymes also contain a number of clinically significant polymorphisms. The 2C9 family is involved in the metabolism of a number of clinically important drugs including several with narrow therapeutic indices such as phenytoin and warfarin. Two of these genetic variants involve amino acid substitutions at the active site of the enzyme that significantly reduce the overall activity of the enzyme. The 2C19 family of enzymes is involved in the metabolism of several commonly used proton-pump inhibitors as well as certain benzodiazepines such as diazepam. Approximately 1% to 3% of Caucasians are poor metabolizers for warfarin and phenytoin and, as a result, are at increased risk of bleeding and phenytoin toxicity, respectively, at therapeutic doses. Poor metabolizers of proton-pump inhibitors might actually have a therapeutic advantage in that reduced inactivation of these agents can lead to higher levels in the gut. In a study by Furata, genetically poor metabolizers of omeprazole had significantly higher cure rates for *H. pylori* than did patients taking similar doses who were normal metabolizers of the drug.[15] A higher prevalence of polymorphisms for these enzymes amongst Asian populations has also resulted in the prescribing of lower doses of diazepam for patients of Asian descent.[16]

Although the CYP3A4 family of liver enzymes accounts for more than half of all hepatic metabolism, few polymorphisms in this family have been reported to date and none appear to be clinically significant. However, activity of this particular group of enzymes can be greatly influenced by numerous drugs that act as inducers (e.g., carbamazepine, phenobarbital, phenytoin) or inhibitors (e.g., cimetidine, erythromycin, ketoconazole) of 3A4.

A number of clinically significant polymorphisms have been reported in a phase II metabolizing enzymes such as N-acetyltransferase (NAT2), glutathione transferases, and thiopurine methyltransferase (TPMT).[13] One particularly relevant clinical example involves the enzyme TPMT that methylates anticancer drugs such as mercaptopurine and azathioprine. Several SNPs have been identified for TPMT, which can alter its activity. Since methylation is involved in both activation and metabolism of mercaptopurine, altered enzyme activity will affect the concentration of both active and toxic metabolites. The therapeutic index for the thiopurine agents is very narrow with life-threatening myelosuppression being the major concern. Patients with polymorphic TPMT will often require significant dose reduction in order to avoid toxicity.

As a result of the demonstrated clinical impact of polymorphisms in CYP2C9 and TPMT, the Food and Drug Administration (FDA) recommends that at-risk patients be tested for the presence of the variants before receiving warfarin or azathioprine, respectively. The availability of rapid and simple genetic testing, such as the hand-held AmpliChip CYP450 microarray system, can greatly facilitate genotypic testing of patients for metabolizing enzyme polymorphisms prior to drug administration.

A second factor that can significantly impact drug pharmacokinetics are polymorphisms in drug transporters. A number of transmembrane transport proteins are present in the walls of the GI tract, hepatocytes, kidney tubules, and blood-brain barrier. These transporters are responsible for selectively transporting substance across biologic membranes. Perhaps the best studied group of transport proteins are the p-glycoproteins (PGP), which function as energy-dependent, multidrug efflux pumps.[17] PGP is widely distributed in normal cells and is involved in the efflux of numerous drugs including digoxin and immunosuppressants, such as tacrolimus and HIV protease inhibitors. The expression of PGP appears to differ significantly from individual to individual. Various degrees of PGP expression also occur in cancer cells and bacteria where they play a key role in anticancer drug and antibiotic resistance. A number of polymorphisms have been identified in the multidrug resistance gene (MDR-1), which codes for PGP. One of these, an SNP in exon 26, is associated with altered intestinal expression of PGP and thus significantly altered absorption of drugs like digoxin or protease inhibitors.

Genetic Variability and Drug Pharmacodynamics

Pharmacodynamic variations in drug response are those that occur due to genetic differences in drug targets (e.g., receptors, enzymes, etc.). A significant number of drug target polymorphisms have been identified thus far (Table 1-2). One clinically relevant example involves a reduced response to asthma medications due to variants in β_2 adrenergic receptors and 5-lipoxygenase. At least 11 SNPs have been identified in the β_2-receptor gene.[18] A number of these polymorphisms appear to alter receptor expression, down-regulation, or second-messenger coupling and therefore patient response.[15] Polymorphisms in the β_1 receptor gene have also been identified, which may alter the responsiveness of certain patients to the cardiovascular effects of beta blockers as well. Serotonin receptor and transporter polymorphisms have likewise been reported, which can alter the efficacy of certain antidepressant and antipsychotic agents. Other drug-target polymorphisms with potential clinical significance include those for various enzymes such as 5-lipoxygenase (altered Zileuton response), HMG-CoA reductase (altered statin response), and angiotensin-converting enzyme.[19]

The anticoagulant warfarin is a particularly interesting case since it is affected by both drug metabolizing enzyme (CYP2C9) polymorphisms and drug target polymorphisms.

Table 1–2
Examples of the Impact of Pharmacogenomics on Drug Pharmacodynamics

Gene Product	Affected Drug	Clinical Impact
Angiotensin Converting Enzyme (ACE)	ACE Inhibitors	Altered efficacy and toxicity of ACE inhibitors
β_2-adrenergic receptors	Albuterol	Variable efficacy
Serotonin Transporters & Receptor	Fluoxetine, clozapine	Altered drug efficacy and toxicity
Thymidylate Synthase	Methotrexate	Altered cancer cell responsiveness
5-Lipoxygenase	Zileuton	Altered response in asthma
HMG-CoA Reductase	"Statin" drugs	Altered efficacy in reducing serum cholesterol

Clinical Pearl

The response of the individual to a drug may be influenced by polygenic factors.

The anticoagulant actions of warfarin are due to its inhibition of vitamin K reductase—an enzyme involved in the regeneration of reduced vitamin K, which is a necessary cofactor for synthesis of clotting factors by the liver. Several SNPs have been identified in the vitamin K epoxide reductase (VKOR) gene, which can reduce its susceptibility to blockade and thus lead to patients who are "warfarin resistant."[20] In 2007, the FDA concluded that there was sufficient evidence to warrant a change in labeling of warfarin to include information about the potential impact of genetic variation on dosing.

Identification of genetic variability in drug targets has also been of great utility in cancer chemotherapy. For example, lung tumor cells with activation mutations in the tyrosine kinase portion of their epidermal growth factor receptors are known to be particularly sensitive to drugs (gefitinib) that inhibit this receptor. A second enzyme, thymidylate synthase, is expressed both in normal cells and cancer cells. Anticancer drugs, such as methotrexate and fluorouracil, inhibit this enzyme in cancer cells in order to interfere with cancer cell nucleic acid metabolism. Polymorphisms in this enzyme have been identified that can affect both the efficacy of these agents in cancer cells as well as their toxicity in normal cells.[21]

Several interesting polymorphisms have also been documented in genes coding for various ion channels in the heart.[22] These polymorphisms can alter the flux of ions like potassium, which in turn may affect cardiac conduction. Some conduction changes such as prolonged QT intervals can predispose an individual to dangerous arrhythmias such as torsades des pointes.

Clinical Applications of Pharmacogenomics and the Role of the Pharmacist

Despite significant expansion of pharmacogenomic research in the past decade, the actual application of PG in daily clinical practice is still relatively limited. There are clearly a number of challenges that need to be considered regarding the comprehensive application of pharmacogenomics to therapeutics. First is the polygenic nature of many drug responses. The example of warfarin highlights just how complex the effects of genetic variation can be with regards to a patients overall drug response. The effect of polymorphisms in a particular drug-disposition pathway may be heightened or blunted by other variations in separate but related pathways. This finding is further complicated by the fact that there are likely a large number of SNPs yet to be identified and characterized. Second, therapeutic options for a number of diseases and conditions may be relatively limited. If pharmacogenomic testing eliminates one or more of the drug options for a patient there may not be any effective alternative therapies available with which to treat the patient. Third is the lack of economic incentive for developing drugs that may only useful in a limited patient population. Since the cost of bringing a new drug to market can be in the range of several hundred million dollars, it would not be worthwhile for a drug company to spend a large amount of money on a new medication if it cannot recoup its initial investment and eventually turn a profit. Finally, healthcare providers will need to receive an extensive education with regards to the fundamentals of pharmacogenomics including various types of pharmacogenomic testing, interpreting these tests, and applying their results in daily practice.

It is perhaps in this last area of clinician and patient education that pharmacists might have the most immediate impact. When compared to other healthcare specialists, pharmacists have the most training with regards to the pharmacology, pharmacokinetics, and pharmacodynamics of various drugs. Clinical pharmacists currently practice a form of individualized medication therapy when they consider the many factors that can alter drug pharmacokinetics and effect from patient to patient. Pharmacists tailor medications to individuals based on their liver function, renal function, age, size, concomitant drug use, etc., so the concept of using another specific trait, namely genetic make-up, should not seem unusual to this group of practitioners.

Clinical Pearl

Pharmacogenomics may be used to optimize drug dose and choice thus improving therapeutic efficacy and reducing side effects.

In addition to their role a healthcare providers, pharmacists currently play an important role as educators and clinical consultants—places where their knowledge and understanding of pharmacogenomics can be invaluable. Pharmacists need not become experts in molecular biology or genetics in order to be competent and comfortable with the applications of pharmacogenomics. They do, however, need to become familiar with the basic terminology that defines this area of study. Pharmacists should understand how genetic data from patients is obtained, along with the significance of such data and how it may be applied clinically. From the authors' own research, it appears that the amount of pharmacogenomic knowledge current pharmacists and students of pharmacy receive is insufficient.[23-25] While the number of educational resources for pharmacists in the area of pharmacogenomics has increased significantly in recent years, there is still a great need for continuing education and training of pharmacists in this area. These educational needs may be met in part through an increased number of specialized CE programs, workshops, and journal articles dedicated to training current and future pharmacists in the fundamentals and applications of pharmacogenomics. Likewise, the amount and type of pharmacogenomics education students of pharmacy receive needs to be evaluated now and in the future.

Clinical Pearl

As a result of their comprehensive training in drug pharmacokinetics and pharmacodynamics, pharmacists are ideally situated to advance the frontiers of pharmacogenomics and facilitate its entry into the mainstream of clinical practice.

While the current role of the pharmacist in pharmacogenomics is not well-defined, there are a number of areas where pharmacists who are knowledgeable in this field might be of great asset. Pharmacists can take the lead in educating physicians and patients about pharmacogenomics. In the near future, it is estimated that nearly one quarter of all prescriptions may contain some pharmacogenomic information as part of their package insert. Inclusion of such information will undoubtedly elicit many questions from both patients and healthcare providers that the trained pharmacist would be ideally suited to answer. Likewise, as pharmacogenomic testing of patients expands, pharmacists will be asked many questions by both patients and healthcare providers about interpreting and applying the results of such tests. Pharmacists in various institutional clinical settings can become the main consultants on pharmacogenomic issues and applications related to drug therapy.

Another important area where pharmacists might take the lead in applying pharmacogenomics is in drug efficacy and safety. Pharmacogenomics has the potential to identify patient populations that will be most likely to experience specific benefits or adverse effects from a particular drug. Such information can be used by pharmacists to guide drug therapy to ensure its maximal efficacy and safety. Examples include the analysis of drug metabolizing enzymes as biomarkers to identify patients who might be "slow-metabolizers" for a certain drug or the use of pharmacogenomic data to optimize the dose of warfarin a patient receives. Pharmacists might also utilize pharmacogenomic information to predict (and thus prevent) potential drug interactions in a specific patient population.

Impact of Pharmacogenomics on Future Drug Development

Despite the fact that the amount of money spent by the pharmaceutical industry on new drug development has essentially doubled in the last decade, the number of new drugs brought to market in this same period has remained the same. Likewise, the success rate of drugs in various phases of clinical development has declined significantly. Starting back in 2003, the FDA has made a concerted effort to promote the use of pharmacogenomics in drug development. In addition to hosting numerous workshops, the FDA has also released written guidelines for the submission of genomic data, and published a table of valid genomic biomarkers that can be included in FDA-approved drug labels.[26,27] In their publication *Guidance for Industry— Pharmacogenomic Data Submissions,* the FDA encouraged pharmacogenomic testing in new drug development and in a follow-up white paper published by the FDA in 2004; the use of pharmacogenomics was identified as a key opportunity for future drug development.[28]

Clinical Pearl

Pharmacogenomics may facilitate the drug development process.

There are several means by which pharmacogenomics can aid the process of future drug development. Pharmacogenomics/pharmacogenetics can provide investigators with a tool for identifying new drug targets. As the use of gene-wide microarrays expands it is likely that researchers will identify numerous changes in gene expression associated specific disease states or conditions. These changes in gene expression might serve as the starting point for the development of drugs targeting the product of these genes or directly modify expression of the genes themselves. However, one main drawback to the genome-wide approach of identifying new candidate genes it that is does not account for the potential interaction of other genes that impact the overall phenotype that is being studied (the polymorphic natures of warfarin is a good example of this). An interesting approach to identifying new potential pharmacogenomic targets involves the concept of examining "disease" or "drug response" pathways. For example, if one looks at the disease of asthma there are a number of documented polymorphisms affecting the response to both beta-2 adrenergic agents and corticosteroids. The polymorphisms occur not only in genes coding the actual drug targets (receptors) but also in genes coding for signaling proteins, second messengers, and other factors that modulate the response of these agents. Polymorphisms in the 5-lipoxygaenase pathway have also been identified that can alter response of asthma medications directed at inhibition of this enzyme pathway. By focusing on the specific pathways of drug response in asthma one might be more likely to identify and characterize not only polymorphisms but also interactions between polymorphic genes in this pathway.

Pharmacogenomics can also assist in developing drugs designed for specific patient populations or subsets of patients that might be most responsive to a particular medication. Such new drugs would potentially have enhanced efficacy in this target population. This selectivity would also potentially reduce the overall occurrence of adverse effects that could occur if the drug were widely used in a population that was not likely to respond to it. The application of pharmacogenomics might actually shift the focus of pharmaceutical drug development to some extent away from broad-market drugs to those targeted more toward specific subpopulations. Targeted drug development may present some economic challenges to drug companies since the profitability of new compounds for select markets may be limited. However, the potential wealth of new drug targets identified by pharmacogenomics could offset this potential drawback.

Pharmacogenomics might also aid the development of new drugs by allowing investigators to identify populations of patients, which might be more likely to exhibit adverse effects from a new drug and thus eliminate this particular population from clinical trials. One can't help but wonder if some of the many drugs removed from the market in recent years due to adverse reactions might not have been if potentially unidentified genetic susceptibilities in a percentage of the patient population had been identified and those patients excluded. Likewise, pharmacogenomics might allow for earlier detection of specific adverse effects before a new drug goes further on in the development process. An interesting example is the cholesterol-lowering drug cervistatin. This agent was removed from the market in 2001 due to the occurrence of rhabdomyolysis (muscle destruction). While all of the statins marketed today have a similar mechanism of action, they differ in their potential for causing rhabdomyolysis. There is some evidence that the risk for this potentially serious adverse effect correlates with the extent by which the individual statins are metabolized by various CYP450 enzymes.[29] In the case of cervistatin, the greatest risk for the occurrence of rhabdomyolysis occurred in patients taking gemfibrozil, a second cholesterol-lowering agent that can inhibit key CYP isoezymes involved in the metabolism of cervistatin. Could some of these instances of rhabdomyolysis have avoided if pharmacogenomic testing were used to identify specific patients who were "slow" metabolizers and avoid use of this agent in this population?

Pharmacists may also play an important role in new drug development as part of a multidisciplinary, collaborative drug-development team. Their expertise in drug formulation, pharmacokinetics, and clinical pharmacotherapy can make pharmacists important contributors to the drug development process at many different phases. A number of pharmacists-researchers are currently at the leading edge of pharmacogenomics research and in some instances even leading major research projects in this area.

Future Promise of Pharmacogenomics

For a number of years the question has been asked, how great an impact will pharmacogenomics have on future drug therapy? Pharmacogenomics is currently impacting several important aspects of clinical practice on a daily basis and the list of polymorphisms with potential clinical significance is steadily growing. With the completion of the human genome project, increased pharmacogenomics research and greater application of pharmacogenomic testing, the next decade will likely be one significant of growth in terms of the amount of clinical practice and drug development impacted by pharmacogenomics. Pharmacogenomics clearly holds significant potential for aiding in the development of drugs that are highly specific and efficacious due to their targeting of specific enzymes, proteins or other cellular targets. Pharmacogenomics might also provide an additional and highly specific means of determining drug dose for an individual, one that goes beyond just weight and age but also considers perhaps a patients' ability to metabolize a drug or respond to it. This individual dose maximization would also improve drug efficacy and reduce side effects. Overall drug safety could likewise be improved by the use of pharmacogenomics since it might allow practitioners to use the best possible drug or dose for a patient the first time. The drug discovery and development process can also benefit greatly from pharmacogenomics. A wide array of potential genomic targets can be readily identified as starting places for new drug development. Multiples genes in pathways involved in a particular disease or drug effect can be studies simultaneously with respect to their relationship and role in the disease process or drug response. The likelihood of a new drug failing in clinical trials might be significantly reduced if studies are conducted in populations that have been identified as more likely to respond to the drug, or less likely to exhibit adverse effects to the drug based on their genetic profile. Finally, the potential economic benefit of pharmacogenomics cannot be overlooked. By improving drug efficacy, reducing adverse drug effects, decreasing drug trial failure, and speeding new drug development, pharmacogenomics can have an unequivocal impact on the overall cost of healthcare (Table 1-3).

Table 1–3
Pharmacogenomics: Benefits and Challenges

Potential Benefits of Pharmacogenomics	Challenges to the Growth & Expansion of Pharmacogenomics
• Optimization of drug choice and dose to improved drug efficacy and reduce drug side-effects.	• Education of various healthcare providers regarding pharmacogenomics.
• Development of highly efficacious drugs for specific target populations.	• Potentially smaller and more specialized drug markets.
• Reduced failure of drugs in clinical trials.	• Complexity of polygenic drug response.
• Identification of numerous potential new drug targets.	• Resistance to genetic testing.
• Identification of polygenic drug effects.	• Ethical & legal issues.
• Overall reduction in health care costs.	• Expense
• More rapid drug development.	
• Advance disease screening.	
• Determining microbial sensitivity and resistance to drugs.	

Clinical Pearl

In the long term, the money spent of pharmacogenomic research and testing could reduce overall healthcare costs by improving drug efficacy, reducing adverse drug effects, decreasing drug trial failure, and speeding new drug development.

If the use of pharmacogenomics is to become fully incorporated into daily clinical practice, pharmacists will need to be an integral part of the process. One day patients may carry around a "super card" that contains all of their medical history and data including a detailed genetic profile. Pharmacists would be able to access this data from the patient instantly at their practice sites and use it to ensure that drug choice and dose was optimal. Pharmacists may also one day play a vital role in performing key genetic tests on patients at their point of contact. Both of the above scenarios would require pharmacists to be well-trained in the fundamentals of pharmacogenomics. They not only need to be able to interpret the results of pharmacogenomic tests, but they also have to be able apply the data obtained to the specific pharmacotherapy of their patient. Pharmacists are currently called on by physicians to optimize patient drug therapy; pharmacogenomic data would simply be another variable or tool that pharmacists could use to do so. It is likely in the future that pharmacists will have to become familiar with other disciplines of study that likewise may utilize genomics to impact clinical care. The "omics" revolution includes other fields of study such as *proteomics,* which explores changes in protein expression of individuals under various conditions; *nutrigenomics,* which studies the potential interaction between dietary nutrients and genotypic expression; *metabolonomics,* which investigates the alteration of metabolites and metabolic pathways under various conditions; and *toxicogenomics,* which studies how genomes are effected by toxins or other environmental factors.

While it is clear that there are still a number of challenges to overcome, the promise of pharmacogenomics remains bright. In order to help this promise become reality, pharmacists must be willing to not embrace this emerging discipline but to take the lead in its future implementation and direction.

References

1. Burton ME, Shaw LM, Schentag JJ, et al. *Applied Pharmacokinetics & Pharmacodynamics.* Baltimore, MD: Lippincott Williams & Wilkins; 2006.
2. Kalow W. Familial incidence of low pseudocholinesterase level. *Lancet.* 1956;2:576-577.
3. Carson PE, Flanagan CL, Ickes CE, et al. Enzymatic deficiency in primaquine-sensitive erythrocytes. *Science.* 1956;124:484-485.
4. Evans DAP, Manley KA, McKusick VA. Genetic control of isoniazid metabolism in man. *Br Med J.* 1960;2:485-491.
5. Vogel F. Moderne Probleme der Humangenetik. *Ergeb Inn Med Kinderheilkd.* 1959;12:52-125.
6. Mahgoub A, Idle JR, Lancaster R, et al. Polymorphic hydroxylation of Debrisoquine in man. *Lancet.* 1977;17:584-586.
7. Weinshilboum RM, Sladek SL. Mercaptopurine pharmacogenetics: Monogenic inheritance of erythrocyte thiopurine methyltransferase activity. *Am J Hum Genet.* 1980;32:651-662.
8. Wedlund PJ, Aslanian WS, McAllister CB. Mephenytoin hydroxylation deficiency in Caucasians: frequency of a new oxidative drug metabolism polymorphism. *Clin Pharmacol Ther.* 1984;36:773-780.
9. Gibaldi M. Pharmacogenetics: part I. *Ann Pharmacother.* 1992;26:121-126.
10. Gibaldi M. Pharmacogenetics: part II. *Ann Pharmacother.* 1992;26:255-261.
11. Collins FS, Gree ED, Guttmacher AE, et al. A vision for the future of genomics research. *Nature.* 2003;422:835-847.
12. Speedie MK. The Impact of Biotechnology upon Pharmacy Education. *Am J Pharm Ed.* 1990;54:55-60.
13. Wilkinson GR. Drug Metabolism and Variability among Patients in Drug Response. *N Engl J Med.* 2005;352:2211-2221.
14. Akullu E, Persson I, Bertilsson L, et al. Frequent distribution of ultrarapid metabolizers of debrisoquine in an Ethiopian population carrying duplicated and multi-duplicated functional CYP2D6 alleles. *J Pharmacol Exp Ther.* 1996;278:441-446.
15. Furata T, Ohashi K, Kamata T, et al. Effect of genetic differences in omeprazole metabolism on cure rates for Helicobacter pylori infection and peptic ulcer. *Ann Intern Med.* 1998;129:1027-1030.
16. Ozawa S, Soyama A, Saeki M. Ethnic differences in genetic polymorphisms CYP2D6, CYP2C19, CYP3A4's and MDR1/ABCB1. *Drug Metab Pharmacokin.* 2004;19:83-95.
17. Kerb R. Implications of genetic polymorphisms in drug transporters for pharmacotherapy. *Cancer Lett.* 2006;234:4-33.
18. Brodde OE, Leineweber K. Beta-2-adrenoceptor gene polymorphisms. *Pharmacogen Gen.* 2005;15:267-275.
19. Evans WE, McLeod HL. Pharmacogenomics-drug disposition, drug targets and side effects. *N Engl J Med.* 2003;348:538-549.
20. Hall AM, Wilkins MR. Warfarin: a case history in pharmacogenetics. *Heart.* 2005;91:563-564.
21. Lee W, Lockhart AC, Kim RB, et al. Cancer pharmacogenomics: powerful tools in cancer chemotherapy and drug development. *The Oncologist.* 2005;10:104-111.
22. Pfeufer A, Jalilzadeh S, Siegfried P. Common Variants in Myocardial Ion Channel Genes Modify the QT Interval in the General Population. *Circ Res.* 2005;96:693-701.

23. Latif DA, Pharmacogenetics and pharmacogenomics instruction in schools of pharmacy in the USA: is it adequate? *Pharmacogenomics.* 2005;6:317-319.

24. Zdanowicz MM, Huston SA, Weston GS. Pharmacogenomics in the Professional Pharmacy Curriculum: Content, Presentation and Importance. *Int J Pharm Ed.* 2006;2:1-12.

25. Koomer A, Dutta AP, Tran HT. Current State of Pharmacogenomics/Pharmacogenetics Information in the schools and colleges of US, Canada and UK. Paper presented at: Annual meeting of the American Association for Colleges of Pharmacy; July 19-23, 2008; Chicago, IL.

26. US Food and Drug Administration. Genomics at FDA. Available at: http://www.fda.gov/cder/genomics/default.htm. Accessed April 30, 2009.

27. US Food and Drug Administration. Table of Valid Genomic Biomarkers in the Context of Approved Drug Labels. Available at: http://www.fda.gov/cder/genomics/genomic_biomarkers_table.htm. Accessed April 30, 2009.

28. US Food and Drug Administration. Innovation, Stagnation. Challenge and opportunity on the critical path to new medical products. Available at: http://www.fda.gov/oc/initiatives/criticalpath/whitepaper.html. Accessed April 30, 2009.

29. Schreiber DH, Anderson T. Statin-induced rhabdomyolysis. *J Emer Med.* 2006;31:177-180.

Chapter 2

The Genetic Basis of Pharmacogenomics

Taimour Y. Langaee, MSPH, Ph.D.; Jaekyu Shin, Pharm.D., MS, BCPS

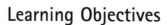

Learning Objectives

After completing this chapter, the reader should be able to

- Define human gene structure and its regulatory sequences.
- Describe the difference between genetic variation and polymorphism and mention a few examples of different polymorphisms.
- Be able to calculate frequencies of genotypes and alleles from genotype data.
- Describe the Hardy-Weinberg Equilibrium, linkage disequilibrium, and haplotype.
- Explain the racial/ethnic genetic differences and their role in pharmacogenomics study.

Key Definitions

Allele—Alternative forms of a gene at a given locus.

Allelic imbalance—Occurs when one allele in a heterozygote shows lower or higher expression than the other allele.

Autologous—Originating within an organism itself.

Autosome (autosomal)—Any chromosome other than the sex chromosomes or the mitochondrial chromosome.

Chimeric gene—Also called fusion gene. A gene constructed from DNA fragments from different genes.

Chromatid—The two parallel identical strands, connected at the centromere, of the doubled chromosome after chromosomal replication but before anaphase.

Genome—The genome includes the total genetic material contained within the chromosomes of an organism, and in humans, the 46 chromosomes that make up our genome.

Heterozygote (heterozygous)—An individual who has two different alleles at a give locus on a pair of homologous chromosomes.

Homologous—Pertaining to a pair of chromosomes.

Homozygote (homozygous)—An individual possessing a pair of identical alleles at a given locus on a pair of homologous chromosomes.

Nonhomologous—Not pertaining to a pair of chromosomes.

Paralogs—The genes that are related by duplication in the genome.

Introduction

The field of molecular biology and genetics has advanced a great deal in the past 10 years. New technologies, assays, and methods are being developed at a fast pace. Although it's a big challenge to collect and present all the genetics related to pharmacogenomics in a single chapter, we tried to focus on key areas that would be of value to practicing pharmacists. In this chapter, we provide the fundamental and essential information that the readers can easily understand and apply to pharmacogenomics study. The first part of this chapter provides a brief introduction to molecular biology and includes information about the structure of deoxyribonucleic acid (DNA), ribonucleic acid (RNA), purine and pyrimidine bases, nucleotide (the building block of DNA), and human genes, as well as a short description of transcription (transfer of genetic information from DNA to messenger ribonucleic acid [mRNA]), and translation (protein synthesis). In the second part, genetic variation (DNA mutations and polymorphisms) genotypes and phenotypes are discussed. In the third part, the Hardy-Weinberg Equilibrium (HWE), linkage disequilibrium (LD), haplotype, and at last, the genetic differences among racial and ethnic groups will be covered. It is the goal of this chapter to provide readers with a sufficient background in genetics to allow them to better understand and apply the fundamental concepts of pharmacogenomics.

Case Study—Warfarin

A.J. is a 56-year-old African-American man who is recently diagnosed with hypertension. He does not have any other comorbidities. He does not smoke. He comes to your pharmacy with a prescription for hydrochlorothiazide. He has been told by his geneticist friend that he is unlikely to receive a prescription for a beta blocker since they generally don't work well in African-Americans because 34% of African-Americans are homozygous for the arginine allele at codon 389 in beta$_1$-adrenergic receptor gene (*ADRB1*).

Questions:

1. What is the frequency of the arginine allele in African-Americans?
2. The *ADRB1* gene contains another important nonsynonymous polymorphism at codon 49. Data suggest that haplotype consisting of SNPs at codons 49 and 389 better predicts genotype at either locus alone. How can A.J.'s haplotype information be obtained?
3. The two loci (codons 49 and 389) are in linkage disequilibrium to some extent. Which measure of linkage disequilibrium is useful to obtain information on past recombination events between the loci? Which measure is helpful to obtain tagging SNP information?
4. Why do African-Americans have more SNPs in *ADRB1* than Caucasians and Asians?

Deoxyribonucleic and Ribonucleic Acids (DNA and RNA)

Deoxyribonucleic acid (DNA) is composed of deoxyribonucleotide subunits. Each deoxyribonucleotide contains a 5-carbon deoxyribose sugar, a phosphate group, and either a purine (adenine or guanine) or a pyrimidine (cytosine or thymine) cyclic nitrogen base (Figures 2-1 and 2-2). In DNA, adenine (A) always base pairs with thymine (T), and cytosine base pairs with guanine (G). DNA exists as double-stranded helix that run antiparallel and is complementary to each other. The two DNA strands are bound together through A-T, and C- G base pairing. During the DNA synthesis, each new nucleotide molecule is added to a hydroxyl group on the carbon 3 of deoxyribose of the existing DNA strand at the 3' end (Figure 2-1).

The transfer of DNA information from parent to daughter cell occurs through a precise process called DNA replication. The synthesis of DNA involves several proteins and enzymes, as well as the DNA polymerases that are equipped with proof reading and repair systems. These DNA polymerases are responsible for catalyzing the synthesis of new strands of DNA and correcting any errors that occur during synthesis. The newly synthesized double-stranded DNA is made of one old and one new strand of DNA from parent and daughter cells, respectively.

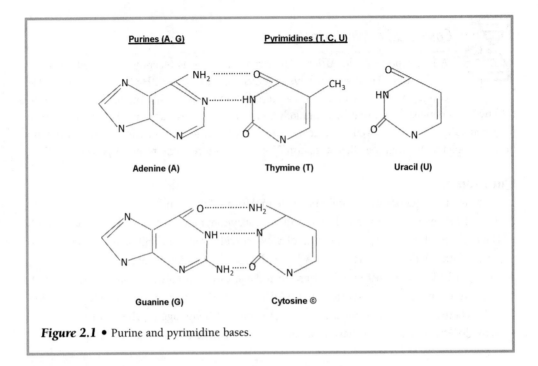

Figure 2.1 • Purine and pyrimidine bases.

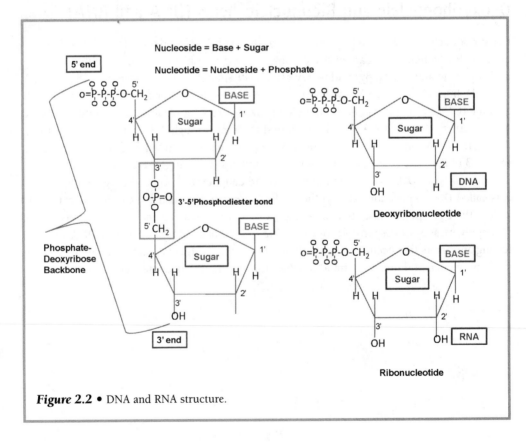

Figure 2.2 • DNA and RNA structure.

Ribonucleic acid (RNA) consists of a long chain of ribonucleotide subunits. Each RNA subunit or nucleotide, like DNA, is made of a nitrogenous base, a phosphate, and a 5-carbon sugar (ribose). There are a few differences between RNA and DNA; DNA is more stable and durable than RNA, RNA nucleotides contain ribose instead of deoxyribose, in RNA the base uracil (U) is used instead of thymine, RNA is usually single-stranded while DNA is double-stranded (Figures 2-1 and 2-2).[1]

The Genetic Code

The genetic code is a set of trinucleotide sequences (codons) encoded in DNA or RNA that are translated into corresponding amino acids to form polypeptide chain (protein). Each three nucleotides or bases designate an amino acid. There are a total of 64 codons of which three codons code for no amino acid but rather act as "stop codons" (UAG, UGA, and UAA), and the rest code for 20 amino acids. The number of codons that code for the 20 amino acids can vary from one codon (AUG that codes for amino acid methionine) to six codons (CGU, CGC, CGA, CGG, AGA, and AGG that code for amino acid arginine). The most common start codon (the first codon on the actual reading frame in the mRNA sequence) is AUG that codes for methionine; as a result, most amino acid chains (polypeptides) start with this amino acid.

To better understand how the reading frame of a particular sequence may vary, we look at an example of a short sequence that starts as CCCGGGAAA. If the reading of the codon starts from the first position, we'll have CCC, GGG, and AAA, which translates into amino acids: proline (Pro), glycine (Gly), and lysine (Lys). If the reading starts from the second position, we'll have CCG and GGA, and if the reading starts from the third position, we'll have CGG and GGA. As seen we can have three possible reading frames for each strand of DNA, and for both forward strand (5'→3') and reverse strand (3'→5'), we can have a total of six possible reading frames each coding for a different sequence of amino acids.[1,2]

Gene Structure

Genes are the basic unit of heredity and are made of DNA. In humans, the genes contain both coding (exons) and noncoding (introns) sequences. In addition to the exons and introns, the genes also have regulatory sequences, located before or upstream (5') of the coding sequence called 5' untranslated region (5' UTR), and after or downstream (3') of the coding sequence called 3' untranslated region (3' UTR). These untranslated regions are transcribed into mRNA, but are not translated into amino acids (Figure 2-3). Regulatory sequences such as enhancers, silencers, insulators, cis and trans-acting elements play important role in the regulation of gene expression at the transcription and translation level. Transcription factors bind to these regulatory sequences that may be located in close proximity or far from the promoters in the introns and cause an increase or decrease in the gene expression. Repressors of translation (during protein synthesis) can also bind to cis and trans-acting elements on the mRNA to repress or inhibit the protein synthesis. The regulation of ferritin (an iron storage protein) by the concentration of iron in the cells is a good example of regulation of translation (protein synthesis). Promoters are sequence on the DNA that are located at 5' or upstream of coding region, and they are the sites where the RNA polymerase II along with transcription factors bind and start the process of transcription (Figure 2-3).[3-5]

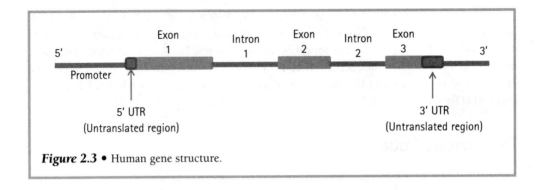

Figure 2.3 • Human gene structure.

Transcription

Transcription is the process of transcribing or copying the DNA nucleotide sequence into RNA for the synthesis of amino acids and from amino acids to proteins that carry out the cell functions. RNA is transcribed in the 5'→3' direction from the complementary or antisense DNA strand running in 3'→5' direction. The RNA strand that is synthesized from DNA is called messenger RNA (mRNA), since it carries the message from DNA to the protein synthesis machinery of the cell.

In eukaryotes, the process of transcription occurs in three steps (initiation, elongation, and termination). The transcription initiation in eukaryotes is very complex, and unlike DNA replication, transcription does not require a primer for RNA synthesis. The RNA polymerase II enzyme does not directly recognize the promoter sequences, but instead binds to a transcription initiation complex, consisting of several proteins (transcription factors), which initiates transcription. The transcription process is ATP-dependent, and the DNA helicase enzyme unzips (unwinds) the DNA template for RNA polymerase to synthesize the RNA through base pairing. The elongation and mRNA synthesis may be performed by many RNA polymerases from a single DNA template depending on the cell's need for production of a particular protein. The sequence of the synthesized mRNA is an exact copy of the forward 5'→3' (sense) DNA strand, except that in mRNA the base uracil is used instead of thymine; hence, this DNA strand is called coding strand. The termination of mRNA synthesis occurs when RNA polymerase reaches the poly A signal (AAUAAA), located after the last exon at the 3' end of RNA that is responsible for polyadenylation (adding a series of adenines) of the newly formed mRNA. It is at this point that RNA polymerase separates from the DNA template and the transcription process is terminated.[1-2,6-7]

For the newly synthesized RNA (pre-mRNA transcripts) to become functional before being transported to the cytoplasm, it requires additional processing. This processing in eukaryotes include 5'-capping, 3'-polyadenylation, and splicing. During RNA transcription, a guanine cap is added to the 5' end of pre-mRNA by RNA polymerase II to protect it from degradative enzymes. In polyadenylation, many adenine (A) nucleotides are added to the 3' end of mRNA transcript after the completion of transcription.[8]

RNA splicing is the most important stage in RNA processing. The noncoding sequence of RNA (introns) is removed, and the coding sequences (exons) are joined together by spliceosome (a complex of small nuclear ribonucleoproteins, snRNPs). The spliceosome cleaves the introns that have a GU sequence at their 5' end (referred to as splice donor site), and an AG sequence at their 3' end (referred to as splice acceptor site). The variation at the splice sites is critical since this results in the formation of different mRNAs and, consequently, various proteins (isoforms) through a process called alternative splicing. Alternative splicing occurs in more than 60% of human genes and is responsible for higher variation and complexity of proteome (all the proteins produced by human genes) derived from limited number of genes (Figure 2-4).[9-10]

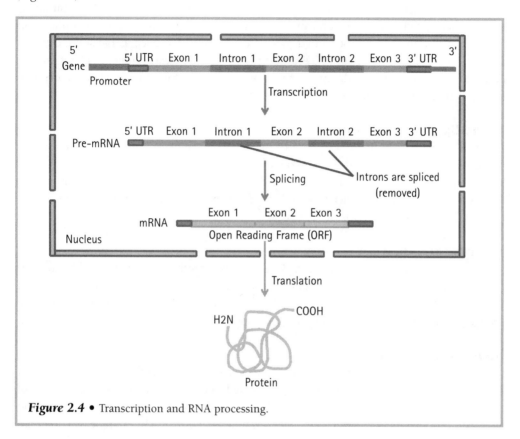

Figure 2.4 • Transcription and RNA processing.

Translation (Protein Synthesis)

Translation is the last step before post-translational modification (e.g., glycosylation) in the process of gene expression, and it involves translation of the genetic codes on the mRNA into corresponding amino acids and eventually proteins. The mRNA formed from the transcription of DNA is transported from nucleus to cytoplasm where the ribosomes are located. Ribosomes are the site of protein synthesis. As the mRNA that serves as the template for proteins synthesis is decoded by ribosomes and tRNAs, the transfer RNAs (tRNAs) carry the correct and designated amino acid (anticodon, an RNA trinucleotides that are complementary to the mRNA codon) to the ribosome for the synthesis of polypeptide chain. The process of translation (protein synthesis) takes place in three steps (initiation, elongation, and termination). In brief, the initiation step involves the binding of small subunit of ribosome to the 5' end of mRNA by initiation factors. The elongation of polypeptide chain occurs in 5'→3' direction, corresponding to the amino terminal (N-terminal) to the carboxy terminal (C-terminal) direction of amino acid sequences in the protein. When the A-site of ribosome faces one of the stop codons (UAA, UAG, or UGA) on the mRNA, no tRNA is able to recognize these codons and the releasing factors recognize these nonsense codons and thus cause the release of newly synthesized polypeptide chain to terminate the process of protein synthesis.[1-2,11-12]

Genetic Variation and Polymorphisms

Mutation

The DNA in living cells is subject to frequent chemical changes (e.g., during DNA replication) that if not corrected by cell's DNA repair system can result in a mutation (a subtle variation in DNA). Mutation in DNA can be caused by environmental factors such as radiation, cigarette smoke, drugs, sunlight, or by copying error during the DNA replication process. Mutations can occur at three genetic levels: the gene, the chromosome, and the genome. Here we describe these different kinds of mutations:

Single-Base or Point Mutation

This is a simple substitution of one base or nucleotide by another. If the substitution occurs between bases of purine (A and G), or pyrimidine (C and T), it is called a transition. If a purine base is replaced by a pyrimidine base, it is called transversion. The C to T transition is more common and frequent than other substitutions. Single-base mutations often occur when DNA is being copied, and the error is not corrected.

Missense Mutation

When a new nucleotide changes the codon in a way that results in it being coded for another amino acid, it's called missense mutation. In sickle-cell anemia, the substation of A in codon GAG to T (GTG) at the nucleotide position 17 of beta chain of hemoglobin gene results in the change of glutamic acid amino acid (GAG) to valine amino acid (GTG).[13]

Nonsense Mutation

A nonsense mutation occurs when one nucleotide in a codon is replaced with another and that replacement results in a stop codon (TAA, TAG, and TGA), which terminates the process of translation or protein synthesis prematurely. This kind of mutation occurs in many genes and results in truncated proteins, which are unable to function normally. An example of a nonsense mutation (TGG codon of tryptophan amino acid at peptide position 1282, and 1316 to stop codon) occurs in the cystic fibrosis transmembrane conductance regulator (CFTR) gene, which results in a premature stop in the protein synthesis of this transporter.[14]

Silent Mutation

When substitution from one nucleotide to a new one (any of the three other bases) takes place on the third position of the codon, it usually does not result in a new amino acid. This is because many amino acids are encoded by more than one codon. For example, if the third base on the CGT codon for arginine is changed to any of the three other possible bases (C, G, A), arginine will still be encoded.

Insertions and Deletion Mutation (Indels)

When nucleotide(s) or base pair(s) are added or deleted from the DNA sequence of a gene, they are called insertions (I) and deletions or indels, respectively. If indels are one or two nucleotides, in many instances they can cause a "frameshift mutation." The following example shows how the shift in the reading frame occurs:

   If the sequence starts as GAA/TTC/AAG/GTT, it is coding for glutamic acid/phenylalanine/ lysine/valine. If there is an addition (insertion) of a C nucleotide at the beginning of the sequence [C]GAA/TTC/AAG/GTT, it changes to CGA/ATT/CAA/GGT, which now codes for arginine/isoleucine/glutamine/glycine. Frameshift mutations often result in stop codons. The frameshift mutation in human cytochrome P450 (CYP) 3A subfamily, *CYP3A5* gene (*CYP3A5*7* allele) that is created by a T insertion in nucleotide position (27131-32) and observed in African descent population is an example of this mutation.[15] If the indels are three nucleotides or multiples of three nucleotides, they may not change the reading frame, but in some cases they can result in genetic human disorders, such as fragile X syndrome or Huntington's disease that are caused by insertion of many copies of three nucleotides (like CGG, and CAG respectively). In Huntington's disease the insertion of CAG that codes for amino acid glutamine creates so-called "Huntingtin protein," which in turn results in abnormal increases of p53 protein level in the brain cells that causes cell death by apoptosis. The genetic mutation in Huntington's disease is also called guanine expansion. While the general population may have from six to 26 of the CAG repeats, patients with Huntington's disease may have from 40 to over 100 CAG repeats.[16]

The fragile X syndrome is another example of indel mutation, caused by insertion and expansion of trinucleotide repeats (CGG) in 5'UTR of the fragile X mental-retardation-1 gene (FMR-1) on the human X chromosome. The number CGG repeats in normal people may range from six to 60 repeats, but in individuals with the disorder the number of repeats go over 200 and may grow up to 1,000 repeats.[17]

Inversion Mutation

Inversion mutations occur when a short (a few bases) fragment or an entire section of DNA is reversed. Inversions in some cases may involve several genes from a large region of chromosome. Inversion of DNA can result in genomic disorders such as Hunter's syndrome (an X-linked recessive disorder with progressive damage of various tissues and organs), and some forms of hemophilia.[18]

Duplications

Duplication occurs when a segment of genome is doubled during the crossing over process in meiosis. This usually happens when the two sister chromatids are not aligned properly, and the breaking and rejoining of DNA is not 100% accurate. This results in one chromosome having more DNA than the other of the pair. Duplicated genes (paralogs) can result in gene loss as redundant genes are usually removed from genome. If duplicated genes persist, they require different function or result in more gene expression, and consequently more protein. An example is the *CYP2D6* gene duplication that results in ultra-rapid metabolism of drugs that are substrate for this genetically polymorphic enzyme. The ultra-rapid genotype occurs in 3% of the northern European white population, 5% to 10% of southern European populations and Arabian, and in 10% to 30% of northeast African populations.[19-20] The chimeric gene duplication occurring during unequal crossing over during meiosis between aldosterone gene and 11 β–hydroxylase gene is another example of gene duplication, which results in formation of the dominant mutant gene that overproduces the steroid hormone aldosterone and leads to high blood pressure (hereditary hypertension).[21]

Translocations

When a segment of one chromosome is transferred (translocated) to another nonhomologous chromosome it is called translocation. Chromosomal translocations join two unlinked pieces of the genome together, which may result in gene fusions and diseases such as leukemia. Translocation of two nonhomologous segments occurs more often and is referred to as reciprocal translocation. Translocations can make a gene nonfunctional if the break takes place within a gene, or it can result in synthesis of a hybrid or fusion gene. If the hybrid genes are translated, they may yield proteins that have an N-terminal of one protein coupled to the C-terminal of another protein. The altered chromosome 22 (also known as Philadelphia chromosome) is the result of translocation that is created by reciprocal fusion of two segments of chromosome 9 and 22. This translocation produces a hybrid or fusion gene that includes two genes called BCR and ABL-1, which in humans may cause hematologic malignancies. The Philadelphia chromosome is often seen in the cancer cells of patient with chronic myelogenous leukemia (CML). In most B-cell tumors, the translocation occurs between chromosome 8 and three other chromosomes (2, 14, and 22). Most patients with the Burkitt's lymphoma (a high grade B-cell neoplasm and a childhood tumor that is also seen in adults) carry translocation of c-myc oncogene from chromosome 8 to either immunoglobulin (Ig) heavy chain region on chromosome 14 or on light chain loci of chromosomes 2 or 22. In this translocation no fusion gene or protein is produced, and the oncogene from chromosome 8 is under transcriptional control of an Ig gene promoter, which causes overexpression of the oncogenic protein involved in Burkitt's tumor.[22-23]

Chromosomal Aberrations (Monosomy and Trisomy)

Chromosomal aberrations may also be referred to as genome mutations. In trisomy, an extra copy of a chromosome is made. An example is in trisomy 21 (Down syndrome, having three chromosome 21 instead of two), which occurs in 1 of 660 newborns. In monosomy, a whole chromosome is absent. An example of monosomy is seen as seen in Turner syndrome (monosomy X, have only one X sex chromosome), which occurs in 1 of 2,500 females.[24-25]

Polymorphisms

Single Nucleotide Polymorphisms (SNPs)

Single nucleotide polymorphisms (SNPs or "snips") are the most common DNA sequence variation in humans, occurring in about one nucleotide of every 300–750 nucleotides in human genomic DNA. When mutation occurs in 1% or more in a population, it is called a polymorphism. The frequency of polymorphisms may vary among different racial/ethnic groups. Some of these gene polymorphisms or variations may only be responsible for small differences among people such as hair and eye color, while some may result in diseases or increase the risk of diseases in people. The SNPs are responsible for more than 90% of genetic variation in the human genome. The most recent data from the largest public SNP database (National Center for Biotechnology Information [NCBI] polymorphism database, dbSNP; available at http://www.ncbi.nlm.nih.gov) shows more than 55,000,000 SNP submissions, of which more than 14,000,000 of them have reference SNP number (rs #). A little over 6,500,000 SNPs have been validated (dbSNP Build 129, Genome Build 36.3, April 2008). SNPs are found and reported from coding, noncoding, and regulatory regions of genes. Based on the locations of SNPs on the genes, they show different effects on gene expression and function. SNPs are bi-allelic genetic markers that replaced the microsatellite (polymorphic tandem repeats of short stretches of 1-4 nucleotides, which occur throughout human genome) DNA markers and are being used extensively in animal and human genetic studies.[26-29]

Coding Region Polymorphisms

The single nucleotide changes in the coding regions of DNA sequence (exonic regions that comprise about 3% of human genome) may change the amino acid sequence and protein function. This kind of polymorphism is referred to as nonsynonymous SNPs or polymorphisms, and they are the most frequently studied SNPs because of their possible functional role in gene expression. The nonsynonymous polymorphisms in the thiopurine methyltransferase (TPMT) gene that result in variant alleles called, TPMT*2, TPMT*3A, and TPMT*3C is an example of this kind of polymorphism.[30,31] These TPMT variants are associated with reduced enzyme activity and increased potential toxicity of drugs such as azathioprine and mercaptopurine. The SNPs that do not lead to the changes in amino acids are referred to as synonymous SNPs (silent polymorphisms). Although the synonymous polymorphisms do not result in change of amino acids, they may affect RNA secondary structure and cause allelic imbalance that could alter gene expression. The synonymous SNP in DNA excision repair gene (ERCC1) associated with altered 5-fluorouracil/oxaliplatin therapy in colorectal cancer is an example of this type of SNP.[32-34]

Noncoding Region Polymorphisms

The noncoding region (introns and regulatory regions) comprise the largest fraction (about 97%) of the human genome. Polymorphisms in these regions can affect altered mRNA stability and degradation, and gene expression and alternative splicing resulting in different protein isoforms. The SNPs that occur in the noncoding, regulatory regions of genes are referred to as regulatory SNPs (rSNPs). The following are examples of noncoding polymorphisms that have functional effects on gene expression.[28,35,36]

Promoter Polymorphisms

Polymorphisms in the promoter region can either increase or decrease the mRNA expression and, consequently, protein expression. One good example is the dinucleotide TA repeat polymorphism in the promoter of *UGT1A1* gene that results in a variant allele called *UGT1A1*28*. This polymorphism (*UGT1A1*28*) decreases expression of UGT1A1 protein and impairs elimination of bilirubin leading to Gilbert syndrome.[37]

5' and 3'UTR Polymorphisms

The 5'UTR of genes harbor regulatory sequences or elements such as promoters and enhancers, which play important roles in gene expression. The regulatory SNP (rSNP) in the promoter region of tumor necrosis factor α (TNF-α) gene creates a new binding site for the Oct-1 transcription factor that results in over expression of TNF-α in monocytes and increased susceptibility to cerebral malaria in affected Africans.[38]

The polymorphisms in the 3'UTR of genes can affect mRNA stability, half-life, and degradation and can result in alteration of gene expression.[39,40] The rSNP in the 3'UTR region of the human dihydrofolate reductase (DHFR) gene transcript results in the increased expression of DHFR protein, which may alter the effectiveness of drugs such as methotrexate that inhibits the DHFR enzyme.[41]

Splice-Site Polymorphisms

Polymorphisms in the splice sites can result in alternative splicing, abnormal protein production, and clinical consequences in some cases. The T to A polymorphism in the GT splice donor sequence of the β globin gene results in an alternative splicing site. Individuals who carry this polymorphism cannot produce β globin polypeptides and suffer from a disease called β⁰ thalassemia (a severe form of anemia).[42]

Short Tandem Repeat (STRs) Polymorphisms

Short tandem repeat (STR) or variable number of tandem repeats (VNTR) polymorphisms are short sequences of DNA, usually from 2–5 base pair long, that are repeated in tandem in the 5'→3' direction and occur in a variable copy number. The STRs are also referred to as microsatellites with one to six number of repeats of dinucleotides. One example of this type of polymorphism is the tandem repeats of multiple nucleotide sequence of 5'-GGCGGG-3' in the promoter region of 5-lipoxygenase (*ALOX5*) gene, which has been implicated as an important marker for inflammatory diseases. The most commonly occurring allele has five repeats (5'-GGCGGG GGCGGG GGCGGG GGCGGG GGCGGG -3'), and the three most common variant alleles have four STRs with deletion of one repeat (5'-GGCGGG GGCGGG GGCGGG GGCGGG -3'), three STRs with deletion of two repeats (5'-GGCGGG GGCGGG GGCGGG -3'), and six STRs with addition or insertion of one repeat (5'-GGCGGG GGCGGG GGCGGG GGCGGG GGCGGG GGCGGG -3'). It has been shown that the variant alleles have decreased promoter activity and, consequently, decreased transcription of *ALOX5* gene. Reduced ALOX5 protein production may in turn affect the clinical response of patients with asthma to drugs such as ABT-761, which target the 5-lipoxygenase pathway.[43]

Insertion Deletions (Indels) Polymorphisms

The insertion/deletion (I/D) polymorphisms (indels), which are the insertion or deletion of one or more nucleotide(s) that may occur anywhere in the DNA sequence of genes, are quite common and widely distributed in the human genome. There are many examples of indel polymorphisms, and a few examples with clinical importance include I/D in angiotensin-I-converting enzyme (ACE), I/D polymorphism of Alpha2B-adrenoceptor (ADRA2B) gene, and I/D polymorphism in NOD1 (CARD4) and its association with susceptibility to inflammatory bowel disease (IBD).[44]

Genotypes and Phenotypes

In 1908, Wilhelm Johannsen proposed the distinction between genotype and phenotype after realizing that the hereditary and developmental pathways had separate causes. The distinction between genotype and phenotype by Johannsen was induced from Mendel's work on inheritance in garden peas in 1900. Mendel's work clearly made the distinction between what we call today the "genome" and the "phenome." The genome includes all of the genes and noncoding sequences. Humans have two different genomes: a nuclear genome (3.2 billion base pairs) and a mitochondrial genome (37,000 base pairs). The phenome refers to all the phenotypes expressed by an organism, including all phenotypic traits caused by either genetic or environmental factors. The association between genotype and phenotype is not always clear and may depend on the interaction between genes, environmental factors, and epigenetic (changes in the gene expression caused by factors other than DNA sequence [nongenetic factors]) processes. In some cases a single phenotype may include many genotypes, as seen in multigenic diseases. Now researchers can acquire individual-level genotype-phenotype data from the database of the Genotype and Phenotype (dbGaP; http://www.ncbi.nlm.nih.gov/entrez/query.fcgi?db=gap). The dbGaP was created and is operated by the National Library of Medicine's National Center for Biotechnology Information (NCBI; http://www.ncbi.nlm.nih.gov/), which receives and archives data from studies that investigated the association between phenotype and genotype such as genome-wide association studies (GWAS). The phenotype and genotype data is provided to researchers at two levels of access: open access that is available to everyone without restriction and controlled access that requires authorization.[45]

Calculation of Genotype and Allele Frequencies from Genotype Data

Many pharmacogenomic studies are an association study, which aims to identify a genetic variation that may predict drug responses. These pharmacogenomic association studies compare frequencies of genotypes and alleles for a drug response phenotype. Thus, it is important to understand how frequencies of genotypes and alleles are calculated.

Let n_{AA}, n_{Aa} and n_{aa} be the number of subjects with corresponding AA, Aa, and aa genotypes in a pharmacogenomic study. The total number of the subjects (N) in the study is $N = n_{AA} + n_{Aa} + n_{aa}$. Let P_{AA}, P_{Aa}, and P_{aa} be the frequencies of the AA, Aa, and aa genotypes in the study. Then, $P_{AA} = n_{AA}/N$, $P_{Aa} = n_{Aa}/N$, and $P_{aa} = n_{aa}/N$. In addition, $P_{AA} + P_{Aa} + P_{aa} = 1$.

If the alleles, A, and a are located on an autosomal (nonsex) chromosome, the frequency of each allele can be calculated by the following formula:

$$P_A = (2n_{AA} + n_{Aa})/2N$$

$$P_a = (2 n_{aa} + n_{Aa})/2N$$

Note that the denominator should be 2N because an individual has a pair of autosomal chromosomes. Table 2-1 shows genotype data obtained from 293 subjects. The frequencies of AA, Aa, and aa genotypes are 0.75 (= 220/293), 0.22 (= 65/293), and 0.03 (=8/293), respectively. The A and a alleles occur in 86% (= (2 × 220 + 65) × 100/(2 × 293)) and 14% (= (2 × 8 + 65) × 100 /(2 × 293)) of the population.

Table 2-1
A Genotype Data from 293 Subjects

	Genotype			
	AA	Aa	Aa	Total
Count	220	65	8	293
Frequency	0.75 (= 220/293)	0.22 (= 65/293)	0.03 (= 8/293)	1.0 (= 0.75 + 0.22 + 0.03)

Hardy-Weinberg Equilibrium

Hardy-Weinberg Equilibrium (HWE) is a fundamental principle in population genetics. In 1908, an English mathematician G.H. Hardy and a German physician W. Weinberg individually described the principle to explain why dominant traits do not automatically replace recessive traits in a population.[46,47] Since pharmacogenomic studies often involve a large number of subjects with a certain phenotype who are genotyped for a particular locus, understanding of the concept of HWE and the potential causes of departure from HWE is very important. HWE states that the genotype and allele frequencies of a large, randomly mating population remain constant from generation to generation unless factors that disrupt the equilibrium have occurred.

Suppose we start with a single genetic locus with two alleles represented by A and a. Let the frequencies of the A and a alleles in a population be p and q, respectively. Since there are only two alleles in the population, the sum of their frequencies is 1 ($p + q = 1$). In addition, suppose mating occurs in the population independent of genotypes (random mating). Then, there will be three genotypes in the second generation (Table 2-2): AA, Aa, and aa. The frequencies of each of the genotypes will be p^2, $2pq$, and q^2, respectively. In addition, $p^2 + 2pq + q^2 = 1$.

Table 2-2
Genotype Frequencies in the Second Generation[a,b]

		Maternal gametes	
		A (p)	a (q)
Paternal gametes	A (p)	AA (p^2)	Aa (pq)
	a (q)	Aa (pq)	aa (q^2)

[a]Parentheses are the frequencies of alleles or genotypes.
[b]Genotype frequency: AA = p^2; Aa=2pq; aa=q^2.

If random mating occurs among the AA, Aa, and aa genotypes in the second generation (Table 2-3), the resultant genotypes and their frequencies (in parenthesis) in the next generation will be

AA × AA = AA (p^4)

AA × Aa = AA ($2p^3q$) and Aa ($2p^3q$)

AA × aa = Aa ($2p^2q^2$)

Aa × Aa = AA (p^2q^2), Aa ($2p^2q^2$) and aa (p^2q^2)

Aa × aa= Aa ($2pq^3$) and aa ($2pq^3$)

aa × aa = aa (q^4)

Table 2-3
Frequency of Type of Mating in the Third Generation[a]

		Maternal genotypes		
		AA (p^2)	Aa ($2pq$)	aa (q^2)
Paternal genotypes	AA (p^2)	AA × AA (p^4)	AA × Aa ($2p^3q$)	AA × aa (p^2q^2)
	Aa ($2pq$)	Aa × AA ($2p^3q$)	Aa × Aa ($4p^2q^2$)	Aa × aa ($2pq^3$)
	aa (q^2)	aa × AA (p^2q^2)	aa × Aa ($2pq^3$)	aa × aa (q^4)

[a]Parentheses are the frequencies of the genotypes.

As a result, the frequencies of the AA, Aa, and aa genotypes in the third generation are

$$AA = p^4 + 2p^3q + p^2q^2 = p^2 (p^2 + 2pq + q^2) = p^2 (p+q)^2 = p^2 \times 1 = p^2$$
$$Aa = 2p^3q + 4p^2p^2 + 2pq^3 = 2pq (p^2 + 2pq + q^2) = 2pq (p+q)^2 = 2pq$$
$$aa = p^2q^2 + 2pq^3 + q^4 = q^2 (p^2 + 2pq + q^2) = q^2 (p+q)^2 = q^2$$

Since from our original equation $p^2 + 2pq + q^2 = 1$, the frequency of each genotype remains constant and stable over successive generations. A population with a stable genotype frequency is said to be in Hardy-Weinberg equilibrium.

Calculation of Genotype and Allele Frequencies Using Hardy-Weinberg Equilibrium

HWE can be used to determine genotype frequencies from allele frequency data and/or allele frequencies from genotype frequency data in a study population. For example, cytochrome P450 2C9*2 (*CYP2C9*2*) is a C to T change at nucleotide position 430 in *CYP2C9* gene. The frequencies of the C and T alleles in Caucasians are 87% and 13%, respectively.[48] According to HWE it is estimated that 76% (= 0.87 × 0.87 × 100) of Caucasians carry CC; 22% (= 2 × 0.87 × 0.13 × 100) are CT and 2% (= 0.13 × 0.13 × 100) have TT. Beta$_1$-adrenergic receptor gene (*ADRB1*) contains an arginine to glycine change at codon 389. Thirty-four percent of African-Americans are homozygous for the arginine allele at codon 389 in *ADRB1*.[49] What are the frequencies of the arginine and glycine alleles in this population? Let the frequencies of the arginine and glycine alleles be p and q, respectively. According to HWE, $p^2 = 0.34$. Therefore, $p = \sqrt{0.34} = 0.58$. Since p + q = 1, q = 1 − 0.58 = 0.42. Thus, 58% and 42% of African-Americans carry arginine and glycine alleles, respectively. In addition, 49% (= 2 × 0.58 × 0.42 × 100) are arginine/glycine heterozygotes, and 17% (= 0.42 × 0.42 × 100) are glycine/glycine homozygotes.

Hardy-Weinberg Equilibrium in Pharmacogenomic Studies

If pharmacogenomic studies assess multiple genetic polymorphisms, HWE should be tested for each polymorphism. Departure from HWE indicates that experimental errors and/or factors that disrupt HWE may have influenced the study (see below). When applied to a cohort study, HWE should be tested in an entire study population. On the other hand, HWE should be tested only in the control population in a case-control study because departure from HWE is expected among cases if a genetic polymorphism is associated with a phenotype.[50] Since HWE assumes random mating independent of genotypes, Pearson's X^2-square test for independence is commonly used to evaluate the equilibrium.[51] The test, which is also called a goodness-of-fit-X^2 test, compares the observed genotype count in the study population with the expected count under HWE. In the example in 2-4, X^2 test statistics= Σ (observed-expected)^2/expected = 1.194 < 3.841, the critical value of $X^2_{\text{degree of freedom=1}}$ at $\alpha = 0.05$. As a result, the genotype frequency in the study population is in HWE. The X^2 test can produce a false-positive result, particularly when the study has a small size and/or a low minor allele frequency because the test assumes an asymptotic distribution of genotypes in the population.[51,52] Thus, an exact test should be used in studies with a small sample size and/or a low minor allele frequency. Alternative exact tests of HWE have been developed, and computer software codes of an exact test of HWE are freely available (http://www.sph.umich.edu/csg/abecasis/Exact/index.html).[53]

Table 2-4
Pearson's X^2-Ttest of the Genotype Data for Hardy-Weinberg Equilibrium[a]

		AA	Aa	aa	Total
Observed	Count	220	65	8	293
	Genotype	0.75	0.22	0.03	
Allele frequency			A: 0.86		
			a: 0.14		
Expected	Genotype	0.74	0.24	0.02	
		(= 0.86 × 0.86)	(= 2 × 0.86 × 0.14)	(= 0.14 × 0.14)	
	Count	216.8	70.3	5.9	
		(= 0.74 × 293)	(= 0.24 × 293)	(= 0.02 × 293)	

[a]Σ (observed-expected)^2/expected = (220-216.8)^2/216.8 + (65-70.3)^2/70.3 + (8-5.9)^2/5.9 = 0.047 + 0.400 + 0.747 = 1.194.

Factors Disrupting Hardy-Weinberg Equilibrium

HWE can be disrupted by biological (or evolutionary) and experimental factors. Biological factors include nonrandom mating, migration, genetic drift, founder effect, mutation, and natural selection.[54] Nonrandom genotyping error and missing genotype data are main experimental causes.[50] In human population, members of a particular subpopulation (social, ethnic, etc.) commonly mate with each other (nonrandom mating).[54] Inbreeding or mating between close relatives increases homozygosity for all genes. Assortative mating or mating between individuals who have a similar or a dissimilar phenotype can also change frequencies of homozygotes.[54] Mating with a similar phenotype increases homozygosity for genes involved in its expression, while mating with a dissimilar phenotype decreases the homozygosity. Migration also influences genotype frequencies in a population.[54,55] If a small population with a certain recessive genotype moves to a geographical region and becomes an isolate, it will have a higher frequency of the genotype. Genetic drift or allelic drift is a process in which genotype frequencies change from one generation to the next due to by chance.[55] Its effect is greater in a small population. Small populations are also more susceptible to founder effect. If founders of a population fail to pass a genetic allele on to the next generation, only the alternative alleles will be found in the successive generations.[54,55] If the founders pass a rare genetic allele to the next generation, its frequency increases in the successive generations. As a result, the founder effect changes the frequency of a certain rare genotype in a genetic isolate. Mutation, a change in the genetic material, occurs at a rate of 10^{-6} to 10^{-4} mutations per locus per gamete per generation.[54,55] At equilibrium, the genotype frequency is a balance between the rates of the introduction of new alleles by mutation and of the removal of the mutated alleles by negative selection.

Environmental factors such as radiation and chemicals that change the mutation rate can influence the balance. Biological fitness may differ by phenotype (hence genotype). A phenotype with low biological fitness has negative selection pressure, which will reduce the frequency of the genotype in the successive generations.[54,55] In contrast, a positive selection pressure will increase the frequency of the phenotype with high biological fitness. As a result, natural selection influences genotype frequencies in the population.

Nonrandom genotyping errors involve a systematic genotyping error, and this error disrupts HWE by misclassifying a particular genotype.[50] A preferentially missing genotype or allele can also break HWE. In addition, nonrandom genotyping error and missing data may lead to a spurious genotype-phenotype association; therefore, pharmacogenomic studies should have certain measures of quality control of genotyping assay to minimize the experimental errors.

Data Deviated from Hardy-Weinberg Equilibrium

In general, genotypes that are not in HWE are excluded from genotype–phenotype association analyses.[50] Often it is difficult to distinguish whether the departure from HWE is due to systematic experimental errors, violations of the assumptions of HWE, or a true association with a phenotype. A thorough examination of data is a key to identifying the cause. For example, data indicating heterozygotes are disproportionately missing relative to homozygotes may suggest a systematic experimental error. Data showing only one genetic marker is not in HWE among the markers in strong linkage disequilibrium (see below) may also imply a systematic experimental error. On the other hand, a consistent pattern of departure from HWE among the genetic markers in strong linkage disequilibrium may suggest violations of the assumptions of HWE. Departure from HWE due to violations of the assumptions may be replicated in an independent cohort, while that due to chance may not.

Haplotype

Haplotype is defined as a group of alleles on a chromosome.[54] Suppose that a pair of homologous chromosomes has three polymorphic loci (C or A at locus 1, T or G at locus 2, and C or G at locus 3) (Figure 2-5). Also, suppose that the dark gray and the light gray chromosomes are passed down from the person's mother and father, respectively. The *genotypes* in Figure 2-5 are CA at locus 1, TG at locus 2, and CG at locus 3. On the other hand the haplotypes, the multiple alleles on the same chromosome, are CTC (on the dark gray chromosome) and AGG (on the light gray chromosome). Individuals who are homozygous for C at locus 1, T at locus 2, and C at locus 3 carry two copies of CTC haplotype and 0 copy of AGG haplotype. Therefore, the maximum number of the copies of a particular haplotype an individual can carry is two and the minimum number is 0.

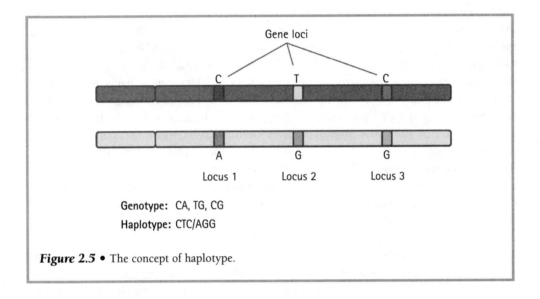

Figure 2.5 • The concept of haplotype.

Haplotypes are more useful than genotypes because haplotypes provide more information on local linkage disequilibrium and historical recombination events (see below).[56,57] Haplotype information can be obtained in two ways. Molecular haplotyping involves direct sequencing of multiple polymorphic loci on a chromosome. This method produces the most accurate information about haplotypes; however, it is often laborious and expensive, and technically challenging, particularly if the genetic loci are far apart.[51] Statistical haplotyping, such as an accelerated expectation maximization method, is more widely used to infer haplotypes in a study population.[51] It is based on the fact that the human genome consists of many genomic regions with a relatively small number of haplotypes due to strong linkage disequilibrium (see below). Various computer software such as PHASE, SNPHAP, and FASTPHASE have been developed to infer haplotypes. These programs are accurate in inferring haplotypes, particularly when they are used in data with high genomic marker density and few missing genotypes.[58]

Clinical Pearl

Haplotypes are more informative than genotypes. They can give information on past recombination events and local linkage disequilibrium.

Linkage Disequilibrium

Linkage disequilibrium is the nonrandom association of alleles at different sites.[54] Alleles in linkage disequilibrium are tightly linked together; as a result, they are more likely found together in a population. Linkage disequilibrium is a key concept in pharmacogenomic association studies, and it is used not only to select genomic markers but also to analyze genomic data in the association studies. It is also important in genome-wide association studies, which survey up to a million single nucleotide polymorphisms (SNPs) to associate a phenotype. As a basis of linkage disequilibrium, we will first review recombination process during meiosis.

Recombination Process

During meiosis, homologous chromosomes are paired together; subsequently, some of the genetic materials are exchanged between the pair. This process is called crossover or recombination.[59] Alleles close to each other on a chromosome are more likely to be passed along together, whereas alleles far apart are more likely to be regrouped during this process. Consider two bi-allelic loci on two different chromosomes (Figures 2-6; A/a and B/b on chromosome 1, and C/c and D/d on chromosome 2). Because the two loci in Figure 2-6 (A) are close, the next generation will have only two haplotypes: AB and ab (recall that a haplotype is a group of alleles on a chromosome). In contrast, the two loci in Figure 2-6 (B) may be regrouped during meiosis because they are far apart; as a result, the next generation will have four haplotypes (CD, cD, Cd, and cd). The recombination process is a basis of linkage disequilibrium and genetic diversity in human population. On average, 30–40 recombination events occur per chromosome during meiosis.[59]

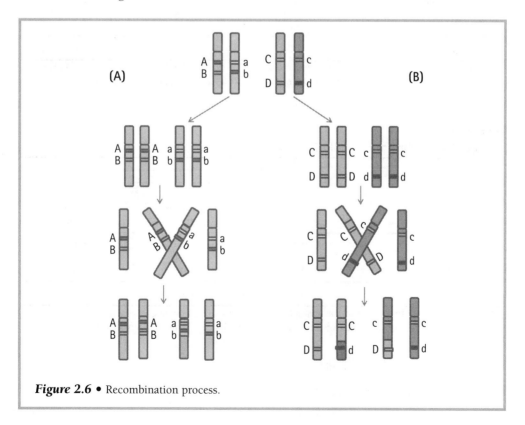

Figure 2.6 • Recombination process.

Mathematical Expression of Linkage Disequilibrium

Mathematical formula are helpful to understand the concept of linkage disequilibrium. Consider two bi-allelic loci (A or a allele at one locus, and B or b allele at the other locus) in a population. Assume the population is in HWE at both loci. Let P_{AB} be the frequency of AB haplotype in the population. In addition, let P_A and P_B be the frequencies of A and B alleles. If the two loci are independent of each other, then $P_{AB} = P_A \times P_B$. If the two loci are correlated with each other or in linkage disequilibrium, $P_{AB} \neq P_A \times P_B$.

Tables 2-5 and 2-6 illustrate this concept. Both tables contain two bi-allelic loci with four haplotypes (AB, Ab, aB, and ab). In Table 2-5, the frequency of the AB haplotype is 0.1 (P_{AB} = 0.1), and it is the product of the frequencies of the two alleles, P_A and P_B ($P_A \times P_B = 0.2 \times 0.5$ = 0.1): $P_{AB} = P_A \times P_B$. In addition, $P_{Ab} = P_A \times P_b$, $P_{aB} = P_a \times P_B$ and $P_{ab} = P_A \times P_b$; as a result, the two loci in Table 2-5 are not in linkage disequilibrium. In contrast, $P_{AB} \neq P_A \times P_B$ in Table 2-6 since $P_{AB} = 0.2$, while $P_A \times P_B = 0.6 \times 0.5 = 0.3$. Also, $P_{Ab} \neq P_A \times P_b$, $P_{aB} \neq P_a \times P_B$ and Pab ≠ $P_a \times P_b$; as a result, the two loci in Table 2-6 are in linkage disequilibrium.

Table 2-5
Linkage Disequilibrium Example 1[a]

			Locus 2		
			Allele		
			B	b	Total
Locus 1	Allele	A	0.1	0.4	0.5
		a	0.1	0.4	0.5
Total			0.2	0.8	1.0

[a]The numbers are the frequencies of haploytpes and alleles. For example, the frequencies of AB and Ab haplotypes are 0.1 and 0.4, respectively. The frequencies of A and B alleles are 0.5 and 0.2, respectively.

Table 2-6
Linkage Disequilibrium Example 2[a]

			Locus 2		
			Allele		
			B	b	Total
Locus 1	Allele	A	0.2	0.4	0.6
		a	0.3	0.1	0.4
Total			0.5	0.5	1.0

[a]The numbers are the frequencies of haplotypes and alleles. For example, the frequencies of AB and Ab haplotypes are 0.2 and 0.4, respectively. The frequencies of A and B alleles are 0.6 and 0.5, respectively.

Measures of Linkage Disequilibrium

Three parameters are commonly used to measure linkage disequilibrium in pharmacogenomic studies: D, D', and R^2. D is how much observed frequency of a haplotype differs from its expected frequency, and D' is a D value adjusted for allele frequency. R^2 is how strongly two variables are correlated.

Suppose two bi-allelic loci (A or a allele at locus 1, and B or b allele at locus 2). P_{AB} is the observed frequency of the haplotype AB formed by the two alleles A and B. D is defined as $D = P_{AB} - P_A \times P_B = P_{Ab} - P_A \times P_b = P_{aB} - P_a \times P_B = P_{ab} - P_a \times P_b$.[60] If the two loci are not in linkage equilibrium, D = 0, since $P_{AB} = P_A \times P_B$. In Table 2-5, the two loci are not in linkage disequilibrium since D = 0 ($P_{AB} - P_A \times P_B = 0.1 - 0.5 \times 0.2 = 0$). In Table 2-6, the two loci are in linkage disequilibrium since D ≠ 0 ($P_{AB} - P_A \times P_B = 0.2 - 0.6 \times 0.5 = -0.1$ or $P_{Ab} - P_A \times P_b = 0.4 - 0.6 \times 0.5 = 0.1$).

D intuitively explains the concept of linkage disequilibrium. However, its numerical value does not quantify the strength of linkage disequilibrium since the value varies as allele frequency changes. D' is defined as $D' = D / |D|_{max}$ where $|D|_{max} = \min (P_A \times P_b, P_a \times P_B)$, if D > 0 or min $(P_A \times P_B, P_a \times P_b)$, if D < 0.[60]

D' accounts for allele frequency since it is a normalized D value relative to the maximum D value achievable given allele frequency.[61] D' ranges between -1 and 1. $|D'| = 1$ suggests the two SNPs have not been separated by recombination. In other words, $|D'| = 1$ indicates perfect linkage disequilibrium between the loci. $|D'| < 1$ suggests the perfect linkage disequilibrium has been disrupted by recombination. The two loci in Table 2-5 are not in linkage disequilibrium since its D' = 0. In Table 2-6, D' = -0.1/min(0.3, 0.2) = -0.1/0.2 = -0.5; as a result, the two loci in Table 2-6 have some degree of linkage disequilibrium. D' has limitations. First, it is not clear how to interpret values of D' between 0 and 1 (e.g., we are not sure how different the two D' values, 0.4 and 0.6, are). In addition, sample size of a study can influence D' value because a small sample size tends to overestimate the value.[51] As a result, D' may not be a good measure to compare between studies with different sample sizes.

r^2 is a statistical coefficient of determination. It is defined as $r^2 = D^2/(P_A \times P_a \times P_B \times P_b)$.[60] It measures the extent of correlation between a pair of variables. r^2 ranges between 0 and 1, and a higher value indicates a higher degree of correlation between the pair. $r^2 = 1$ indicating perfect correlation is said to have "perfect linkage disequilibrium" between the loci. Since two bi-allelic loci can be perfectly correlated only if minor allele frequencies are identical at both loci, r^2 does not give information on recombination between the loci. In Table 2-5, $r^2 = 0$. In Table 2-6, $r^2 = (-0.1)^2/(0.6 \times 0.4 \times 0.5 \times 0.5) = 0.17$. Though D value in Table 2-6 suggests linkage disequilibrium, the r^2 value indicates that the degree of correlation between the two loci in the population is weak. r^2 is used to calculate the sample size of a pharmacogenomic association study since the sample size is inversely related to a r^2 value given a fixed effect size.[62] Suppose three polymorphic loci (locus 1, 2, and 3) with different r^2 values: $r^2 = 0.5$ between loci 1 and 2, and $r^2 = 1.0$ between 1 and 3. If a study selects the locus 1 to cover the locus 2, it requires twice as many subjects as a study that genotypes for the locus 1 to represent the locus 3. As with D, r^2 value is influenced by allele frequency since its calculation does not require normalization of allele frequency. Finally, r^2 is more useful to select "tagging SNPs" from a set of the potential SNPs since r^2 represents a degree of correlation between the SNPs.[63]

Which linkage disequilibrium measure should be used? Choice of a measure depends on the purpose of the study. In a pharmacogenomics association study, r^2 is more useful since it helps calculate the sample size and selection of tagging SNPs. In general, an r^2 value between the two loci ≥0.8 is considered as a strong correlation.[63]

Clinical Pearl

r^2 is more often used to obtain tag SNPs than the other measures of linkage disequilibrium.

Linkage Disequilibrium in Pharmacogenomic Association Studies

How is linkage disequilibrium used in a pharmacogenomic association study? Let's consider Figure 2-7. Suppose that the locus A in the gene harbors a SNP that causes variable drug response by changing an amino acid of a protein. If the loci B and C are in strong linkage disequilibrium with the locus A, then the SNPs at either the locus B or C can be chosen to represent the locus A. An SNP that represents the other SNPs, such as the SNPs at the loci B and C, is called a tagging SNP. The tagging SNPs may not cause phenotype variability among individuals. It is often hard to pinpoint a causal SNP that changes phenotype. Since tagging SNPs are highly correlated with a causal SNP, they can be used to identify the causal SNP or to narrow down the genomic region where the causal SNPs might be located. For example, the population in Table 2-7 has only two haplotypes: AB and ab. If a person carries the A allele, then the individual never carries the b allele but always the B allele on the same chromosome. As a result, genotyping for either locus 1 or 2 instead of both of the loci will obtain the allelic information of the other locus. Either one of the SNPs can be used to tag the other SNP. On the other hand, neither of the SNPs in Table 2-6 can be used as a tagging SNP since its population has four haplotypes (AB, Ab, aB, and ab). Note the SNPs in Table 2-6 are in weak linkage disequilibrium since D = 0.1, D' = 0.5, and r^2 = 0.17. In contrast, the SNPs in Table 2-7 are in strong linkage disequilibrium:

$D = P_{AB} - P_A \times P_B = 0.7 - 0.7 \times 0.7 = 0.21$

$D' = D/ |D| max = 0.21/min\ ((0.7)(0.3), (0.3)(0.7)) = 0.21/0.21 = 1$

$r^2 = D2/(PA \times Pa \times PB \times P_b) = (0.21)^2/(0.7 \times 0.3 \times 0.7 \times 0.3) = 1$

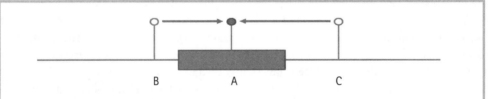

B   A   C

Figure 2.7 • Locus A is located in a gene while loci B and C are in nongenetic region. The loci B and C are in linkage disequilibrium with locus A. Because of linkage disequilibrium, genotyping at either locus B or C can give the genotype information on locus A. SNP refers to single nucleotide polymorphism.

Table 2-7
Linkage Disequilibrium Example 3[a]

			Locus 2		
			Allele		
			B	b	Total
Locus 1	Allele	A	0.7	0	0.7
		a	0	0.3	0.3
Total			0.7	0.3	1.0

[a]The numbers are the frequencies of haplotypes and alleles. For example, the frequencies of AB and Ab haplotypes are 0.7 and 0, respectively. The frequencies of A and B alleles are 0.7 and 0.7, respectively.

Note $r^2 \geq 0.8$ in Table 2-7, suggesting a strong correlation. These examples that show a pharmacogenomic association study can be more efficiently conducted if the SNPs in the study are in strong linkage disequilibrium.

Clinical Pearl

Linkage disequilibrium is a basis for genetic association studies including genome-wide association studies.

International HapMap Project

International HapMap Project is a multinational study to identify and catalog human genetic diversities.[64] In this ongoing Project, which started in 2002, DNA samples from four representative populations (Yoruba in Ibadan, Nigeria; Caucasians in Utah, USA; Han Chinese in Beijing, China; and Japanese in Tokyo, Japan) were sequenced to discover and map over 6 million SNPs as of October 1, 2008. The data are publicly available at www.hapmap.org. According to the HapMap data, most recombination events have occurred at short genomic regions called hotspots.[64] Linkage disequilibrium is often broken down at around hotspots due to their high recombination rate; as a result, the human genome has discontinuous linkage disequilibrium patterns and can be considered a block-like structure of linkage disequilibrium. Each block has limited numbers of common haplotypes due to its strong linkage disequilibrium. In fact, the average number of the common haplotypes in a block is four to five, even if each block contains 30–70 SNPs on average.[64] In addition, only a limited number of tag SNPs are required to obtain genetic variations in a block. The block-like linkage disequilibrium structure of human genome and the strong linkage disequilibrium within a block are an important basis for design and analysis of pharmacogenomic association studies, including genome-wide association studies.

Linkage Disequilibrium and Genome-wide Association Study

The human genome is estimated to have about 12 million common SNPs (minor allele frequency (MAF) >5%). The genome-wide association studies survey these SNPs to correlate a drug response (phenotype) to a genetic variant. Genotyping of all of these SNPs is technically feasible but laborious and time-consuming. Genome-wide association studies genotype 100,000 to 1,000,000 SNPs in the entire human genome.[65] Even if these numbers are smaller than the total number of the common SNPs, the information obtained from the tagging SNPs would be similar to that from all the common SNPs; as a result, genome-wide association studies are efficient. In addition, genome-wide association studies are expected to provide new biological information of a gene involved in drug response phenotypes since the studies have no hypothesis regarding a potential role of a gene in the phenotypes. For example, a genome-wide association study identified a genomic marker that is associated with statin-induced myopathy (phenotype).[66] The study, which enrolled 85 cases of statin-induced myopathy and 80 controls (no statin-induced myopathy), genotyped over 300,000 SNPs to associate a genetic marker with the risk of the phenotype. An SNP, rs4363657, located in the solute carrier organic anion transporter family member 1B1 gene (*SLCO1B1*) was strongly associated with the phenotype. The *SLCO1B1* gene encodes for organic anion transporting polypeptide, which mediates cellular uptake of various drugs including statins. Because the SNP was located in the intron, the exons of the *SLCO1B1* gene were resequenced to discover SNPs, which were in strong linkage disequilibrium with rs4363657 and may influence the functions of the protein by changing an amino acid. The rs4363657 SNP was found to be in strong linkage disequilibrium ($r^2 > 0.95$) with a nonsynonymous SNP, rs4149056, which changes valine to alanine at codon 174. This discovery may lead to better understanding of pathogenesis of the statin-induced myopathy. If it is replicated and the pathophysiological roles of *SLCO1B1* and its SNPs in the statin-induced myopathy are elucidated, then the SNPs may be used to identify patients who are at a high risk of this adverse event when treated with a statin.

Clinical Pearl

Genome-wide association studies will help discover new functions of a gene. The number of publications on the genome-wide association studies has recently dramatically increased.

Linkage Disequilibrium and Clinical Practice

Linkage disequilibrium is also used to select SNPs to genotype in clinical practice. The vitamin K epoxide reductase complex subunit 1 (*VKORC1*) gene encodes for a target protein of warfarin, an anticoagulant. Although the gene contains several nonsynonymous SNPs, their frequencies are low (minor allele frequency < 5%) in the population.[67] The gene also includes about 30 SNPs in the noncoding regions. Ten noncoding SNPs with a minor allele frequency ≥5% have been studied for an association with interindividual variability in warfarin dose requirements.[67] SNPs with a minor allele frequency <5% are often excluded in a pharmacogenomic study because they usually give inadequate power to the study and may be clinically unimportant.[65] Five of the 10 SNPs in strong linkage disequilibrium form two common haplotypes have been identified as a genetic factor, which influences the interindividual variability in warfarin dose requirements (Table 2-8): C at -4931 always occurs with A at -1639, T at 1173, C at 1542, and T at 2255.[67] Likewise, T is always associated with G at -1639, C at 1173, G at 1542, and C at 2255. As such, all of the five SNPs need not be genotyped to predict a patient's warfarin dose. Instead, only one locus can be chosen to infer alleles at the other four loci. For example, if a patient has C at 1173, the other alleles should be T at -4931, G at -1639, G at 1542, and C at 2255. Thus, strong linkage disequilibrium can decrease the number of the SNPs to be genotyped for clinical practice.

Table 2-8
Five Noncoding Single Nucleotide Polymorphisms in *VKORC1* Gene That Have Been Associated with Interindividual Variability in Warfarin Dose Requirements[a]

Locus	−4931	−1639	1173	1542	2255
SNPs	C	A	T	C	T
	T	G	C	G	C

[a]Because of strong linkage disequilibrium, SNPs in the first row (CATCT) occur together as the SNPs in the second row (TGCGC).

Clinical Pearl

Tagging SNPs can be used to predict drug therapy outcomes: *VKORC1 -1639G/A* is a tag SNP to predict warfarin dose.

Linkage Disequilibrium Plot

A linkage disequilibrium plot is often used to visualize pairwise linkage disequilibrium between SNPs. In addition, it helps identify haplotype blocks in a genomic region. Computer software such as Haploview are employed to construct a linkage disequilibrium plot from genotype data.[68] Figures 2-8a and 2-8c are linkage disequilibrium plots in beta2-adrenergic receptor (*ADRB2*) gene region in Caucasians, Yoruban Africans, and Chinese/Japanese. The haplotype blocks in Figures 2-8a, 2-8b, and 2-8c are defined based on 95% confidence bounds on D'.[56] The Caucasians have seven common SNPs with minor allele frequency >5%, and two haplotype blocks in the region (Figure 2-8a). Haplotype block 1 includes rs2400707, rs12654778, rs1042713, rs1042714, and rs1042717, and block 2 consists of rs1042718 and rs1042719. Linkage disequilibrium plots can display values of the various measures of linkage disequilibrium. In Figures 2-8a through 2-8c, r^2 values are shown since r^2 is used to select tagging SNPs. The two SNPs (rs2400707 and rs1042714) have a strong correlation because their r^2 value is ≥80. As a result of this strong correlation (one, between rs2400707 and rs1042714, and two, between rs12654778 and rs1042713) in the haplotype block 1, only three SNPs (rs1042717, either rs2400707 or rs1042714, and either rs12654778 or rs1042713) are required to cover the block. Since the two SNPs (rs1042718 and rs1042719) in the haplotype block 2 have r^2

<80, both of them may need to be genotyped. However, due to a strong correlation between rs1042717 and rs1042718 (r^2=80), only one of them can be selected. As a result, the total number of the tagging SNPs in the Caucasian population is four.

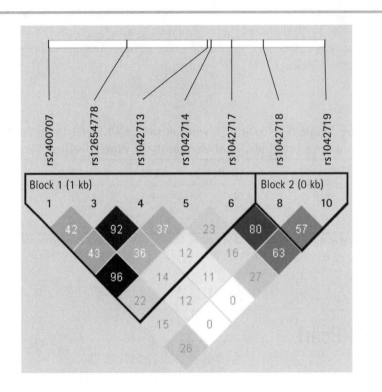

Figure 2.8a • The linkage disequilibrium plot is obtained from single nucleotide polymorphisms (SNPs) genotyped in the HapMap Project. The plot is generated by Haploview. The bars in the long white box in the upper part of the figure indicate the locations of the seven SNPs with minor allele frequency >5% in the Caucasian population. Note the region contains two haplotype blocks: block 1 (SNPs 1, 3, 4, 5, and 6) and block 2 (SNPs 8 and 10). Pairwise r^2 values are shown in the diamond boxes.

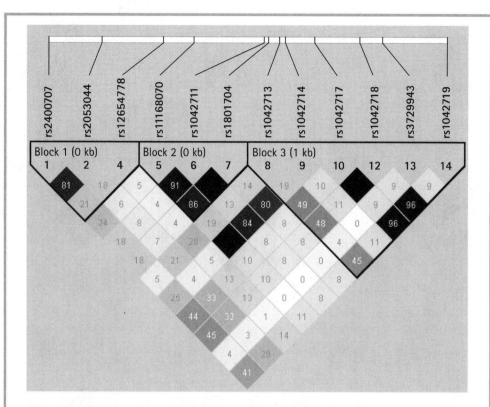

Figure 2.8b • The linkage disequilibrium plot is obtained from single nucleotide polymorphisms (SNPs) genotyped in the HapMap Project. The plot is generated by Haploview. The bars in the long white box in the upper part of the figure indicate the locations of the 12 SNPs with minor allele frequency >5% in the Yoruban population. Note the region contains three haplotype blocks: block 1 (SNPs 1, 2, and 4), block 2 (SNPs 5, 6, and 7), and block 3 (SNPs 8, 9, 10, 12, 13, and 14). Pairwise r^2 values are shown in the diamond boxes.

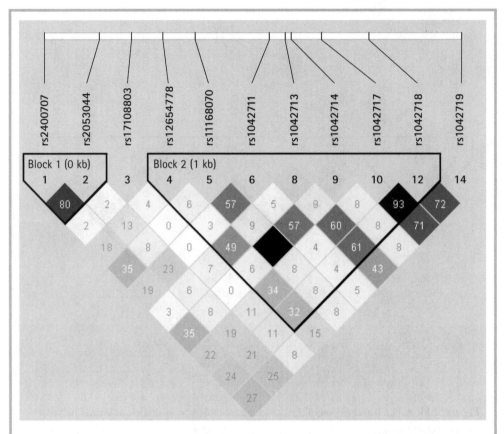

Figure 2.8c • The linkage disequilibrium plot is obtained from single nucleotide polymorphisms (SNPs) genotyped in the HapMap Project. The plot is generated by Haploview. The bars in the long white box in the upper part of the figure indicate the locations of the 11 SNPs with minor allele frequency >5% in the Chinese/Japanese population. Note the region contains two haplotype blocks: block 1 (SNPs 1 and 2) and block 2 (SNPs 4, 5, 6, 8, 9, 10, and 12). Pairwise r^2 values are shown in the diamond boxes.

In contrast to Caucasians, Yoruban Africans have 12 common SNPs with three haplotype blocks in the region (Figure 2-8b). Because of strong correlations between some of the SNPs, information on the *ADRB2* variations can be obtained with only six SNPs (rs2053044, rs12654778, rs1042711, rs1042713, rs1042718, and rs3729943).

The Chinese/Japanese populations have two haplotype blocks with 11 common SNPs in *ADRB2* (Figure 2-8c). Linkage disequilibrium data suggest the region requires eight tagging SNPs (rs2053044, rs17108803, rs12654778, rs1042711, rs1042713, rs1042714, rs1042717, and rs1042719).

Genetic Differences Among Racial and Ethnic Groups

Study populations with different ancestral history should be considered when pharmacogenomic studies are designed and interpreted as shown in the linkage disequilibrium plots of the three distinct populations in *ADRB2*. First, the number of the common SNPs in a genomic region may differ by study population. In *ADRB2*, the numbers are 7, 12, and 11 in Caucasians, Yoruban Africans, and Chinese/Japanese, respectively. The number of the genetic variations depends on how long ago a population was formed. The population with a longer history has more opportunity to develop new genetic variations such as mutation and recombination. Since African-descent populations were formed prior to the establishment of European- or Asian-descent populations, they have the largest number of genetic variations.[55] In addition, African-descent populations have shorter haplotype blocks and more haplotypes within a block than the other populations because of their higher genetic variability.[56,64] Populations living in close geographic regions have a similar pattern of genetic variations compared with those living far away from each other.[55] For example, Japanese and Chinese populations are genetically closer than Japanese and Europeans. Japanese and Chinese have similar frequencies of the minor allele (G) of rs1042714 (8 and 12%), while those in Caucasians and Yoruban Africans are 47% and 18%. Since study populations with different ancestral history may have differences in allele frequency, it should be checked for each population studied. Linkage disequilibrium patterns may also differ by study population. In *ADRB2*, for example, Yoruban Africans have three haplotype blocks while Caucasians and Chinese/Japanese have two blocks. In addition, the structures of the haplotype blocks are different between the Caucasian and the Chinese/Japanese populations despite their having the same number of the blocks. Finally, study populations may have distinct degrees of pairwise linkage disequilibrium. For example, Caucasians have strong linkage disequilibrium between rs1042714 and rs2400707 ($r^2 = 96$); in contrast, it is weak in Yoruban Africans and Chinese/Japanese ($r^2 = 25$ and 35).

Common *ADRB2* haplotypes, defined as its frequency >5% in each study population, are estimated based on an accelerated expectation maximization algorithm (Table 2-9a, 2-9b, and 2-9c).[68] Caucasians have four common haplotypes (Table 2-9a). Because of the eight common SNPs, Caucasians can have up to 256 ($=2^8$) potential haplotypes; however, the four common haplotypes account for about 93% of the total haplotype variability in Caucasians. Significant portions of the total variability in Yoruban Africans and Chinese/Japanese are also explained by the small number of the common haplotypes (Table 2-9b and 2-9c). The frequencies of the haplotype that occurs most often are 0.442, 0.291, and 0.337 in Caucasians, Yoruban Africans, and Chinese/Japanese, respectively. Because African-descent populations have higher genetic variability than the other populations, Yoruban Africans have the lowest frequency of the haplotype (0.291). The higher genetic variability in African-descent population also explains the lowest contribution (87%) of the total haplotype variability by the common haplotypes in Yoruban Africans.

Table 2–9a
Common *ADRB2* Haplotypes in Caucasians[a,b]

Haplotype block #		1				2		
SNP #	1	3	4	5	6	8	10	Frequency
Haplotype	A	G	G	G	G	C	G	0.442
	G	A	A	C	G	C	G	0.240
	G	G	G	C	A	A	C	0.175
	G	A	A	C	G	C	C	0.069

[a]SNP #1= rs2400707; SNP #3= rs12654778; SNP #4= rs1042713; SNP #5= rs1042714; SNP #6= rs1042717; SNP #8= rs1042718; SNP #10= rs1042719.

[b]rs numbers are reference SNP accession IDs in dbSNP (single nucleotide polymorphism database in National Center for Biotechnology Information). Genotype data are obtained from www.HapMap.org. AGGGGCG is a haplotype with a frequency of 0.442. Haplotypes are inferred by an accelerated expectation maximization method on Haploview software.

Table 2–9b
Common *ADRB2* Haplotypes in Yoruban Africans[a]

Haplotype block #		1		2				3					
SNP #	1	2	4	5	6	7	8	9	10	12	13	14	Frequency
	G	G	G	C	T	T	G	C	A	A	C	C	0.291
	A	A	G	C	T	T	A	C	G	C	C	G	0.267
Haplotype	G	G	A	C	T	T	A	C	G	C	C	G	0.192
	A	A	G	G	C	C	G	G	G	C	C	G	0.122

SNP #1= rs2400707; SNP #2= rs2053044; SNP #4= rs12654778; SNP #5= rs11168070; SNP #6= rs1042711; SNP #7= rs1801704; SNP #8= rs1042713; SNP #9= rs1042714; SNP #10= rs1042717; SNP #12= rs1042718; SNP #13= rs3729943; SNP #14= rs1042719.

[a]rs numbers are reference SNP accession IDs in dbSNP (single nucleotide polymorphism database in National Center for Biotechnology Information). Genotype data are obtained from www.HapMap.org. Haplotypes are inferred by an accelerated expectation maximization method on Haploview software.

Table 2-9c
Common *ADRB2* haplotypes in Chinese/Japanese[a]

Haplotype block #	1						2					Frequency
SNP #	1	2	3	4	5	6	8	9	10	12	14	
	G	G	T	G	C	T	G	C	A	A	C	0.337
	G	G	T	A	C	T	A	C	G	C	G	0.253
	A	A	T	G	C	T	A	C	G	C	G	0.139
Haplotype	G	G	G	G	C	T	G	C	A	A	C	0.079
	G	G	T	A	C	T	A	C	G	C	C	0.057
	A	A	T	G	G	C	G	G	G	C	G	0.056

SNP #1= rs2400707; SNP #2= rs2053044; SNP #3= rs17108803; SNP #4= rs12654778; SNP #5= rs11168070; SNP #= rs1042711; SNP #8= rs1042713; SNP #9= rs1042714; SNP #10= rs1042717; SNP #12= rs1042718; SNP #14= rs1042719.

[a]rs numbers are reference SNP accession IDs in dbSNP (single nucleotide polymorphism database in National Center for Biotechnology Information). Genotype data are obtained from www.HapMap.org. Haplotypes are inferred by an accelerated expectation maximization method on Haploview software.

Clinical Pearls

African-descent populations are genetically more diverse than European-descent and Asian-descent population: African-descent populations may need more SNPs to predict drug response compared with the other populations.

Population Stratification and Admixture

Pharmacogenomic association studies are often carried out as a case-control study. Cases are those who have a particular drug response phenotype and controls are the patients who do not have the particular phenotype. This design aims to discover the differences in allele frequency between cases and controls. Population stratification and admixture should be considered as potential confounders of these studies.[69] A study involving two or more unevenly distributed populations with differences in allele frequency between cases and controls can produce a false association. Such a study is said to have population stratification because differences in the allele frequency between cases and controls are not related to the phenotype but attributable to the uneven distribution of the background populations.[70] For example, a study found that a certain haplotype in human leukocyte antigen gene was associated with the risk of type II diabetes mellitus in Pima Indians. Since the haplotype has been more common in Caucasians, the data were reanalyzed according to Pima Indian ancestry. After adjustment for Pima Indian ancestry, it was not associated with an increased risk for the disease.[71]

Population admixture can also confound pharmacogenomic studies. Since allele frequency in an admixed population will be changed when two populations with differences in the allele frequency are admixed, comparing such populations for a phenotype difference may lead to a spurious association. Hispanics, for example, are an admixture of Caucasians, Africans, and Native Americans. Ancestral history in Hispanics differs by geographic region. Puerto Ricans are mainly an admixture of Caucasians and Africans, whereas Mexicans are of Caucasians and Native Americans. As a result, comparison of Puerto Ricans with Mexicans may produce a false association between an allele and a phenotype. A spurious association can also be found in a seemingly homogenous population if the population has genetically distinct subpopulations due to nonrandom mating.[69]

Careful matching strategies and sampling can minimize the confounding effects of population stratification and admixture in a pharmacogenomic case-control study.[70] In addition, the difference in population structure can be adjusted by using anonymous genetic markers and/or ancestral information markers.[70,71] A set of anonymous genetic markers scattered throughout the genome can be selected as an indicator of the amount of diversity in cases and controls. Ancestral information markers are genetic markers, often SNPs, which help identify a distinct population (e.g., Europeans, Africans, Asians, etc.) because these markers have differences in their frequencies between populations.[72] The ancestral information markers may be useful in distinguishing complex admixed populations, such as Hispanic populations in pharmacogenomics studies.

Clinical Pearl

Population structure and admixture can produce false associations between genes and drug responses.

Summary

The field of pharmacogenomics has burgeoned in recent years due rapid advances in molecular biology and expanded knowledge of human genomics. As pharmacogenomics begins to impact clinical practice, a fundamental understanding of human genetics will be essential for applying pharmacogenomics and to interpret the results of pharmacogenomic testing data on patients. The fact that multiple genetic variations can impact the actions of a single drug, as in the case of warfarin, adds a layer of complexity to our understanding of the impact of pharmacogenomics in clinical practice. While pharmacists and clinicians need not become geneticists to benefit from the application of pharmacogenomics, their knowledge of human genomics and the fundamental principles of pharmacogenomics will need to be enhanced and updated on a regular basis.

Case Study Answers

1. 58% (p^2=0.34. p=0.58).
2. Molecular haplotyping.
3. D' is useful for past recombination events and r^2 for obtaining tag SNPs.
4. African-descent populations have more genetic diversity since they are thought to have lived longer than the other populations.

References

1. Strachan T, Read AP. DNA structure and gene expression. In: Strachan T, Read AP, eds. *Human Molecular Genetics.* 3rd ed. Oxford: Garland Science; 2003:4-32.
2. Langaee TY, Zineh I. Applied molecular and cellular biology. In: *Pharmacogenomics: Applications to Patient Care.* Lenexa, KS: American College of Clinical Pharmacy (ACCP); 2004:53-116.
3. Kornberg RD. Eukaryotic transcriptional control. *Trends Cell Biol.* 1999;9:M46-M49.
4. Burgess-Beusse B, Farrell C, Gaszner M, et al. The insulation of genes from external enhancers and silencing chromatin. *Proc Natl Acad Sci USA.* 2002;99(Suppl 4):16433-16437.
5. Goessling LS, Daniels-McQueen S, Bhattacharyya-Pakrasi M, et al. Enhanced degradation of the ferritin repressor protein during induction of ferritin messenger RNA translation. *Science.* 1992;256:670-673.
6. Dvir A, Conaway JW, Conaway RC. Mechanism of transcription initiation and promoter escape by RNA polymerase II. *Curr Opin Genet Dev.* 2001;11:209-214.
7. Korzheva N, Mustaev A. Transcription elongation complex: structure and function. *Curr Opin Microbiol.* 2001;4:119-125.
8. Herbert A, Rich A. RNA processing and the evolution of eukaryotes. *Nat Genet.* 1999;21:265-269.
9. Kornblihtt AR. Chromatin, transcript elongation and alternative splicing. *Nat Struct Mol Biol.* 2006;13:5-7.
10. Lander ES, Linton LM, Birren B, et al. Initial sequencing and analysis of the human genome. *Nature.* 2001;409:860-921.
11. Sachs AB, Sarnow P, Hentze MW. Starting at the beginning, middle, and end: translation initiation in eukaryotes. *Cell.* 1997;89:831-838.
12. Nakamura Y, Ito K, Isaksson LA. Emerging understanding of translation termination. *Cell.* 1996;87:147-150.
13. Ingram VM. Sickle-cell anemia hemoglobin: the molecular biology of the first "molecular disease"—the crucial importance of serendipity. *Genetics.* 2004;167:1-7.
14. Rolfini R, Cabrini G. Nonsense mutation R1162X of the cystic fibrosis transmembrane conductance regulator gene does not reduce messenger RNA expression in nasal epithelial tissue. *J Clin Invest.* 1993;92:2683-2687.
15. Kuehl P, Zhang J, Lin Y, et al. Sequence diversity in CYP3A promoters and characterization of the genetic basis of polymorphic CYP3A5 expression. *Nat Genet.* 2001;27:383-391.
16. Snell RG, MacMillan JC, Cheadle JP, et al. Relationship between trinucleotide repeat expansion and phenotypic variation in Huntington's disease. *Nat Genet.* 1993;4:393-397.
17. Crawford DC, Schwartz CE, Meadows KL, et al. Survey of the fragile X syndrome CGG repeat and the short-tandem-repeat and single-nucleotide-polymorphism haplotypes in an African American population. *Am J Hum Genet.* 2000;66:480-493.
18. Korneev S, O'Shea M. Evolution of nitric oxide synthase regulatory genes by DNA inversion. *Mol Biol Evol.* 2002;19:1228-1233.
19. Kirchheiner J, Schmidt H, Tzvetkov M, et al. Pharmacokinetics of codeine and its metabolite morphine in ultra-rapid metabolizers due to CYP2D6 duplication. *Pharmacogenomics J.* 2007;7:257-265.
20. Kawanishi C, Lundgren S, Agren H, et al. Increased incidence of CYP2D6 gene duplication in patients with persistent mood disorders: ultrarapid metabolism of antidepressants as a cause of nonresponse. A pilot study. *Eur J Clin Pharmacol.* 2004;59:803-807.

21. Lifton RP, Dluhy RG, Powers M, et al. Hereditary hypertension caused by chimaeric gene duplications and ectopic expression of aldosterone synthase. *Nat Genet.* 1992;2:66-74.

22. Mitelman F, Johansson B, Mertens F. The impact of translocations and gene fusions on cancer causation. *Nat Rev Cancer.* 2007;7:233-245.

23. Neri A, Barriga F, Knowles DM, et al. Different regions of the immunoglobulin heavy-chain locus are involved in chromosomal translocations in distinct pathogenetic forms of Burkitt lymphoma. *Proc Natl Acad Sci USA.* 1988;85:2748-2752.

24. Korenberg JR, Chen XN, Schipper R, et al. Down syndrome phenotypes: the consequences of chromosomal imbalance. *Proc Natl Acad Sci USA.* 1994;91:4997-5001.

25. Hook EB, Warburton D. The distribution of chromosomal genotypes associated with Turner's syndrome: livebirth prevalence rates and evidence for diminished fetal mortality and severity in genotypes associated with structural X abnormalities or mosaicism. *Hum Genet.* 1983;64:24-27.

26. Sherry ST, Ward MH, Kholodov M, et al. dbSNP: the NCBI database of genetic variation. *Nucleic Acids Res.* 2001;29:308-311.

27. Marsh S, Kwok P, McLeod HL. SNP databases and pharmacogenetics: great start, but a long way to go. *Hum Mutat.* 2002;20:174-179.

28. Prokunina L, Alarcón-Riquelme ME. Regulatory SNPs in complex diseases: their identification and functional validation. *Expert Rev Mol Med.* 2004;6:1-15.

29. Vignal A, Milan D, SanCristobal M, et al. A review on SNP and other types of molecular markers and their use in animal genetics. *Genet Sel Evol.* 2002;34:275-305.

30. Relling MV, Hancock ML, Rivera GK, et al. Mercaptopurine therapy intolerance and heterozygosity at the thiopurine S-methyltransferase gene locus. *J Natl Cancer Inst.* 1999;91:2001-2008.

31. McLeod HL, Siva C. The thiopurine S-methyltransferase gene locus—implications for clinical pharmacogenomics. *Pharmacogenomics.* 2002;3:89-98.

32. Nackley AG, Shabalina SA, Tchivileva IE, et al. Human catechol-O-methyltransferase haplotypes modulate protein expression by altering mRNA secondary structure. *Science.* 2006;314:1930-1933.

33. Wang D, Sadée W. Searching for polymorphisms that affect gene expression and mRNA processing: example ABCB1 (MDR1). *AAPS J.* 2006;8:E515-E520.

34. Viguier J, Boige V, Miquel C, et al. ERCC1 codon 118 polymorphism is a predictive factor for the tumor response to oxaliplatin/5-fluorouracil combination chemotherapy in patients with advanced colorectal cancer. *Clin Cancer Res.* 2005;11:6212-6217.

35. Marsh S. Pharmacogenomics. *Ann Oncol.* 2007;18(Suppl 9):ix24-ix28.

36. Roden DM, Altman RB, Benowitz NL, et al. Pharmacogenetics Research Network—pharmacogenomics: challenges and opportunities. *Ann Intern Med.* 2006;145:749-757.

37. Ratain MJ. From bedside to bench to bedside to clinical practice: an odyssey with irinotecan. *Clin Cancer Res.* 2006;12:1658-1660.

38. Knight JC, Udalova I, Hill AV, et al. A polymorphism that affects OCT-1 binding to the TNF promoter region is associated with severe malaria. *Nat Genet.* 1999;22:145-150.

39. Jacobson A, Peltz SW. Interrelationships of the pathways of mRNA decay and translation in eukaryotic cells. *Annu Rev Biochem.* 1996;65:693-739.

40. Decker CJ, Parker R. Mechanisms of mRNA degradation in eukaryotes. *Trends Biochem Sci.* 1994;19:336-340.

41. Goto Y, Yue L, Yokoi A, et al. A novel single-nucleotide polymorphism in the 3'-untranslated region of the human dihydrofolate reductase gene with enhanced expression. *Clin Cancer Res.* 2001;7:1952-1956.

42. Divoky V, Bissé E, Wilson JB, et al. Heterozygosity for the IVS-I-5 (G-->C) mutation with a G-->A change at codon 18 (Val-->Met; Hb Baden) in cis and a T-->G mutation at codon 126 (Val-->Gly; Hb Dhonburi) in trans resulting in a thalassemia intermedia. *Biochim Biophys Acta.* 1992;1180:173-179.

43. Drazen JM, Yandava CN, Dubé L, et al. Pharmacogenetic association between *ALOX5* promoter genotype and the response to anti-asthma treatment. *Nat Genet.* 1999 Jun;22:168-170.

44. McGovern DP, Hysi P, Ahmad T, et al. Association between a complex insertion/deletion polymorphism in NOD1 (CARD4) and susceptibility to inflammatory bowel disease. *Hum Mol Genet.* 2005;14:1245-1250.

45. Rasmuson M. The genotype-phenotype link. *Hereditas.* 2002;136:1-6.

46. Hardy GH. Mendelian proportions in a mixed population. *Science.* 1908;28:49-50.

47. Weinberg W. Über den nachweis der vererbung beim menschen. *Jahreshefte des Vereins für vaterländische Naturkunde in Württemberg.* 1908;64:368-382.

48. Gage BF, Lesko LJ. Pharmacogenetics of warfarin: Regulatory, scientific, and clinical issues. *J Thromb Thrombolysis.* 2008;25:45-51.

49. Shin J, Johnson JA. Pharmacogenetics of beta-blockers. *Pharmacotherapy.* 2007;27:874-887.

50. Lunetta KL. Genetic association studies. *Circulation.* 2008;118:96-101.

51. Balding DJ. A tutorial on statistical methods for population association studies. *Nat Rev Genet.* 2006;7:781-791.

52. Emigh TH. A comparison of tests for Hardy-Weinberg equilibrium. *Biometrics.* 1980;36:627-642.

53. Wigginton JE, Cutler DJ, Abecasis GR. A note on exact tests of Hardy-Weinberg equilibrium. *Am J Hum Genet.* 2005;76:887-893.

54. Strachan T, Read AP. *Human Molecular Genetics.* 3rd ed. Oxford: Garland Science/Taylor & Francis Group; 2003.

55. Cavalli-Sforza LL. Human evolution and its relevance for genetic epidemiology. *Annu Rev Genomics Hum Genet.* 2007;8:1-15.

56. Gabriel SB, Schaffner SF, Nguyen H, et al. The structure of haplotype blocks in the human genome. *Science.* 2002;296:2225-2229.

57. de Bakker PI, Yelensky R, Pe'er I, et al. Efficiency and power in genetic association studies. *Nat Genet.* 2005;37:1217-1223.

58. Marchini J, Cutler D, Patterson N, et al. A comparison of phasing algorithms for trios and unrelated individuals. *Am J Hum Genet.* 2006;78:437-450.

59. Gelehrter TD, Collins FS, Ginsburg DG. *Principles of Medical Genetics.* 2nd ed. Baltimore, MD: Williams & Wilkins; 1998.

60. Devlin B, Risch N. A comparison of linkage disequilibrium measures for fine-scale mapping. *Genomics.* 1995;29:311-322.

61. Lewontin RC. The interaction of selection and linkage. ii. optimum models. *Genetics.* 1964;50:757-782.

62. Pritchard JK, Przeworski M. Linkage disequilibrium in humans: Models and data. *Am J Hum Genet.* 2001;69:1-14.

63. Carlson CS, Eberle MA, Rieder MJ, et al. Selecting a maximally informative set of single-nucleotide polymorphisms for association analyses using linkage disequilibrium. *Am J Hum Genet.* 2004;74:106-120.

64. International HapMap Consortium. A haplotype map of the human genome. *Nature.* 2005;437:1299-1320.

65. Hirschhorn JN, Daly MJ. Genome-wide association studies for common diseases and complex traits. *Nat Rev Genet.* 2005;6:95-108.

66. SEARCH Collaborative Group, Link E, Parish S, et al. *SLCO1B1* variants and statin-induced myopathy—a genomewide study. *N Engl J Med.* 2008;359:789-799.

67. Rieder MJ, Reiner AP, Gage BF, et al. Effect of *VKORC1* haplotypes on transcriptional regulation and warfarin dose. *N Engl J Med.* 2005;352:2285-2293.

68. Barrett JC, Fry B, Maller J, Daly MJ. Haploview: Analysis and visualization of LD and haplotype maps. *Bioinformatics.* 2005;21:263-265.

69. Hu D, Ziv E. Confounding in genetic association studies and its solutions. In: Qing Y, ed. *Pharmacogenomics in Drug Discovery and Development.* New York, NY: Humana Press; 2008:31-39.

70. Cardon LR, Palmer LJ. Population stratification and spurious allelic association. *Lancet.* 2003;361:598-604.

71. Knowler WC, Williams RC, Pettitt DJ, et al. Gm3;5,13,14 and type 2 diabetes mellitus: an association in American Indians with genetic admixture. *Am J Hum Genet.* 1988;43:520-526.

72. Halder I, Shriver MD. Measuring and using admixture to study the genetics of complex diseases. *Hum Genomics.* 2003;1:52-62.

Chapter 3

Methodologies in Pharmacogenomics

Christina L. Aquilante, Pharm.D.

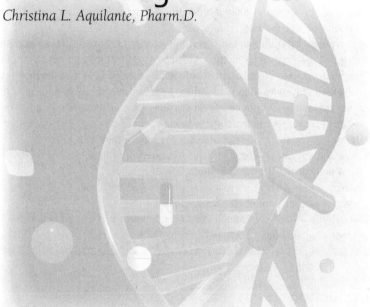

Learning Objectives

After completing this chapter, the reader should be able to

- Describe the processes of DNA collection and DNA isolation.
- Describe the chemistry used in the polymerase chain reaction (PCR).
- Explain the difference between the principles of allele discrimination and allele detection.
- Specify factors that may influence the selection of a particular genotyping method.
- Compare and contrast the chemistries used in common genotyping methods, such as restriction fragment length polymorphism (RFLP) analysis, Pyrosequencing, TaqMan®, mass spectrometry, and microarrays.
- Discuss how Food and Drug Administration-approved clinical genotyping tests, such as the Roche AmpliChip CYP450 test and the Invader UGT1A1 Molecular Assay, are used to determine an individual's genetic makeup.

Key Definitions

Allele—Alternative DNA sequences at a particular site in the DNA.

Allele detection—Method used in a genotyping reaction to capture the information from the allele discrimination step.

Allele discrimination—Method used in a genotyping reaction to differentiate between wild-type and polymorphic alleles.

Allele specific hybridization—A common allele discrimination method used in genotyping procedures whereby probes are designed to bind complementary to specific DNA sequences and are used to interrogate the polymorphism of interest.

Assay—In the setting of pharmacogenomics, a general procedure or test used to determine a person's genetic makeup.

Genotyping—Determination of a person's genetic make-up at a particular site in the DNA.

Multiplexing—Analysis of multiple polymorphisms in the same genotyping reaction.

Oligonucleotides—Short fragments of single-stranded DNA that are designed to bind to specific DNA sequences. Oligonucleotides are often referred to as primers or probes.

Primer extension—A common allele discrimination method used in genotyping procedures whereby a single-stranded oligonucleotide is bound complementary to the sequence of interest and the strand is extended over the polymorphism of interest.

Restriction enzymes—Enzymes that recognize a specific short sequence of nucleotides in the DNA and cut the DNA at that site.

Restriction sites—Short nucleotide sequences (generally four to eight base pairs in length) that are present throughout the genome.

Throughput—Number of samples or polymorphisms that can be genotyped with a particular genotyping method.

Introduction

The field of pharmacogenomics is aimed at understanding the influence of interindividual genetic variability on drug disposition and response.[1] Pharmacogenomic studies have heavily populated the scientific literature in recent years, and this pharmacogenomic information is starting to migrate into clinical practice.[2,3] One of the key factors driving pharmacogenomic research, and the subsequent incorporation of this information into clinical practice, is the increased number of sophisticated technologies that are available to determine a person's genetic makeup (i.e., genotyping).[4] Until a few years ago, the lack of sophisticated genotyping technology was considered a significant obstacle in the field.[4] However, genotyping technology has rapidly evolved in the last few years. As a result of these advances, the accurate and timely determination of a person's genetic makeup is no longer the rate-limiting step in the field of pharmacogenomics.

Although clinicians will rarely be asked to perform laboratory-based genetic tests, an understanding of how genetic information is obtained, processed, and analyzed is crucial for the successful clinical application of pharmacogenomic information.[5] Moreover, an understanding of the principles underlying common genotyping methods will allow for the appropriate analysis and interpretation of pharmacogenomic studies that are published in the literature. The goal of this chapter is to highlight the most common methodological procedures used in the field of pharmacogenomics. From DNA sample collection to genotype determination, the basic laboratory steps involved in the pharmacogenomic process will be discussed including (1) DNA sample collection; (2) DNA isolation; (3) DNA target sequence amplification via polymerase chain reaction (PCR); and (4) genotyping methods such as restriction fragment length polymorphisms (RFLP) analysis, pyrosequencing, TaqMan®, mass spectrometry, and microarrays.

 ## Case Study

Cytochrome P450 (CYP) 2D6 is an oxidative enzyme that is responsible for the hepatic metabolism of a wide variety of clinically-used drugs such as antidepressants, antipsychotics, antiarrhythmics, opiates, antiemetics, and beta-adrenergic receptor blockers.[6] CYP2C19 is also an oxidative enzyme that is responsible for the hepatic metabolism of drugs such as anticonvulsants, proton pump inhibitors, anticoagulants, benzodiazepines, and antimalarials.[6] The *CYP2D6* gene is highly polymorphic, with over 70 polymorphisms identified in the gene thus far. Functional polymorphisms in the *CYP2D6* gene are associated with altered metabolizing enzyme activity and result in different CYP2D6 metabolizing enzyme phenotypes such a poor metabolizers, intermediate metabolizers, extensive metabolizers, and ultrarapid metabolizers. Two common polymorphisms in the *CYP2C19* gene are associated with a poor metabolizer phenotype. Knowledge of an individual's *CYP2D6* and *CYP2C19* genotype and phenotype may help predict CYP2D6 and CYP2C19 drug metabolizing enzyme activity and may help clinicians select the most safe and effective medications for a particular disease.[6] Recently, the Food and Drug Administration approved the Roche AmpliChip CYP450 test. This test is intended to identify a patient's *CYP2D6* and *CYP2C19* genotype. The package insert for the Roche AmpliChip CYP450 test states that information about *CYP2D6* and *CYP2C19* genotype may be used as an aid to clinicians in determining therapeutic strategy and treatment dose for therapeutics that are metabolized by the *CYP2D6* or *CYP2C19* gene product.[6] The Roche AmpliChip CYP450 test can be prescribed by a physician and processed at a participating laboratory. The *CYP2D6* and *CYP2C19* genotype and phenotype results are sent back to the provider usually within a week.

Questions:
1. In clinical practice, what are the most common ways to collect human genomic DNA?
2. Explain the process by which DNA is isolated from nucleated cells.
3. What role does polymerase chain reaction play in the genotyping process?
4. What factors influence the choice of a genotyping method for a particular laboratory or pharmacogenomic application?
5. The Roche AmpliChip CYP450 test is a DNA microarray. Explain how genotyping by a microarray is different than genotyping with other methods, such as PCR-RFLP, pyrosequencing, or TaqMan®.

DNA Sample Collection

Pharmacogenomics is based on the accurate determination of an individual's genetic makeup at a particular site in their genomic DNA. While nonhuman genetic information (e.g., tumor, bacteria, and virus) can be used to guide pharmacologic therapy, the processes described hereafter are focused on the collection, isolation, and interrogation of human genomic DNA. Human genomic DNA can be obtained from any cell in the body that contains a nucleus, most commonly blood lymphocytes or buccal (cheek) cells. Genomic DNA cannot be obtained from non-nucleated cells, such as red blood cells or platelets. The gold standard method to obtain a DNA sample is through collection of peripheral whole blood.[7] Whole blood collection is the preferable method because it yields a large amount of DNA. For example, a 5-mL whole blood sample yields enough DNA (approximately 150 mcg) to perform thousands of genotyping reactions.[8] Although clinical genetic tests usually only require a few genotyping reactions, whole blood collection is advantageous because it allows for the storage of an ample amount of DNA for future pharmacogenomic investigations. Furthermore, some studies suggest that the DNA obtained from whole blood is of superior quality than DNA obtained from other sources, such as buccal cells or saliva.[9] The disadvantage of whole blood collection is that it involves an intravenous blood draw. The venipuncture procedure may be resource-, time-, or cost-prohibitive in certain patient care settings, and it may pose challenges or discomfort in certain patient populations (e.g., pediatrics).

Another common method for DNA sample collection is through the collection of buccal epithelial cells using a cheek swab, cheek brush, or oral rinse.[7,10,11] The cheek swab and brush methods involve rubbing a foam-tipped swab or cytobrush against the inside of the cheek for approximately 30 seconds.[12] The swab or brush is then placed in a sterile container. For the oral rinse method, patients are asked to vigorously swish approximately 10 to 30 mL of commercially available mouthwash for 30 to 60 seconds and then expectorate into a sterile collection container.[10,11,13] Some studies have shown that the oral rinse method produces higher DNA yields than the swab or brush methods (e.g., 55 mcg of DNA oral rinse method versus 12 mcg of DNA brush or swab methods).[10,12,14] In terms of advantages, buccal cell methods are noninvasive, easy to perform, and relatively painless. However, buccal cell methods may be disadvantageous because they result in lower DNA yields than whole blood collection, often have nonhuman DNA contamination (e.g., bacteria), and may not be ideal for certain patient groups. For example, in children, cytobrushes may be painful, and the oral rinse technique may be difficult for children to execute without swallowing or aspirating the liquid.[15] Additionally, some data suggest that DNA obtained from buccal cell methods may be of lower quality than DNA obtained from whole blood, and thus may not perform as well in subsequent genotyping reactions.[16]

The newest method of DNA collection involves obtaining a whole saliva sample, which includes both buccal epithelial cells and white blood cells found in the mouth. In this method, patients are asked to expectorate approximately 2 mL of saliva into a sterile container. The whole saliva method yields more DNA (i.e., approximately 35 mcg per 2-mL saliva sample) than other buccal cell collection methods; however, the amount of nonhuman DNA is high.[17] A commercial whole saliva collection kit is available (Oragene® DNA self-collection kit, DNA Genotek Inc.), whereby once a patient expectorates into the container and closes the cap, the contents in the container initialize the beginning phases of DNA isolation and stabilization. This type of collection kit lends itself well to situations where DNA needs to be stored for long periods of time, or shipped at room temperature.[12]

DNA Isolation

After DNA collection, the next step in the process is to extract, isolate, and purify the DNA from the cells in the sample. This process will be hereafter referred to as *DNA isolation*. There are many commercially available kits to aid in the DNA isolation process, and the methods used in these kits differ based on the type of sample that is collected, the chemicals used in the DNA isolation process, and the quantity of DNA that needs to be isolated. In general, the process of genomic DNA isolation involves the following steps: (1) disruption and lysis of cells in order to release genomic DNA; (2) removal of proteins and cellular debris; and (3) recovery of purified DNA.[18] In terms of DNA isolation from whole blood, the first step in the process is to lyse the red blood cells (which do not contain genomic DNA), while keeping the white blood cells (which contain genomic DNA) intact. The white blood cells are then collected in a pellet through centrifugation, and the cellular membranes are lysed with a detergent. During the disruption and lysis process, protease is added to the sample in order to digest proteins contained in the cells.[18] In some DNA isolation protocols, organic solvents (e.g., phenol, chloroform, or isoamyl alcohol) or high concentrations of salts (e.g., potassium acetate or ammonium acetate) are used to extract the proteins from the lysed cells.[18] These methods have some limitations in that they are time-consuming and often require the use of toxic substances (e.g., organic solvents). In most commercially available DNA isolation kits, the use of protease is preferred because it is easy, reliable, and relatively nontoxic. Following treatment with protease, the digested cellular proteins are collected in a pellet by centrifugation, and the supernatant, which contains the genomic DNA, is collected. The genomic DNA in the supernatant is then recovered from the sample by an alcohol precipitation step using ethanol or isopropanol.[18] The precipitated DNA is collected in a pellet by centrifugation and is resuspended in an appropriate buffer for long-term storage.[18]

The process of isolating DNA from buccal cells varies slightly from the isolation process of whole blood samples because it does not require a red blood cell lysis step. Instead, buccal cell samples are centrifuged to concentrate the cells in a pellet. This pellet is then resuspended and the processes of cell lysis, protein removal, DNA precipitation, and DNA recovery are performed.[14] Following the DNA isolation process, the purity and concentration of DNA can be measured by spectrophotometry. The concentration of DNA is determined by measuring the absorbance at 260 nm. The purity of DNA is determined by measuring the ratio of absorbances at 260 nm and 280 nm. A ratio of 1.7 to 1.9 indicates that the DNA sample is pure and free of protein contaminants.[18]

DNA Amplification via Polymerase Chain Reaction

The human genome contains approximately 3 billion base pairs. Thus, most clinical pharmacogenomic tests require that a specific region of DNA within the genome be targeted and amplified. A specific region of DNA that contains the gene or polymorphism of interest is often referred to as a target sequence. Target sequences can vary in size depending on the subsequent genotyping method to be used, but in general, target sequences are usually a few hundred base pairs in length. PCR is the method that is used to target and amplify a specific sequence of DNA within the genome.[19, 20]

PCR was developed based on the inherent physiochemical properties of DNA. DNA consists of two strands bound together in antiparallel form (5' to 3' and 3' to 5').[21] The nucleotide bases (adenine, thymine, cytosine, and guanine) in the two strands are bound complementary to each other by hydrogen bonds such that adenine binds with thymine and cytosine binds with guanine.[21] The major steps of the PCR process are shown in Figure 3-1 and include (1) denaturation (i.e., strand separation); (2) primer annealing; and (3) strand extension.[5,19] The hallmark of PCR is the cycling of different temperatures, in the presence of key reaction components, to target and exponentially amplify a specific DNA target sequence. A PCR mixture generally contains the following reaction components: genomic DNA, deoxynucleoside triphosphates (dATP, dCTP, dGTP, and dTTP), buffer, cations (e.g., magnesium or potassium), primers, and DNA polymerase.[22]

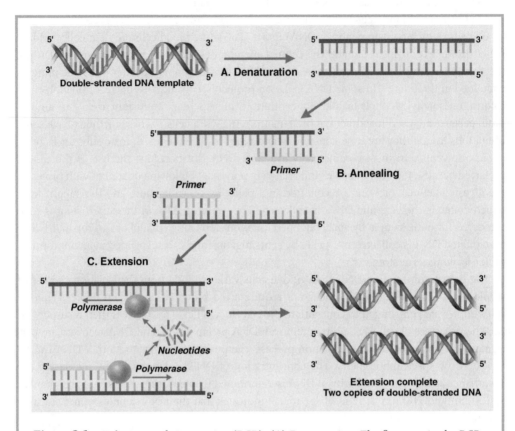

Figure 3.1 • Polymerase chain reaction (PCR). (A) Denaturation: The first step in the PCR process is to separate the double-stranded DNA into two single-stranded template molecules. Denaturation is typically accomplished at 95 °C. (B) Annealing: Following strand separation, the reaction is cooled to allow the primers present in the reaction mixture to hybridize to the single-stranded DNA templates. One primer binds complementary to one strand in the forward direction, while the second primer binds complementary to the other strand in the reverse direction. (C) Extension: DNA polymerase catalyzes the addition of deoxynucleotides to the 3' end of each hybridized primer. Extension is typically accomplished at 72 °C. Following extension, the complementary strand of each of the single-stranded products is built up to form two double-stranded replicates. These replicates then serve as templates in the next series of temperature cycles. This series of cycles (denaturation, annealing, and extension) is repeated 30–40 times, and the number of double-stranded replicates increases in an exponential fashion. Originally published in Aquilante CL, Zineh I, Beitelshees AL, et al. Common laboratory methods in pharmacogenomics studies. *Am J Health-Syst Pharm.* 2006;63:2101-2110. Illustration by Marie Dauenheimer, CMI.

During the process of denaturation, the hydrogen bonds holding the double-stranded DNA molecule together are broken, and the double-stranded DNA molecule is separated into two single-stranded molecules. This typically occurs at a temperature of approximately 95°C. Following denaturation, two single-stranded primers (also known as oligonucleotides) are annealed to the single-stranded DNA molecules. A primer is a short sequence of nucleotides (generally 17 to 30 base pairs in length) that is designed to bind complementary to a specific sequence of nucleotides in the single-stranded DNA molecule.[20] One primer is designed to bind complementary to one strand of the DNA molecule in the forward direction (5' to 3'), while the second primer is designed to bind complementary to the other strand of the DNA molecule in the reverse direction (3' to 5').[20] The temperature required for the primers to anneal to the single-stranded DNA molecule is highly dependent on the sequence of nucleotides in the template DNA. However, in general, annealing temperatures range from 40°C to 70°C. Once the two primers are annealed to the single-stranded DNA molecules, the process of extension can occur. The extension step of the PCR reaction is typically carried out at 72°C and is catalyzed by an enzyme called DNA polymerase, which promotes the synthesis of a complementary strand of DNA in the 5' to 3' direction.[22] Specifically, DNA polymerase functions to add deoxynucleoside triphosphates (dATP, dCTP, dGTP, and dTTP) to the 3' end of each primer that is annealed to the single-stranded DNA molecule. In this way, each single-stranded DNA template strand is built up to form a double-stranded DNA replicate. There are many different types of DNA polymerases that may be used in the DNA process; however, the most common is Taq polymerase, a heat-stable DNA polymerase that comes from the bacterium, *Thermus aquaticus*.[19] The cycle of denaturation, annealing, and extension is repeated 30 to 40 times resulting in an exponential increase in the number of DNA replicates. At the end of the PCR process, millions of copies of the DNA target sequence are present in the reaction mixture.

Once PCR is complete, a small amount of the PCR product is often subjected to gel electrophoresis to verify that the PCR worked correctly and that the amplified target sequence (also referred to as an amplicon) is the correct size (Figure 3-2).[5,22] In gel electrophoresis, a portion of the PCR product is mixed with a tracking dye and injected onto an agarose gel, along with a DNA molecular weight marker (also called a "ladder"). The agarose gel is placed in an electrophoresis unit, where an electric current is then passed through the unit. The electric current prompts the negatively charged DNA to pass through the gel towards the positive electrode. The agarose gel is porous, and the speed at which the PCR product moves through the gel is dependent on the size of the PCR product.[23] For example, large PCR products move slowly through the gel, whereas small PCR products move quickly through the gel.[5] The agarose gel is typically stained with ethidium bromide, a substance which intercalates into DNA and can be visualized under ultraviolet light. After completion of electrophoresis, the gel can be viewed under ultraviolet light and the position of the PCR product (i.e., band) is compared to the position of the bands of the DNA molecular weight marker. This allow the size of the PCR product to be estimated.[5]

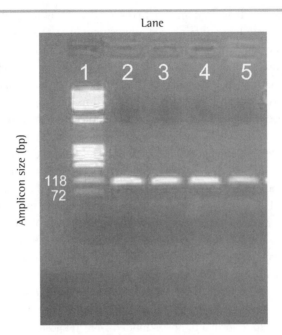

Figure 3.2 • Gel electrophoresis. A 106 base pair target sequence in human genomic DNA was amplified by PCR. The PCR product underwent electrophoresis on a 1.5% agarose gel and was stained with ethidium bromide to allow for visualization under ultraviolet light. Lane 1 shows the DNA molecular weight marker ("ladder"). Lanes 2 through 5 show the PCR product (highlighted bands) from four patient samples. The expected size of the PCR product (106 base pairs) can be verified by comparing the band position on the gel in relation to the band positions of the DNA ladder (118 bp and 72 bp). Originally published in Aquilante CL, Zineh I, Beitelshees AL, et al. Common laboratory methods in pharmacogenomics studies. *Am J Health-Syst Pharm.* 2006;63:2101-2110. © 2006, American Society of Health-System Pharmacists, Inc. All rights reserved. Reprinted with permission (R0932).

Principles of Genotype Determination

Once the DNA sequence of interest is targeted and amplified, the next step in the pharmacogenomic process is to determine a person's genetic makeup (i.e., genotype) at a particular site within that DNA sequence. There are many genotyping methods and technologies available to accomplish this goal. The two overarching principles that differ between genotyping methods are (1) allele discrimination and (2) allele detection.[24,25] Allele is a term that refers to alternative DNA sequences at a particular site in DNA. At each site in DNA, a person has two alleles, one from their mother and one from their father. The term *allele discrimination* refers to the chemistry that is used to distinguish between polymorphic (i.e., variant) and nonpolymorphic (i.e., wild-type) alleles that are present at a particular locus in a person's DNA sample. The term *allele detection* refers to the chemistry that is used to detect the information obtained from the allele discrimination reaction.

Beyond differences in allele discrimination and detection chemistries, the choice of genotyping method can be influenced by a number of other factors such as the number of samples and polymorphisms that can be genotyped at one time (also referred to as *throughput*); the type of polymorphism that can be genotyped using the method (e.g., single nucleotide polymorphisms versus insertion/deletion polymorphisms); equipment acquisition and genotyping costs (i.e., labor, consumables); turn-around-time; required technical expertise; and the ability of the method to genotype more than one polymorphism at one time (i.e., multiplex genotyping).[5,24-26] Ideally, the chosen method should be able to determine a genotype in one attempt, and if a second attempt is necessary, it should be fast and inexpensive.[5,27] Given the millions of polymorphisms present in the human genome, the genotyping method should also allow for fast and easy assay development and validation.[28] The ability to set up a new genotyping assay is a key component for productivity in the field of pharmacogenomics. The genotyping method should also provide genetic results in a manner that is software-driven and easy to interpret.[29] This decreases the chance for errors in human interpretation and ambiguous genotype determinations.

As pharmacogenomic tests begin to make their way into the clinical arena, additional analytical parameters such as specificity, sensitivity, reproducibility, and accuracy are also important considerations in the genotyping process.[29,30] The challenge associated with evaluating genetic test performance characteristics is that many tests arise out of academic laboratories and are not Food and Drug Administration-approved diagnostic tests.[30] As such, analytical test performance characteristics may be unpublished, or may differ between or within a laboratory.[30] Analytical test characteristics that should be considered in the genotyping method selection process include analytical sensitivity, analytical specificity, reproducibility, and accuracy.[29,31] In the context of genetic testing, analytical sensitivity refers to the probability that a test will be positive when a particular DNA sequence is present, while analytical specificity refers to the probability that a test will be negative when a particular DNA sequence is absent.[32] Reproducibility refers to the probability of the test repeatedly producing the same results in the same person.[31,32] Accuracy is the degree to which the observed genotype matches the true genotype.[29]

Many different methods are available to determine a person's genetic makeup, and the list grows substantially each year as genomic technologies become more sophisticated and less expensive. This chapter will focus on the most widely used genotyping methods. For each method, the principle allele discrimination and allele detection chemistries are presented, along with a discussion of pertinent factors (e.g., throughput, cost) that might influence the choice of that particular genotyping method. An abbreviated summary of the described methods is presented in Table 3-1. A presentation of the primary advantages and disadvantages of the more popular genotyping methodologies is presented in Table 3-2. The discussion of genotyping methods is focused on their ability to genotype single nucleotide polymorphisms. However, it is important to point out that in many cases the genotyping method can be engineered to detect other polymorphisms, such as insertions/deletions and nucleotide repeats.

Table 3-1
Summary of Genotyping Methods Discussed in the Text

Genotyping Method	Allele Discrimination Method	Allele Detection Method	Throughput	Cost Estimates per SNP[a]
Traditional Sanger DNA sequencing	Chain terminator chemistry	Capillary gel electrophoresis	Low	Medium
PCR-RFLP	Restriction endonucleases	Gel electrophoresis	Low	High
Pyrosequencing	Primer extension	Light	Medium	Medium
TaqMan®	Allele-specific hybridization	Fluorescence	Medium to high	Low
Mass spectrometry	Various (e.g., allele-specific hybridization or primer extension)	Molecular weight	Medium to high	Low
SNaPshot	Primer extension	Fluorescence and capillary gel electrophoresis	Medium to high	Low
Ligation	Allele-specific hybridization and Ligase enzyme	Fluorescence	Medium to high	Low
Invader assay	Endonuclease enzyme (e.g., Cleavase®)	Fluorescence	Medium to high	Low
DNA microarrays (e.g., Affymetrix GeneChip or Illumina BeadArray)	Allele-specific hybridization	Fluorescence	High	Low

SNP = single nucleotide polymorphism; PCR = polymerase chain reaction; RFLP = restriction fragment length polymorphism.

[a]Cost Estimates: high = greater than $4.00 per SNP; medium = $1.00 to $4.00 per SNP; low = less than $1.00 per SNP.

Table 3–2
Notable Advantages and Disadvantages of the Most Popular Genotyping Methods

Genotyping Method	Advantages	Disadvantages
PCR-RFLP	Low equipment acquisition costs	Low throughput Lengthy sample processing times High per SNP cost Limited multiplexing capability Requires user to assign genotype calls, which can introduce error
Pyrosequencing	Provides sequence information for the region surrounding the SNP, thus providing a specificity measure in each reaction High sensitivity Software assigns genotype calls	Higher per SNP cost Difficulty interrogating regions that contain long stretches of the same nucleotide (i.e., homopolymeric regions) Lower order multiplexing capability
TaqMan®	Combines PCR and allele discrimination in a single reaction, which results in time and cost savings Software assigns genotype calls	Less amenable to multiplexing Fluorescent-labeled probes can be expensive Lower order multiplexing capability
Mass spectrometry	High sensitivity High throughput Higher order multiplexing capability Software assigns genotype calls	High equipment acquisition costs Requires technical expertise Requires labor-intensive purification procedures
Invader assay	Does not require a PCR amplification step Highly accurate Software assigns genotype calls	Requires large quantities of genomic DNA Limited multiplexing capability
DNA microarray	Capable of genotyping hundreds of thousands of polymorphisms Utilized in genome wide association studies	High cost per chip may be cost-prohibitive for studies involving thousands of patients

SNP = single nucleotide polymorphism; RFLP = restriction fragment length polymorphism.

Genotyping Methods

DNA Sequencing

Before the recent advent of sophisticated high-throughput genotyping technologies, direct DNA sequencing (i.e., determination of the sequence of nucleotides along a DNA strand) was one of the most popular methods used to determine a person's genetic makeup. Although other genotyping modalities are often used today, direct DNA sequencing is still considered a gold standard genotyping method. Furthermore, many advances in sequencing technology have resulted in faster, less cumbersome methods that are more amenable to high-throughput genomic analyses.[33]

The origins of direct DNA sequencing are largely based on a method developed by Dr. Fred Sanger in 1975. The Sanger method is often referred to as the chain termination method, and the foundation of this method is the use of dideoxynucleotides (also known as chain terminators). Dideoxynucleotides are similar to nucleotides, except they do not have a hydroxyl group at the 3' carbon position of the molecule (Figure 3-3).[34] In order to elongate a DNA chain, a phosphodiester bond must form between the 3' carbon of the nucleotide that is already incorporated into the DNA sequence and the 5' carbon of the nucleotide that is being added to the DNA sequence. When added to a sequencing reaction, dideoxynucleotides can incorporate into the DNA sequence; however, because they lack a 3' hydroxyl group, no additional nucleotides can be added to the growing DNA chain (i.e., no phosphodiester bond can be formed). Thus, the DNA chain is terminated (Figure 3-3).[34]

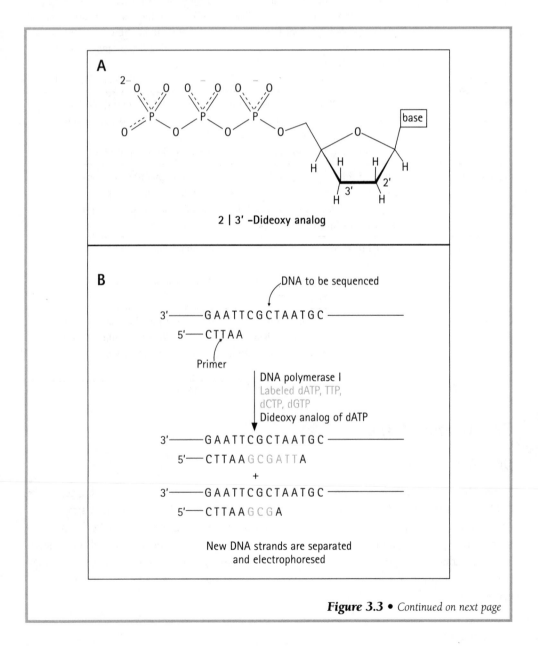

Figure 3.3 • *Continued on next page*

Continued

Figure 3.3 • Principles of the Sanger method of DNA sequencing. Dideoxynucleotides (also known as *chain terminators*) are similar to deoxynucleotides, except they lack a hydroxyl group at the 3' carbon position, as shown in part A of the figure. In part B of the figure, the strategy of the chain-termination method for DNA sequencing is depicted. A primer is annealed to a single-stranded DNA molecule. In each reaction mixture, DNA polymerase catalyzes the incorporation of deoxynucleotides or dideoxynucleotides into the growing complementary DNA chains. Deoxynucleotides are present at a higher concentration than dideoxynucleotides. If a dideoxynucleotide gets randomly incorporated into the DNA sequence, the chain elongation reaction is terminated because the dideoxynucleotide lacks a 3' hydroxyl group (i.e., a phosphodiester bond cannot form with the 5'carbon of the next incoming nucleotide). In part B of the figure, the dideoxynucleotide that is present in the reaction mixture is ddATP. The random incorporation of ddATP into the growing DNA chains results in chain termination and produces a mixture of DNA fragments of different lengths. The different fragments can be separated based on size on a gel and the DNA sequence can be reconstructed. Reprinted with minor modifications from Berg JM, Tymoczko JL, Stryer L. *Biochemistry.* 5th ed. © 2002, W. H. Freeman and Company. Used with permission of W. H. Freeman and Company.

Sanger used the chain-terminating chemistry of dideoxynucleotides to develop a novel DNA sequencing method. In this method, DNA is separated into single stranded molecules and a primer is annealed to the strand. The mixture is divided into four separate sequencing reactions that contain DNA polymerase, all four deoxynucleotides (dATP, dCTP, dGTP, and dTTP), and one dideoxynucleotide (e.g., ddATP in reaction mixture 1, ddCTP in reaction mixture 2, etc).[35] In each reaction mixture, DNA polymerase catalyzes the incorporation of deoxynucleotides or dideoxynucleotides into the growing complementary DNA chain. In the reaction mixture, deoxynucleotides are present at a higher concentration than dideoxynucleotides, thus the deoxynucleotides and the dideoxynucleotides compete for incorporation into the growing DNA chain.[35] If a dideoxynucleotide gets randomly incorporated into the complementary DNA sequence and the chain elongation reaction is terminated, this results in a mixture of DNA fragments of different lengths.[35,36] These fragments all have a common 5' end, but because of variable chain termination, will have different 3' ends, and thus different sizes.[35,36] The fragments in each of the four sequencing reaction mixtures can then be sized using capillary gel electrophoresis and the DNA sequence can be read from the position of bands on the gel.[35,36] In many automated DNA sequencing systems, the primers or dideoxynucleotides are labeled with a fluorescent dye. As the DNA fragments move through the gel and pass a laser, the fragments fluoresce and the output is recorded as peaks on a chromatogram. The chromatogram is recorded and serves as the basis from which the DNA sequence can be reconstructed.[35,36] When used for genotyping purposes, the direct DNA sequencing output can be used to determine if an individual has polymorphic or wild-type alleles at a particular site in the DNA sequence (Figure 3-4).[37]

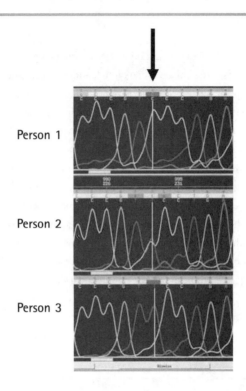

Figure 3.4 • DNA sequencing output. A portion of a DNA sequencing trace is shown for three individuals, 1, 2, and 3. The arrow shows the position where a polymorphism is located (C or T). Person A: At the site shown by the arrow, there is a clear, tall peak in the C trace. Thus, person 1's genotype is C/C. Person 2: At the site shown by the arrow, there is a smaller peak in the C trace and a peak in the T trace. Thus, person 2's genotype is C/T. Person 3: At the site shown by the arrow, there is a tall peak in the T trace. Thus, Person 3's genotype is T/T. Adapted by permission from Stephens M, Sloan JS, Robertson PD, et al. Automating sequence-based detection and genotyping of SNPs from diploid samples. *Nat. Gen.* 2006;38:375-381. © 2006, Macmillian Publishers Ltd.

Like many genotyping technologies, DNA sequencing has become high throughput in nature. Many researchers are moving away from the traditional Sanger method of DNA sequencing and are opting to use newer, more sophisticated instruments.[38] In general, these newer instruments (e.g., Roche's [454] GS FLX Genome Analyzer, Illumina's Solexa sequencer, and Applied Biosystems's SOLiD system) have circumvented the challenges associated with older sequencing instruments by eliminating the need for individual DNA sample preparation and electrophoretic gel separation.[33,39] Instead, many of these next-generation sequencing technologies are carried out on solid phase support structures (e.g., beads, or a solid surface known as a flow cell) with nongel detection systems that allow several hundred thousand sequencing reactions to be carried out in parallel, as compared to only 96 to 384 sequencing reactions with traditional Sanger sequencing.[33,38,39] As a result, next-generation sequencing systems are being used in whole genome resequencing efforts because of their high throughput capabilities, improved depth of sequencing coverage, low cost, and high resolution.[33,39]

PCR-Restriction Fragment Length Polymorphism Analysis

One of the oldest, nonautomated genotyping methods is PCR coupled with restriction fragment length polymorphism (RFLP) analysis. The PCR-RFLP genotyping method uses restriction enzymes to discriminate between polymorphic and wild-type alleles.[25] Subsequently, this method uses gel electrophoresis to detect the alleles present in a given sample. The hallmark of RFLP is the use of restriction enzymes, which recognize specific sequences of nucleotides in DNA, called restriction sites. Restriction sites are short nucleotide sequences (generally four to eight base pairs in length) that are present throughout the genome. When a specific restriction enzyme recognizes a specific restriction site, it cuts the DNA at that site. In pharmacogenomics, investigators are interested in whether an individual carries a polymorphic or wild-type allele at a particular site in the DNA. Oftentimes, a specific allele will either result in the presence or absence of a restriction site. As such, a restriction enzyme can be chosen based on this knowledge.[40,41] Subsequently, when the restriction enzyme is mixed with a PCR product (that contains the target sequence of interest), the restriction enzyme will recognize either the wild-type or polymorphic allele and cut the DNA at that site. The restriction digest reaction is then electrophoretically separated on a gel, and different fragment patterns are produced based on the size of the fragments resulting from the digest.[42] An individual's genotype can then be visually assigned based on these restriction digest fragment patterns (Figure 3-5).[5]

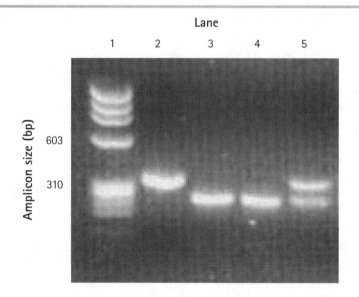

Figure 3.5 • Polymerase chain reaction (PCR)-restriction fragment length polymorphism (RFLP). The $G_s\alpha$ gene contains a single nucleotide polymorphism (T→C) at position 393 in exon 5. PCR was performed to generate a 345 base pair product. The C allele creates a restriction site for the restriction enzyme, *Fok*I. Subsequently, the PCR product was digested with this enzyme. Lane 1 is the DNA ladder; lane 2 represents a patient with a T/T genotype (uncut band; 345 bp); lane 3 and 4 represent patients with the C/C genotype (cut band; 259 bp); and lane 5 represents a patient with a heterozygous T/C genotype (both bands; 345 and 259 bp). Originally published in Aquilante CL, Zineh I, Beitelshees AL, et al. Common laboratory methods in pharmacogenomics studies. *Am J Health-Syst Pharm.* 2006;63:2101-2110. © 2006, American Society of Health-System Pharmacists, Inc. All rights reserved. Reprinted with permission (R0932).

The PCR-RFLP genotyping technique was used frequently in the pregenomic era because it was easy to perform and the equipment acquisition costs (e.g., gel electrophoresis chamber) were low. However, since the completion of the Human Genome Project, and the emergence of more sophisticated genotyping technologies, PCR-RFLP as a primary genotyping method has fallen out of routine use. PCR-RFLP is not well-suited for most genotyping laboratories for the following reasons: (1) it is an intensive process which can result in high labor costs; (2) it is associated with long turnaround times (e.g., restriction digests can take between 3 to 12 hours, and electrophoretic separation of the digest can take between 2 to 4 hours); (3) it is a low throughput method, capable of genotyping only a limited number of samples at one time; (4) it is typically not amenable to genotyping more than one polymorphism at a time (i.e., it is difficult to multiplex RFLP assays); and (5) it is associated with observer bias during visual analysis of the gel fragment patterns.[5,27] Nonetheless, PCR-RFLP may be an appropriate method for laboratories that genotype small numbers of samples for a few polymorphisms.

Pyrosequencing

An automated genotyping method that is used in many laboratories is pyrosequencing. This method uses primer extension as the principal allele discrimination method and the capture of light as the principal allele detection method. Pyrosequencing is sometimes referred to as *real-time sequencing by synthesis* because it uses some of the concepts of traditional DNA sequencing and provides information about the polymorphism and the surrounding sequence in the genotyping reaction.[43,44]

Prior to performing pyrosequencing, the target sequence of DNA that contains the polymorphism of interest is amplified by PCR. The PCR product is then immobilized onto beads and denatured to form single-stranded PCR molecules. An illustration of the chemistry used in the pyrosequencing method is shown in Figure 3-6.[43] The first step in the pyrosequencing method is a primer extension reaction whereby a sequencing primer is hybridized to the single-stranded PCR product either next to, or a few bases upstream of, the polymorphism of interest. Next, the reaction mixture is placed in an automated instrument and DNA polymerase and nucleotides are added to initiate the sequencing reaction. With the pyrosequencing method, nucleotides are added in a sequential fashion based on the known DNA template sequence.[45] If an added nucleotide is complementary to the template sequence, it is incorporated by DNA polymerase into the complementary DNA strand, starting from the 3' end of the hybridized sequencing primer. When a nucleotide gets incorporated into the DNA sequence, a pyrophosphate molecule is released. This release of pyrophosphate drives a series of enzymatic reactions that result in the production of visible light.[44] Specifically, the pyrophosphate molecule reacts with ATP sulfurylase in the reaction mixture and produces ATP. The ATP then reacts with luciferase enzyme and D-luciferin, and light is produced. This light is captured on a camera and appears as a peak on the pyrosequencing output (also called a pyrogram). If the nucleotide that was added does not bind complementary to the template sequence, it is degraded by another enzyme in the reaction mixture called apyrase. Thus, the amount of light produced during the pyrosequencing reaction is proportional to the number of nucleotides that have been incorporated into the DNA strand. The process of nucleotide addition and degradation is repeated in an iterative fashion culminating in the synthesis of a DNA strand that is complementary to the template sequence of interest.[46] As such, the pyrogram provides real-time sequencing data regarding the polymorphism of interest and the surrounding DNA sequence. An example of a patient pyrogram is shown in Figure 3-7.[5]

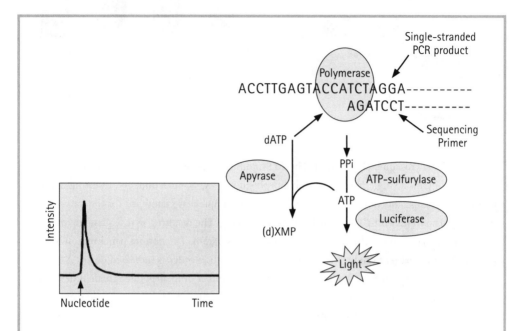

Figure 3.6 • Principles of pyrosequencing chemistry. In pyrosequencing chemistry, a sequencing primer is bound complementary to a single-stranded PCR product. In the presence of DNA polymerase, nucleotides are added in a sequential fashion based on the known DNA sequence. In this example, dATP was added to the reaction mixture. It bound complementary to the sequence (i.e., A bound to T of the single-stranded PCR product) and a pyrophosphate molecule was released (depicted in the figure as PPi). The pyrophosphate reacts with the enzyme ATP-sulfurylase to produce ATP, and the ATP reacts with the enzyme luciferase to produce light. Light emission and intensity are then captured on a camera and appear as a peak on a pyrogram. If a nucleotide does not bind complementary to the single-stranded PCR product, it is degraded by the enzyme apyrase. This is shown in the figure as (d) XMP (i.e., degradation of nonincorporated nucleotides). Reprinted with permission from Ronaghi M. Pyrosequencing sheds light on DNA sequencing. *Genome Res.* 2001;11:3-11. © 2001.

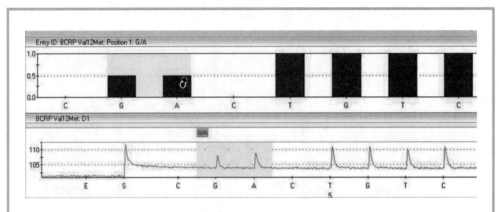

Figure 3.7 • Pyrosequencing output. The ATP-binding cassette subfamily G, member 2 gene (*ABCG2*) contains a single nucleotide polymorphism (G→A) at nucleotide 34, resulting in an amino acid change at codon 12 (Val→Met). A patient sample was genotyped for the Val^{12}Met polymorphism in the *ABCG2* gene using pyrosequencing. The resulting pyrosequencing output is shown. The top panel represents a theoretical histogram. The bottom panel represents a pyrogram from a patient sample. The nucleotide dispensation order is indicated on the X axis. The peak height, denoted on the Y axis, indicates the number of incorporated nucleotides. On the top panel, peak height values of 0.5 suggest heterozygosity, while values of 1 indicate the incorporation of 1 base (no polymorphism). Letters E and S on the pyrogram denote the addition of enzyme and substrate to the reaction mixture. The C nucleotides, located before and after the G and A nucleotides (in the shaded region), have no peaks because they are negative controls assigned by the software. The sequence analyzed in this example was G/ATGTC. The patient's genotype was G/A (Val/Met). Val = Valine; Met = Methionine. Originally published in Aquilante CL, Zineh I, Beitelshees AL, et al. Common laboratory methods in pharmacogenomics studies. *Am J Health-Syst Pharm.* 2006;63:2101-2110. © 2006, American Society of Health-System Pharmacists, Inc. All rights reserved. Reprinted with permission (R0932).

Compared to PCR-RFLP, where the observer visually assigns a genotype, the pyrosequencing method relies on pattern recognition software to automatically assign a genotype for the polymorphic site of interest.[46] Specifically, the software compares the light pattern and peak heights produced on the pyrogram to the light pattern and peak heights of a theoretical histogram (i.e., the expected light pattern and peak heights based on the known dispensation of nucleotides and the interrogated DNA sequence).[46] Based on the match between the observed pyrogram and the theoretical pyrogram, the software then scores the quality of the pyrosequencing reaction and assigns a genotype for the polymorphism of interest. Thus, the automated pyrosequencing recognition software removes observer bias, which has often plagued older genotyping methods such as PCR-RFLP.

Pyrosequencing is considered a medium throughput genotyping method, with some users estimating that approximately 1,000 to 2,000 genotypes can be performed per day.[26,47] The turnaround time associated with this method is also relatively fast. For a 96-sample plate, the post-PCR processing step takes between 30 minutes to 1 hour and the automated genotyping portion of the assay takes between 10 to 20 minutes.[48] The technology is typically used in the simplex format (i.e., the interrogation of one polymorphism in a single well of the plate). However, the technology does allow the user to run different simplex assays for different polymorphisms on the same plate. Thus, a number of different polymorphisms can be genotyped in a single pyrosequencing run. Furthermore, the technology is capable of genotyping multiple polymorphisms in the same reaction mixture (i.e., multiplex genotyping). As such, pyrosequencing is a relatively versatile technology for many clinical pharmacogenomic applications. This technology does have limitations, one being cost. The equipment acquisition costs for this system are expensive, ranging from $75,000 to $100,000.[5] Furthermore, the labor costs associated with the post-PCR processing step, and the reagent costs for the enzymatic reaction mixture, may be prohibitive for some laboratories.[5] The technology can also be problematic for sequences that have long stretches of the same nucleotide (i.e., homopolymeric regions). Recent advances in pyrosequencing technology have attempted to improve the system by using 384 well plates, decreasing the required PCR sample volume, and increasing the sequencing read length by adding a binding protein that stabilizes single-stranded DNA.[44] As such, pyrosequencing will likely remain a useful genotyping method for medium throughput laboratories that genotype a moderate number of polymorphisms.

TaqMan®

TaqMan® is an automated, medium-to-high throughput genotyping system that relies on allele-specific hybridization as the allele discrimination method, and fluorescence as the allele detection method.[25,49,50] Figure 3-8 provides an illustration of TaqMan® chemistry.[5] The foundation of TaqMan® is the use of fluorescence-labeled probes, which drive the allele-specific hybridization reaction.[51] These probes are short stretches of nucleotides that are designed to bind complementary to the template sequence of interest. For biallelic polymorphisms, one probe is designed to bind complementary to the wild-type allele and one probe is designed to bind complementary to the polymorphic allele. Each probe is labeled with a reporter dye on the 5' end and a quencher dye on the 3' end. The reporter dye is responsible for releasing a fluorescent signal while the quencher dye neutralizes the fluorescent signal.[52] When the probes are intact, the close proximity of the reporter dye to the quencher dye prevents fluorescence. However, when the probe is disrupted or cleaved, the reporter dye and quencher dye become separated and fluorescence is emitted.[52]

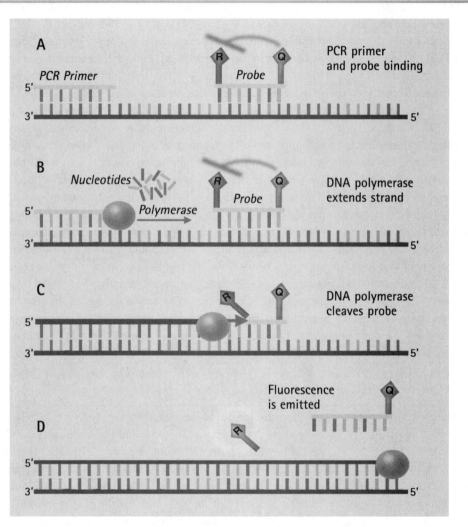

Figure 3.8 • Principles of TaqMan® chemistry. The TaqMan® assay combines both PCR amplification and allele discrimination in a single reaction Two fluorescence-labeled probes are used for allele discrimination, one of which is complementary to the wild-type allele and one that is complementary to the variant allele. Each probe is labeled on the 5' end with a reporter dye (R) and on the 3' end with a quencher (Q) dye. When the probes are intact, the quencher dye neutralizes the fluorescence emitted by the reporter dye, thus no fluorescence is emitted. This figure depicts the binding of a single probe that is complementary to a single strand of DNA. (A) During the PCR reaction, the PCR primer and fluorescence-labeled probe anneal complementary to the DNA. Because the probe is complementary to the sequence of interest, it forms a stable structure on the single strand of DNA. (B) Following primer and probe annealing, DNA polymerase catalyzes the addition of deoxynucleotides to the 3' end of the hybridized PCR primer, resulting in extension of the strand. (C) When the DNA polymerase encounters the fluorescence-labeled probe

Continued on next page

Figure 3.8 • Continued

that is bound securely to the DNA strand, it cleaves the probe at the 5' end. This separates the 5' reporter dye from the 3' quencher dye. (D) Because the reporter dye and quencher dye are no longer intact, the quencher dye is no longer able to neutralize the fluorescent signal from the reporter dye. Thus, there is an increase in the fluorescence released by the reporter dye. Fluorescence measurements are made using commercially available systems. Originally published in Aquilante CL, Zineh I, Beitelshees AL, et al. Common laboratory methods in pharmacogenomics studies. *Am J Health-Syst Pharm.* 2006;63:2101-2110. Illustration by Marie Dauenheimer, CMI.

TaqMan® is different than other genotyping methods because the PCR amplification step and the allele discrimination step are conducted in the same reaction, rather than in separate steps as in PCR-RFLP and pyrosequencing.[51] As such, TaqMan® consists of both PCR primers and two allele-specific fluorescence-labeled probes in the reaction mixture. During the annealing step of the amplification process, both the PCR primers and fluorescence-labeled probes bind complementary to the DNA target sequence. The probe that binds perfectly to the target sequence (i.e., contains no nucleotide mismatches) forms a stable duplex, while the probe that contains a mismatch does not form a stable duplex.[26,51] During the extension step of the amplification process, DNA polymerase extends the complementary DNA strand from the 3' end of the PCR primer. When the DNA polymerase encounters the probe that is bound tightly to the strand (i.e., a perfect match), it cleaves the probe at the 5' end. The resulting cleavage results in the separation of the 5' reporter dye from the 3' quencher dye on the probe. As a result, fluorescence is emitted and subsequently measured. Software is used to process the fluorescence data and assign a genotype.

TaqMan® is considered to be a medium-to-high throughput genotyping method with the capability of determining approximately 1,000 to 10,000 genotypes per day.[26] Many laboratories find the TaqMan® system to be particularly well-suited for pharmacogenomic analyses, as it incorporates both PCR amplification and genotype determination into one step and does not require post-PCR processing or gel electrophoresis.[53] Compared to other methods, TaqMan® is associated with lower sample processing times and reduced labor costs. The primary limitation of this method is the high fixed cost of the fluorescence-labeled probes, which must be designed and optimized for each polymorphism.[53,54] Thus, for laboratories that want to genotype a large number of different polymorphisms, the TaqMan® method may be costly during the assay design and validation phases. The equipment acquisition costs may also be prohibitive in some settings. The TaqMan® system uses a real-time PCR thermal cycler, which is more expensive than a traditional thermal cycler ($30,000 to $100,000 versus $4,000 to $10,000, respectively).[5]

Mass Spectrometry

Mass spectrometry has become a useful allele detection method in the genotyping process. The technique of matrix-assisted laser desorption-ionization time-of-flight (MALDI-TOF) mass spectrometry is used to measure the molecular mass of DNA molecules.[41,55,56] While other allele detection methods rely on light, electrophoresis, or fluorescence, mass spectrometry differentiates between alleles based on mass alone. As such, the technology obviates the need for expensive primer labeling or lengthy gel electrophoresis runs.[57,58] Additionally, mass spectrometry has excellent precision and high throughput capabilities. The primary drawbacks of mass spectrometry as an allele detection method are the high equipment acquisition costs, high level of required technical expertise, and rigorous sample purification procedures.

Because mass spectrometry is used primarily as an allele detection method, it is typically coupled with allele discrimination methods, such as single primer extension or allele-specific hybridization.[59] For example, the MassARRAY® system (manufactured by Sequenom) uses primer extension whereby primers are annealed upstream of the polymorphism of interest and are extended to yield products that differ in molecular weight.[25] The mass of the different extension products is measured by MALDI-TOF mass spectrometry, and genotypes are assigned accordingly.

Other Genotyping Methodologies

Primer extension, a common methodology for allele discrimination, is a versatile tool that can be coupled with various allele detection methods (e.g., light, mass, fluorescence) in order to discriminate between polymorphic and wild-type alleles. In this chapter, primer extension as an allele discrimination method was described in the context of genotyping methods such as pyrosequencing and the MassARRAY® system. In pyrosequencing, the allele detection method is light, whereas in the MassARRAY® system the allele detection method is mass. Primer extension can also be coupled with the allele detection method of fluorescence for genotype determination. An example of this type of genotyping method is the SNaPshot kit which is manufactured by Applied Biosystems. In the SNaPshot technology, primers are designed to bind to a PCR product, immediately upstream of the polymorphism of interest.[25] Fluorescent-ly-labeled dideoxynucleotides are added to the reaction mixture and these dideoxynucleotides bind complementary to the template to extend the DNA strand.[25] The different sized extension products, which are fluorescently-labeled, are separated by capillary gel electrophoresis (i.e., the same type of electrophoresis that is used in automated DNA sequencing reactions). As the DNA fragments pass through the gel and a laser, the fragments fluoresce and the output is recorded as peaks on a chromatogram and genotypes can be determined.

While primer extension and allele-specific hybridization are common allele discrimination methods, a technique that is increasingly being employed to discriminate between polymorphic and wild-type alleles is ligation. This method relies on the use of a ligase enzyme, which is used to join two primers that have been bound to the DNA strand. In most ligation reactions, two allele-specific probes (i.e., one probe that binds complementary to the sequence containing the polymorphic allele, and one probe that binds complementary to the sequence containing the wild-type allele) are used to interrogate the polymorphism of interest. A common probe is also used in the reaction.[25] The common probe binds next to the allele-specific probes, regardless of the alleles that are present in the sample. When the ligase enzyme is added to the reaction, it joins the common probe to the allele-specific probe that has bound perfectly to the sequence of interest.[25] The probes are most commonly labeled with fluorescent markers. As such, the different fluorescence patterns that are produced during the ligation reaction can be measured and genotypes can be assigned.

Another technique that is used as a genotyping method is enzymatic cleavage. This concept was previously discussed in the context of PCR-RFLP, whereby restriction endonucleases are used to discriminate between polymorphic and wild-type alleles. The disadvantages of PCR-RFLP (e.g., low throughput, high cost) have made this methodology somewhat outdated in the current genomic environment. However, the principal of using enzymes to discriminate between different alleles has been applied to automated, high throughput genotyping systems.[25] For example, in the Invader assay (Third Wave Technologies) the principal allele discrimination method is an endonuclease enzyme, called Cleavase®. The chemistry of the Invader assay is shown in Figure 3-9.[60] In this technology, two allele-specific probes and one common probe are used in the reaction mixture. The common probe (also called an invader) forms a three-dimensional structure with the allele-specific probe that has bound perfectly to the sequence of interest. An endonuclease enzyme is then added, which recognizes and cleaves the three-dimensional structure.[25] The nucleotide "flap" (i.e., overlapping structure) that is cleaved in the reaction then participates in a second reaction where it serves as the invader.[60] It binds complementary and forms a three-dimensional structure to one of two fluorescent-labeled molecules in the reaction mixture in an allele-specific manner. The endonuclease enzyme recognizes and cleaves the three-dimensional structure. This results in the release of fluorescence in an allele-specific manner such that a genotype can be determined. Notably, the Invader assay can be used to directly genotype from genomic DNA, without a PCR amplification step.[25] The Invader assay is highly accurate; however, it is limited by the need for large amounts of template DNA per reaction, and it is difficult to multiplex Invader assays.

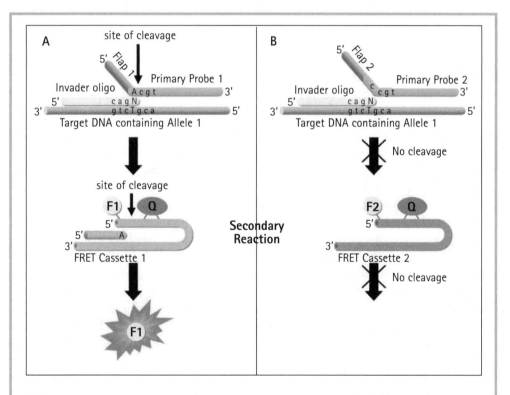

Figure 3.9 • Principles of the Invader assay. In part A of this figure, an allele specific probe (Probe 1) and a common probe (invader oligo) behind complementary to the sequence of interest. A three-dimensional, invasive structure forms as a result of the single-base overlap between the invader oligo and Probe 1. An endonuclease enzyme is then added which recognizes and cleaves the three-dimensional structure. The nucleotide "flap" (i.e., overlapping structure) that is cleaved in the reaction then participates in a secondary reaction where it

Continued on next page

Figure 3.9 • *Continued*

serves as the invader. It binds complementary to, and forms a three-dimensional structure with, one of two fluorescent-labeled molecules in the reaction mixture in an allele-specific manner (in part A of the figure, the fluorescence molecule is shown as FRET Cassette 1). The endonuclease enzyme recognizes and cleaves the three-dimensional structure that has formed between the flap and the fluorescence molecule. This results in the release of fluorescence in an allele-specific manner, shown in this figure as the release of fluorescence 1 (F1). In part B of the figure, a second probe (Probe 2) and a common probe (invader oligo) are added to the mixture. However, Probe 2 is not specific to the allele present in the reaction mixture and does not behind complementary to the sequence of interest. As a result, a three-dimensional structure does not form because there is not a single-base overlap between Probe 2 and the invader oligo. This results in no cleavage when the endonuclease is added to the mixture, and a nucleotide "flap" is not released and cannot participate in the secondary fluorescence reaction. Thus, no fluorescence is released. Reprinted, with minor modifications, from Olivier M. The Invader assay for SNP genotyping. *Mutation Research*. 2005;573:103-110. © 2005, used with permission from Elsevier.

DNA Microarrays

One of the more recent advances in genotyping methodologies is the use of DNA microarrays in pharmacogenomic research. The move to DNA microarrays has changed the pharmacogenomic landscape in terms of the way researchers address hypotheses. Traditionally, pharmacogenomic hypotheses have been tested using a candidate-gene approach, whereby a select number of genes or polymorphisms are chosen based on proteins known to influence the pharmacology of drug disposition and drug response.[28] For example, in the treatment of asthma, significant interindividual variability exists in response to β_2 agonists (e.g., albuterol). If one takes a candidate gene approach to investigate interindividual variability in albuterol response, the β_2 adrenergic receptor gene (which encodes the β_2 adrenergic receptor) would be a logical starting point because the β_2 adrenergic receptor is the target of albuterol's action. However, with the completion of the Human Genome Project, many pharmacogenomic researchers are moving away from the candidate-gene approach and are now taking a genome-wide approach. In the genome-wide approach, thousands of polymorphisms across the genome are interrogated for their association with drug disposition or response.[28] The move from the candidate-gene approach to the genome-wide approach is due, in large part, to the availability of DNA microarrays.

DNA microarrays are a collection of probes that are bound in a grid-like pattern to a solid phase support structure, such as a nylon membrane, glass slide, or silicon chip.[61,62] As such, microarrays are often referred to as *gene chips*. For genotyping purposes, the probes that are bound to the chip are oligonucleotides—short fragments of single-stranded DNA that are designed to bind to specific sequences in the DNA. For pharmacogenomic applications, these oligonucleotides are designed to interrogate the polymorphisms of interest. Depending on the type of microarray, between 1,000 to 500,000 polymorphisms can be interrogated at one time.[28] There are several gene chips that are commercially available, one of which is the Affymetrix Genechip®. For the Affymetrix technology, the patient's DNA sample is digested into smaller pieces, attached to an adaptor sequence, and then PCR-amplified.[25,63,64] The amplified

PCR product is then fluorescently-labeled and hybridized onto the chip. Each polymorphism on the chip is represented by different allele-specific oligonucleotide probe sets containing a perfect match probe and a mismatch probe.[25] Thus, in the Affymetrix Genechip®, the allele discrimination method is allele-specific hybridization. The binding of the patient's DNA to a particular probe results in the release of fluorescence. The fluorescence patterns following probe binding are analyzed and a genotype is assigned by automated software.

Another microarray technology that is being used in genome-wide association studies is the Illumina BeadChip platform.[65] This platform employs the Illumina BeadArray technology, whereby 3-micron silica beads are randomly assembled in microwells of a substrate (such as a fiber optic bundle or silica slide).[25,65] Attached to each bead are thousands of copies of a specific oligonucleotide sequence that are specific to the sequences containing the polymorphisms that are to be interrogated. Prior to adding genomic DNA to the beads, the sample is subjected to PCR and an allele discrimination reaction that involves both allele-specific hybridization and ligation.[25] When the processed PCR product is added to the beads, the oligonucleotide sequences on the beads will bind complementary to the PCR product in an allele-specific manner and the information from this reaction is captured and genotypes are assigned.[25]

While the focus of this chapter has been on genotyping methodologies used to interrogate polymorphisms in the DNA sequence, it is also important to note that microarrays are available to determine the gene expression profiles of certain types of cancers (e.g., lymphoid malignancies). This information can be used to categorize the cancer and help guide treatment.

FDA–Approved Genotyping Tests in Clinical Practice

In the past, genotyping technologies were largely limited to academic laboratories. However, the Food and Drug Administration (FDA) has recently approved several pharmacogenomic diagnostic tests for use in clinical practice. One of these clinical pharmacogenomic diagnostic tests is the Roche AmpliChip CYP450 test. The intended use of the Roche AmpliChip CYP450 test is to identify a patient's *CYP2D6* and *CYP2C19* genotypes from genomic DNA extracted from a whole blood sample.[6] In the clinic, a patient's blood sample is drawn and the specimen is sent to a participating laboratory that has the required equipment to perform the pharmacogenomic test. The Roche AmpliChip CYP450 test is a DNA microarray that uses Affymetrix gene chip technology. The DNA microarray is designed to interrogate 27 alleles in the *CYP2D6* gene and three alleles in the *CYP2C19* gene.[6] The five steps involved in the AmpliChip test are PCR amplification of purified DNA; fragmentation and labeling of the amplified PCR product; hybridization of the amplified product to the microarray; scanning of the microarray; and determination of CYP450 genotype and assignment of a predicted phenotype.[6] As discussed previously, numerous oligonucleotide probes, which are designed to be complementary to the wild-type or polymorphic sequences, are bound to the microarray. When the patient's DNA is added to the microarray, the pattern of hybridization to the specific probes is analyzed and a genotype is determined.[6] The genotype information is compiled by a software program and a report is provided that summarizes the identified alleles and genotypes. This information is used to predict an individual's CYP2D6 and CYP2C19 metabolizing enzyme phenotype (Figure 3-10).[6] This phenotype information can then be used by providers to help guide drug therapy. In general the Roche AmpliChip assay takes 1 to 2 days to complete. Compared to DNA sequencing, the Roche AmpliChip is accurate, with observed genotype call agreements of 99.2% for CYP2D6 and 99.6% for CYP2C19.[6] The interlaboratory reproducibility of this assay is reported to be 99.9%.[6]

A. Predicted phenotypes of the *CYP2D6* genotypes detected by the AmpliChip CYP450 test

Allele	1	2	3	4	5	6	7	8	9	10	11	15	17	19	20	29	35	36	40	41	1XN	2XN	4XN	10XN	17XN	35XN	41XN
1	E	E	E	E	E	E	E	E	E	E	E	E	E	E	E	E	E	E	E	E	U	U	E	E	E	U	E
2		E	E	E	E	E	E	E	E	E	E	E	E	E	E	E	E	E	E	E	U	U	E	E	E	U	E
3			P	P	P	P	P	P	—	—	P	P	—	P	P	—	E	—	P	—	E	E	P	—	—	E	—
4				P	P	P	P	P	—	—	P	P	—	P	P	—	E	—	P	—	E	E	P	—	—	E	—
5					P	P	P	P	—	—	P	P	—	P	P	—	E	—	P	—	E	E	P	—	—	E	—
6						P	P	P	—	—	P	P	—	P	P	—	E	—	P	—	E	E	P	—	—	E	—
7							P	P	—	—	P	P	—	P	P	—	E	—	P	—	E	E	P	—	—	E	—
8								P	—	—	P	P	—	P	P	—	E	—	P	—	E	E	P	—	—	E	—
9									—	—	—	—	—	—	—	—	E	—	—	—	E	E	—	—	—	E	—
10										—	—	—	—	—	—	—	E	—	—	—	E	E	—	—	—	E	—
11											P	P	—	P	P	—	E	—	P	—	E	E	P	—	—	E	—
15												P	—	P	P	—	E	—	P	—	E	E	P	—	—	E	—
17													—	—	—	—	E	—	—	—	E	E	—	—	—	E	—
19														P	P	—	E	—	P	—	E	E	P	—	—	E	—
20															P	—	E	—	P	—	E	E	P	—	—	E	—
29																—	E	—	—	—	E	E	—	—	—	E	—
35																	E	E	P	E	E	E	E	E	E	E	E
36																		E	—	—	E	E	—	E	E	U	E
40																			P	—	E	E	P	—	—	P	—
41																				—	E	E	—	—	—	E	E

B. Predicted phenotypes of the *CYP2C19* genotypes detected by the AmpliChip CYP450 test

Allele	1	2	3
1	E	E	E
2		P	P
3			P

Figure 3.10 • *Continued on next page*

Continued

Figure 3.10 • Roche AmpliChip CYP450 microarray. The Roche AmpliChip CYP450 test is a DNA microarray that is used to identify a patient's *CYP2D6* and *CYP2C19* genotypes. CYP2D6 and CYP2C19 drug metabolizing enzyme phenotypes can then be predicted based on the genotypes identified by the AmpliChip CYP450 test. Part A of the figure shows predicted phenotypes of the *CYP2D6* genotypes detected by the AmpliChip CYP450 test. E = extensive metabolizer; I = intermediate metabolizer; P =poor metabolizer; U = ultrarapid metabolizer. Part B of the figure shows predicted phenotypes of the *CYP2C19* genotypes detected by the AmpliChip CYP450 test. E = extensive metabolizer; P = poor metabolizer. Reprinted with permission from AmpliChip CYP450 [test package insert]. Pleasanton, CA: Roche Molecular Systems; Doc Rev. 6.0 dated 01/2009.

Another Food and Drug Administration-approved pharmacogenomic diagnostic test that is available for use in clinical practice is the Invader® UGT1A1 Molecular Assay. UDP glucuronosyltransferase 1A1 (UGT1A1) is an enzyme that is responsible for the glucuronidation of the active metabolite of the anticancer drug, irinotecan.[66] Furthermore, UGT1A1 is responsible for the glucuronidation of bilirubin.[66] Several common polymorphisms exist in the *UGT1A1* gene. The most widely studied polymorphism is a TA repeat in the *UGT1A1* promoter. Individuals with seven TA repeats at this position (designated as the *28 allele) have reduced glucuronidating capacity of the enzyme compared to wild-type individuals who possess only six TA repeats at this position (designated as the *1 allele).[66] In terms of irinotecan, the active metabolite, SN-38, is inactivated by UGT1A1 through glucuronidation. Carriers of a *UGT1A1*28 allele are less able to inactivate SN-38, resulting in increased SN-38 plasma concentrations which can be associated with side effects such as neutropenia and diarrhea.[66] The intended use of the Invader® UGT1A1 Molecular Assay is for the detection and genotyping of the *1 and *28 alleles in the *UGT1A1* gene in genomic DNA obtained from whole blood.[66] The genotyping method used in this diagnostic test is the Invader assay (described previously in Other Genotyping Methods). When compared to bidirectional DNA sequencing, the Invader® UGT1A1 Molecular Assay has been shown to be highly accurate, with an observed genotype call agreement of 100%.[66] The interlaboratory reproducibility of this assay is reported to be 98.1%.[66]

Summary

Over the past few years, the field of pharmacogenomics has witnessed an explosion in the technologies and resources available to conduct genomic analyses. Pharmacogenomic tests have also begun to move out of the academic laboratory and into mainstream medicine. Currently, there are several FDA-approved diagnostic pharmacogenomic tests available for clinical use. Undoubtedly, in coming years, genotyping technology for pharmacogenomic applications will become more sophisticated in nature, less costly, and with higher throughput. Additionally, as sequencing technologies continue to mature, it is estimated that in the future, it will cost only $1,000 to sequence an individual's entire genome. This represents 0.1% of the current cost of whole genome sequencing.[67] With the growing availability of clinical pharmacogenomic diagnostic tests, and as clinical evidence documenting improved patient outcomes with genotype-guided pharmacotherapy mounts, pharmacogenomics will serve as a useful tool to aid in the safe and rationale use of drug therapy.

References

1. Ginsburg GS, Konstance RP, Allsbrook JS, et al. Implications of pharmacogenomics for drug development and clinical practice. *Arch Intern Med.* 2005;165:2331-2336.
2. Collins FS, Green ED, Guttmacher AE, et al. A vision for the future of genomics research. *Nature.* 2003;422:835-847.
3. Zineh I, Gerhard T, Aquilante CL, et al. Availability of pharmacogenomics-based prescribing information in drug package inserts for currently approved drugs. *Pharmacogenomics J.* 2004;4:354-358.
4. Tsongalis GJ, Coleman WB. Clinical genotyping: the need for interrogation of single nucleotide polymorphisms and mutations in the clinical laboratory. *Clin Chim Acta.* 2006;363:127-137.
5. Aquilante CL, Zineh I, Beitelshees AL, et al. Common laboratory methods in pharmacogenomics studies. *Am J Health-Syst Pharm.* 2006;63:2101-2110.
6. AmpliChip CYP450 [test prescribing information]. Pleasanton, CA: Roche Molecular Systems Inc; 2007.
7. Feigelson HS, Rodriguez C, Robertson AS, et al. Determinants of DNA yield and quality from buccal cell samples collected with mouthwash. *Cancer Epidemiol Biomarkers Prev.* 2001;10:1005-1008.
8. Lench N, Stanier P, Williamson R. Simple non-invasive method to obtain DNA for gene analysis. *Lancet.* 1988;1:1356-1358.
9. Philibert RA, Zadorozhnyaya O, Beach SR, et al. Comparison of the genotyping results using DNA obtained from blood and saliva. *Psychiatr Genet.* 2008;18:275-281.
10. Garcia-Closas M, Egan KM, Abruzzo J, et al. Collection of genomic DNA from adults in epidemiological studies by buccal cytobrush and mouthwash. *Cancer Epidemiol Biomarkers Prev.* 2001;10:687-696.
11. Lum A, Le Marchand L. A simple mouthwash method for obtaining genomic DNA in molecular epidemiological studies. *Cancer Epidemiol Biomarkers Prev.* 1998;7:719-724.
12. Rogers NL, Cole SA, Lan HC, et al. New saliva DNA collection method compared to buccal cell collection techniques for epidemiological studies. *Am J Hum Biol.* 2007;19:319-326.
13. Andrisin TE, Humma LM, Johnson JA. Collection of genomic DNA by the noninvasive mouthwash method for use in pharmacogenetic studies. *Pharmacotherapy.* 2002;22:954-960.
14. Heath EM, Morken NW, Campbell KA, et al. Use of buccal cells collected in mouthwash as a source of DNA for clinical testing. *Arch Pathol Lab Med.* 2001;125:127-133.
15. Milne E, van Bockxmeer FM, Robertson L, et al. Buccal DNA collection: comparison of buccal swabs with FTA cards. *Cancer Epidemiol Biomarkers Prev.* 2006;15:816-819.
16. Hansen TV, Simonsen MK, Nielsen FC, et al. Collection of blood, saliva, and buccal cell samples in a pilot study on the Danish nurse cohort: comparison of the response rate and quality of genomic DNA. *Cancer Epidemiol Biomarkers Prev.* 2007;16:2072-2076.
17. Ng DP, Koh D, Choo S, et al. Saliva as a viable alternative source of human genomic DNA in genetic epidemiology. *Clin Chim Acta.* 2006;367:81-85.
18. QIAGEN Genomic DNA Handbook 2001. Available at: www1.qiagen.com/HB/QIAGENGenomicDNA. Accessed November 30, 2008.
19. Eisenstein BI. The polymerase chain reaction. A new method of using molecular genetics for medical diagnosis. *N Engl J Med.* 1990;322:178-183.
20. Markham AF. The polymerase chain reaction: a tool for molecular medicine. *BMJ.* 1993;306:441-446.
21. DNA structure and gene expression. In: Strachan T, Read A. Human Molecular Genetics. New York: Wiley; 1999:1-26.
22. Baumforth KR, Nelson PN, Digby JE, et al. Demystified ... the polymerase chain reaction. *Mol Pathol.* 1999;52:1-10.
23. Miesfeld RL. Applied Molecular Genetics. New York: Wiley; 1999:18-19.

24. Kwok PY. Methods for genotyping single nucleotide polymorphisms. *Annu Rev Genomics Hum Genet.* 2001;2:235-258.

25. Kim S, Misra A. SNP genotyping: technologies and biomedical applications. *Annu Rev Biomed Eng.* 2007;9:289-320.

26. Chen X, Sullivan PF. Single nucleotide polymorphism genotyping: biochemistry, protocol, cost and throughput. *Pharmacogenomics J.* 2003;3:77-96.

27. Aquilante CL, Lobmeyer MT, Langaee TY, et al. Comparison of cytochrome P450 2C9 genotyping methods and implications for the clinical laboratory. *Pharmacotherapy.* 2004;24:720-726.

28. Hernandez-Boussard T, Klein TE, Altman RB. Pharmacogenomics: The relevance of emerging genotyping technologies. *MLO Med Lab Obs.* 2006;38:24, 26-30.

29. Isler JA, Vesterqvist OE, Burczynski ME. Analytical validation of genotyping assays in the biomarker laboratory. *Pharmacogenomics.* 2007;8:353-368.

30. Flockhart DA, O'Kane D, Williams MS, et al. Pharmacogenetic testing of CYP2C9 and VKORC1 alleles for warfarin. *Genet Med.* 2008;10:139-150.

31. Weiss ST, McLeod HL, Flockhart DA, et al. Creating and evaluating genetic tests predictive of drug response. *Nat Rev Drug Discov.* 2008;7:568-574.

32. Promoting safe and effective genetic testing in the United States. Available at: http://www.genome.gov/10002404. Accessed November 30, 2008.

33. Mardis ER. Next-generation DNA sequencing methods. *Annu Rev Genomics Hum Genet.* 2008;9:387-402.

34. Berg, Tymoczko, Stryer. *Biochemistry.* New York: WH Freeman and Company; 2002.

35. The principles of DNA sequencing. Available at: http://depts.washington.edu/pceut/pceut_services/DNA-Sequencing-NCBI.pdf. Accessed December 1, 2008.

36. DNA sequencing. In: Strachan T, Read A. *Human Molecular Genetics.* New York: Wiley; 1999:129-134.

37. Stephens M, Sloan JS, Robertson PD, et al. Automating sequence-based detection and genotyping of SNPs from diploid samples. *Nat Genet.* 2006;38:375-381.

38. Schuster SC. Next-generation sequencing transforms today's biology. *Nat Methods.* 2008;5:16-18.

39. Morozova O, Marra MA. Applications of next-generation sequencing technologies in functional genomics. *Genomics.* 2008;92:255-264.

40. Gut IG. Automation in genotyping of single nucleotide polymorphisms. *Hum Mutat.* 2001;17:475-492.

41. Shi MM. Technologies for individual genotyping: detection of genetic polymorphisms in drug targets and disease genes. *Am J Pharmacogenomics.* 2002;2:197-205.

42. Daly AK. Development of analytical technology in pharmacogenetic research. *Naunyn Schmiedebergs Arch Pharmacol.* 2004;369:133-140.

43. Ronaghi M. Pyrosequencing sheds light on DNA sequencing. *Genome Res.* 2001;11:3-11.

44. Ahmadian A, Ehn M, Hober S. Pyrosequencing: history, biochemistry and future. *Clin Chim Acta.* 2006;363:83-94.

45. Alderborn A, Kristofferson A, Hammerling U. Determination of single-nucleotide polymorphisms by real-time pyrophosphate DNA sequencing. *Genome Res.* 2000;10:1249-1258.

46. Fakhrai-Rad H, Pourmand N, Ronaghi M. Pyrosequencing: an accurate detection platform for single nucleotide polymorphisms. *Hum Mutat.* 2002;19:479-485.

47. Ronaghi M, Karamohamed S, Pettersson B, et al. Real-time DNA sequencing using detection of pyrophosphate release. *Anal Biochem.* 1996;242:84-89.

48. Eriksson S, Berg LM, Wadelius M, et al. Cytochrome p450 genotyping by multiplexed real-time dna sequencing with pyrosequencing technology. *Assay Drug Dev Technol.* 2002;1:49-59.

49. Jenkins S, Gibson N. High-throughput SNP genotyping. *Comp Funct Genomics.* 2002;3:57-66.

50. Livak KJ. SNP genotyping by the 5'-nuclease reaction. *Methods Mol Biol.* 2003;212:129-147.

51. Livak KJ. Allelic discrimination using fluorogenic probes and the 5' nuclease assay. *Genet Anal.* 1999;14:143-149.

52. Livak KJ, Flood SJ, Marmaro J, et al. Oligonucleotides with fluorescent dyes at opposite ends provide a quenched probe system useful for detecting PCR product and nucleic acid hybridization. *PCR Methods Appl.* 1995;4:357-362.

53. Ranade K, Chang MS, Ting CT, et al. High-throughput genotyping with single nucleotide polymorphisms. *Genome Res.* 2001;11:1262-1268.

54. McGuigan FE, Ralston SH. Single nucleotide polymorphism detection: allelic discrimination using TaqMan. *Psychiatr Genet.* 2002;12:133-136.

55. Sauer S, Gut IG. Genotyping single-nucleotide polymorphisms by matrix-assisted laser-desorption/ionization time-of-flight mass spectrometry. *J Chromatogr B Analyt Technol Biomed Life Sci.* 2002;782:73-87.

56. Tost J, Gut IG. Genotyping single nucleotide polymorphisms by mass spectrometry. *Mass Spectrom Rev.* 2002;21:388-418.

57. Gut IG. DNA analysis by MALDI-TOF mass spectrometry. *Hum Mutat.* 2004;23:437-441.

58. Storm N, Darnhofer-Patel B, van den Boom D, et al. MALDI-TOF mass spectrometry-based SNP genotyping. *Methods Mol Biol.* 2003;212:241-262.

59. Lechner D, Lathrop GM, Gut IG. Large-scale genotyping by mass spectrometry: experience, advances and obstacles. *Curr Opin Chem Biol.* 2002;6:31-38.

60. Olivier M. The Invader assay for SNP genotyping. *Mutat Res.* 2005;573:103-110.

61. Meloni R, Khalfallah O, Biguet NF. DNA microarrays and pharmacogenomics. *Pharmacol Res.* 2004;49:303-308.

62. Villeneuve DJ, Parissenti AM. The use of DNA microarrays to investigate the pharmacogenomics of drug response in living systems. *Curr Top Med Chem.* 2004;4:1329-1345.

63. Maresso K, Broeckel U. Genotyping platforms for mass-throughput genotyping with SNPs, including human genome-wide scans. *Adv Genet.* 2008;60:107-139.

64. Grant SF, Hakonarson H. Microarray technology and applications in the arena of genome-wide association. *Clin Chem.* 2008;54:1116-1124.

65. Illumina BeadArray Technology. Available at: http://www.illumina.com. Accessed December 1, 2008.

66. Invader UGT1A1 Molecular Assay [prescribing information]. Madison, WI: Third Wave Technologies; 2005.

67. Wheeler DA, Srinivasan M, Egholm M, et al. The complete genome of an individual by massively parallel DNA sequencing. *Nature.* 2008;452:872-876.

Chapter 4

The Pharmacogenetics of Drug Metabolism

G. Scott Weston, R.Ph., Ph.D.

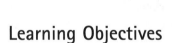

Learning Objectives

After completing this chapter, the reader should be able to

- Briefly explain the potential impact of pharmacogenetic differences on the rate of adverse drug reactions (ADRs) that occur in patients receiving drug therapy.
- List and discuss several commonly used therapeutic agents whose safe and effective usage is impacted by pharmacogenetic differences in drug metabolic enzymes.
- Give an example of a diagnostic test (targeted at drug metabolic enzymes) that is commonly used with a specific therapeutic agent.
- List the major commercial tests available to determine patient genotypes for drug metabolic enzymes and the enzymes covered by each test.
- Briefly discuss the potential usefulness of each of the major commercially available metabolic genotyping and phenotyping tests in initiating or modifying pharmacotherapeutic regimens.

Key Definitions

Adverse drug reaction (ADR)—A response to a medicine, which is noxious, unintended, and occurs at doses normally used in man.[1]

Cytochrome P450s (CYP450s, microsomal mixed function oxidases)—A family of heme-containing monooxygenase enzymes, many of which are polymorphic, that are major players in drug metabolism.

Isoform—A protein having a similar function and sequence as another protein, but arising from a different gene (or from a splice variant of the same gene).

Narrow therapeutic index (or ratio) (NTI) agent—An agent for which there is less than a twofold difference in median lethal dose (LD50) and median effective dose (ED50) values, or there is less than a twofold difference in the minimum toxic concentrations and minimum effective concentrations in the blood, and for which the safe and effective use of the drug products require careful titration and patient monitoring.[2]

Xenobiotic—A substance foreign to the human body.

Introduction

The safe and effective use of therapeutic agents by patients is the goal of every healthcare professional. The advent of personalized medicine allows this goal to be made even more specific—namely, to determine which patients are most likely to **benefit** from a given therapy, for which patients a given therapy would be **inappropriate**, and what the **appropriate dosing regimen** of a therapeutic agent should be.[3-5] However, patient-to-patient differences in responses to drug therapy that impact these therapeutic objectives are common. Some studies indicate that the most commonly used pharmaceuticals are effective in only 25% to 60% of patients.[6] In addition, between 770,000 and 2 million cases of adverse drug reactions (ADRs) occur in the U.S. each year, leading to at least 100,000 fatalities and costs of up to $5.6 million per hospital.[7,8] One report estimates that the total number of drug-related deaths may be as high as 3% of the total fatalities in the general population.[9] Differences in patient responses to medications, including those differences that lead to potential ADRs, may arise from many sources, including environmental, genetic, and disease-based factors. Of the many genetic factors that may influence the way patients respond to therapeutic agents, differences in the enzymes involved in drug metabolism are known to play a major role. Many studies have suggested that the majority of ADRs might be preventable with the appropriate use of pharmacogenetic profiling of drug metabolic enzymes.[10-14] For example, antithrombotic agents are involved in most of the fatal ADRs.[9] Warfarin is one of the most commonly used antithrombotic drugs in the world, but individual patient responses to this agent vary widely. A large part of the interpatient variability in the response to warfarin therapy is believed to be due to pharmacogenetic differences in two key polymorphic enzymes: the CYP450 2C9 (CYP2C9, one of the primary metabolic enzymes responsible for inactivating warfarin) and the vitamin K epoxide reductase complex subunit 1 (VKORC1, the target through which warfarin exerts its therapeutic effects).[15,16] Increasing evidence suggests that the use of pharmacogenetic profiling of these two polymorphic enzymes, in combination with other clinical data, results in more appropriate dosing regimens that may reduce potential ADRs.[17-19]

Clinical Pearl

A majority of ADRs might be preventable with the appropriate use of pharmacogenetic profiling, for example, the use of CYP2C9 and VKORC1 genotyping in patients prior to the initiation of warfarin therapy.

It is important to note that there are several complicating factors in understanding the impact of pharmacogenetic differences in drug metabolizing enzymes on a patient's responses to pharmaceutical therapy. First, metabolism is only one of the many things that occur *in vivo* upon exposure to a therapeutic agent. Other biochemical processes— including absorption, distribution, and elimination, as well as the sensitivity and number of drug targets available (in addition to other factors such as disease state, age, etc.)—also have a direct impact on a patient's response to drug therapy. Focusing only on the contribution of metabolism-to-drug reponse variability, it is important to note that any specific therapeutic agent may be metabolized by a number of different enzymes in the body. For example, tamoxifen (a common anti-estrogen agent used in the treatment of hormone-dependent breast cancer) is metabolized by the CYP450 isoforms 1B1, 2A6, 2B6, 2C8, 2C9, 2C19, 2D6, 2E1, and 3A4, and also by the flavin monooxygenases (FMOs).[20,21] Conversely, each of the enzymes involved in human drug metabolism may be involved in the metabolism of more than one therapeutic agent.[20-26] For example, it is estimated that CYP2D6 is responsible for the metabolism of approximately 15% to 30% of the currently used drugs (specific literature estimates differ by the date and the set of drugs evaluated) (Figure 4-1).[20-22] Pharmacogenetically-based metabolic differences in drug responses are typically most pronounced in cases where (1) the elimination of the pharmaceutical agent is primarily due to metabolism, **and** (2) the metabolism of the drug is primarily due to a single polymorphic enzyme. These differences are of the most significance to clinicians in situations involving either commonly used therapeutic agents (e.g., the use of the opioid codeine for analgesia) or pharmaceutical agents with a narrow therapeutic index (or ratio, NTI) (e.g., the anticoagulant warfarin).

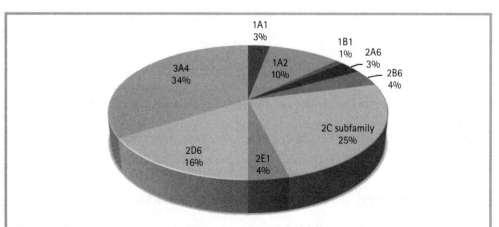

Figure 4.1 • Relative involvement of individual CYP450 isoforms in CYP-mediated phase I human drug metabolism.[20] (Adapted from substrate data from reference 20, Table 6, page 362.)

Clinical Pearl

Pharmacogenetic differences in drug metabolism are of particular significance to clinicians when they involve either commonly used therapeutic agents (e.g. the use of the opioid codeine for analgesia) or pharmaceutical agents with an NTI (e.g., the anticoagulant warfarin).

Case Study—Analgesic Failure with Post-Operative Codeine Usage

J.M., a 17-year-old Caucasian male, had oral surgery for the removal of his third molars ("wisdom teeth") and received a postoperative prescription for a combination analgesic containing 300 mg of acetaminophen and 30 mg of codeine phosphate per tablet with instructions for taking one tablet every 4–6 hours as needed for pain. All of J.M.'s vital signs and lab values were within normal ranges. He reported being on no other OTC or prescription medications, and he had no other concomitant diseases. Several hours after surgery, J.M. reported that he was in excruciating pain, and the prescriber recommended increasing the dosage of his medication to two tablets every 4–6 hours. The next morning, J.M.'s mother brought him into the prescriber's office, explaining that he was still in great pain and had not been able to rest at all following the surgery.

Questions:

1. What is the primary reason that J.M. was unable to achieve symptom relief, even at higher doses of his analgesic medication?
2. What is the major human metabolic enzyme involved in the biotransformation of codeine to the active analgesic morphine?
3. What are the clinical implications for patients who have a deficiency in the activity of this enzyme and are prescribed a codeine-containing product for analgesia?
4. What genotypic or phenotypic tests are currently available for determining the level of activity of the major codeine biotransformation enzyme present in a patient?
5. Propose an alternative analgesic regimen for a patient who is unable to obtain pain relief using a codeine-based agent.

Discussion:

Codeine, a narcotic antitussive agent, is also commonly used as an analgesic agent for the relief of mild-to-moderate pain. However, some patients experience no pain relief when using codeine-based products. The analgesic effects of codeine depend on the biotransformation (specifically, the O-demethylation) of this compound to morphine (see the section on CYP2D6 below for additional information).[27-29]

Enzymes Involved in Human Drug Metabolism

Both the enzymes and the types of biochemical reactions involved in human drug metabolism have historically been divided into two major classes or phases: Phase I and Phase II (Table 4-1).[21-25] In general, Phase I metabolic reactions involve the oxidative, reductive, or hydrolytic exposure or addition of chemical functional groups that frequently act as "handles" (or attachment sites) for subsequent Phase II conjugation reactions. Phase II reactions, such as glucuronidation and sulfation, involve the transfer of additional chemical moieties onto the functional group "handles" present either in the original compound or added in Phase I. Phase II reactions usually, but not always (e.g., methylation), result in making a compound more polar or hydrophilic in order to facilitate its elimination from the body. However, it should be noted that not all therapeutic agents go through **both** Phase I and Phase II metabolism. For example, some pharmaceuticals (e.g., digoxin, isoflurane) do not undergo any significant metabolism in the human body and are excreted primarily as the unchanged drug, while others may primarily undergo only Phase I metabolism (e.g., succinylcholine) or only Phase II metabolism (e.g., lorazepam), but not both (Figure 4-2).[30-33]

Table 4-1
Enzymes Involved in the Major Phases of Human Drug Metabolism[21-25]

Phase I	Phase II
Alcohol dehydrogenase	Glutathione-S-transferases (GSTs)
Aldehyde dehydrogenase	Methyltransferases (MTs)
Cytochrome P450s (CYP450s)	N-acetyltransferases (NATs)
Epoxide hydrolases	Sulfotransferases (SULTs)
Esterases	UDP-glucuronosyltransferases (UGTs)
Flavin-containing monooxygenases (FMOs)	
NADPH-quinone oxidoreductase (NQO)	
Peptidases/proteases	

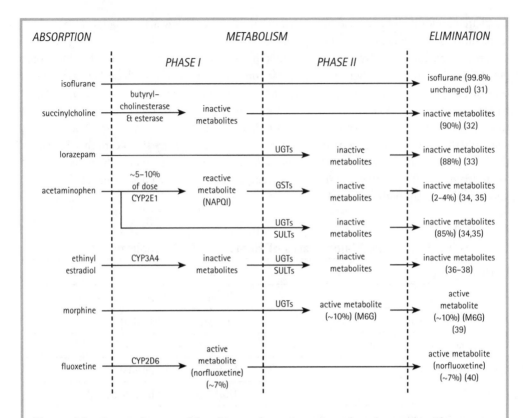

Figure 4.2 • Potential routes of drug biotransformation using selected examples. The examples given here are not exhaustive, but are intended to be illustrative of the many possible paths of biotransformation taken by different pharmaceutical agents. Percentages, where noted, refer to the percent of the original dose of the compound administered. Literature references are noted in parentheses. GSTs = glutathione-S-transferases; M6G = morphine-6-beta-glucuronide; NAPQI = N-acetyl-*p*-benzoquinone imine; SULTs = sulfotransferases; UGTs = UDP-glucuronosyltransferases.

Types of Phase I biotransformations include oxidation, reduction, and hydrolysis reactions (Figure 4-2).[21-25] Specific enzymes in Phase I include the CYP450 superfamily, various dehydrogenases, epoxide hydrolases, esterases, amidases, and the FMO superfamily. The largest and most notable subgroup of Phase I enzymes is the CYP450 enzymes (microsomal mixed function oxidases), a superfamily of heme-containing monooxygenases involved in the metabolism of not only drugs, but also other xenobiotics and endogenous compounds (Table 4-1 and Figure 4-3).[21-25] At least 18 different families of CYP450s, including more than 50 individual enzymes, have been identified in humans, but only four families (CYP450s 1, 2, 3, and 4—although there is scant information about the CYP4 family's role available at this time) are currently known to play a major role in drug metabolism (Figure 4-1 and Figure 4-3).[43-45]

There are multiple CYP450s isoforms and many individual CYP450 enzymes have the ability to metabolize a wide variety of types of substrates. The nomenclature used for cytochrome P450s (CYP450s), which is based on gene sequence analysis, uses a number to designate each family followed by a letter to denote the appropriate subfamily and is concluded by a number that identifies the specific gene product.[44,45] For example, CYP2D6, one of the well-studied polymorphic members of this metabolic enzyme superfamily, is in CYP family 2, subfamily D, and was the 6th gene product to be identified within this group.

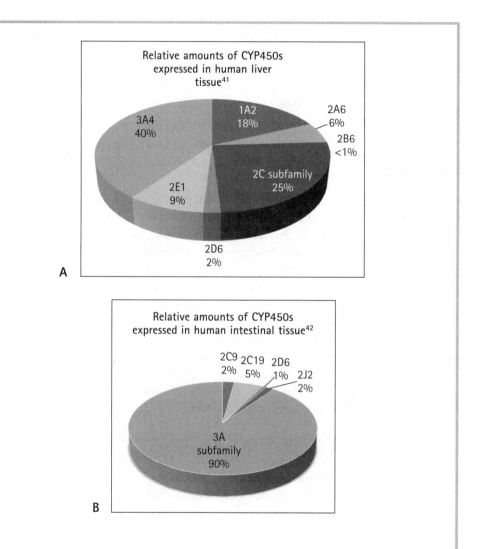

Figure 4.3 • Relative percentages of human hepatic CYP450 enzymes expressed in human liver (A) and intestinal (B) tissue.[41,42]

Clinical Pearl

CYP450s, the major type of Phase 1 biotransformation enzymes, are the group of most interest to clinicians regarding both potential drug-drug interactions and pharmacogenetic influences on drug metabolism.

Phase II metabolic biotransformations involve transfer or conjugation reactions (Figure 4-2).[20-26] Most, but not all (e.g., methylation), Phase II reactions result in the formation of a more polar (or hydrophilic) product that is easier to eliminate in the urine. Metabolic enzymes included in the Phase II group include the glutathione-S-transferases (GSTs), the methyltransferases (MTs), the N-acetyltransferases (NATs), the sulfotransferases (SULTs), and the UDP-glucuronosyltransferases (UGTs) (Table 4-1 and Figure 4-2).[21-26]

Specific Examples of Pharmacogenetic Differences in Drug Metabolism

As noted earlier, pharmacogenetically-based metabolic differences in drug responses are typically most pronounced in cases where the elimination of the pharmaceutical agent is primarily due to metabolism **and** the metabolism of the drug is primarily due to a single polymorphic enzyme. In more practical terms, as healthcare providers we are primarily concerned with cases in which these metabolic differences may lead to potentially serious, or even lethal, outcomes and cases that involve the most commonly used pharmaceutical agents. In most, but not all, cases in which pharmacogenetic differences in drug metabolic enzymes are known to exist, these differences lead to a lower rate of activity (i.e., a "poor metabolizer [PM]" phenotype) of the enzyme. A lower rate of biotransformation of a pharmaceutical agent typically causes reduced deactivation and clearance of the agent, which may lead to higher concentrations of the drug being present in the body. Higher concentrations of the drug in the body may ultimately cause a higher rate of ADRs or toxicities, especially for agents with an NTI, such as warfarin and the hydantoin anticonvulsants. Exceptions to this trend of genetic mutations causing decreased metabolic activity exist, including pharmacogenetic differences in CYP2D6 and the NATs, which lead to higher rates of activity (i.e., "rapid," "ultrarapid," or "fast" metabolizer phenotypes) for each of these biotransformation enzymes in some patients.[21-25] In the case of faster metabolizers, the increased rate of clearance may lead to the need for more frequent or larger doses in order to achieve an optimal therapeutic effect.

Clinical Pearl

Most cases, but not all (e.g., the CYP2D6 and NAT2 ultrarapid or "fast" metabolizer phenotypes), of pharmacogenetic variations in drug metabolic enzymes lead to a lower rate of metabolism of the drug substrate, increasing the risk of ADRs for patients and necessitating consideration of modified dosing regimens.

At a molecular level, phenotypes that display reduced metabolic enzyme activity are sometimes due to amino acid residue changes (including, but not limited to, SNPs), which lead to reduced drug substrate binding, reduced enzymatic activity, or both. For example, the E mutation (*CYP2D6*7* allele, 1.5% frequency in Caucasians) in CYP2D6 is based on a single nucleotide change (3023A>C in exon 6) in the *CYP2D6* gene that results in a histidine to proline change at residue 324 (His324Pro or H324P) in this enzyme.[46] This solitary change in the identity of an amino acid residue near the active site of the 2D6 isoform leads to the complete loss of activity of this important drug metabolic enzyme. Many other changes (including multiple residue mutations, deletions (of entire genes, domains, or specific residues), splicing defects, crossovers, gene duplications, and frameshift mutations) in the CYP2D6 gene are known to occur with most, but not all, having a similar negative impact on this enzyme's metabolic activity (see reference 44 for current and complete list). The distribution of 2D6 alleles that give rise to reduced or no enzymatic activity varies across ethnic groups, with European Caucasians, for example, having a significant but relatively lower frequency (~27% to 30%) compared to patients of Asian and African descent (each ~50%) (Table 4-2).[47,48]

Table 4–2
CYP2D6 Phenotypes and Characteristics[a,47–50]

Phenotype	Freq.	Genetic Bases	Implications for Pharmacotherapeutic Agents	
			Activated by 2D6	Deactivated by 2D6
Poor metabolizer (PM)	~5% to 10%	No functional alleles present	Lack of therapeutic effects may be observed	Reduced dosing may be needed
Intermediate metabolizer (IM)	~20% to 40%	Either one functional and one mutant/ deficient allele or two partially active/ deficient alleles present	May show reduced effects	May be able to achieve therapeutic effects at lower than normal doses
Extensive metabolizer (EM)	~60% to 80%	Either two active alleles or a combination of one active and one partially active allele present	Should be able to achieve therapeutic effects with normal dosing	Should be able to achieve therapeutic effects with normal dosing
Ultrarapid metabolizer (UM)	~1% to 5%	Three or more active alleles present	Increased risk of toxicity (for any agents with active, toxic, or reactive metabolites); lower doses may be required	Increased risk of therapeutic failure (beta-blockers[46]); higher doses may be required

[a]In order of increasing enzymatic activity; frequency (freq.) of occurrence in a sample ethnic population (Caucasians).

At the genetic level, different combinations (e.g., homozygous or heterozygous) of the various possible alleles of each polymorphic metabolic enzyme are possible. These different genotypic combinations can produce a spectrum of phenotypes, from a lack of enzymatic activity (the PM that carries no functional alleles), to enhanced enzymatic activity (the "extensive metabolizer" [EM] with two functional alleles and the "ultrarapid metabolizer" [UM] with more than two functional alleles), and those that fall in between (the "intermediate metabolizer" [IM] that has either one defective and one functional allele or one or two reduced function alleles).[47-50] For the CYP2D6 enzyme, at least four different phenotypes have been identified (Table 4-2).

Although there is an increasing number of genotypic assays available to profile one or more polymorphic drug metabolizing enzymes (Table 4-3 and Table 4-4), it is important for clinicians to note the current limitations of such genetic tests. First, genotypic testing determines only the patient's gene profile (genotype), not the patient's actual metabolic enzyme activity (phenotype). Also, genotype assays are aimed at testing for the presence of specific SNPs or alleles, typically the most common polymorphisms (e.g., CYP2D6*4 PM allele found in ~12–20% of Caucasians) or those that are known to be associated with deficits in enzyme activity.[52] Other polymorphisms that are not detected by the assay, but which may still influence the activity of the metabolic enzymes being probed, may be present but not detected by genotypic testing. Finally, commercial clinical tests for many of the polymorphisms that impact drug metabolism are either not yet available or are costly, limiting access to objective data that might be used to adjust pharmacotherapeutic regimens. For example, one recent study found that polymorphisms in the *CYP4F2* gene can impact warfarin clearance, but there are currently no commercial genotypic or phenotypic assays available for this CYP isoform.[53] In many cases, however, an indirect phenotypic approach using either the serum blood levels of a therapeutic agent or a different surrogate molecule metabolized by the same polymorphic enzyme or, alternatively, a representative marker of drug action (e.g., international normalized ratios [INRs] for anticoagulants or blood glucose levels for antidiabetic agents) may be used as an indirect indicator of the pharmacogenetic profile of a patient's drug metabolic enzymes.[54,55]

Table 4-3
Examples of Polymorphic Drug Metabolizing Enzymes of Clinical Importance[21-26]

Phase I	Phase II
CYP1A2	N-acetyltransferase 2 (NAT2)
CYP2B6	Thiopurine S-methyltransferase (TPMT)
CYP2C9	UDP-glucuronosyltransferase 1A1 (UGT1A1)
CYP2C19	
CYP2D6	
Dihydropyrimidine dehydrogenase (DPD)	
Butyrylcholinesterase (BChE)	

Table 4-4
Examples of Current Commercially Available *in Vitro* Genotyping Tests for Polymorphic Drug Metabolizing Enzymes of Clinical Importance[51,227]

Test	Genes Profiled	Manufacturer
AmpliChip™ CYP450 test	CYPs 2C19 & 2D6	Roche Diagnostics (Indianapolis, IN)
eSensor® XT-8 system for warfarin sensitivity	CYP2C9, VKORC1	Osmetech Molecular Diagnostics, (Pasadena, CA)
Infiniti™ 2C9-VKORC1 multiplex assay	CYP2C9, VKORC1	AutoGenomics (Carlsbad, CA)
Invader® UGT1A1 molecular assay	UGT1A1	Third Wave Technologies (Madison, WI)
Paragon Dx rapid genotyping assay	CYP2C9, VKORC1	Paragon Dx, LLC (Morrisville, NC)
TheraGuide 5-FU™	DPYD, TYMS	Myriad Genetic Laboratories (Salt Lake City, UT)
Verigene® Warfarin Metabolism Nucleic Acid Test	CYP2C9, VKORC1	Nanosphere (Northbrook, IL)

CYP = cytochrome P450; *DPYD* = dihydropyrimidine dehydrogenase; *TYMS* = thymidylate synthetase; *UGT1A1* = UDP-glucuronosyltransferase 1A1; *VKORC1* = vitamin K epoxide reductase complex subunit 1 (the target of warfarin).

The polymorphic Phase I metabolic enzymes of the most clinical relevance include several members of the CYP450 superfamily (CYP1A2, CYP2B6, CYP2C9, CYP2C19, CYP2D6), dihydropyrimidine dehydrogenase (DPD), and butyrylcholinesterase (BChE) (Table 4-3). [20-26,42-45,56,57] Phase II polymorphic enzymes of the most clinical importance include N-acetyltransferase 2 (NAT2), the thiopurine S-methyltransferase (TPMT), and UDP-glucuronosyltransferase 1A1 (UGT1A1).[20-26,58-60] It should be noted that this is not an exhaustive list, as many other polymorphic members of both groups of metabolic enzymes are known, and more are being discovered every year. However, for purposes of this chapter, we will focus only on the most current clinically relevant examples.[20-26]

Phase I Metabolic Enzymes

Cytochrome P450s (CYP450s)
The aryl hydrocarbon hydroxylase CYP1A2 (EC 1.14.14.1), although having one of the higher expression levels of the P450 isoforms in the human liver (Figure 4-3), is estimated to be involved in the metabolism of only about 10% of therapeutic agents.[20,41] The 1A2 isoform plays a major role in the metabolic clearance (N-demethylation and aromatic hydroxylation) of the bronchodilator theophylline and the atypical antipsychotics clozapine (N-demethylation) and olanzapine (N-demethylation and aromatic hydroxylation).[55,61-63] CYP450 1A2 preferentially binds substrates that are polar heterocyclic compounds (e.g., theophylline) and aryl amines (e.g., clozapine and olanzapine).[20,64-66]

While over 15 variant *CYP1A2* alleles are currently known to exist, there are two major single nucleotide polymorphisms (SNPs) that have been identified in humans.[44,67] The *CYP1A2*1C* allele (resulting from the single point mutation -3860G>A) is associated with decreased metabolic enzyme activity relative to the wild-type *1A* allele, while the *CYP1A2*1F* allele (resulting from the single point mutation -163C>A) is associated with increased enzyme induction compared to the wild-type (or nonmutated) allele.[68] Population studies done to date indicate that the homozygous and heterozygous *1F* allele combinations are more prevalent, suggesting that high CYP1A2 induction is the most common phenotype here.[69]

Of particular importance to clinicians is the predominant role that CYP1A2 plays in the clearance of clozapine, an atypical antipsychotic agent with several potentially fatal toxicities, including agranulocytosis, seizures, and myocarditis.[70,71] Patients who are poor 1A2 metabolizers are at greater risk of clozapine toxicity due to their reduced clearance of this agent. For example, recent research has highlighted the increased risk of side-effects such as tardive dyskinesia in clozapine-treated patients who have both reduced CYP1A2 activity (homozygous *1C* genotype) and mutations in the D_3 dopaminergic receptor (although conflicting studies have also been published).[72-74] Conversely, patients with higher-than-normal levels of CYP1A2 activity, presumably due to a combination of a high induction phenotype along with exposure to a 1A2 inducer (such as cigarette smoke), are at increased risk of treatment failure with clozapine due to their rapid clearance of this agent.[75,76]

There is currently at least one commercial clinical company (Genelex Corporation, Seattle, WA) that provides CYP1A2 genotyping services to healthcare providers. At the time of this writing, there are currently no commercially available *in vitro* genotyping tests for the 1A2 isozyme. However, as an alternative to direct genotype testing, several researchers have suggested the use of a simple caffeine (another agent that is a CYP1A2 substrate) metabolism profile as an indirect means of assessing 1A2 phenotypes.[55,63,77,78]

Clinical Pearl

Patients taking clozapine, an atypical antipsychotic agent with several potentially fatal toxicities, may benefit from CYP1A2 genotypic or phenotypic testing in order to modify dosing regimens, if needed.

CYP2B6 (EC 1.14.14.1) is another example of a polymorphic enzyme involved in Phase I biotransformation reactions. The cytochrome P405 2B6 enzyme is involved in the metabolism of approximately 4% of current pharmaceuticals, including the antidepressant bupropion, the anticancer agents ifosfamide and cyclophosphamide, the opioid analgesic methadone, and the non-nucleoside reverse transcriptase inhibitors (NNRTIs) efavirenz and nevirapine.[20,79-85] The substrate preferences observed for this CYP isoform are for nonplanar structures, usually containing at least one aromatic ring with relatively high lipophilicity and one or two hydrogen bond-forming groups.[64-66] Although less well-studied than some of the better-known CYP isoforms, the *CYP2B6* gene appears to be one of the more polymorphic cytochrome genes in man, with well over 100 different SNPs identified to date.[86,87] The most frequently occurring mutant allele, *CYP2B6*6* (which gives rise to Q172H & K262R mutations in the 2B6 enzyme), has a variable distribution across different ethnic groups ranging from a 14% frequency in Koreans to over 40% in West Africans to 62% in Papua New Guineans.[86,88-90] Most of the mutant alleles identified to date seem to contribute to lower expression levels and/or lower activity rates of CYP2B6, particularly when present in a homozygous combination, although the genotype-phenotype relationships in this case are especially complicated and additional studies of larger patient groups are needed.[86]

One area of potential clinical importance regarding agents metabolized by CYP2B6 is the interpatient variation in the pharmacokinetic parameters of the anticancer agents ifosfamide and cyclophosphamide.[91] Each of these nitrogen mustard derivatives is administered as a prodrug and is dependent on the 2B6 isoform to help create the therapeutically-active species (initially, 4-hydroxycyclophosphamide/aldophosphamide (4-OH-CP) and, subsequently, the phosphoramide mustard) in vivo.[92] Most studies have shown a lower level of formation of the active 4-OH-CP metabolite and a higher rate of elimination (each of which may potentially lead to a lower therapeutic benefit) of these agents in patients with variant CYP2B6 alleles (e.g., see reference 93). However, given the number of enzymes involved in cyclophosphamide metabolism, the inducibility of CYP2B6, and the relatively small sample sizes used in most clinical studies to date, larger studies are needed to more fully elucidate the association between the 2B6 PM phenotype and cyclophosphamide treatment outcomes.[86] There are currently no commercially available clinical assays for either CYP2B6 genotypes or phenotypes, but the measurement of the hydroxylation of bupropion has been proposed as a means of profiling a patient's 2B6 activity level.[94]

The polymorphic CYP450 enzyme 2C9 (EC 1.14.13.80), with several different alleles identified in man, is the major human isoform of the CYP2C subfamily (CYPs 2C8, 2C9, 2C18, and 2C19).[44,95,96] Together, CYP2C9 and CYP2C19 are involved in the metabolism of approximately 25% of currently used therapeutic agents (Figure 4-1).[20] Drug substrates (e.g., phenytoin) for CYP2C9 usually are weakly acidic and have one or more aromatic rings (Table 4-5 and Figure 4-4).[20,64-66] There are two major inherited SNPs of the 2C9 gene, leading to the alleles CYP2C9*2 (430C>T, resulting in the enzyme mutation R144C) and CYP2C9*3 (1075A>C, resulting in the enzyme mutation I359L), each of which decreases 2C9 function.[95,96] Patients having one of these alleles maintain CYP2C9 activity, but at a reduced rate (i.e., the PM phenotype), and thus may require lower than normal doses of 2C9-metabolized agents (especially NTI agents such as the hydantoin anticonvulsants and warfarin) in order to optimize therapeutic response and minimize toxicity (Figure 4-5). Population-based studies indicate that the CYP2C9 PM phenotype is more common (~14% frequency) in Caucasian patients than in Asians or Africans (~4% in each group).[95,96]

Table 4-5

Selected Examples of CYP2C9 Substrates from the Top 200 Drugs (as ranked by sales) in the U.S. Market from 2008[a,97]

Generic Name	Brand Name(s)	Reaction(s) Catalyzed by CYP2C9 (metabolites inactive unless otherwise specified)	Clinical Implications of Reduced CYP2C9 Activity
Carvedilol	Coreg®, Coreg® CR	*O*-methylation (of the *S*(-)-isomer)[98]	Probably minimal (2D6 is the major metabolic enzyme for carvedilol)[98]
Celecoxib	Celebrex®	Oxidation of methyl group to primary alcohol and continued oxidation to carboxylic acid (Figure 4-4)[99]	Greater risk of adverse cardiovascular events[100,101]
Losartan	Cozaar®, part of Hyzaar®	Oxidation of primary alcohol to carboxylic acid (active metabolite (E-3174) that is 10–40 times more potent than parent compound)[102,103]	Lower therapeutic effects due to lower levels of the active metabolite[104]
Montelukast	Singulair®	Hydroxylation of methyl group[105]	Greater potential risk of neuropsychiatric events[105]
Rosiglitazone	Avandia®, part of Avandaryl®, part of Avandamet®	*N*-demethylation[106]	Minimal (2C8 is the primary isoform involved in deactivation)[106]
Valsartan	Diovan®, part of Diovan HCT®	4-hydroxylation[107]	Minimal (4-hydroxy metabolite represents ~9% of dose; 80% eliminated as unchanged drug)[107]

[a]Salt information not shown. Not all possible metabolic reactions for CYP2C9 or for each of the selected compounds are shown. The 2C9 isoform may not be the only enzyme involved in the biotransformation of the drugs shown here.

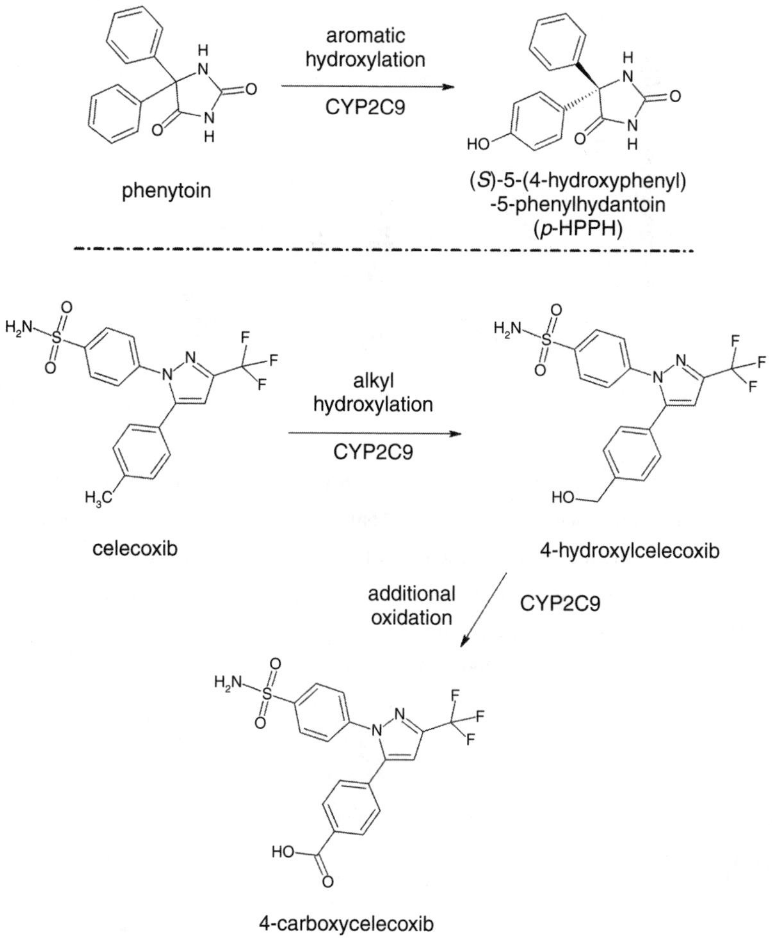

Figure 4.4 • CYP2C9-mediated metabolism of phenytoin (top) and celecoxib (bottom) in man.[21,99,108-110]

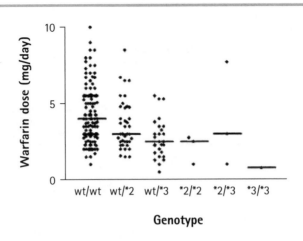

Figure 4.5 • Relationship between CYP2C9 genotype and warfarin dose requirement for 200 randomly selected Caucasian individuals.[50,288] Samples were genotyped only for *CYP2C9*2* and *CYP2C9*3*. The median dose for each genotype is indicated by the horizontal bars. A significant difference in dosing requirements between genotypes was found (p = 0.0002, Kruskal-Wallis test). Used with permission from Daly AK, King BP. Pharmacogenetics of oral anticoagulants. *Pharmacogenetics.* 2003;13:247-252.

Clinical Pearl

Population-based studies indicate that ~14% of Caucasian patients are deficient in the activity of CYP2C9, a metabolic enzyme that plays a key role in the biotransformation of several oral sulfonylurea hypoglycemic agents, nonsteroidal anti-inflammatory drugs (NSAIDs), and NTI drugs such as the hydantoin anticonvulsants and warfarin. When these patients are treated with therapeutics that are metabolized by CYP2C9, dosage adjustments may be required in order to avoid side-effects and toxicity.

CYP2C9 plays a key role in drug metabolism due to its involvement in the biotransformation of more than 100 currently used therapeutic agents, including several oral sulfonylurea hypoglycemic agents, NSAIDs (including the COX-2 inhibitor celecoxib), angiotensin II receptor blockers (ARBs), and NTI agents such as the hydantoin anticonvulsants and warfarin (Figure 4-4).[15-19,99,102-104,108-112] There are several potential issues of clinical importance regarding 2C9 polymorphisms, including the potential adverse reactions that are possible with some of the more commonly used therapeutic agents such as the NSAIDs and the sulfonylurea antidiabetic agents. For example, patients deficient in CYP2C9 activity are up to five times more likely to experience hypoglycemia on initiation of antidiabetic pharmacotherapy with sulfonylureas at "normal" doses due to their decreased clearance of these agents.[111] Similarly, patients having at least one of the two major 2C9 SNPs (who are thus 2C9 PMs) have a much higher risk of gastrointestinal bleeding associated with NSAID therapy.[112]

Of particular interest to clinicians here are the potential ADRs arising from the use of NTI agents such as warfarin and the hydantoin anticonvulsants in patients who have decreased levels of CYP2C9 activity. Antithrombotic agents, such as warfarin, are involved in a majority of fatal ADRs.[9] Warfarin is currently the second most common cause of emergency room visits (after insulin) due to adverse drug events for patients who are 65 and older.[113] In order to avoid potential toxicities, dosage adjustments for both warfarin and the hydantoin anticonvulsants may be needed in patients who are deficient in 2C9 activity. This issue has attracted the attention of the FDA, which in 2007 approved new pharmacogenetic tests to measure the activity of CYP2C9 (which plays a key role in the metabolism of warfarin) and the vitamin K epoxide reductase complex subunit 1 (VKORC1, the enzymatic target of warfarin *in vivo*).[114] At the same time, the FDA also updated the prescribing information for this drug to encourage the use of these tests by healthcare professionals in order to optimize warfarin pharmacotherapy.[115] The FDA also currently recommends that clinicians consider the CYP2C9 phenotype of patients receiving the COX-2 inhibitor celecoxib, another agent whose metabolic clearance is dependent on this CYP450 isoform (Figure 4-4).[116] Given the known cardiovascular adverse events of the COX-2 inhibitors that have led to the removal of most of the members of this class of agents from the market, this advice seems particularly prudent.[101]

It should be noted that warfarin and celecoxib are not the only therapeutic agents that include pharmacogenetic information in their labeling. One recent study of FDA-approved drugs from 1945–2005 found that 69 different agents from this period contained human genomic information as a part of the prescribing information, with a majority (62%) of these cases referring specifically to CYP enzymes.[117] The FDA's own estimates are that approximately 10% of drugs currently approved in the U.S. contain pharmacogenomic information as part of their labeling.[116] Recent FDA guidance in this area suggests that this trend is likely to increase.[118]

In spite of the recognized therapeutic importance of genetic variation in this enzyme, several factors have slowed the adoption of *2C9* genotypic testing by clinicians as a standard of care.[119] One major factor currently limiting the more widespread adoption of these tests (and pharmacogenomic tests, in general) is the lack of long-term studies demonstrating their clinical benefits across a variety of patient groups.[120,121] Another factor is cost. Currently, it may cost up to several hundred dollars to obtain CYP2C9 genotyping test results from a commercial clinical laboratory for a patient and insurance coverage for these tests varies. An additional concern is that 2C9 testing alone is not sufficient for optimizing the dosing regimens of therapeutic agents, because, in many cases, CYP2C9 is not the only metabolic enzyme involved in the clearance of these drugs. For example, in different studies, the CYP2C9 genotype alone accounted for only 10% to 32% of the observed variation in the maintenance doses of warfarin.[122,123] In this case, it is clear that other information, such as a patient's VKORC1 phenotype or the activity level of other CYP450 enzymes, must also be taken into account in order to more accurately design warfarin dosing regimens.[15-19]

Because of its importance in the metabolism of multiple NTI drugs, *CYP2C9* genotyping is currently available from several commercial clinical laboratories, including DNA Direct, Inc. (San Francisco, CA) and Genelex Incorporated (Seattle, WA). In addition, there are now at least four commercially available clinical testing systems that have been approved by the FDA for use in warfarin pharmacotherapy (Table 4-4), including the Verigene® system (Nanosphere, Inc., Northbrook, IL), the Infiniti™ assay and analyzer (AutoGenomics, Inc., Carlsbad, CA), the Rapid Genotyping Assay (ParagonDx LLC, Morrisville, NC), and eSensor® XT-8 system (Osmetech Molecular Diagnostics, Pasadena, CA). While *CYP2C9* genotyping certainly provides additional objective data for use in optimizing dosing regimens, clinicians should be aware of the general limitations of such testing, as noted earlier.

Another member of the CYP450 2C subfamily that demonstrates polymorphism (with at least seven different alleles known) in humans is the 2C19 isoform (ECs 1.14.13.48, 1.14.13.49, and 1.14.13.80) (Figure 4-1 and Figure 4-3).[44,124] CYP2C19 (previously referred to as the S-mephenytoin hydroxylase) is known to be involved in the biotransformation of a number of commonly used therapeutic agents, including the antiplatelet agent clopidogrel, the hydantoin anticonvulsants, and the proton pump inhibitors (PPIs) (Table 4-6 and Figure 4-6).[108-110,125-134,136] This CYP450 isoform displays a preference for aromatic, heteroaromatic, and heteroalkyl drug substrates, with aromatic hydroxylation and O- and N-dealkylations as prototypical 2C19-catalyzed biotransformation reactions.[20,64-66] As with many of the other CYP450 enzymes, the major 2C19 polymorphic alleles, *CYP2C19*2* (681G>A and 3-4 additional SNPs) and *CYP2C19*3* (636G>A and two additional variant positions), that have been reported result in a PM phenotype.[124] Population-based studies suggest a higher frequency of the 2C19-deficient phenotype in patients of Asian and Pacific Islander ancestry (~14% of Chinese and up to 70% of some Pacific Islander populations) than in other ethnic groups.[124]

Table 4-6

Selected Examples of CYP2C19 Substrates from the Top 200 Drugs (as ranked by sales) in the U.S. Market from 2008[a,97]

Generic Name	Brand Name(s)	Reaction(s) Catalyzed by CYP2C19 (metabolites inactive unless otherwise specified)	Clinical Implications of Reduced CYP2C19 Activity
Clopidogrel	Plavix®	Prodrug is transformed first to the inactive 2-oxo metabolite and, subsequently, to the active thiol form[126-132]	Greater risk of adverse cardiovascular events due to lower levels of active form of drug[126-132]
Escitalopram	Lexapro®	N-demethylation to S-desmethylcitalopram (active metabolite with $\frac{1}{7}$ of the activity of the parent compound)[135]	Minimal (the 2D6 and 3A4 isoforms also metabolize escitalopram)[135]
Esomeprazole	Nexium®	O-demethylation[133,134,136]	Greater acid inhibition and higher *H. pylori* eradication rates[133,134,136]
Formoterol	Foradil®, part of Symbicort®	O-demethylation[137]	Minimal (glucuronidation is the major metabolic route)[137]

[a]Salt information not shown. Not all possible metabolic reactions for CYP2C19 or for each of the selected compounds are shown. The 2C19 isoform may not be the only enzyme involved in the biotransformation of the drugs shown here.

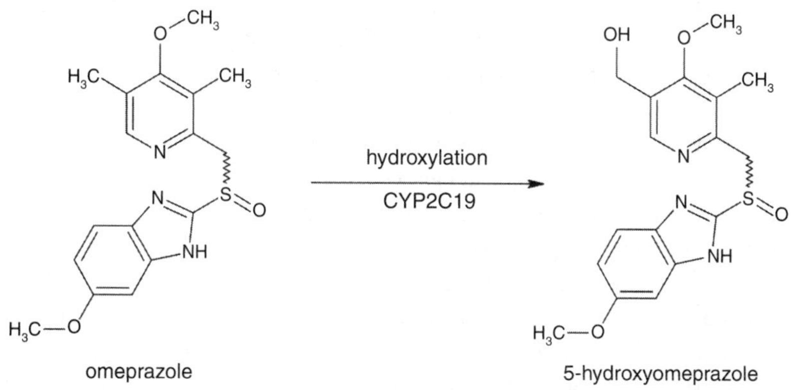

Figure 4.6 • CYP2C19-mediated metabolism of omeprazole (or esomeprazole) in man.[133,134,136]

There are several issues of clinical importance regarding 2C19 polymorphisms. The most notable of these include the potential adverse reactions that are possible with the anticonvulsant NTI agent phenytoin and with the commonly used anticoagulant clopidogrel. For phenytoin (and also for its prodrug fosphenytoin), the clinical implications of being a 2C19 PM are most pronounced in patients who are **also** 2C9 deficient or are receiving another medication that acts as a competitive substrate (or inhibitor) of either CYP450 2C9 or 2C19. Both CYP2C9 and CYP2C19 are involved in the metabolism and clearance of phenytoin, so dosage adjustments may be required in patients who have lower activity (due either to genetic reasons or the presence of competitive substrates or inhibitors) of **both** of these biotransformation enzymes.

The impact of CYP2C19 polymorphisms on the adverse effects experienced by patients being treated with the widely used antiplatelet agent clopidogrel has recently been receiving increasing clinical attention.[126-132] In part, this is due to the fact that, as an anticoagulant, clopidogrel (like warfarin) can cause serious ADRs that lead to hospitalization and even death.[129,130] Clopidogrel is administered in the form of a prodrug that requires action by CYP2C19 to produce the active form of this agent (Table 4-6).[129,130] Thus, patients who are 2C19 PMs may produce less of the active form of clopidogrel and display resistance to the antiplatelet effects of this agent.[126-132] Given the widespread usage of clopidogrel as a blood-thinning agent for acute coronary syndrome and following myocardial infarction or ischemic stroke, failure to achieve a full therapeutic effect may have significant deleterious consequences for the patient. For example, in one recent study among patients who underwent percutaneous coronary interventions during hospitalization and received clopidogrel, the rate of cardiovascular events among patients with two *CYP2C19* loss-of-function alleles was 3.58 times the rate in individuals with no deficient alleles.[129]

The impact of CYP2C19 deficiency on the effectiveness of clopidogrel therapy is magnified with the concurrent use of other agents that compete for this metabolic enzyme. For example, the PPIs, a family of therapeutic agents frequently used to reduce the production of stomach acid, act as competitive substrates or inhibitors of the CYP450 2C19 isoform.[133,134] Due to the increased risk of gastrointestinal bleeding in patients receiving anticoagulants such as clopidogrel, PPIs have been commonly prescribed as concurrent therapy for the prevention of gastric ulcers. Increasing clinical evidence from a number of large studies shows that the concurrent use of clopidogrel with a PPI leads to a higher rate of clopidogrel treatment failures.[138-140] For example, one recent report shows that the 1-year risk of adverse cardiovascular events is increased more than 50% in patients taking a PPI concurrently with clopidogrel.[140] Interestingly, the new thienopyridine anticoagulant prasugrel, although both structurally and mechanistically related to clopidogrel, doesn't appear to require CYP2C19 for activation *in vivo*.[141-143] Prasugrel, therefore, may represent a new and viable option for patients who are deficient in 2C19 activity but need to be on concurrent anticoagulant and PPI therapy. Another therapeutic option would be to use the H$_2$-receptor antagonists in place of PPIs as concomitant antiulcer therapy in patients receiving clopidogrel.

With regard to other therapeutic agents, clinicians should be aware that the FDA has also issued guidance suggesting the usefulness of *2C19* genotyping for patients receiving the azole antifungal voriconazole.[116] Also, in contrast to the concerns about genotype testing increasing healthcare costs, Desta and colleagues have suggested that CYP2C19 genotype testing of Asian patients (who are more likely to be poor 2C19 metabolizers) with gastric or duodenal ulcers could actually save up to $5,000 for every 1,000 patients tested as a result of the use of lower doses of the relatively expensive PPIs to achieve the same therapeutic outcomes.[124]

CYP2C19 genotyping is currently available from several commercial clinical laboratories, including DNA Direct, Inc. (San Francisco, CA) and Genelex Incorporated (Seattle, WA). The commercially available AmpliChip™ P450 assay (Table 4-4) also profiles *CYP2C19* (and *CYP2D6*) genotypes. Although *CYP2C19* genotype testing provides useful data for use in optimizing therapeutic regimens, clinicians should be aware of the general limitations of such genetically-targeted testing, as noted earlier.

Clinical Pearl

Patients who are deficient in CYP2C19 activity are at greater risk for adverse cardiovascular events when placed on clopidogrel therapy, especially when being treated concurrently with a PPI. Clinicians should consider prasugrel as an alternative antiplatelet agent or H$_2$-receptor antagonists as an alternative group of antiulcer agents in order to minimize the risk of adverse cardiovascular events in these patients.

CYP2D6 (EC 1.14.14.1), which was formerly known as the debrisoquine/sparteine hydroxylase, was the first specific human drug metabolic enzyme identified as being polymorphic.[144-147] Another distinctive feature of the P450 2D6 isoform is that it is among the most prolific with regard to the number of different alleles (currently over 15) that have been identified in man.[44] Population studies indicate that reduced function alleles (such as *CYP2D6*9*, *CYP2D6*10*, and *CYP2D6*17*) are more common in African Americans and Asians, while completely nonfunctional alleles (such as *CYP2D6*3*, *CYP2D6*4*, *CYP2D6*5*, and *CYP2D6*6*) are more common in Caucasians.[52] However, with regard to drug metabolism, the specific phenotype that exists in a patient is dependent on the combination of alleles that are present, as previously noted.

CYP2D6 displays a preference for lipophilic amine substrates.[20,52] Due to the large number of drugs that fit this structural pattern, the 2D6 isoform plays a key role in the biotransformation of an estimated 15% to 50% of commonly used therapeutic agents (Figure 4-1).[20-22,52] Specific metabolic reactions catalyzed by the CYP450 2D6 include aromatic hydroxylation and

O- and N-dealkylations.[20-22,52] CYP2D6 drug substrates include agents used as antidepressants, antipsychotics, antihypertensives, and antiarrhythmics (Table 4-7 and Figure 4-7).[148-158] As noted earlier, the multiplicity of CYP2D6 alleles results in the existence of at least four major phenotypes[47-50,179]:

1. PM—No functional alleles present, resulting in a lack of CYP2D6 activity.
2. IM—Either one functional and one mutant/deficient allele or two partially active/deficient alleles present, resulting in diminished CYP2D6 activity.
3. EM—Either two active alleles or a combination of one active and one partially active allele present, resulting in normal CYP2D6 activity.
4. UM—Three or more active alleles present due to gene duplication, resulting in higher than normal CYP2D6 activity.

Table 4-7
Selected Examples of CYP2D6 Substrates from the Top 200 drugs (as ranked by sales) in the U.S. Market from 2008[a,97]

Generic Name	Brand Name(s)	Reaction(s) Catalyzed by CYP2D6 (metabolites inactive unless otherwise specified)	Clinical Implications of Reduced CYP2D6 Activity
Atomoxetine	Strattera®	4-hydroxylation[159] (4-hydroxyatomoxetine reported to be equipotent to parent compound[160]), N-demethylation[160]	Higher rates of adverse reactions[159]
Carvedilol	Coreg®, Coreg® CR	4'-hydroxylation (produces an active metabolite with 13 times the β-blocking potency of the parent compound[98]) and 5'-hydroxylation (both isomers)[98]	Greater risk of hypotension, due to decreased clearance
Darifenacin	Enablex®	Hydroxylation[161] (primarily on dihydrobenzofuran ring,[162,163] to produce a metabolite with 1/9 the potency of the parent compound)[164]	Minimal (also metabolized by 3A4 isoform)
Duloxetine	Cymbalta®	Hydroxylation of naphthyl ring (at least two active metabolites reported, with one having 1/5 the potency of the parent compound)[165-169]	Probably minimal (also metabolized by 1A2 isoform)[165]
Olanzapine	Zyprexa®	Hydroxylation of 2-methyl group[170]	Minimal (glucuronidation and 1A2-mediated N-demethylation are the major pathways)[171]

Continued on next page

Table 4–7 *(Continued)*

Generic Name	Brand Name(s)	Reaction(s) Catalyzed by CYP2D6 (metabolites inactive unless otherwise specified)	Clinical Implications of Reduced CYP2D6 Activity
Oxycodone	OxyContin®	*O*-demethylation (to the 40-fold[172] more active compound oxymorphone)[173,174]	Potentially lower analgesia[175,176] (due to less formation of the more active metabolite, but this is not the major metabolic pathway)
Venlafaxine	Effexor®, Effexor XR®	*O*-demethylation (to the equipotent active metabolite desvenlafaxine [O-desmethylvenlafaxine])[177]	None (the PM phenotype shifts the ratios of the parent compound and active metabolite, but the two compounds are equipotent and the total amounts of the two are similar)[177]

[a]Salt information not shown. Not all possible metabolic reactions for CYP2C19 or for each of the selected compounds are shown. The 2C19 isoform may not be the only enzyme involved in the biotransformation of the drugs shown here.

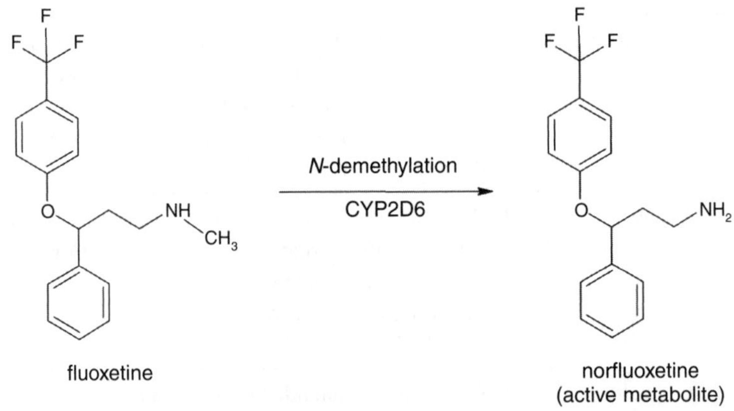

Figure 4.7 • CYP2D6-mediated metabolism of fluoxetine in man.[178]

The frequency of CYP2D6 phenotypes varies across different ethnic groups, with the PM phenotype reported to be more common (~5% to 14%) in Caucasians, while UMs are found more frequently among Saudi Arabians (~15% to 21%) and Ethiopians (~30%).[47-50,179-181] PMs and UMs are of the most clinical interest, due to the potential for either treatment failure or adverse events on exposure to agents metabolized by CYP2D6. For example, codeine, a narcotic antitussive agent, is also commonly used as an analgesic agent for the relief of mild-to-moderate pain. However, the analgesic effects of codeine depend on the 2D6-catalyzed biotransformation (specifically, the *O*-demethylation) of this compound to morphine.[27-29] Patients who are deficient in 2D6 activity are biochemically unable to convert codeine into the active analgesic morphine and are thus highly likely to experience treatment failure (a lack of pain relief, in this case).[27-29] Even in the absence of explicit genotype or phenotype information, in cases of analgesic treatment failure with codeine clinicians should consider the use of pain-relieving agents that do not require activation by CYP2D6, such as tramadol (which is metabolized by 2D6 and other CYPs, so lower doses may be required to avoid potential side-effects in PMs), morphine (which is metabolized primarily by glucuronidation), or diclofenac (which is metabolized by other CYPs and UGT2B7).[39,182-185]

Conversely, patients who have the UM phenotype will convert codeine to morphine more quickly than normal, resulting in higher exposure to morphine occurring more quickly. Even though UMs occur much less frequently than the other CYP2D6 phenotypes in most ethnic groups (with the apparent exceptions of some Middle Eastern and North African populations), this is a clinical issue that has resulted in patient deaths.[180,181] For example, mothers who are nursing and are also 2D6 UMs that take codeine-containing products may inadvertently cause the nursing infant to overdose on the morphine contained in their breast milk.[186,187] Other cases of life-threatening or fatal opioid intoxication in patients due to the ultrarapid metabolism of codeine have also been reported.[188-190]

Clinical Pearl

Even in the absence of explicit genotype or phenotype information, when patients experience analgesic treatment failure with codeine, clinicians should consider the use of pain-relieving agents that do not require activation by CYP2D6, such as tramadol, morphine, or diclofenac.

Another clinically relevant example of a therapeutic agent that is dependent on the polymorphic CYP2D6 enzyme for its bioactivation is the anticancer agent tamoxifen, which is converted to the major active metabolite (4-hydroxy-*N*-desmethyl tamoxifen /endoxifen) *in vivo*.[191] Tamoxifen is currently the most widely used antiestrogen agent for the treatment of hormone-dependent breast cancer.[192] Because this agent relies on the 2D6 isoform for the production of its therapeutically active form(s) *in vivo*, patients who are CYP2D6 PMs are at greater risk for treatment failures with tamoxifen. Although the FDA has not yet issued any formal guidance for the use of *2D6* genotyping in patients receiving tamoxifen therapy, an increasing number of clinical reports have shown a correlation between the CYP2D6 PM phenotype and both a shorter time to recurrence and a worsening of relapse-free survival in breast cancer patients treated with tamoxifen.[193-195] Genotypic or phenotypic testing of patients receiving tamoxifen therapy may improve therapeutic outcomes.

Clinical Pearl

An increasing number of clinical reports have shown a correlation between the CYP2D6 PM phenotype and both a shorter time to recurrence and a worsening of relapse-free survival in breast cancer patients treated with tamoxifen. Genotypic or phenotypic testing of patients receiving tamoxifen therapy may improve therapeutic outcomes.

For patients being treated with therapeutic agents whose metabolic clearance, rather than bioactivation (e.g., codeine use for analgesia), is dependent on 2D6 activity (such as the serotonin-selective reuptake inhibitor [SSRI] paroxetine and the tricyclic antidepressants [TCAs] nortriptyline and desipramine), the potential clinical issues are reversed.[196-198] In these cases, patients who are deficient in CYP2D6 activity will metabolize these agents more slowly, leading to potential ADRs due to increased drug levels over longer periods of time in the body. UMs, on the other hand, are at greater risk of experiencing treatment failures with these drugs, in most cases, due to the rapid clearance of these agents from the body. For drugs that are activated by the 2D6 isozyme to produce active metabolites, such as fluoxetine, risperidone, and venlafaxine (Table 4-7 and Figure 4-7), the impact of either deficient or overactive CYP2D6 activity becomes more complicated and is determined by both the relative levels of the administered drug and the active metabolite in the body, and the relative activity ratios of these two compounds.[177-178,199] In any case, given multiple clinical reports of both patient deaths and treatment failures with agents that are converted to active metabolites *in vivo* by CYP2D6, caution in this area is still warranted.[200-202] With regard to specific agents, the FDA currently suggests that 2D6 genotyping may be useful in patients being treated with either fluoxetine or atomoxetine, a selective norepinephrine reuptake inhibitor (SNRI) that is a nonstimulant agent used in the treatment of attention-deficit hyperactivity disorder (ADHD).[116,159,160] CYP2D6 genotype testing is currently available from several commercial clinical laboratories, including DNA Direct, Inc. (San Francisco, CA) and Genelex Incorporated (Seattle, WA). Common 2D6 polymorphisms may also be determined by use of the AmpliChip assay (Roche Diagnostics) (Table 4-4).

Other Polymorphic Phase I Enzymes

In addition to the CYP450 enzymes discussed above, there are also other Phase I metabolic enzymes that are known to be polymorphic in man. The two examples of the most current clinical relevance are the dihydropyrimidine dehydrogenase (DPD) and butyrylcholinesterase (BChE) (Table 4-3).[22,56,57]

Dihydropyrimidine dehydrogenase (DPD, EC 1.3.1.2) catalyzes the initial and rate-limiting step in the catabolism of pyrimidines (uracil and thymine) of both endogenous and exogenous origin.[203] This polymorphic enzyme is of clinical importance because it plays a key role in the degradation of the fluoropyrimidine-based anticancer agents 5-fluorouracil (5-FU), floxuridine (fluorodeoxyuridine), and capecitabine (each of which is a prodrug that requires bioactivation by other enzymes *in vivo*) (Figure 4-8).[21,56,204-206] Both floxuridine and capecitabine are derivatives of 5-FU, which are eventually converted to 5-fluorouracil in the body.[21] More than 80% of the amount of 5-fluorouracil ultimately present in the body (regardless of the specific fluoropyrimidine agent administered) is metabolized by DPD.[207] 5-FU is a mainstay in the treatment of numerous types of solid tumors and is frequently used in combination with other agents (e.g., the FOLFOX [leucovorin/5-FU/oxaliplatin] and FOLFIRI [leucovorin/5-FU/irinotecan] chemo-therapy regimens used in the treatment of advanced colorectal cancer).[208,209] Capecitabine, an orally-administered prodrug of 5-fluorouracil, is also seeing increasing usage as evidenced by its ranking on the list of the top 200 most-prescribed therapeutic agents.[97]

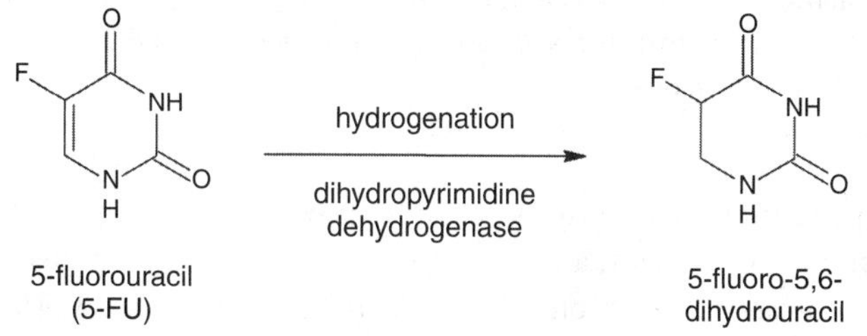

Figure 4.8 • The dihydropyrimidine dehydrogenase (DPD)-mediated metabolism of 5-fluoro-uracil in man.[21]

While the number of large-scale pharmacogenomic studies currently available for the *DYPD* gene is more limited than the number of *CYP* gene studies, there are more than 40 sequence variants of the *DYPD* gene that have been identified to date, and it appears that the *DYPD*2A* (the IVS14+1G>A change at the 5'-splice site of intron 14) mutation is the one most commonly associated with DPD deficiency.[210,211] Regarding genotypic frequency, it has been estimated that ~3.5% of the population is heterozygous for, and 0.1% is homozygous for, *DYPD* alleles with low DPD activity.[212,213] The dihydropyrimidine dehydrogenase phenotype has been found to vary by both ethnicity and gender.[214] For example, one recent study suggest that African-American women have a higher prevalence (~12.3%) of genetic DPD activity deficits than do either African-American males (~4%) or the general Caucasian population (~2% to 5%).[215]

Deficiencies in the level of dihydropyrimidine dehydrogenase activity are of clinical impor-tance due to the serious (and potentially lethal) side-effects and toxicities associated with the fluoropyrimidine-based anticancer agents.[56,204,205] As many as one in three patients receiving 5-FU-based therapeutics experience dose-limiting ADRs, ranging from mucositis, diarrhea, and leukopenia to more severe hematological, gastrointestinal, and neurological toxicities.[210,216] While it is clear that the level of DPD activity is not the only factor involved in all 5-FU toxici-ties, multiple reports have made it clear that it that there is a strong association between dihy-dropyrimidine dehydrogenase deficiency and fluoropyrimidine-related ADRs for a significant number of patients.[56,217-225] For example, Raida and colleagues reported that individuals with the *DYPD* polymorphism IVS14+1G>A (the *DYPD*2A* allele) have a sevenfold increased risk of Grade 3 or 4 toxicity during 5-FU therapy.[226] Separately, Morel et al. found that 60% of patients with either of two SNPs (IVS14+1G>A or 2846A>T) in the *DYPD* gene experienced early grade 3 or 4 toxicity upon treatment with 5-fluorouracil.[56] Recognizing this association, the FDA cur-rently suggests that clinicians evaluate a patient's DPD status with regard to fluoropyrimidine therapy.[116] However, it is clear that additional, large-scale studies are needed to fully elucidate the specific factors (including the influence of various genes, gender, epigenetic contributions, and common concurrent drug therapy regimens) that contribute to and influence fluoropy-rimidine toxicity.[214,215,221]

Clinical Pearl

For cancer patients eligible for treatment with fluoropyrimidine-based agents, early determination of dihydropyrimidine dehydrogenase (DPD) status (through either genotypic or phenotypic testing) should allow for the identification of those individuals who are at the greatest risk for fluoropyrimidine-associated toxicities and assist in subsequent dose adjustments or in the selection of other treatment modalities.

DPYD genotype testing is currently available from several commercial clinical laboratories, including Specialty Laboratories (Valencia, CA) and Genelex Incorporated (Seattle, WA). In addition, there is currently at least one clinical *DYPD* genotyping assay, TheraGuide 5-FU™, available for use by healthcare professionals (Table 4-4).[227] Finally, other approaches, such as the use of a C-labeled uracil breath test and the assay of DPD activity in peripheral blood mononuclear cells, have also been proposed as a means of measuring a patient's DPD activity levels.[13,228,229]

Butyrylcholinesterase (BChE, EC 3.1.1.8; formerly known as pseudocholinesterase) is another example of a non-CYP450 Phase I enzyme known to exhibit polymorphism.[21-26,57,230] This mutation was among the earliest variation in drug metabolic enzymes to be recognized, dating back to the work of Kalow and colleagues in the 1950s.[231,233] Interpatient differences in the activity of butyrylcholinesterase are of clinical interest due to the involvement of this enzyme in the metabolism of ester-based therapeutic agents, including some neuromuscular blockers (e.g., succinylcholine/suxamethonium), local anesthetics (e.g., procaine), drugs of abuse (e.g., cocaine), and prodrugs (Figure 4-9).[32,234-239] For example, individuals who have lower levels of BChE activity are known to experience slower clearance of ester-based neuromuscular blocking agents (such as succinylcholine/suxamethonium), leading to prolonged apnea and muscle paralysis when these medications are used.[32] In addition, there is evidence that suggests that butyrylcholinesterase-deficient patients may receive less of a therapeutic benefit from ester-based prodrugs such as irinotecan.[239,240] Finally, individuals who have a PM phenotype for butyrylcholinesterase may be at greater risk for toxicity upon exposure to ester-containing drugs of abuse, such as cocaine.[241]

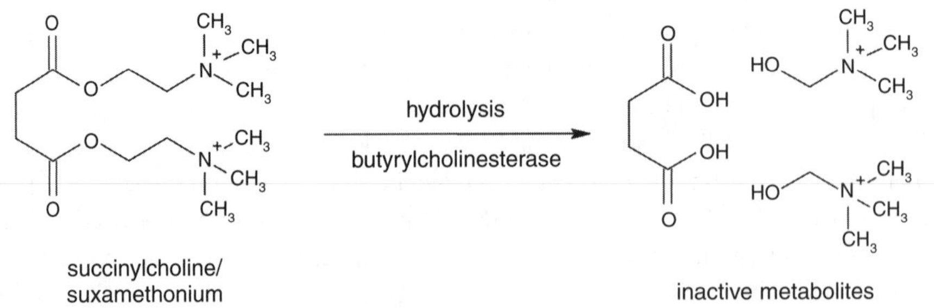

Figure 4.9 • The butyrylcholinesterase-mediated metabolism of succinylcholine/suxamethonium in man.[32]

Clinical Pearl

Patients with a PM phenotype for butyrylcholinesterase are more likely to experience slower clearance of ester-based neuromuscular blocking agents (such as succinylcholine/suxamethonium), leading to prolonged apnea and muscle paralysis when these medications are used. Butyrylcholinesterase PMs may also be at greater risk for treatment failure with the use of ester-based prodrugs and for toxicity upon exposure to cocaine.

As with most of the metabolic enzymes discussed earlier, the majority of the 67 or more variants in the *BCHE* gene that have been identified are associated with either a reduction in, or the complete absence of, butyrylcholinesterase activity.[242,243] There are two major *BCHE* alleles: the A (atypical) form (leading to the D70G residue change in BChE and virtually no amount of active enzyme present); and the K form (a quantitative variant leading to the A539T residue change in BChE, resulting in both lower enzyme activity and lower levels of enzyme present). The A form, while found less frequently, may be of more clinical relevance because the resulting mutant BChE enzyme displays only ~30% of the activity of the wild-type enzyme and thus has more of a potential impact on pharmacotherapeutic agents. [244-246] While few, if any, large-scale population studies of butyrylcholinesterase genotype or phenotype distribution have been conducted, it has been estimated that approximately 1 in 2,500 Caucasian patients have the homozygous AA *BCHE* genotype.[244-246] Standard clinical *in vitro* butyrylcholinesterase phenotyping methods involve the measurement of BChE activity along with the assessment of the degree of BChE inhibition by sodium fluoride, dibucaine, and the dimethylcarbamate, RO-02-0683.[247]

Phase II Metabolic Enzymes

Phase II metabolic biotransformations involve transfer or conjugation reactions, and most Phase II reactions result in the formation of a more polar (or hydrophilic) product that is easier to eliminate in the urine (Figure 4-2).[20-26] The phase II polymorphic enzymes of the most clinical importance include NAT2, TPMT, and UGT1A1.[20-26,58-60]

N-acetyltransferase 2 (NAT2, arylamine N-acetyltransferase, EC 2.3.1.5) is involved in the metabolism of a variety of therapeutic agents, including several hydrazine-based drugs (e.g., hydralazine, isoniazid) and arylamine-containing agents (e.g., procainamide, dapsone) (Figure 4-10).[21-26] Like CYP2D6, NAT2 is one of the few examples of drug metabolic enzymes identified to date that has multiple phenotypes—in this case, "fast/rapid," "intermediate," and "slow" metabolizers.[21-26] The recognition of interpatient variations in the activity level of NAT2 date back to pharmacokinetic studies with isoniazid in the 1960s (prior to the identification of the NAT2 enzyme or the idea of genotyping).[248,249]

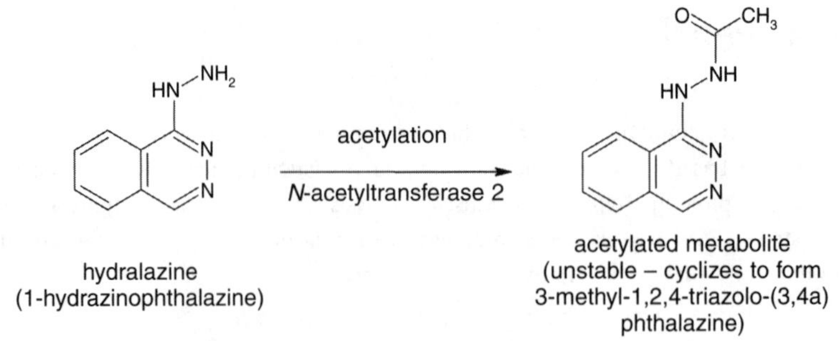

Figure 4.10 • The NAT2-mediated metabolism of hydralazine in man.[21]

In addition to the wild-type allele (*NAT2*4*, in this case), at least 20 genetic variations of the *NAT2* gene have been reported to date.[250] Patients carrying "fast/rapid" *NAT2* alleles (*NAT2*12*, *NAT2*13*) are "fast acetylators" who are capable of clearing NAT2 drug substrates more quickly than individuals who are "slow acetylators."[251] The NAT2 alleles most commonly associated with the "slow acetylator" phenotype are *NAT2*5, NAT2*6, NAT2*7*, and *NAT2*14*.[251] Phenotype distribution studies indicate that more than 50% of Europeans and Africans are slow acetylators, while <20% of Asians fit this profile.[22,252] Fast acetylators are found more commonly in Asians (80% to 90%) and less frequently in Caucasians (30% to 45%).[22] NAT2 phenotypes directly impact the pharmacokinetics of substrates metabolized by this enzyme. For example, one pharmacokinetic study on the use of isoniazid (INH) in children found that the *in vivo* half-live of this agent in slow acetylators was more than double that in fast acetylators.[253] Another study reported that NAT2 slow acetylators were 3.8-fold more likely to develop isoniazid-associated hepatotoxicity as compared to rapid acetylators, presumably due to reduced clearance of this agent and corresponding higher drug levels over longer periods of time in the body.[254]

With regard to specific therapeutic agents, the FDA currently suggests that *NAT2* genotyping may be useful in tuberculosis patients being treated with a combination of rifampin, isoniazid, and pyrazinamide.[116] *NAT2* genotype testing is currently available through multiple commercial clinical laboratories, including Genelex Incorporated (Seattle, WA) and PGXL Laboratories (Louisville, KY).

Clinical Pearl

Genotypic or phenotypic profiling of NAT2 may be helpful in optimizing the dosing regimens of tuberculosis patients receiving combination therapy with rifampin, isoniazid, and pyrazinamide.

Patient-to-patient variations in the activity level of TPMT (EC 2.1.1.67) are of clinical importance due to the involvement of this enzyme in the deactivation of thiopurine-based therapeutic agents (6-mercaptopurine [6-MP], azathioprine [a prodrug of 6-MP], thioguanine [6-TG]) (Figure 4-11).[59,255,256] Thiopurines, which serve as antimetabolites of endogenous purine nucleic acid bases, are used in the treatment of solid organ transplant rejection, some auto-immune diseases (e.g., rheumatoid arthritis), and various types of cancer.[257-259] The toxicities, including myelosuppression and hepatotoxicity, associated with the use of thiopurine-based pharmaceutical agents are serious and can be life-threatening. Patients who have lower levels of TPMT activity are at greater risk for experiencing ADRs when exposed to these agents.[260,261] The FDA, recognizing these safety issues, currently recommends that clinicians determine the TPMT activity levels of patients (through either genotypic or phenotypic assays) before beginning treatment with a thiopurine in order to adjust dosing regimens and minimize the number of potential ADRs.[116]

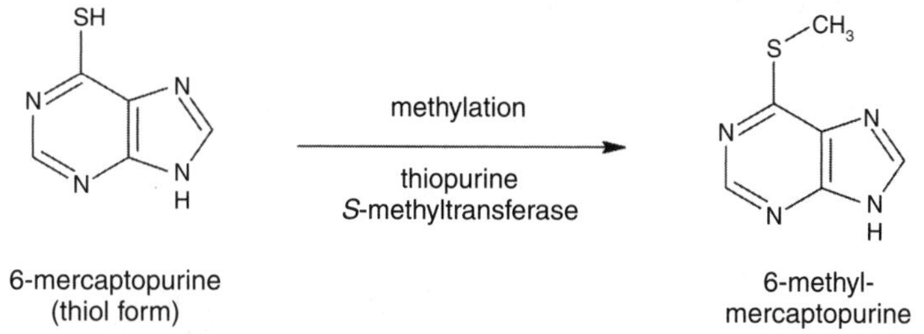

Figure 4.11 • The TPMT-mediated metabolism of 6-mercatopurine in man.[59]

Clinical Pearl

The toxicities, including myelosuppression and hepatotoxicity, associated with the use of thio-purine-based pharmaceutical agents are serious and can be life-threatening. Patients who have lower levels of TPMT activity are at greater risk for experiencing ADRs when exposed to these agents.

As with other drug metabolic enzymes, most of the known *TPMT* allelic variants lead to a lower level of TPMT activity. Variations in the frequencies of the most common *TPMT* alleles across different ethnic groups have also been noted. For example, the *TPMT*3A* allele (G460>A and A719>G) has been reported to be the most common (4.5%) reduced function variant in Caucasians (contributing to a PM phenotype in 0.6% of this ethnic group), while the *TPMT*3C* allele (A719>G) seems to be more common (2.3%) in Asians.[262,263] *TPMT* genotype testing is currently available through multiple commercial clinical laboratories, such as Sonora Quest Laboratories (Tempe, AZ) and Specialty Laboratories (Valencia, CA). Some laboratories, such as Prometheus Therapeutics & Diagnostics (San Diego, CA) offer both *TPMT* genotypic and TPMT phenotypic testing.

In terms of drug substrates, the UGT enzymes are second only to the CYPs in the number of pharmaceutical agents that are biotransformed by this group of enzymes.[264,265] The human UGT superfamily is comprised of two families (UGT1 and UGT2) and three subfamilies (UGT1A, UGT2A, and UGT2B).[264,265] Genetic polymorphism has been described for at least six of the 16 functional human UGT genes.[266-270] Within this metabolic enzyme family, the major clinical interest is in the polymorphism of the UDP-glucuronosyltransferase (UGT) 1A1 isoform (UGT1A1, EC 2.4.1.17) due to its role in the inactivation of the active form (SN-38) of the anticancer prodrug irinotecan (Figure 4-12).[271-274] A frequent UGT1A1 polymorphism, the *UGT1A1*28* allele, involves a specific mutation ($[TA]_6 \rightarrow [TA]_7$) in the promoter region (the *TATA* box) of this gene that leads to reduced gene expression and results in impaired enzyme activity.[275] This variant allele is common in many ethnic groups, ranging from a frequency of 26% to 39% in Caucasians to 9% to 16% in Asians and 42% to 56% in Africans.[276-278] Multiple studies have shown that impaired UGT1A1 activity in patients who are homozygous for the *UGT1A1*28* allele results in severe, dose-limiting toxicity (diarrhea, neutropenia) during irinotecan therapy. [271-274,279-282] These findings led to a recent update in the irinotecan labeling information to include dosing recommendations based on the presence of a *UGT1A1*28* allele.[282] The FDA currently recommends an assessment of a patient's level of UGT1A1 activity prior to the initiation of irinotecan therapy.[116]

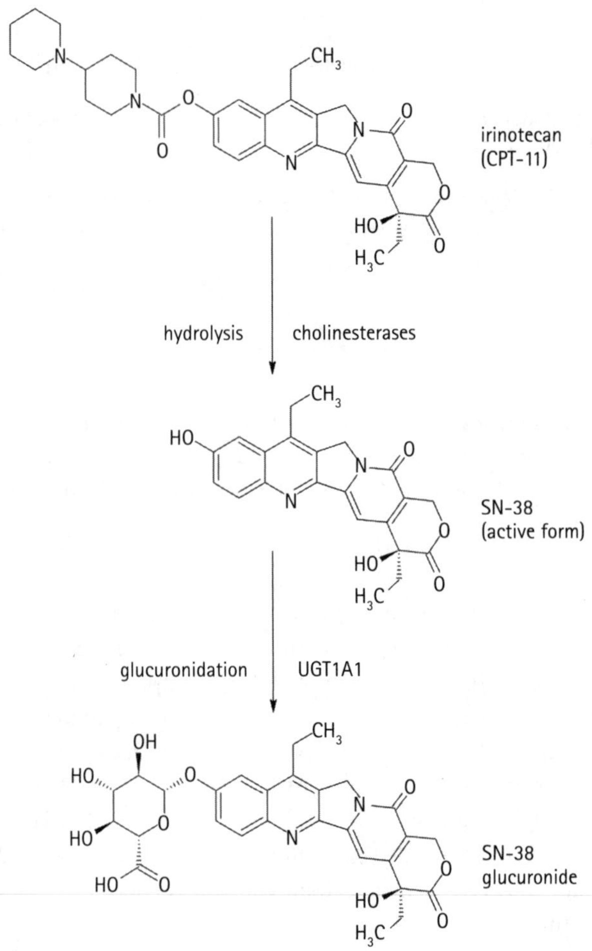

Figure 4.12 • The UGT1A1-mediated metabolism of irinotecan in man.[271]

Clinical Pearl

Patients who are homozygous for the *UGT1A1*28* allele have impaired metabolism of the active form (SN-38) of the anticancer agent irinotecan that results in severe, dose-limiting toxicity (diarrhea, neutropenia). The FDA currently recommends an assessment of a patient's level of UGT1A1 activity prior to the initiation of irinotecan therapy.

UGT1A1 genotype testing is currently available through multiple commercial clinical laboratories, including Genelex Incorporated (Seattle, WA), Arup Laboratories (Salt Lake City, UT), and Molecular Diagnostics Laboratories (Cincinnati, OH). In addition, the Invader® UGT1A1 Molecular Assay (Third Wave Technologies, Madison, WI) is commercially available for clinics and healthcare professionals who wish to do pharmacogenetic testing for patients who are homozygous for the *UGT1A1*28* allele (Table 4-4) .

The development and use of the Invader® UGT1A1 Molecular Assay (Third Wave Technologies, Madison, WI) for screening patients for potential irinotecan toxicity illustrates an important and growing trend in drug development—the rise of companion diagnostics.[283,284] This trend has been driven by the increasing recognition that personalized medicine can improve patient care and decrease healthcare costs. Over a dozen different companion diagnostic tests, several of which are targeted at specific drug metabolic enzymes, have been approved by the FDA for use by clinicians in order to guide and inform pharmacotherapeutic regimens (Table 4-4). Several of these diagnostic tests, including assays for HER2 protein overexpression for candidates for trastuzumab therapy, are considered required for treatment decisions.[116] Pharmaceutical companies are increasingly developing companion diagnostics in the early stages of the drug development process.[285,286] Oncology, in particular, has become an area of intense development of companion diagnostics, due to the relatively high costs of many of the agents, the risks of potential treatment failures, and the possibility of serious ADRs that occur with many anticancer agents. Several FDA initiatives, including the Critical Path Initiative and the Drug-Diagnostic Co-Development Concept Paper, have sought to promote and encourage the identification and use of valid biomarkers to help guide therapeutic decisions.[118,287]

Future Developments

As noted at the beginning of this chapter, the safe and effective use of therapeutic agents by patients is the goal of every healthcare professional. The advent of personalized medicine allows this goal to be made even more specific, namely, to determine which patients are most likely to **benefit** from a given therapy, for which patients a given therapy would be **inappropriate,** and what the **appropriate dosing regimen** of a therapeutic agent should be. [3-5] In selected cases (e.g., the use of *UGT1A1* genotyping for patients who are candidates for irinotecan therapy), the use of pharmacogenetic profiling of drug metabolic enzymes has already contributed to this goal. However, in order for the potential of this approach to be more fully realized, more work is required. Rigorous large-scale studies evaluating multiple nongenetic factors, including gender, concomitant disease states, and concurrent pharmacotherapy, along with the pharmacogenetic profiling of drug transporters, drug metabolic enzymes, and drug targets (and off-targets) for specific pharmaceutical agents are needed to fully elucidate what combinations of factors should be taken into account with regard to patient selection and dosing regimens. If the example of warfarin is illustrative, it is likely that more than solely the level of activity of a single drug metabolic enzyme will be required to optimize results in this area. In addition, the widespread acceptance of pharmacogenetic testing by both clinicians and insurance providers will largely rest on the demonstration that such testing improves clinically meaningful outcomes.

References

1. World Health Organization. Safety of Medicines: A Guide to Detecting and Reporting Adverse Drug Reactions. Geneva, Switzerland: World Health Organization; 2002. Available at: http://whqlibdoc.who.int/hq/2002/WHO_EDM_QSM_2002.2.pdf.
2. US Office of the Federal Register. 21 CFR 320.33(c).
3. Burke W, Psaty BM. Personalized medicine in the era of genomics. *JAMA*. 2007;298:1682-1684.
4. Evans WE, Relling MV. Moving towards individualized medicine with pharmacogenomics. *Nature*. 2004;429:464-468.
5. Sadée W, Dai Z. Pharmacogenetics/genomics and personalized medicine. *Human Molecular Genetics*. 2005;14(Review Issue 2):R207-R214.
6. Spear BB, Heath-Chiozzi M, Huff J. Clinical application of pharmacogenetics. *Trends Mol Med*. 2002;7:201-204.
7. Agency for Healthcare Research and Quality, US Department of Health & Human Services. Reducing and preventing adverse drug events to decrease hospital costs. Available at: http://www.ahrq.gov/qual/aderia/aderia.htm. Accessed September 20, 2009.
8. Lazarou J, Pomeranz BH, Corey PN. Incidence of adverse drug reactions in hospitalized patients: a meta-analysis of prospective studies. *JAMA*. 1998;279:1200-1205.
9. Wester K, Jönsson AK, Spigset O, et al. Incidence of fatal adverse drug reactions: A population based study. *Br J Clin Pharmacol*. 2007;65:573-579.
10. Phillips KA, Veenstra DL, Oren E, et al. Potential role of pharmacogenomics in reducing adverse drug reactions. *JAMA*. 2001;286:2270-2279.
11. Severino G, Del Zompo M. Adverse drug reactions: role of pharmacogenomics. *Pharm Res*. 2004;49:363-373.
12. Pirmohamed M, Park BK. Cytochrome P450 enzyme polymorphisms and adverse drug reactions. *Toxicol*. 2003;192:23-32.
13. Ingelman-Sundberg M. Pharmacogenetic biomarkers for prediction of severe adverse drug reactions. *N Eng J Med*. 2008;358:638.
14. Wilke RA, Lin DW, Roden DM, et al. Identifying genetic risk factors for serious adverse drug reactions: current progress and challenges. *Nat Rev Drug Discov*. 2007;6:904-916.
15. Hirsh J, Fuster V, Ansell J, et al. American Heart Association/American College of Cardiology Foundation guide to warfarin therapy. *J Am Coll Cardiol*. 2003;41:1633-1652.
16. Hall AM, Wilkins MR. Warfarin: a case history in pharmacogenetics. *Heart*. 2005;91:563-564.
17. Klein TE, Altman RB, Eriksson N, et al. Estimation of the warfarin dose with clinical and pharmacogenetic data. *N Eng J Med*. 2009;360:753-764.
18. Gage BF, Eby C, Milligan PE, et al. Use of pharmacogenetics and clinical factors to predict the maintenance dose of warfarin. *Thromb Haemost*. 2004;91:87-94.
19. Gage BF, Eby C, Johnson JA, et al. Use of pharmacogenetics and clinical factors to predict the therapeutic dose of warfarin. *Clin Pharm Ther*. 2008;84:326-331.
20. Rendic, S. Summary of information on human CYP enzymes: human metabolism data. *Drug Metab Rev*. 2002;34:83-448.
21. Williams DA. Drug Metabolism. In: Williams DA, Lemke TL, eds. Foye's Principles of Medicinal Chemistry. 6th ed. Philadelphia, PA: Lippincott Williams & Wilkins; 2008:253-326.
22. Kramer SD, Testa B. The biochemistry of drug metabolism—an introduction. Part 6. Inter-individual factors affecting drug metabolism. *Chem Biodiv*. 2008;5:2465-2578.

23. Gonzalez FJ, Tukey RH. Drug metabolism. In: Brunton LL, Lazo JS, Parker KL, eds. Goodman and Gilman's The Pharmacological Basis of Therapeutics. 11th ed. New York, NY: McGraw-Hill Professional; 2006:71-92.

24. Taniguchi C, Guengerich FP. Drug metabolism. In: Golan DE, Tashjian AH, Armstrong EJ, et al., eds. Principles of Pharmacology: The Pathophysiological Basis of Drug Therapy. 2nd ed. Philadelphia, PA: Lippincott Williams & Wilkins; 2008:49-61.

25. Correia MA. Drug biotransformation. In: Katzung BG, ed. Basic and Clinical Pharmacology. 11th ed. New York, NY: McGraw-Hill Medical; 2009:53-66.

26. Smith DA, van de Waterbeemd H, Walker DK. Pharmacokinetics and Metabolism in Drug Design. Weinheim, Germany: Wiley-VCH; 2006.

27. Williams DG, Patel A, Howard RF. Pharmacogenetics of codeine metabolism in an urban population of children and its implications for analgesic reliability. *Br J Anaesth.* 2002;89:839-845.

28. Drendel A. Pharmacogenomics of analgesic agents. Clin Ped Emerg Med. 2007;8:262-267.

29. Flores CM, Mogil JS. The pharmacogenomics of analgesia: toward a genetically-based approach to pain management. *Pharmacogenomics.* 2001;2:177-194.

30. Marcus FI, Kapadia GJ, Kapadia GG. The metabolism of digoxin in normal subjects. *J Pharmacol Exp Ther.* 1964;145:203-209.

31. Forane® [prescribing information/package insert]. Deerfield, IL: Baxter Healthcare Corporation; 2006.

32. Anectine® [prescribing information/package insert]. Research Triangle Park, NC: GlaxoSmith-Kline; 1999.

33. Elliott HW. Metabolism of lorazepam. *Br J Anesth.* 1976;48:1017-1023.

34. Brodie BB, Axelrod J. The fate of acetanilide in man. *J Pharmacol Exp Ther.* 1948;94:29-38.

35. Gelotte CK, Auiler JF, Lynch JM, et al. Disposition of acetaminophen at 4, 6, and 8 g/day for 3 days in healthy young adults. *Clin Pharm Ther.* 2007;81:840-848.

36. Helton ED, Williams MC, Goldzieher JW. Human urinary and liver conjugates of 17-alphaethinylestradiol. *Steroids.* 1976;27:851-867.

37. Ebner T, Remmel RP, Burchell B. Human bilirubin UDP-glucuronosyltransferase catalyzes the glucuronidation of ethinylestradiol. *Mol Pharm.* 1993;43:649-654.

38. Orme MLE, Back DJ, Ball S. Interindividual variation in the metabolism of ethinylestradiol. *Pharmacol Ther.* 1989;43:251-260.

39. Skarke C, Lotsch J. Morphine metabolites: clinical implications. Seminars in Anesthesia. *Perioperative Medicine and Pain.* 2002;21:258-264.

40. DeVane CL. Metabolism and pharmacokinetics of selective serotonin reuptake inhibitors. *Cell Mol Neurobiol.* 1999;19:443-466.

41. Shimada T, Yamazaki H, Mimura M, et al. Interindividual variations in human liver cytochrome P-450 enzymes involved in the oxidation of drugs, carcinogens and toxic chemicals: studies with liver microsomes of 30 Japanese and 30 Caucasians. *J Pharmacol Exp Ther.* 1994;270:414-423.

42. Paine MF, Hart HL, Ludington SS, et al. The human intestinal cytochrome P450 "pie." *Drug Metab Disp.* 2006;34:880-886.

43. Nelson DR. Human Cytochrome P450s. Available at: http://drnelson.utmem.edu/human.P450. Chapter 4 - Table.html. Accessed September 20, 2009.

44. Human Cytochrome P450 (CYP) Allele Nomenclature Committee. Allele nomenclature for Cytochrome P450 enzymes. Available at: http://www.cypalleles.ki.se. Accessed September 20, 2009.

45. Nelson DR, Koymans L, Kamataki T, et al. P450 superfamily: update on new sequences, gene mapping, accession numbers and nomenclature. *Pharmacogenetics.* 1996;6:1-42.

46. Evert B, Griese E-U, Eichelbaum M. A missense mutation in exon 6 of the CYP2D6 gene leading to a histidine 324 to proline exchange is associated with the poor metabolizer phenotype of sparteine. *Naunyn-Schmiedeberg's Arch Pharmacol.* 1994;350:434-439.

47. Bradford LD. CYP2D6 allele frequency in European Caucasians, Asians, Africans, and their descendants. *Pharmacogenomics.* 2002;3:229-243.

48. Bradford LD, Kerlin WG. Polymorphism of CYP2D6 in black populations: implications for psychopharmacology. *Int J Neuropsychopharmacol.* 1988;1:173-185.

49. Yengi LG. Pharmacogenetics and pharmacogenomics. In: Nassar AF, ed. *Drug Metabolism Handbook: Concepts and Applications.* New York, NY: John F. Wiley & Sons; 2009:65-88.

50. Daly AK. Pharmacogenetics. In: Pearson PG, Wienkers LC, eds. *Handbook of Drug Metabolism*. 2nd ed. (Drugs and the Pharmaceutical Sciences). New York, NY: Informa Healthcare; 2008:179-202.

51. Shin J, Kayser SR, Langaee TY. Pharmacogenetics: from discovery to patient care. *Am J Health-Syst Pharm*. 2009;66:625-637.

52. Ingelman-Sundberg M. Genetic polymorphisms of cytochrome P450 2D6 (CYP2D6): clinical consequences, evolutionary aspects and functional diversity. *Pharmacogenomics J*. 2005;5:6-13.

53. Caldwell MD, Awad T, Johnson JA, et al. CYP4F2 genetic variant alters warfarin dose. *Blood*. 2008;111:4106-4112.

54. Crettol S, Deglon JJ, Besson J, et al. Methadone enantiomer plasma levels, CYP2B6, CYP2C19, and CYP2C9 genotypes, and response to treatment. *Clin Pharmacol Ther*. 2005;78:593-604.

55. Ozdemir V, Kalow W, Posner P, et al. CYP1A2 activity as measured by a caffeine test predicts clozapine and active metabolite norclozapine steady-state concentration in patients with schizophrenia. *J Clin Psychopharmcol*. 2001;21:398-407.

56. Morel A, Boisdron-Celle M, Fey L, et al. Clinical relevance of different dihydropyrimidine dehydrogenase gene single nucleotide polymorphisms on 5-fluorouracil tolerance. *Mol Cancer Ther*. 2006;5:2895-2904.

57. Jensen FS, Schwartz M, Viby-Mogensen J. Identification of human plasma cholinesterase variants using molecular biological techniques. *Acta Anaesth Scand*. 1995;39:142-149.

58. Agundez JAG. Polymorphisms of human N-acetyltransferases and cancer risk. *Curr Drug Metab*. 2008;9:520-531.

59. Reuther LO, Vainer B, Sonne J, et al. Thiopurine methyltransferase (TPMT) genotype distribution in azathioprine-tolerant and -intolerant patients with various disorders. The impact of TPMT genotyping in predicting toxicity. *Eur J Clin Pharmacol*. 2004;59:797-801.

60. Argikar UA, Upendra A, Iwuchukwu OF, et al. Update on tools for evaluation of uridine diphosphoglucuronosyltransferase polymorphisms. *Exp Opin Drug Metab Toxicol*. 2008;4:879-894.

61. Ha HR, Chen J, Freiburghaus AU, et al. Metabolism of theophylline by cDNA-expressed human cytochromes P-450. *Br J Clin Pharmacol*. 1995;39:321-326.

62. Doude van Troostwijk LJAE, Koopmans RP, Vermeulen HDB, et al. CYP1A2 activity is an important determinant of clozapine dosage in schizophrenic patients. *Eur J Pharm Sci*. 2003:20:451-457.

63. Shirley KL, Hon YY, Penzak SR, et al. Correlation of cytochrome P450 (CYP) 1A2 activity using caffeine phenotyping and olanzapine disposition in healthy volunteers. *Neuropsychopharmacology*. 2003;28:961-966.

64. Lewis, DFV. Guide to Cytochromes P450: Structure and Function. London, UK: Taylor and Francis; 2001.

65. Brown CM, Reisfeld B, Mayeno AN. Cytochromes P450: a structure-based summary of biotransformations using representative substrates. *Drug Metabolism Reviews*. 2008;40:1-100.

66. Guengerich FP. Human Cytochrome P450 Enzymes. In: Ortiz de Montellano PR, ed. *Cytochrome P450: Structure, Mechanism, and Biochemistry*. 3rd ed. New York, NY: Kluwer Academic; 2005:377-382.

67. Skarke C, Kirchhof A, Geisslinger G, et al. Rapid genotyping for relevant CYP1A2 alleles by pyrosequencing. *Eur J Clin Pharmacol*. 2005;61:887-892.

68. Genelex Corporation. Cytochrome P450 1A2 Genotyping. Available at: http://www.healthanddna.com/1A2tech.pdf. Accessed September 20, 2009.

69. Solus JF, Arietta BJ, Harris JR, et al. Genetic variation in eleven phase I drug metabolism genes in an ethnically diverse population. *Pharmacogenomics*. 2004;5:895-931.

70. Doude van Troostwijk LJAE, Koopmans RP, Vermeulen HDB, et al. CYP1A2 activity is an important determinant of clozapine dosage in schizophrenic patients. *Eur J Pharm Sci*. 2003;20:451-457.

71. Clozaril® [prescribing information/package insert]. East Hanover, NJ: Novartis Pharmaceuticals Corporation; 2009.

72. Basile VS, Masellis M, Potkin SG, et al. Pharmacogenomics in schizophrenia: the quest for individualized therapy. *Human Mol Genetics*. 2002;11:2517-2530.

73. Sachse C, Brockmoller J, Baue S, et al. Cytochrome P450 2D6 variants in a Caucasian population: allele frequencies and phenotypic consequences. *Am J Hum Genet*. 1997;60:284-295.

74. Schulze TG, Schumacher J, Muller DJ, et al. Lack of association between a functional polymorphism of the cytochrome P450 1A2 (CYP1A2) gene and tardive dyskinesia in schizophrenia. *Am J Med Genet.* 2001;105:498-501.

75. Bender S, Eap CB. Very high cytochrome P4501A2 activity and nonresponse to clozapine. *Arch Gen Psychiatry.* 1998;55:1048-1050.

76. Bozikas VP, Papakosta M, Niopas I, et al. Smoking impact on CYP1A2 activity in a group of patients with schizophrenia. *Eur Neuropsychopharmacol.* 2004;14: 39-44.

77. Webster E, McIntyre J, Choonara I, et al. The caffeine breath test and CYP1A2 activity in children. *Paediatric and Perinatal Drug Ther.* 2004;5:28-33.

78. Bertilsson L, Carrillo JA, Dahl ML, et al. Clozapine disposition covaries with CYP1A2 activity determined by a caffeine test. *Br J Clin Pharmacol.* 1994;38:471-473.

79. Faucette SR, Hawke RL, Lecluyse EL, et al. Validation of bupropion hydroxylation as a selective marker of human cytochrome P450 2B6 catalytic activity. *Drug Metab Dispos.* 2000;28:1222-1230.

80. Chang TK, Weber GF, Crespi CL, et al. Differential activation of cyclophosphamide and ifosphamide by cytochromes P-450 2B and 3A in human liver microsomes. *Cancer Res.* 1993;53:5629-5637.

81. Crettol S, Deglon JJ, Besson J, et al. Methadone enantiomer plasma levels, CYP2B6, CYP2C19, and CYP2C9 genotypes, and response to treatment. *Clin Pharmacol Ther.* 2005;78:593-604.

82. Totah RA, Sheffels P, Roberts T, et al. Role of CYP2B6 in stereoselective human methadone metabolism. *Anesthesiology.* 2008;108:363-374.

83. Haas DW, Smeaton LM, Shafer RW, et al. Pharmacogenetics of long-term responses to antiretroviral regimens containing efavirenz and/or nelfinavir: an Adult AIDS Clinical Trials Group study. *J Infect Dis.* 2005;192:1931-1942.

84. Haas DW, Ribaudo HJ, Kim RB, et al. Pharmacogenetics of efavirenz and central nervous system side effects: an Adult AIDS Clinical Trials Group study. AIDS 2004;18:2391-2400.

85. Rotger M, Colombo S, Furrer H, et al. Influence of CYP2B6 polymorphism on plasma and intracellular concentrations and toxicity of efavirenz and nevirapine in HIV-infected patients. *Pharmacogenet Genomics.* 2005;15:1-5.

86. Zanger UM, Klein K, Saussele T, et al. Polymorphic CYP2B6: molecular mechanisms and emerging clinical significance. *Pharmacogenomics.* 2007;8:743-759.

87. Mo SL, Liu YH, Duan W, et al. Substrate specificity, regulation, and polymorphism of human cytochrome P450 2B6. *Curr Drug Metab.* 2009;10:730-753.

88. Klein K, Lang T, Saussele T, et al. Genetic variability of CYP2B6 in populations of African and Asian origin: allele frequencies, novel function variants, and possible implications for anti-HIV therapy with efavirenz. *Pharmacogenet Genomics.* 2005;15:861-873.

89. Cho JY, Lim HS, Chung JY, et al. Haplotype structure and allele frequencies of CYP2B6 in a Korean population. *Drug Metab Disp.* 2004;32:1341-1344.

90. Mehlotra RK, Ziats MN, Bockarie MJ, Zimmerman PA. Prevalence of CYP2B6 alleles in malaria-endemic populations of West Africa and Papua New Guinea. *Eur J Clin Pharmacol* 2006;62:267-275.

91. Yule SM, Boddy AV, Cole M, et al. Cyclophosphamide pharmacokinetics in children. *Br J Clin Pharmacol.* 1996;41:13-19.

92. de Jonge ME, Huitema ADR, van Dam, SM, et al. Population pharmacokinetics of cyclophosphamide and its metabolites 4-hydroxycyclophosphamide, 2-dechloroethylcyclophosphamide, and phosphoramide mustard in a high-dose combination with thiotepa and carboplatin. *Ther Drug Monitoring.* 2005;27:756-765.

93. Afsharian P, Terelius Y, Hidestrand M, et al. The role of human CYP2B6 polymorphism in the bioactivation of cyclophosphamide using cDNA expressed enzymes. *Biol Blood Marrow Trans.* 2007;13(Suppl.1):70-71.

94. Faucette SR, Hawke RL, Lecluyse EL, et al. Validation of bupropion hydroxylation as a selective marker of human cytochrome P450 2B6 catalytic activity. *Drug Metab Dispos.* 2000;28:1222-1230.

95. Kirchheiner J, Tsahuridu M, Jabrane W, et al. The CYP2C9 polymorphism: from enzyme kinetics to clinical dose recommendations. *Personalized Med.* 2004;1:63-84.

96. Kirchheiner J, Brockmuller J. Clinical consequences of cytochrome P450 2C9 polymorphisms. *Clin Pharmacol Ther.* 2005;77:1-16.

97. Lamb E. Top 200 drugs by sales. *Pharmacy Times*. Published online May 15, 2009.

98. Coreg® CR [prescribing information/package insert]. Research Triangle Park, NC: GlaxoSmith-Kline; 2009.

99. Sandberg M, Yasar U, Strömberg P, et al. Oxidation of celecoxib by polymorphic cytochrome P450 2C9 and alcohol dehydrogenase. *Br J Clin Pharmacol*. 2002;54:423-429.

100. Celebrex® [prescribing information/package insert]. New York, NY: Pfizer; 2009.

101. Psaty BM, Furberg CD. COX-2 inhibitors—lessons in drug safety. *N Eng J Med*. 2005;352:1133-1135.

102. Yasar U, Tybring G, Hidestrand M, et al. Role of CYP2C9 polymorphism in losartan oxidation. *Drug Metab Disp*. 2001;29:1051-1056.

103. Sica DA, Gehr TWB, Ghosh S. Clinical pharmacokinetics of losartan. *Clinical Pharmacokinetics*. 2005;44:797-814.

104. Joy MS, Dornbrook-Lavender K, Blaisdell J, et al. CYP2C9 genotype and pharmacodynamic responses to losartan in patients with primary and secondary kidney diseases. *Eur J Clin Pharmacol*. 2009;65:947-953.

105. Chiba M, Xu X, Nishime JA, et al. Hepatic microsomal metabolism of montelukast, a potent leukotriene D4 receptor antagonist, in humans. *Drug Metab Disp*. 1997;25:1022-1031.

106. Baldwin SJ, Clarke SE, Chenery RJ. Characterization of the cytochrome P450 enzymes involved in the in vitro metabolism of rosiglitazone. *Br J Clin Pharmacol*. 1999;48:424-432.

107. Nakashima A, Kawashita H, Masuda N, et al. Identification of cytochrome P450 forms involved in the 4-hydroxylation of valsartan, a potent and specific angiotensin II receptor antagonist, in human liver microsomes. *Xenobiotica*. 2005;35:589-602.

108. Giancarlo GM, Venkatakrishnan K, Granda BW, et al. Relative contributions of CYP2C9 and 2C19 to phenytoin 4-hydroxylation in vitro: inhibition by sulfaphenazole, omeprazole, and ticlopidine. *Eur J Clin Pharmacol*. 2001;57:31-36.

109. Karlen B, Garle M, Rane A, et al. Assay of the major (4-hydroxylated) metabolites of diphenylhydantoin in human urine. *Eur J Clin Pharmacol*. 1975;8:359-363.

110. Eadie MJ, Tyrer JH, Bochner F, et al. The elimination of phenytoin in man. *Clin Exp Pharmacol Physiol*. 2007;3:217-224.

111. Holstein A, Plaschke A, Ptak M, et al. Association between CYP2C9 slow metabolizer genotypes and severe hypoglycemia with sulfonylurea hypoglycemic agents. *Br J Clin Pharmacol*. 2005;60:103-106.

112. Pilotto A, Seripa D, Franceschi M, et al. Genetic susceptibility to nonsteroidal anti-inflammatory drug–related gastroduodenal bleeding: role of cytochrome P450 2C9 polymorphisms. *Gastroenterology*. 2007;133:465-471.

113. Budnitz DS, Shehab N, Kegler SR, et al. Medication use leading to emergency department visits for adverse drug events in older adults. *Ann Internal Med*. 2007;147:755-765.

114. News briefs. *Am J Health-Syst Pharm*. 2007;64:2220.

115. Coumadin® [prescribing information/package insert]. Princeton, NJ: Bristol-Myers Squibb; 2007.

116. US Food and Drug Administration. Chapter 4: Table of Valid Genomic Biomarkers in the Context of Approved Drug Labels. Available at http://www.fda.gov/Drugs/ScienceResearch/ResearchAreas/Pharmacogenetics/ucm083378.htm. Accessed September 15, 2009.

117. Frueh FW, Amur S, Mummaneni P, et al. Pharmacogenomic biomarker information in drug labels approved by the United States Food and Drug Administration: Prevalence of related drug use. *Pharmacotherapy*. 2008;28:992-998.

118. US Department of Health and Human Services. Guidance for industry: Definitions for genomic biomarkers, pharmacogenomics, pharmacogenetics, genomic data, and sample coding categories. Washington, DC: US Department of Health and Human Services; 2008. Available at: http://www.fda.gov/downloads/RegulatoryInformation/Guidances/ucm129296.pdf.

119. Bylander J. Personalized medicine not paying the bills yet; more science needed. *The Pink Sheet*. July 7, 2008;18-19.

120. Allingham-Hawkins D. Successful genetic tests are predicated on clinical utility. *Gen Eng News*. August, 2008;6-9.

121. Bylander J. Clinicians split on warfarin testing as a new standard of care. *The Pink Sheet Daily*. August 6, 2008.

122. Hillman MA, Wilke RA, Caldwell MD, et al. Relative impact of covariates in prescribing warfarin according to CYP2C9 genotype. *Pharmacogenetics.* 2004;14:539-547.

123. Wadelius M, Sorlin K, Wallerman O, et al. Warfarin sensitivity related to CYP2C9, CYP3A5, ABCB1 (MDR1) and other factors. *Pharmacogenomics J.* 2004;4:40-48.

124. Desta Z, Zhao X, Shin J-G, et al. Clinical significance of the cytochrome P450 2C19 genetic polymorphism. *Clin Pharmacokinet.* 2002;41:913-958.

125. Goldstein JA, Faletto MB, Romkes-Sparks M, et al. Evidence that CYP2C19 is the major (S)-mephenytoin 4'-hydroxylase in humans. *Biochemistry.* 1994;33:1743-1752.

126. Xie HG, Kim RB, Wood AJ, et al. Molecular basis of ethnic differences in drug disposition and response. *Annu Rev Pharmacol Toxicol.* 2001;41:815-850.

127. Mega JL, Close SL, Wiviott SD, et al. Cytochrome P-450 polymorphisms and response to clopidogrel. *N Engl J Med.* 2009;360:354-362.

128. Collet JP, Hulot JS, Pena A, et al. Cytochrome P450 2C19 polymorphism in young patients treated with clopidogrel after myocardial infarction: a cohort study. *The Lancet.* 2009;373:309-317.

129. Simon T, Verstuyft C, Mary-Krause M, et al. Genetic determinants of response to clopidogrel and cardiovascular events. *N Engl J Med.* 2009;360:363-375.

130. Plavix® [prescribing information/package insert]. Bridgewater, NJ: Bristol-Myers Squibb/Sanofi Pharmaceuticals; 2009.

131. Shuldiner AR, O'Connell JR, Bliden KP, et al. Association of cytochrome P450 2C19 genotype with the antiplatelet effect and clinical efficacy of clopidogrel therapy. *JAMA.* 2009;302:849-857.

132. Kim KA, Park PW, Hong SJ, et al. The effect of CYP2C19 polymorphism on the pharmacokinetics and pharmacodynamics of clopidogrel: a possible mechanism for clopidogrel resistance. *Clin Pharmacol Ther.* 2008;84:236-242.

133. Chong E, Ensom MHH. Pharmacogenetics of the proton pump inhibitors: A systematic review. *Pharmacotherapy.* 2003;23:460-471.

134. Furuta T, Shirai N, Sugimoto M, et al. Pharmacogenomics of proton pump inhibitors. *Pharmacogenomics.* 2004;5:181-202.

135. von Moltke LL, Greenblatt DJ, Giancarlo GM, et al. Escitalopram (S-citalopram) and its metabolites in vitro: cytochromes mediating biotransformation, inhibitory effects, and comparison to R-citalopram. *Drug Metab Disp.* 2001;29:1102-1109.

136. Andersson T, Hassan-Alin M, Hasselgren G, et al. Pharmacokinetic studies with esomeprazole, the (S)-isomer of omeprazole. *Clin Pharmacokinetics.* 2001;40:411-426.

137. Foradil® Aerolizer [prescribing information/package insert]. Basel, Switzerland: Novartis Pharma AG; 2002.

138. Aubert RE, Epstein RS, Teagarden JR, et al. Proton pump inhibitors effect on clopidogrel effectiveness: The clopidogrel Medco outcomes study. *Circulation.* 2008;118:S815.

139. Khalique SC, Cheng-Lai A. Drug interaction between clopidogrel and proton pump inhibitors. *Cardiol Rev.* 2009;17:198-200.

140. Stanek EJ. Possible "class effect" for proton-pump inhibitors on top of clopidogrel therapy. Oral presentation at: Society for Cardiovascular Angiography and Interventions (SCAI) 2009 Meeting; May 6, 2009; Las Vegas, NV.

141. Mega JL, Close SL, Wiviott SD, et al. Cytochrome P450 genetic polymorphisms and the response to prasugrel: relationship to pharmacokinetic, pharmacodynamic, and clinical outcomes. *Circulation.* 2009;119:2553-2560.

142. Petersen KU. Relevance of metabolic activation pathways: the example of clopidogrel and prasugrel. *Arzneimittelforschung.* 2009;59:213-227.

143. Jakubowski JA, Winters KJ, Naganuma H, et al. Prasugrel: a novel thienopyridine antiplatelet agent. A review of preclinical and clinical studies and the mechanistic basis for its distinct antiplatelet profile. *Cardiovasc Drug Rev.* 2007;25:357-374.

144. Mahgoub A, Idle JR, Dring DG, et al. Polymorphic hydroxylation of debrisoquine in man. *Lancet.* 1977;2:584-586.

145. Tucker GT, Silas JH, Iyun AO, et al. Polymorphic hydroxylation of debrisoquine in man. *Lancet.* 1977;2:718.

146. Eichelbaum M, Spannbrucker N, Steinke B, et al. Defective N-oxidation of sparteine in man: a new pharmacogenetic defect. *Eur J Clin Pharmacol.* 1979;16:183-187.

147. Eichelbaum M, Bertilsson L, Säwe J, et al. Polymorphic oxidation of sparteine and debrisoquine. Related pharmacogenetic entities. *Clin Pharmacol Ther.* 1982;31:184-186.

148. Kirchheiner J, Nickchen K, Bauer M, et al. Pharmacogenetics of antidepressants and antipsychotics: the contribution of allelic variations to the phenotype of drug response. *Mol Psychiatry.* 2004;9:442-473.

149. Olesen OV, Linnet K. Metabolism of the tricyclic antidepressant amitriptyline by cDNA-expressed human cytochrome P450 enzymes. *Pharmacology.* 1997;55:235-243.

150. Stahl SM. *Essential Psychopharmacology of Depression and Bipolar Disorder.* Cambridge, UK: Cambridge University Press; 2000.

151. Scordo MG, Spina E, Facciolà G, et al. Cytochrome P450 2D6 genotype and steady state plasma levels of risperidone and 9-hydroxyrisperidone. *Psychopharmacology* (Berl). 1999;147:300-305.

152. Laika B, Leucht S, Heres S, et al. Intermediate metabolizer: increased side effects in psychoactive drug therapy. The key to cost-effectiveness of pretreatment CYP2D6 screening? *Pharmacogenomics J.* 2009;9:1-10.

153. Bijl MJ, Visser LE, van Schaik RH, et al. Genetic variation in the CYP2D6 gene is associated with a lower heart rate and blood pressure in beta-blocker users. *Clin Pharmacol Ther.* 2009;85:45-50.

154. Holtzman NA. Clinical utility of pharmacogenetics and pharmacogenomics. In: Rothstein MA, ed. *Pharmacogenomics: Social, Ethical, and Clinical Dimensions.* Hoboken, NJ: John Wiley & Sons; 2003:163-186.

155. Shin J, Johnson JA. Pharmacogenetics of beta-blockers. *Pharmacotherapy.* 2007;27:874-887.

156. Kirchheiner J, Heesch C, Bauer S, et al. Impact of the ultrarapid metabolizer genotype of cytochrome P450 2D6 on metoprolol pharmacokinetics and pharmacodynamics. *Clin Pharmacol Ther.* 2004;76:302-312.

157. Buchert E, Woosley RL. Clinical implications of variable antiarrhythmic drug metabolism. *Pharmacogenetics.* 1992;2:2-11.

158. Siddoway LA, Thomspon KA, McAllister CB, et al. Polymorphism of propafenone metabolism and disposition in man: clinical pharmacokinetic consequences. *Circulation.* 1987;75:785-791.

159. Strattera® [prescribing information/package insert]. Indianapolis, IN: Eli Lilly & Company; 2009.

160. Witcher JW, Long A, Smith B, et al. Atomoxetine pharmacokinetics in children and adolescents with attention deficit hyperactivity disorder. *J Child Adolesc Psychopharmacol.* 2003;13:53-63.

161. Enablex® [prescribing information/package insert]. Stein, Switerland: Novartis Pharma AG; 2006.

162. Beaumont KC, Cussans NJ, Nichols DJ, et al. Pharmacokinetics and metabolism of darifenacin in the mouse, rat, dog and man. *Xenobiotica.* 1998;28:63-75.

163. Skerjanec A. The clinical pharmacokinetics of darifenacin. *Clin Pharmacokinet.* 2006;45:325-350.

164. Assessment of the relative in vivo potency of the hydroxylated metabolite of darifenacin in its ability to decrease salivary flow using pooled population pharmacokinetic–pharmacodynamic data. *Br J Clin Pharmacol.* 2004;57:170-180.

165. Cymbalta® [prescribing information/package insert]. Indianapolis, IN: Eli Lilly & Company; 2009.

166. Karpa KA, Cavanaugh JE, Lakoski JM. Duloxetine pharmacology: profile of a dual monoamine modulator. *CNS Drug Reviews.* 2002;8:361-376.

167. Bymaster FP, Thomas CL, Knadler MP, et al. The dual transporter inhibitor duloxetine: A review of its preclinical pharmacology, pharmacokinetic profile, and clinical results in depression. *Curr Pharm Design.* 2005;11:1475-1493.

168. Caccia S. Metabolism of the newest antidepressants: comparisons with related predecessors. *IDrugs.* 2004;7:143-150.

169. Kuo F, Gillespie TA, Kulanthaivel P, et al. Synthesis and biological activity of some known and putative duloxetine metabolites. *Bioorg Med Chem Lett.* 2004;14:3481-3486.

170. Ring BJ, Catlow J, Lindsay TJ, et al. Identification of the human cytochromes P450 responsible for the in vitro formation of the major oxidative metabolites of the antipsychotic agent olanzapine. *J Pharmacol Exp Ther.* 1996;27:658-666.

171. Zyprexa® [prescribing information/package insert]. Indianapolis, IN: Eli Lilly & Company; 2009.

172. Chen ZR, Irvine RJ, Somogyi AA, et al. Mu receptor binding of some commonly used opioids and their metabolites. *Life Sci.* 1991;48:2165-2171.

173. Lalovic B, Phillips B, Risler LL, et al. Quantitative contribution of CYP2D6 and CYP3A to oxycodone metabolism in human liver and intestinal microsomes. *Drug Metab Disp.* 2004;32:447-454.

174. Lalovic B, Kharasch E, Hoffer C, et al. Pharmacokinetics and pharmacodynamics of oral oxycodone in healthy human subjects: role of circulating active metabolites. *Clin Pharmacol Ther.* 2006;79:461-479.

175. Susce MT, Murray-Carmichael E, de Leon J. Response to hydrocodone, codeine and oxycodone in a CYP2D6 poor metabolizer. *Prog Neuro-Psychopharmacol Biol Psych.* 2006;30:1356-1358.

176. Foster A, Mobley E, Wang Z. Complicated pain management in a CYP450 2D6 poor metabolizer. *Pain Practice.* 2007;7:352-356.

177. Effexor XR® [prescribing information/package insert]. Philadelphia, PA: Wyeth Pharmaceuticals; 2009.

178. Fluoxetine: clinical pharmacology and physiologic disposition. *J Clin Psychiatry.* 1985;46:14-19.

179. Zhou S-F, Liu J-P, Chowbay B. Polymorphism of human cytochrome P450 enzymes and its clinical impact. *Drug Metab Rev.* 2009;41:89-295.

180. Aklillu E, Persson I, Bertilsson L, et al. Frequent distribution of ultrarapid metabolizers of debrisoquine in an Ethiopian population carrying duplicated and multiduplicated functional CYP2D6 alleles. *J Pharmacol Exp Ther.* 1996;278:441-446.

181. McLellan RA, Oscarson M, Seidegard J, et al. Frequent occurrence of CYP2D6 gene duplication in Saudi Arabians. *Pharmacogenetics.* 1997;7:187-191.

182. Subrahmanyam V, Renwick AB, Walters DG, et al. Identification of cytochrome P-450 isoforms responsible for cis-tramadol metabolism in human liver microsomes. *Drug Metab Disp.* 2001;29:1146-1155.

183. Ultram® ER [prescribing information/package insert]. Raritan, NJ: Ortho-McNeil Inc; 2007.

184. Christup LL. Morphine metabolites. *Acta Anaesthesiol Scand.* 1997;41:116-122.

185. Tang W. The metabolism of diclofenac—enzymology and toxicology perspectives. *Curr Drug Metab.* 2003;4:319-329.

186. Madadi P, Koren G, Cairns J, et al. Safety of codeine during breastfeeding: Fatal morphine poisoning in the breastfed neonate of a mother prescribed codeine. *Can Fam Physician.* 2007;53:33-35.

187. Madadi P, Ross CJD, Hayden MR, et al. Pharmacogenetics of neonatal opioid toxicity following maternal use of codeine during breastfeeding: a case–control study. *Clin Pharmacol Ther.* 2008;85:31-35.

188. Gasche Y, Daali Y, Fathi M, et al. Codeine intoxication associated with ultrarapid CYP2D6 metabolism. *N Engl J Med.* 2004;351:2827-2831.

189. Ferreiros N, Dresen S, Hermanns-Clausen M, et al. Fatal and severe codeine intoxication in 3-year-old twins—interpretation of drug and metabolite concentrations. *Int J Legal Med.* Published online: 07 April 2009.

190. Hermanns-Clausen M, Weinmann W, Auwarter V, et al. Drug dosing error with drops—severe clinical course of codeine intoxication in twins. *Eur J Pediatr.* 2009;168:819-824.

191. Lim YC, Desta Z, Flockhart DA, et al. Endoxifen (4-hydroxy-N-desmethyl-tamoxifen) has antiestrogenic effects in breast cancer cells with potency similar to 4-hydroxy-tamoxifen. *Cancer Chemother Pharmacol.* 2005;55:471-478.

192. Tamoxifen (2009). In Encyclopædia Britannica. Retrieved September 19, 2009, from Encyclopædia Britannica Online: http://www.britannica.com/EBchecked/topic/582056/tamoxifen.

193. Goetz MP, Knox SK, Suman VJ, et al. The impact of cytochrome P450 2D6 metabolism in women receiving adjuvant tamoxifen. *Breast Cancer Res Treat.* 2007;101:113-121.

194. Higgins MJ, Rae JM, Flockhart DA, et al. Pharmacogenetics of tamoxifen: who should undergo CYP2D6 genetic testing? *J Natl Compr Canc Netw.* 2009;7:203-213.

195. Hoskins JM, Carey LA, McLeod HL. CYP2D6 and tamoxifen: DNA matters in breast cancer. *Nat Rev Cancer.* 2009;9:576-586.

196. Greenblatt DJ, von Moltke LL, Harmatz JS, et al. Human cytochromes and some newer antidepressants: kinetics, metabolism, and drug interactions. *J Clin Psychopharmacol.* 1999;19(suppl 1);23S-35S.

197. Caccia S. Metabolism of newer antidepressants: an overview of the pharmacological and pharmacokinetic implications. *Clin Pharmacokin.* 1998;34:281-302.

198. Paxil® [prescribing information/package insert]. Research Triangle Park, NC: GlaxoSmithKline; 2009.

199. Mannens G, Huang ML, Meuldermans W, et al. Absorption, metabolism, and excretion of risperidone in humans. *Drug Metab Dispos*. 1993;21:1134-1141.

200. Sallee FR, DeVane CL, Ferrell RE. Fluoxetine-related death in a child with cytochrome P-450 2D6 genetic deficiency. *J Child Adolesc Psychopharmacol*. 2000;10:27-34.

201. de Leon J, Susce MT, Pan RM, et al. The CYP2D6 poor metabolizer phenotype may be associated with risperidone adverse drug reactions and discontinuation. *Eur J Pediatr*. 2009;168:819-824.

202. Lessard E, Yessine MA, Hamelin BA, et al. Influence of CYP2D6 activity on the disposition and cardiovascular toxicity of the antidepressant agent venlafaxine in humans. *Pharmacogenetics*. 1999;9:435-443.

203. Gonzalez FJ, Fernandez-Salguero P. Diagnostic analysis, clinical importance and molecular basis of dihydropyrimidine dehydrogenase deficiency. *Trends Pharmacol Sci*. 1995;16:325-327.

204. FUDR® [prescribing information/package insert]. Paramus, NJ: Faulding Pharmaceutical Company; 2002.

205. Xeloda® [prescribing information/package insert]. Nutley, NJ: Roche Laboratories Inc; 2006.

206. Soong R, Diasio RB. Advances and challenges in fluoropyrimidine pharmacogenomics and pharmacogenetics. *Pharmacogenomics*. 2005;6:835-847.

207. Ho DH, Townsend L, Luna MA, et al. Distribution of dihydrouracil dehydrogenase activities using 5-fluorouracil as a substrate. *Anticancer Res*. 1986;6:781-784.

208. Goldberg RM. Therapy for metastatic colorectal cancer. *The Oncologist*. 2006;11:981-987.

209. Pasetto LM, Jirillo A, Iadicicco G, et al. FOLFOX versus FOLFIRI: a comparison of regimens in the treatment of colorectal cancer metastases. *Anticancer Res*. 2005;25(1B):563-576.

210. Podoltsev NA, Saif MW. Dihydropyrimidine dehydrogenase gene (DPD) polymorphism among Caucasian patients (pts) with 5-FU and capecitabine (CAP)-related toxicity. *J Clin Oncol*. 2009;27(May 20 Supplement):e14588.

211. Saif MW, Ezzeldin H, Vance K, et al. DPD*2A mutation: the most common mutation associated with DPD deficiency. *Cancer Chemother Pharmacol*. 2007;60:503-507.

212. Milano G, Etienne MC. Potential importance of dihydropyrimidine dehydrogenase (DPD) in cancer chemotherapy. *Pharmacogenetics*. 1994;4:301-306.

213. Milano G, Etienne MC. Dihydropyrimidine dehydrogenase (DPD) and clinical pharmacology of 5-fluorouracil. *Anticancer Res*. 1994;14:2295-2297.

214. Amstutz U, Farese S, Aebi S, et al. Dihydropyrimidine dehydrogenase gene variation and severe 5-fluorouracil toxicity: a haplotype assessment. *Pharmacogenomics*. 2009;10:931-944.

215. Mattison LK, Fourie J, Desmond RA, et al. Increased prevalence of dihydropyrimidine dehydrogenase deficiency in African-Americans compared with Caucasians. *Clin Cancer Res*. 2006;12:5491-5495.

216. Harris BE, Carpenter JT, Diasio RB. Severe 5-fluorouracil toxicity secondary to dihydropyrimidine dehydrogenase deficiency. *Cancer*. 1991;68:499-501.

217. Lecomte T, Ferraz J-M, Zinzindohoué F, et al. Thymidylate synthase gene polymorphism predicts toxicity in colorectal cancer patients receiving 5-fluorouracil-based chemotherapy. *Clin Cancer Res*. 2004;10:5880-5888.

218. Pullarkat ST, Stoehlmacher J, Ghaderi V, et al. Thymidylate synthase gene polymorphism determines response and toxicity of 5-FU chemotherapy. *Pharmacogenomics J*. 2001;1:65-70.

219. Ichikawa W, Takahashi T, Suto K, et al. Orotate phosphoribosyltransferase gene polymorphism predicts toxicity in patients treated with bolus 5-fluorouracil regimen. *Clin Cancer Res*. 2006;12:3928-3934.

220. Schwab M, Zanger UM, Marx C, et al. Role of genetic and non-genetic factors for fluorouracil treatment related severe toxicity: a prospective clinical trial by the German 5-FU toxicity study group. *J Clin Oncology*. 2008;26:2131-2138.

221. Ezzeldin HH, Diasio RB. Predicting fluorouracil toxicity: can we finally do it? *J Clin Oncology*. 2008;26:2080-2082.

222. Gross E, Busse B, Riemenschneider M, et al. Strong association of a common dihydropyrimidine dehydrogenase gene polymorphism with fluoropyrimidine-related toxicity in cancer patients. *PLoS One*. 2008;3:e4003.

223. Omura K. Clinical implications of dihydropyrimidine dehydrogenase (DPD) activity in 5-FU-based chemotherapy: mutations in the DPD gene, and DPD inhibitory fluoropyrimidines. *Int J Clin Oncol.* 2003;8:132-138.

224. van Kuilenburg AB, Vreken P, Beex LV, et al. Severe 5-fluorouracil toxicity caused by reduced dihydropyrimidine dehydrogenase activity due to heterozygosity for a G-->A point mutation. *J Inherit Metab Dis.* 1998;21:280-284.

225. Wei X, McLeod HL, McMurrough J, et al. Molecular basis of the human dihydropyrimidine dehydrogenase deficiency and 5-fluorouracil toxicity. *J Clin Invest.* 1996;98:610-615.

226. Raida M, Schwabe W, Hausler P, et al. Prevalence of a common point mutation in the dihydropyrimidine dehydrogenase (DPD) gene within the 5'-splice donor site of intron 14 in patients with severe 5-fluorouracil (5-FU)-related toxicity compared with controls. *Clinical Cancer Research.* 2001;7:2832.

227. Myriad Genetics Laboratories Inc. About TheraGuide 5-FU. Available at: http://www.myriadtests.com/hcp/about_theraguide.php. Accessed September 20, 2009.

228. Mattison LK, Fourie J, Hirao Y, et al. The uracil breath test in the assessment of dihydropyrimidine dehydrogenase activity: pharmacokinetic relationship between expired 13CO2 and plasma [2-13C]dihydrouracil. *Clin Cancer Res.* 2006;12:549-555.

229. Furuhata T, Kawakami M, Okita K, et al. Plasma level of a 5-fluorouracil metabolite, fluoro-beta-alanine correlates with dihydropyrimidine dehydrogenase activity of peripheral blood mononuclear cells in 5-fluorouracil treated patients. *J Exp Clin Cancer Res.* 2006;25:79-82.

230. iHOP (information linked over proteins) web site. Butyrylcholinesterase. Available at: http://www.ihop-net.org/UniPub/iHOP/gs/86703.html. Accessed September 24, 2009.

231. Kalow W, Staron N. On distribution and inheritance of atypical forms of human serum cholinesterase, as indicated by dibucaine number. *Can J Biochem.* 1957;35:1306-1317.

232. Kalow W, Gunn DR. Some statistical data on atypical cholinesterase of human serum. *Ann Hum Genet.* 1959;23:239-250.

233. Kalow W, Gunn DR. The relation between dose of succinylcholine and duration of apnea in man. *J Pharmacol Exp Ther.* 1957;120:203-214.

234. Ostergaard D, Viby-Mogensen J, Rasmussen SN, et al. Pharmacokinetics and pharmacodynamics of mivacurium in patients phenotypically homozygous for the atypical plasma cholinesterase variant—effect of injection of human cholinesterase. *Anesthesiology.* 2005;102:1124-1132.

235. Barta C, Sasvari-Szekely M, Devai A, et al. Analysis of mutations in the plasma cholinesterase gene of patients with a history of prolonged neuromuscular block during anesthesia. *Mol Genet Metab.* 2001;74:484-488.

236. Jensen FS, Viby-Mogensen J. Plasma cholinesterase and abnormal reaction to succinylcholine—20 years experience with the Danish Cholinesterase Research Unit. *Acta Anaesthesiol Scand.* 1995;39:150-156.

237. Wood M. Pharmacogenetics and anesthetic toxicity. In: Rice SA, Fish KJ, eds. *Anesthetic Toxicity.* New York, NY: Raven Press Ltd; 1994:199-218.

238. Hoffman RS, Henry GC, Wax PM, et al. Decreased plasma cholinesterase activity enhances cocaine toxicity in mice. *Pharmacol Exp Ther.* 1992;263:698-702.

239. Morton CL, Wadkins RM, Danks MK, et al. The anticancer prodrug CPT-11 is a potent inhibitor of acetylcholinesterase but is rapidly catalyzed to SN-38 by butyrylcholinesterase. *Cancer Research.* 1999;59:1458-1463.

240. Leiderer BM, Borchardt RT. Enzymes involved in the bioconversion of ester-based prodrugs. *J Pharm Sci.* 2006;95:1177-1195.

241. Hoffman RS, Henry GC, Howland MA, et al. Association between life-threatening cocaine toxicity and plasma cholinesterase activity. *Ann Emerg Med.* 1992;21:247-253.

242. Souza RLR, Mikami LR, Maegawa EA, et al. Four new mutations in the BCHE gene of human butyrylcholinesterase in a Brazilian blood donor sample. *Mol Genet Metab.* 2005;84:349-353.

243. Parmo-Follani F, Nunes K, Lepienski LM, et al. Two new mutations of the human BCHE gene (IVS3-14T>C and L574fsX576). *Chemico-Biological Interactions.* 2008;175:135-137.

244. Lando G, Mosca A, Bonora R, et al. Frequency of butyrylcholinesterase gene mutations in individuals with abnormal inhibition numbers: an Italian population study. *Pharmacogenetics.* 2003;13:265-270.

245. Pestel G, Sprenger H, Rothhammer A. Frequency distribution of dibucaine numbers in 24,830 patients. *Anaesthesist.* 2003;52:495-499.

246. Bartels CF, Jensen FS, Lockridge O, et al. DNA mutation associated with the human butyrylcholinesterase K-variant and its linkage to the atypical variant mutation and other polymorphic sites. *Am J Hum Genet.* 1992;50:1086-1103.

247. Evans RT. Cholinesterase phenotyping: clinical aspects and laboratory applications. *CRC Crit Rev Clin Lab Sci.* 1986;23:35-64.

248. Price Evans DA, Manley KA, McKusick VA. Genetic control of isoniazid metabolism in man. *Br Med J.* 1960;2:485-491.

249. Price Evans DA, Storey PB, Wittstadt FB. Determination of the isoniazid inactivator phenotype. *Am Respir Dis.* 1960;82:853-861.

250. Agundez JAG, Golka K, Martinez C, et al. Unraveling ambiguous NAT2 genotyping data. *Clinical Chemistry.* 2008;54:1390-1394.

251. Genelex Corporation. N-Acetyltransferase 2 Genotyping. Available at: http://www.healthanddna.com/healthcare-professional/nat2-genotyping.html. Accessed September 25, 2009.

252. Lin HJ, Han CY, Lin BK, et al. Ethnic distribution of slow acetylator mutations in the polymorphic N-acetyltransferase (NAT2) gene. *Pharmacogenetics.* 1994;4:125-134.

253. Rey E, Gendrel D, Treluyer JM, et al. Isoniazid pharmacokinetics in children according to acetylator phenotype. *Fund Clin Pharmacol.* 2001;15:355-359.

254. Cho H-J, Koh W-J, Ryu Y-J, et al. Genetic polymorphisms of NAT2 and CYP2E1 associated with antituberculosis drug-induced hepatotoxicity in Korean patients with pulmonary tuberculosis. *Tuberculosis.* 2007;87:551-556.

255. Coulthard SA, Hogarth LA, Little M, et al. The effect of thiopurine methyltransferase expression on sensitivity to thiopurine drugs. *Mol Pharmacol.* 2002;62:102-109.

256. McLeod HL, Siva C. The thiopurine S-methyltransferase gene locus— implications for clinical pharmacogenomics. *Pharmacogenomics.* 2002;3:89-98.

257. Purinethol® [prescribing information/package insert]. Sellersville, PA: Gate Pharmaceuticals; 2007.

258. Imuran® [prescribing information/package insert]. San Diego, CA: Prometheus Laboratories Inc; 2008.

259. Tabloid® [prescribing information/package insert]. Research Triangle Park, NC: GlaxoSmithKline; 2009.

260. Weinshilboum R. Thiopurine pharmacogenetics: clinical and molecular studies of thiopurine methyltransferase. *Drug Metab Dispos.* 2001;29:601-605.

261. Teml A, Schaeffeler E, Schwab M. Pretreatment determination of TPMT—state of the art in clinical practice. *Eur J Clin Pharmacol.* 2009;65:219-221.

262. Schaeffeler E, Fischer C, Brockmeier D, et al. Comprehensive analysis of thiopurine S-methyltransferase phenotype-genotype correlation in a large population of German-Caucasians and identification of novel TPMT variants. *Pharmacogenetics.* 2004;14:407-417.

263. Xin HW, Xiong H, Wu XC, et al. Relationships between thiopurine S-methyltransferase polymorphism and azathioprine-related adverse drug reactions in Chinese renal transplant recipients. *Eur J Clin Pharmacol.* 2009;65:249-255.

264. King CD, Rios GR, Green MD, et al. UDP-glucuronosyltransferases. *Curr Drug Metab.* 2000;1:143-161.

265. Kiang TK, Ensom MH, Chang TK. UDP-glucuronosyltransferases and clinical drug-drug interactions. *Pharmacol Ther.* 2005;106:97-132.

266. De Wildt SN, Kearns GL, Leeder JS, et al. Glucuronidation in humans. Pharmacogenetic and developmental aspects. *Clin Pharmacokin.* 1999;36:439-452.

267. Mackenzie PI, Miners JO, McKinnon RA. Polymorphisms in UDP glucuronosyltransferase genes: functional consequences and clinical relevance. *Clin Chem Lab Med.* 2000;38:889-892.

268. Miners JO, McKinnon RA, Mackenzie PI. Genetic polymorphisms of UDP-glucuronosyltransferases and their functional significance. *Toxicology.* 2002;181:453-456.

269. Burchell B. Genetic variation of human UDP-glucuronosyltransferase: implications in disease and drug glucuronidation. *Am J Pharmacogenomics.* 2003;3:37-52.

270. Gullemette C. Pharmacogenomics of human UDP-glucuronosyltransferase enzymes. *Pharmacogenomics J.* 2003;3:136-158.

271. Mani S. UGT1A1 polymorphism predicts irinotecan toxicity: evolving proof. *AAPS PharmSci.* 2001;3:1.
272. Innocenti F, Iyer L, Ratain MJ. Pharmacogenetics of anti-cancer agents: lessons from amonafide and irinotecan. *Drug Metab Dispos.* 2001;29:596-600.
273. Ando Y, Saka H, Ando M, et al. Polymorphisms of UDP-glucuronosyltransferase gene and irinotecan toxicity: a pharmacogenetic analysis. *Cancer Res.* 2000;60:6921-6926.
274. Iyer L, King CD, Whitington PF, et al. Genetic predisposition to the metabolism of irinotecan (CPT-11). *J Clin Invest.* 1998;101:847-854.
275. Bosma PJ, Chowdhury JR, Bakker C, et al. The genetic basis of the reduced expression of bilirubin UDP-glucuronosyltransferase 1 in Gilbert's syndrome. *N Engl J Med.* 1995;333:1171-1175.
276. Hall D, Ybazeta G, Destro-Bisol G, et al. Variability at the uridine diphosphate glucuronosyltransferase 1A1 promoter in human populations and primate. *Pharmacogenetics.* 1999;9:591-599.
277. Beutler E, Gelbart T, Demina A. Racial variability in the UDP-glucuronosyltransferase 1 (UGT1A1) promoter: a balanced polymorphism for regulation of bilirubin metabolism? *Proc Natl Acad Sci USA.* 1998;95:8170-8174.
278. PharmGKB: The Pharmacogenomics Knowledge Base. Important Variant Information for UGT1A1. Available at: http://www.pharmgkb.org/search/annotatedGene/ugt1a1/variant.jsp#ImportantVariantInformationforUGT1A1-28. Accessed September 26, 2009.
279. Rouits E, Boisdron-Celle M, Dumont A, et al. Relevance of different UGT1A1 polymorphisms in irinotecan-induced toxicity: a molecular and clinical study of 75 patients. *Clin Cancer Res.* 2004;10:5151-5159.
280. Iyer L, Das S, Janisch L, et al. UGT1A1*28 polymorphism as a determinant of irinotecan disposition and toxicity. *Pharmacogenomics J.* 2002;2:43-47.
281. Kim TW, Innocenti F. Insights, challenges, and future directions in irinogenetics. *Ther Drug Monit.* 2007;29:265-270.
282. Camptosar® [prescribing information/package insert]. New York, NY: Pharmacia & Upjohn Co; 2008.
283. Batchelder K, Miller P. A change in the market—investing in diagnostics. *Nature Biotechnology.* 2006;24:922-926.
284. Boggs J. Companion diagnostics gaining ground, but slowly. *Bioworld Financial Watch.* June 16, 2008.
285. Kuhlmann J. The applications of biomarkers in early clinical drug development to improve decision-making processes. *Ernst Schering Res Found Workshop.* 2007;59:29-45.
286. Bakhtiar R. Biomarkers in drug discovery and development. *J Pharm Tox Methods.* 2008;57:85-91.
287. US Food and Drug Administration. Critical Path Initiative. Available at http://www.fda.gov/ScienceResearch/SpecialTopics/CriticalPathInitiative/default.htm. Accessed September 28, 2009.
288. Daly AK, King BP. Pharmacogenetics of oral anticoagulants. *Pharmacogenetics.* 2003;13:247-252.

Chapter 5

Pharmacogenomics and Drug Transport/Efflux

Arthur G. Cox, Ph.D.

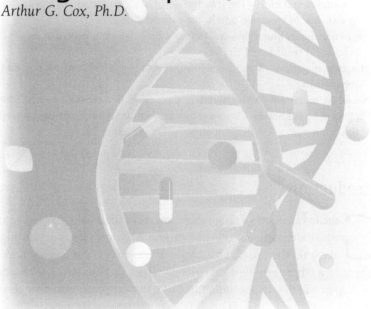

Learning Objectives

After completing this chapter, the reader should be able to

- Classify drug transport proteins by their location in tissues and cells and by their physiological function.
- Discuss the general clinical relevance of the transporters and their inhibitors.
- Describe classes of drugs whose pharmacokinetics are affected by individual transporters.
- Relate genetic variants of transport proteins to variations in drug action.

Key Definitions

Transporter—A protein embedded in a cell membrane responsible for either removing substances from a cell or bringing them into the cell or membrane-bound vesicle within the cell.

Single nucleotide polymorphism (SNP)—A point mutation occurring in >1% of the population.

Syncytiotrophoblast—Multinucleated cells in the placenta that contain transport proteins serving a protective function for the fetus.

Enterocyte—Cells lining the intestine that contain transport proteins with protective roles.

Synonymous mutation—The substitution of a nucleotide within a gene that does not result in a change in an amino acid in the expressed protein.

Nonsynonymous mutation—Nucleotide substitution in a gene that results in a change in the amino acid sequence of a protein.

Missense mutation—A polymorphism that results in a different amino acid being expressed in the protein.

Nonsense mutation—A polymorphism that results in a premature stop codon.

Linkage disequilibrium—A nonrandom association of alleles, causing a certain combination to occur more or less frequently than otherwise expected.

Introduction

Genetic variability of drug metabolizing enzymes has long been recognized as a factor in both differing therapeutic response and adverse effects in individuals and patient populations. The cytochrome family of enzymes is particularly important in this regard. Another area where genotype can strongly affect drug response is that of transport proteins. This chapter will discuss the importance of transport proteins in drug absorption and response and review recent information on the effect of genetic variability on these transporters.

Transporters are those proteins that carry either endogenous compounds or xenobiotics across biological membranes. They can be classified into either efflux or uptake proteins, depending on the direction of transport. The extent of expression of genes coding for transport proteins can have a profound effect on the bioavailability and pharmacokinetics of various drugs. Additionally, genetic variation such as single-nucleotide polymorphisms (SNPs) of the transport proteins can cause differences in the uptake or efflux of drugs. In terms of cancer chemotherapy, tumor cells expressing these proteins can have either enhanced sensitivity or resistance to various anticancer drugs.[1] Transporters that serve as efflux pumps on a cell membrane can remove drugs from the cell before they can act. Transport proteins that are responsible for the vital influx of ions and nutrients such as glucose can promote growth of tumor cells if overexpressed, or lead to increased susceptibility for a drug if the transporter carries that drug into the cell. Additionally, genetic variants of transport proteins can cause or contribute to a number of diseases, such as cystic fibrosis, retinal degeneration, hypercholesterolemia, bile transport defects, and anemia.[2]

There are two superfamilies of transport proteins that have important effects on the absorption, distribution, and excretion of drugs. These are the ATP-binding cassette (ABC) and the solute-carrier (SLC) superfamilies. With the advent of high-throughput screening methods in recent years, screening of large volumes of samples for SNPs has become viable. Public databases of the genetic variants that have been discovered are available and include those maintained by the Human Genome Gene Nomenclature Committee (HGNC), National Center for Biotechnology Information (NCBI) SNP database (dbSNP), the National Human Genome Research Institute haploid map (HapMap), the Japanese SNP database (JSNP), and the pharmacogenetics and pharmacogenomics knowledge base at Stanford University (PharmGKB).

Case Study—Irinotecan

Irinotecan is widely used in cancer chemotherapy but has been associated with unpredictable severe toxic reactions such as myelosuppression and delayed-type diarrhea. Polymorphism of the drug-metabolizing enzyme family UGT1A is a known contributor to varied response and toxicity of irinotecan in different individuals. Polymorphism of multiple drug transport proteins, such as ABCB1, ABCC1, ABCC2, ABCG2, and SLC01B1 have been suggested to have additive or synergistic effects with UGT1A1.[3-6]

Questions:

1. What are the patient parameters normally considered when determining the correct dose for irinotecan?
2. Discuss how genetic polymorphisms can affect patient response to irinotecan.
3. How can knowledge of pharmacogenomics improve the therapeutic use and safety profile of irinotecan?

Individual Transporters of Pharmacogenomic Interest

ABC Transporters

ATP-binding cassette (ABC) transporters are present in cellular and intracellular membranes and can be responsible for either importing or removing (efflux) of substances from cells and tissues. They often transport substances against a concentration gradient by using the hydrolysis of ATP to drive the transport. There are at least 49 ABC transporter genes, which are divided into seven different families (A-G) based on sequence similarity. Three of these seven gene families are particularly important for drug transport and multiple drug resistance in tumor cells[7]: (1) the *ABCB1* gene, encoding MDR1 (also known as P-glycoprotein); (2) *ABCG2* (breast cancer resistance protein); and (3) the *ABCC* family (*ABCC1* through *ABCC6*) or multidrug resistance proteins (MRP).

ABC transporters are characterized as such by the homology of their ATP binding regions. All families but one (ABCG2) contain two ATP binding regions and two transmembrane domains. The transmembrane domains contain multiple alpha helices, which span the lipid bilayer. The number of alpha helices in a transmembrane domain differs depending on the family. The ATP binding regions are located on the cytoplasmic side of the membrane (Figure 5-1). As well as being important mediators of resistance in human chemotherapy, ABC transporters are also found in bacteria and can contribute to the development of resistance to multiple antibiotics. The localization of the proteins depends on the cell type, such as hepatocyte, enterocyte, and renal proximal tubule (Figure 5-2). The majority of ABC transporters move compounds from the cytoplasm to the outside of a cell, although some move compounds into an intercellular compartment such as the endoplasmic reticulum, mitochondria, or peroxisome.

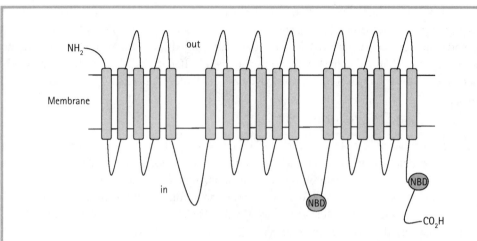

Figure 5.1 • General structure of ATP binding cassette transporters (ABC), showing trans-membrane and nucleotide binding domains (NBD). Individual members of the superfamily contain differing numbers of transmembrane helices within the transmembrane domains. The example shown here illustrates MRP1 (ABCC1). ABCG2 transporters differ from the rest of the members of the superfamily in that they have only one ATP binding domain. The alpha helices making up the transmembrane segments, and the nucleotide binding regions are critical to the function of ABCs (see Figure 5-3). Figure adapted from reference 12.

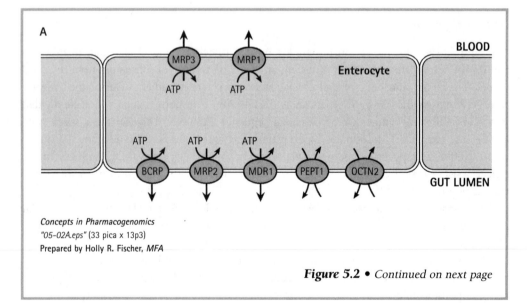

Concepts in Pharmacogenomics
"05-02A.eps" (33 pica x 13p3)
Prepared by Holly R. Fischer, MFA

Figure 5.2 • Continued on next page

Figure 5.2 • *Continued*

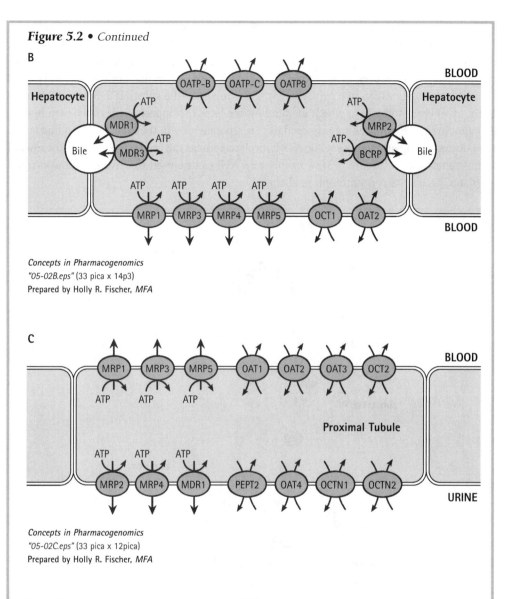

Concepts in Pharmacogenomics
"05-02B.eps" (33 pica x 14p3)
Prepared by Holly R. Fischer, *MFA*

Concepts in Pharmacogenomics
"05-02C.eps" (33 pica x 12pica)
Prepared by Holly R. Fischer, *MFA*

Figure 5.2 • Localization of transporters in differing cell types. A) small intestine enterocyte, B) hepatocyte with canaliculi, and C) renal proximal tubule. In addition to those transporters discussed in the text, other transport proteins with protective and possible pharmacogenomic relevance are shown. OCTN1 and OCTN2: novel organic cation transporters-1 and 2 (*SLC22A4*, *SLC22A5*), OATP-B: organic anion transporting polypeptide-B (*SLCO2B1*), OATP-C (*SLCO1B1*), OATP8 (*SLCO1B3*), OCT1 (*SLC22A1*), OAT2 (*SLC22A7*). Figure adapted from reference 15.

The exact mechanism by which ABC transporters function has not been fully elucidated. It has been proposed that there is an ATP-dependant conformational change in the protein, which causes the substrate to be pumped across the membrane. This hypothesis has been supported by recent x-ray crystallographic studies, which have shown that both import and export proteins oscillate between two conformations: one in which the substrate binding site is open to the cytoplasm, and one in which the binding site faces the opposite side of the membrane.[8] ATP binding and hydrolysis are proposed to play separate roles in the cycle. ATP binding favors the outward facing orientation, while ATP hydrolysis returns the transporter back to the inward facing conformation (Figure 5-3).[8,9] In this way, ATP can be used to drive the transport of a substance against its concentration gradient.

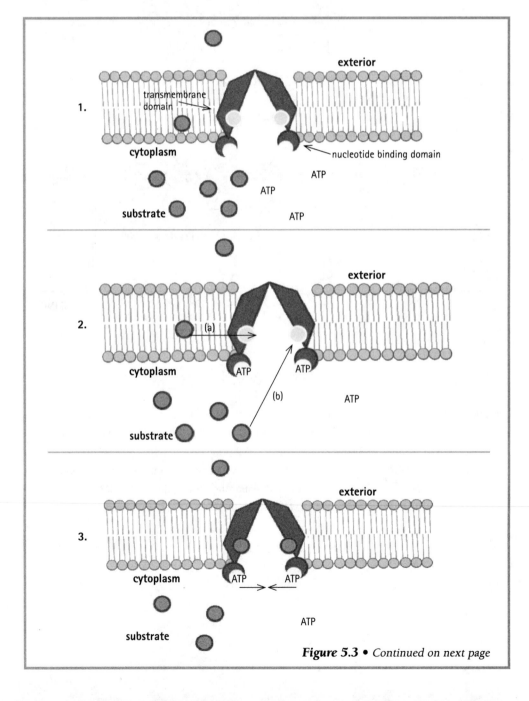

Figure 5.3 • *Continued on next page*

Figure 5.3 • *Continued*

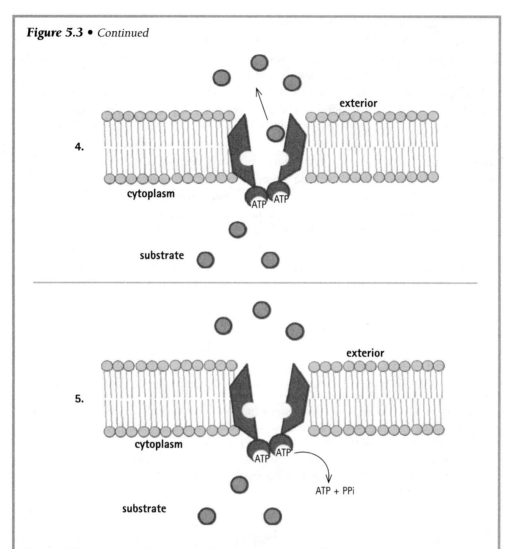

Figure 5.3 • Schematic illustration of the function of ATP efflux transporters. Step 1: The two transmembrane domains that make up the functional protein are attached to nucleotide-binding domains that are widely separated. Step 2: ATP and the substrate bind to their domains. Highly lipophilic substrates may diffuse through the plasma membrane (a). Otherwise, they can diffuse from the cytoplasm to the binding pocket (b). Step 3: The nucleotide binding regions containing ATP undergo a conformational shift, bringing them close together. Step 4: The conformational shift of the NBDs has caused a change in the conformation of the substrate binding pocket, which opens a pocket to the outside of a cell and allows efflux of the substrate. Step 5: ATP is hydrolyzed to ADP and pyrophosphate (PPi). The protein can then return to its resting state, with the substrate binding site directed inward. Figure adapted from reference 9.

ABCB1 Transporters: P-glycoprotein

The *ABCB1* gene codes for a glycosylated membrane protein originally detected in cells that had developed resistance to cancer chemotherapy agents. The protein is commonly referred to as P-glycoprotein (P-gp), PGY1, or multidrug resistance protein-1 (MDR1). It is designated as a multidrug resistance protein due to the fact that its expression in a cell may confer resistance to multiple classes of drugs with differing chemical structures and mechanisms of action. Various cancers tend to display low initial levels of P-gp with levels of expression increasing after chemotherapy and relapse. Of the wide variety of transport proteins that have been discovered and studied, P-gp is the best characterized in terms of distribution and function. Some drugs (e.g., cyclosporine) act as both substrates and inhibitors of P-gp. Other drugs act only as substrates or as inhibitors. The substrates for P-gp are often hydrophobic drugs with a polyaromatic skeleton and a neutral or positive charge.[10] P-gp functions as a dimer of 1280 residue polypeptides, forming a pore across the cell membrane. In addition to cytotoxic chemotherapeutic agents, many other drugs are transported across membranes by P-gp. These include protease inhibitors, immunosuppressants, calcium channel blockers, beta blockers, statins, steroids, antihistamines, anticonvulsants, and antidepressants. The importance of P-gp for pharmacotherapy has led to great interest in its pharmacogenomics.[11-13]

Clinical Pearl

P-glycoprotein translocates multiple structurally unrelated drugs out of cells, including anticancer drugs, immunosuppressants, HIV protease inhibitors, cardiac drugs, and β-adrenoreceptor antagonists. Expression of P-gp in a cell may result in resistance to the effects of a wide variety of drugs, and genetic variation of the protein may result in differing susceptibility to pharmacotherapy. Ethnic background can also increase or decrease the likelihood of interaction between P-gp and a drug.

Besides being expressed in cancer cells, P-glycoprotein is expressed in multiple normal tissues with excretory or protective function including intestine, kidney, liver, blood-brain barrier, spinal cord, testes and placenta. P-gp has an important role in forming a protective barrier against absorption of xenobiotics in these tissues. The broad substrate specificity of P-gp is shared with cytochrome P450 3A4 (CYP3A4), which is well known to metabolize a diverse set of drugs. This broad specificity, coupled with the tissue localization and function of both proteins, has led to the hypothesis that they work in concert, protecting the body from absorption of harmful compounds by acting synergistically in the small intestine.

Significant interindividual variability of the amount of P-gp expressed (two- to eightfold) has been demonstrated in healthy volunteers during intestinal biopsy, suggesting the possibility of variable bioavailability of its substrates. Numerous SNPs of the human *MDR1* gene have been discovered and studied during systematic screening. The frequencies of these SNPs in a population can vary according to racial/ethnic background.[14] At least 29 SNPs have been found, 19 of them located in exonic regions and 11 of them coding for nonsynonymous mutations.[15] Interest in the clinical and functional relevance of polymorphisms of *MDR1* has led to a number of recent reviews.[15-17] Two SNPs of particular interest are a mutation in exon 26 at position 3435 (3435C>T) and a mutation in exon 21 (2677G>T/A). 3435C>T has been extensively studied since it is associated with differences in expression or function of P-gp. Change in nucleotide sequence from C to T at position 3435 does not result in a change of amino acids but is a silent mutation located in the wobble position of the codon. Although there is no change in the expressed protein, both the level of its expression and function can be variable. For instance, a twofold reduction of intestinal P-gp was observed in patients who were homozygous for 3435T.[18] In a number of studies, reduction in P-gp level has been correlated with differences in pharmacokinetic parameters for substrates such as digoxin. There are several possible explanations for the reduction in P-gp expression with homozygous 3435T genotype. One is that there may be a reduction in translation of the protein in this polymorphism.[19]

Other studies have probed the relationship of SNPs with various anticancer agents that are substrates for P-gp transport. For example, one recent study investigated the correlation of *MDR1* polymorphisms with clinical response to docetaxel-cisplatin in nonsmall cell lung cancer (NSCLC) in Han Chinese patients. This study found the 2677 GG genotype was associated with significantly better response to chemotherapy compared with the combined 2677 GT and TT genotypes.[20] The haplotype of 2677G-3435C was also found to be a significant predictor of treatment response in this same study. A demonstrated linkage disequilibrium between the synonymous SNP C3435T and the nonsynonymous SNP 2677G>T/A may explain observed functional differences in P-gp that have previously been attributed to the 3435C>T.[21]

The variation in frequency of SNPs for MDR1 has been studied in different racial/ethnic populations. It has been found that the allelic frequency can differ among these groups. The incidence of C/T and C/C genotypes at position 3435 has been found to be much higher in African than Caucasian or Asian populations. For instance, in one study 83% of Ghanaians and 61% of African Americans were homozygous for the C allele, while only 26% of Caucasians and 34% of Japanese shared this trait.[22] Individuals that are homozygous for the T allele have substantially lower intestinal P-gp than those that are homozygous for the C allele.[18] Lower intestinal P-gp may increase the bioavailability of P-gp substrates. This seems to be supported by studies that show that the maximum plasma concentrations of the P-gp substrate cyclosporine is substantially lower in African Americans than Caucasians.[23] It has been hypothesized that the higher frequency of the C/C genotype in African populations compared to Japanese or Caucasians could result from a selective advantage of this genotype against gastrointestinal-tract infections endemic to tropical regions.[22] On the other hand, the high frequency of the C3435 allele in African populations may explain a high prevalence of more aggressive tumors in breast cancer and the high incidence of resistance to cancer chemotherapy seen in African populations.[14,24,25]

The effect of MDR1 polymorphism on digoxin absorption has been probed in a number of studies.[26,27] Since digoxin is not subject to metabolic transformation, it has been used as a model substrate for the study of phenotype-genotype relationships of *MDR1* polymorphs. A sizable Dutch study (195 elderly patients) involving chronic dosing of digoxin rather than single dose kinetics examined the effect of *MDR1* genotype on digoxin levels.[26] The 3435C>T, 1236C>T, and 2677G>T/A SNPs were identified in peripheral blood DNA. All three variants were associated with serum digoxin concentration of 0.18-0.21 mcg/L per additional T allele. The association was even stronger for the 1236-2677-3435 TTT haplotype and absent from other haplotypes examined. The results of this study agree with another study in healthy Japanese subjects.[28] In this study, a single oral dose of digoxin was administered and the serum concentration of digoxin was monitored. Individuals harboring a T allele at 3435 had significantly lower AUC_4 than those homozygous for C at this position.

It should be noted that not all studies support the association of the 3435C>T SNP with reduced P-gp function or clinical outcome of patients treated with known P-gp substrates. For instance, in a study conducted in Korea of 200 patients with acute myeloid leukemia (AML) undergoing a standard induction chemotherapeutic regimen, no correlation was found between 3435C>T polymorphism and P-glycoprotein function in leukemic blasts or in clinical outcomes.[29] This inconsistency in correlating clinical outcomes with 3435C>T polymorphism in AML and other diseases suggests that other genetic or nongenetic factors also play an important role.

In addition to race and ethnicity, the patient gender can also significantly affect the expression of P-gp. For instance, hepatic P-gp levels are 2- to 2.4-fold lower in females than males.[30] In the case of antineoplastics such as vinca alkaloids, etoposide, doxorubicin, and docetaxel, this means increased risk for myelosuppression and gastrointestinal toxicity in females, as well as prolonged drug exposure.[31] Thus females may have an increased response to a drug, as well as increased toxicity.

Clinical Pearl

Patient gender can influence the rate of clearance and efficacy for drugs that are transported by P-glycoprotein.

Another anticancer drug that has been extensively studied with respect to pharmacogenomics is irinotecan.[3-6] Irinotecan is a prodrug, transformed to the active metabolite 7-ethyl-10-hydroxycamptothecan (SN-38) by carboxylesterase enzymes. SN-38 is thought to be responsible for most of the activity of irinotecan. SN-38 is transformed in phase II metabolism to the glucuronide conjugate by UDP-glucuronosyltransferase (UGT) enzymes. The resultant conjugate is more hydrophilic than the parent and is subsequently eliminated in the bile or urine by transport proteins. These proteins include ABCB1, ABCC1, ABCC2, ABCG2, and SLCO1B1 (OATP1B1). Standard dosing regimens of irinotecan rely on calculation of patient body surface area, which correlates with blood volume. However, it has been found that there is tremendous interindividual variability of response to irinotecan, with some patients developing severe life-threatening diarrhea and neutropenia. Correct dosing is critical since reduced plasma levels will not provide effective treatment, while elevated levels produce toxicity. Modifications of dosing regimens are recommended based on the observed individual toxicity. Polymorphisms of UGT1A1 that reduce glucuronidation and thus increase plasma levels have been definitively identified. Because of this, in 2005 the package labeling was revised to recommend reduced dosing in patients known to be homozygous for the *UGT1A1*28* allele. This includes approximately 10% of the North American population. In 2005 the FDA also approved a genetic test to aid the detection and identification of *UGT1A1*28* (Invader UGT1A1 by Third Wave Technologies Inc.). Polymorphisms of transport proteins with reduced activity would naturally be expected to further modify pharmacokinetics and possibly increase toxicity. This supposition has been supported for *ABCB1* (1236C>T), *ABCC2* (3972T>C), *ABCG2* (delCTCA -19572-19576 and 421C>A), and *SLCO1B1*1b* in various ethnic groups.[32-38] This data indicates that testing for transporter polymorphisms may further improve quality of treatment for irinotecan.

ABCC Transporter Family

The protein product of ABCC genes are commonly known as MRPs or multidrug resistance proteins. In contrast to the neutral and cationic hydrophobic compounds that P-gp transports, MRPs often transport anionic compounds. Ten members of the MRP family are known and at least seven may be involved in conferring resistance to cancer chemotherapeutics (MRP1 to MRP7).[12] MRP1 has the most likely significance in clinical anticancer drug resistance. MRPs are located in various tissues with protective and excretory function such as the brain, liver, kidney, and intestines. They transport a structurally diverse set of endogenous substances, xenobiotics, and metabolites. Genetic polymorphisms of ABCC1-5 have been subject to intensive study recently.[39]

ABCC1 Transporters

The ABCC1 (MRP1) transport protein has broad substrate specificity and is expressed in many tissues of the body. It was originally discovered in small-cell lung cancer cells that showed multidrug resistance without overexpressing ABCB1 (MDR1). Similarly to MDR1, it is able to confer resistance to anthracyclines and vinca alkaloids. MRP1 transports primarily neutral and anionic hydrophobic compounds and their glutathione, sulfate, and glucuronide conjugates. A few cationic substances can also be transported. Many unconjugated substances are cotransported with reduced glutathione (G-SH). The oxidized form of glutathione (G-SS-G) is also transported by MRP1. In most polarized cells, localization of the protein is on basolateral membranes for efflux of substrates into the blood. It occurs in many epithelial tissues, such as the testes, skeletal muscle, heart, kidney, and lung, and may have a protective role for the central nervous system. Physiologically relevant endogenous compounds that are transported by MRP1 include leukotriene C4, which is important for inflammatory reactions.

There are a number of nonsynonymous genetic variants of the transporter that have been studied for functional significance by in vitro methods. For instance, Arg433Ser decreased the transport of leukotriene C4 and estrone sulfate but not estradiol 17-β glucuronide.[40] This same SNP conferred a 2.1-fold resistance to doxorubicin compared to cells expressing the wild type MRP1. Another SNP, Cys43Ser, has been associated with a decrease in vincristine resistance. In this case, the polymorphism led to loss of localization to the correct cell membrane.[41] Polymorphisms in the promoter region of ABCC1 have also been found, raising the possibility of differences in promoter activity and gene expression.[42]

ABCC2 Transporters

The ABCC2 transporter is also known as multidrug resistance protein-2 (MRP2) or canalicular multispecific organic anion transporter (cMOAT). It is the most studied member of the ABCC family. This protein is expressed in the liver, kidneys, and intestines. It plays an important role in chemoprotection by transporting the products of phase II metabolism out of cells. Thus glucuronide, glutathione, and sulfate conjugates of drugs are predominant substrates of MRP2. These conjugates are transported from hepatic cells into the canaliculi and then to the bile for excretion. Unconjugated drugs are also transported, as are the conjugates of bilirubin. Unlike other members of the ABCC family, ABCC2 is expressed in apical membranes of absorptive and excretory cells, such as hepatocytes, enterocytes, renal proximal tubules, and syncytiotrophoblasts of the placenta.

Mutations in the *ABCC2* gene are associated with the rare autosomal recessive disorder Dubin-Johnson syndrome (DJS). These mutations may cause DJS through a variety of mechanisms. The most obvious is the formation of nonfunctional forms of the protein, which results in the inability for hepatocytes to secrete conjugated bilirubin into the bile. Many of the mutations associated with DJS occur on the ATP binding region, which is critical for protein function. Other mutations result in impaired transcription and localization of the protein or reduced substrate binding. The results of the dysfunction are conjugated hyperbilirubinemia and consequent deposition of pigment into hepatocytes. Occurrence of DJS is most common in males, but in women pregnancy or oral contraceptive use may result in jaundice. The prevalence of DJS varies among racial/ethnic populations, and it is most commonly seen in Iranian Jewish patients. Besides modification of hepatic function, DJS patients have been thought to have reduced expression and function of intestinal MRP2, although there is little evidence of this.[43] Wide ranging studies concerning the effect of DJS polymorphisms on drug pharmacokinetics are not yet available, but some small scale studies have been completed.

In a case study of a patient with DJS being treated for large B-cell lymphoma with methotrexate, a threefold reduction in methotrexate elimination rate was observed, resulting in severe overdosing and reversible nephrotoxicity. Genetic analysis of the *ABCC2* gene revealed a heterozygous SNP Arg412Gly, which occurs in a region of the protein associated with substrate binding. Functional analysis revealed that this mutation conferred loss of transport activity.[44] This case is illustrative of a situation where effective pharmacogenomic screening might be successfully applied to improve patient care.

Other studies have attempted to correlate the expression of MRP2 with both intrinsic and acquired resistance to other cancer chemotherapeutics, for instance cisplatin in the treatment of pancreatic cancer.[45] In resected pancreatic cancer tissues only MRP2 mRNA, and not MRP1 or MRP3, was expressed, and it was overexpressed compared to normal pancreatic tissue. In this same study when pancreatic cancer cells were cultured in the presence of cisplatin, they began to overexpress MRP2 but not MRP1 or MRP3 proteins.

ABCC3 Transporters

The *ABCC3* gene, which codes for MRP3, has not been studied as extensively as either MDR1 or MDR2. In contrast to the MDR1, MRP3 does not transport glutathione and is a poor transporter for glutathione conjugates.[46] Glucuronide conjugates are transported, such as estradiol-17-β-glucuronide. MRP3 is localized in the liver, kidneys, and intestines. Location in polarized cells is in basolateral membranes, similar to MRP1. A number of different polymorphs have been investigated for their effect on MRP3 expression levels. One of the SNPs frequently found in the promoter region, 211C>T, has possible relevance for pharmacotherapy and disease progression.[47] Individuals homozygous or heterozygous for this SNP showed significantly lower MRP3 mRNA levels than individuals with a wild-type allele. This SNP has been studied for its association with adult acute myelogenous leukemia (AML) as a predictor for disease predisposition or prognosis.[48] It was found that 211C>T had a negative effect on prognosis. Conflicting results have been obtained for the correlation of 211C>T with treatment outcome in childhood AML.[49]

ABCC4 and ABCC5 Transporters

These proteins, also known as MRP4 and MRP5, respectively, are much less studied than MRP1, MRP2, and MRP3. Tissue localization is shown in Table 5-1. Substrates for both transporters are anticancer/antiviral nucleoside and nucleotide analogs as well as various organic anions. A number of SNPs have been identified for these transporters. Some of these have been suggested to have relevance for pharmacotherapy. For instance, the SNP in MRP4 (rs3765534) was found to dramatically reduce MRP4 function through impairment of membrane localization.[50] This SNP is relatively common in Japanese patients (>18%) and may play a role in the high sensitivity that some patients have for thiopurines.

Table 5-1
Transporter Localizations and Polymorphisms

Transporter (common name)	Gene Name (systematic protein name)	Tissue Localization and Position in Polarized Cells	Representative Substrates	Example Polymorphisms and Phenotype Effect
MDR1, P-gp	ABCB1	Apical: kidney, liver, brain, intestine, placenta	Anthracyclines, cyclosporine, taxanes, vinca alkaloids, doxorubicin[82]	3435C>T (↓ intestinal expression, ↓ substrate bioavailability)[18] 2677G>T/A (↑ response to docetaxel/cisplatin)[20]
MRP1	ABCC1	Lung, ubiquitous on basolateral membrane epithelial: e.g., choroid plexus (blood-cerebrospinal fluid barrier), testes	Anthracyclines, vinca alkaloids, methotrexate, glutathione conjugates, leukotriene C4, bilirubin, glutathione, saquinavir, ritonavir, difloxacin	Arg433Ser (↑ doxorubicin resistance)[40] Cys433Ser (↓ vincristine resistance)[41]
MRP2, cMOAT	ABCC2	Apical: liver, proximal tubule, small intestine, placenta	Bilirubin conjugates, glucuronide, sulfate & glutathione conjugates of various drugs, unconjugated anionic drugs (e.g., methotrexate): broad substrate specificity	↑ cisplatin resistance[45] 2302C>T, 2439T>C (Dubin-Johnson syndrome)[83] c.3972C>T (↑ hepatocellular carcinoma)[84]

Continued on next page

Table 5-1 *(Continued)*

Transporter (common name)	Gene Name (systematic protein name)	Tissue Localization and Position in Polarized Cells	Representative Substrates	Example Polymorphisms and Phenotype Effect
MRP3	ABCC3	Basolateral: liver, kidneys, intestines	Glucuronidated substrates (acetaminophen,[85] morphine,[86] estradiol, bilirubin)	-211C>T (↓ expression),[47] (worsen prognosis: lung cancer)[87] Arg1381Ser, Ser-346Phe, & Ser607Asn (↓ transport activity)[88]
MRP4 and MRP5	ABCC4 and ABCC5	Prostate[89] (asolateral), kidney,[90] lung,[91] brain,[92] pancreas,[93] lymphocytes,[94] platelets,[95] heart (MRP5)[96]	Azidothymidine, mercaptopurine, thioguanine, cladribine, abacavir[39]	MRP4: rs3765534 (↑ thiopurine sensitivity), Gly187Trp, Gly487Glu (↓ azidothymidine transport),[97] A3463G (↓ tenofovir efflux)[98]
MRP6	ABCC6	Basolateral: liver, kidney	Glutathione conjugates, leukotriene C_4	Many: e.g., c.3421C>T (pseudoxanthoma elasticum)[99]
BCRP, MXR, ABCP	ABCG2	Placenta syncytiotrophoblasts, hepatocyte canalicular, apical intestinal epithelia, vascular endothelia	Doxorubicin, daunorubicin, mitoxantrone, topotecan, prazosin, uric acid[58]	↑ anthracyclines, mitoxantrone, SN-38 resistance 421C>A (worsen prognosis: lung cancer & cisplatin),[87] (↑ gefitinib-induced diarrhea)[57] Gln141Lys (↑ chemotherapy-induced diarrhea)[100]
Serotonin transporter	SLC6A4	Neurons, heart valve, intestine (apical)[101]	Serotonin	"l" allele (↑ psychopathology)[102] "s" allele (↓ antidepressant efficacy, citalopram-induced diarrhea)[65]
Reduced folate carrier (RFC-1)	SLC19A1	Apical: kidney, leukemic cells, wide distribution	Methotrexate, leucovorin, pemetrexed	80AA (↑ methotrexate polyglutamation)[103]

Continued on next page

Table 5-1 *(Continued)*

Transporter (common name)	Gene Name (systematic protein name)	Tissue Localization and Position in Polarized Cells	Representative Substrates	Example Polymorphisms and Phenotype Effect
OATP1B1	SLCO1B1	Basolateral: liver, brain	Pravastatin, atorvastatin, lovastatin, cerivastatin, bilirubin, digoxin, estradiol, thyroid hormones, mycophenolate	521T>C (↓ pravastatin AUC)[104]
OATP1B3	SLCO1B3	Basolateral: liver	Methotrexate, glucuronidated estradiol, mycophenolate	334T>G (GG ↑ mycophenolate AUC)[105]
PEPT1 and PEPT2	SLC15A1, SLC15A2	PEPT1: small intestine, duodenum (apical) PEPT2: broad distribution[106]	Cephalexin, other β-lactam antibiotics, ACE inhibitors, valacyclovir, peptides	Arg57His (transport function loss)[107]
RFC-1	SLC19A1	Broad distribution	Methotrexate	80A>G (AA ↑ plasma folate)[77] (↑ remission of rheumatoid arthritis with methotrexate)[78]
CNT1, CNT2, CNT3	SLC28A1, SLC28A2, SLC28A3	Intestinal/renal epithelia, liver, macrophages, leukemic cells[1]	Didanosine, idoxuridine, zidovudine, cladribine, fludarabine, gemcitabine, capecitabine[1]	Unclear relevance for polymorphisms
ENT1, ENT2, ENT3, ENT4	SLC29A1, SLC29A2, SLC29A3, SLC28A4	Intestine, liver, kidney, placenta[108]	Pyrimidine and/or purine nucleosides, adenosine, gemcitabine, cladribine, fludarabine	Unclear relevance for polymorphisms

ABCC6 Transporters

ABCC6 encodes MRP6 protein, also known as MRP-like protein 1 (MLP-1), anthracycline resistance associated protein (ARA), and multispecific organic anion transporter-E (MOAT-E). It is expressed primarily in the liver and kidneys. Mutations in the ABCC6 gene are associated with pseudoxanthoma elasticum, a disease that causes mineralization of elastic fibers in some tissues.

ABCG2 Transporters

ABCG2 is alternatively known as Breast Cancer Resistance Protein (BCRP), placenta-specific ABC transporter (ABCP), and mitoxantrone resistance protein (MTX). It was originally identified in a resistant breast cancer cell line. It is very important in limiting bioavailability of certain drugs, concentrating drugs in breast milk, and protecting the fetus from drugs in maternal circulation.[7] It is highly expressed in the gastrointestinal tract, liver, and placenta, and influences the absorption and distribution of a wide variety of drugs and organic anions.[51-53] The substrate specificity for ABCG2 is broad and overlaps that of P-glycoprotein but is distinct from it. In contrast to the rest of the ABC transporter family, ABCG2 contains only one binding site for ATP and one transmembrane domain, rather than two of each. It is assumed to function as a dimer and is therefore referred to as a *half-transporter.* ABCG2 confers resistance to a broad range of hydrophobic anticancer drugs, similar to P-gp and MDR1, and is considered one of the most important ABC transporters mediating multidrug resistance in cancer cells. Resistance can be brought about by either reduced absorption or increased biliary excretion of the drug.

Various polymorphisms of ABCG2 are known to exist, some of which are associated with increased resistance to anticancer drugs such as mitoxantrone, the anthracyclines, and camptothecin derivatives. Some SNPs that have been associated with altered transport activity are Arg428Gly and Arg428Thr, Cys421Ala, Val12Met, Gln141Lys, Gln126X.[54,55] Other drugs that act as inhibitors of ABCG2 are antiviral nucleoside analogs such as zidovudine (AZT), lopinavir, nelfinavir, etc.[56] One SNP of ABCG2 has been associated with adverse reactions in patients treated with gefitinib, an inhibitor of the epidermal growth factor receptor tyrosine kinase used in nonsmall-cell lung cancer.[57] Thus, 44% of patients that were heterozygous for the Cys421Ala polymorphism developed diarrhea after treatment with gefitinib, versus 12% of patients homozygous for the wild type protein.

Besides being associated with adverse drug reactions and variations in therapeutic efficacy, SNPs of ABCG2 have been found to be highly predictive of plasma uric acid levels in one large study.[58] In this study a genome-wide scan was made for SNPs associated with serum uric acid concentration and gout. The study used phenotype and genotype results from a cohort of the Framingham Heart Study as well as a Rotterdam cohort. SNPs identified as being associated with uric acid concentration and gout were identified in ABCG2, SLC17A3, and SLC2A9. The results of this study were used to calculate a risk score for an individual based on whether they have the polymorphisms associated with hyperuricemia. The risk score was generated based on the number of alleles associated with high uric acid concentration. Mean uric acid concentration rose linearly with the number of risk alleles. For individuals with no risk alleles, prevalence of gout was 1% to 2% across the cohorts examined. The prevalence increased to 8% to 12% with six risk alleles. Individual common genetic variants were found to confer only a modest risk of gout, but their combination resulted in a large association with uric acid and gout. Ultimately the risk score may be used to help identify patients with asymptomatic hyperuricemia and guide therapeutic intervention.

One of the primary tissues in which ABCG2 is expressed in humans is in the placenta. The precise physiological function of the protein in this location is not clear, but it likely plays a strong role in protecting the fetus from xenobiotics, toxins, and metabolites by expelling them across the placental barrier.[59] Wide variations in the expression level of BCRP has been found in human placenta, which may lead to considerable variation in fetal exposure to drugs and xenobiotics. Such variation may be caused by polymorphisms in BCRP.[60]

Solute Carrier Proteins

Solute carrier proteins (SLCs) are important in transport of ions and organic substances across biological membranes in the maintenance of homeostasis. Members of the SLC superfamily consist of membrane channels, facilitative transporters, and secondary active transporters. Examples of some of the endogenous solutes that are transported include steroid hormones, thyroid hormones, leukotrienes, and prostaglandins. Additionally, SLCs are important in the transport of a large number of drugs. The solute carrier protein class includes the transporters known as OATs (organic anion transporters), the OATPs (organic anion transporting polypeptides, which are structurally different from OATs), OCTs (organic cation transporters), and PepTs (peptide transport proteins). In all, more than 40 families of transporters make up the SLC superfamily. Members within an individual SLC family have >20% to 25% sequence homology. However, the homology between families is low or nonexistent. Thus inclusion of a family into the SLC group is not dependent on evolutionary or structural relationship, but rather is a functional classification. Individual members of the SLCs are expressed in a variety of tissues such as liver, kidney, brain, and intestine and transport substances either into or out of cells.

SLCO1B1

Genetic variants of solute carrier proteins, such as SLCO1B1, have been associated with pharmacogenomic relevance. For example, a genome-wide scan of 300,000 genetic markers in a study of statin-induced myopathy found a strong correlation with the rs4363657 SNP located within the SLCO1B1 gene.[61] SLCO1B1 encodes the sodium-independent organic anion transporting peptide OATP1B1. An increased risk of myopathy was associated with simvastatin use in patients expressing this particular variation. Polymorphisms of solute transporter genes have also been associated with pharmacokinetic variance for other statin drugs. For example, altered uptake of pravastatin into the liver has been associated with polymorphisms of SLC21A6 (OATP-C) and SLC22A8 (OAT3).[62] A variant of SLCO1B1 has also been associated with functionally relevant SNPs important for the pharmacokinetics of other drugs, such as the irinotecan metabolite SN-38, estrone 3-sulfate, and estradiol 17-beta glucuronide. Methods have been developed to rapidly identify the relevant SNPs.[63]

SLC6 Family

Members of the SLC6 family are sodium-dependant transporters for neurotransmitters such as dopamine, serotonin, norepinephrine, glycine, and GABA. The *SLC6A4* gene codes for the serotonin transporter (SERT). The best evidence for pharmacogenomic relevance within the SLC6 family has been found for SERT, which is a cotransporter for serotonin and sodium ions. Its physiological function at the synapse is serotonin reuptake and thus termination of the signal. Since this protein is the site of action of the serotonin reuptake inhibitors, there has been much interest in the effect of polymorphisms of SERT on drug action and pathology.

The 5HTTLPR (serotonin transporter linked promoter region) of the *SLC6A4* gene has been extensively studied for association with neuropsychiatric disorders. This polymorphism occurs in the promoter region of the gene rather than in the protein coding region. It is associated with short *s* and long *l* repeats in this region. The short variation contains fourteen repeats of a particular sequence, while the long version contains sixteen repeats. The short version leads to reduced promoter activity and less transcription of *SLC6A4*, while the *l* allele has the opposite effect. A number of studies and meta-analyses have found that the ss genotype or s allele is predictive of reduced antidepressant efficacy, while the LL genotype is associated with better response to therapy. Other studies have found that presence of the s allele is associated with greater numbers of side effects during treatment of depression with selective serotonin reuptake inhibitors.[64] For instance, in one large study, adverse effects of citalopram were strongly associated with the 5HTTLPR s allele and ss genotype. Interestingly, in this study there was no differentiation between therapeutic responses for the different alleles.[65] In summary, there is mounting evidence that genetic screening may soon become useful for predicting if a given antidepressant will be effective or produce adverse effects in a patient. This would be a major advancement for individualizing the pharmacotherapy of depression.

The *SLC6A3* gene encodes for the dopamine transporter DAT1. Polymorphisms have been found for this transporter, and an attempt has been made to correlate genotype with neuropsychiatric disorders, such as attention deficit hyperactivity disorder (ADHD). One study suggested an association of a particular haplotype with adult ADHD.[66] The haplotype implicated was the 9-6 *SLC6A3*-haplotype, formed by the 9-repeat allele of the variable number of tandem repeat (VNTR) polymorphism in the 3' untranslated region of the gene and the 6-repeat allele of the VNTR in intron 8 of the gene. Polymorphisms of DAT1 have also been implicated in variability of response to methylphenidate in ADHD, although there has been conflicting results presented by a number of studies. In one meta-analysis, a significant relationship was seen between low rates of methylphenidate response and a homozygotic 10R VNTR polymorphism.[67]

The *SLC6A2* gene encodes for the norepinephrine transporter (NET). Because of the wide implications of this neurotransmitter in neuropsychiatric disorders and drug action, a number of studies have focused on finding polymorphisms for this gene and correlating them to therapeutic response. One study that examined predictive antidepressant response to the mixed serotonin/norepinephrine reuptake inhibitor milnacipran found that a polymorphism of NET was associated with superior response.[68] Substantially more research is needed in this area to make firm predictions regarding antidepressant response.

SLC15 Family
The PEPT1 and PEPT2 transporters (SLC15A1 and SLC15A2) are proton-coupled oligopeptide transporters. They carry small peptides of two to three residues, as well as peptide-like drugs that would otherwise not cross lipid membranes. Intestinal PEPT1 is involved in uptake of cephalexin and other -lactams. The nucleoside prodrugs valacyclovir and valganciclovir have enhanced bioavailability due to transport by PEPT1.[69] Significant interindividual variation in intestinal absorption of valacyclovir suggests the presence of genetic factors.[70] Angiotensin-converting enzyme inhibitors are also often considered to be substrates for PEPT1 and PEPT2; however, data supporting this claim is inconsistent.[71,72] Besides being localized in the intestine, PEPT transporters are found in the kidney and liver, and in the case of PEPT2, in the central and peripheral nervous system, lung, heart, and mammary glands.

Clinical relevance for genetic variation of PEPT1 or PEPT2 remains murky, but several researchers have studied polymorphisms of these loci. In one study, in a panel of 44 ethnically diverse individuals, nine nonsynonymous and four synonymous polymorphisms were identified in PEPT1.[73] When transfected into an immortal cell line and analyzed for transport capacity, only one rare SNP (Pro586Leu) was found to be associated with reduced activity, which resulted from post-translational reduction of protein expression in the plasma membrane. The results of this study have been confirmed and extended to 247 individuals of various ethnic origins.[74] This study found that there were additional genetic variants of PEPT1, but concluded genetic factors played only a small role in determining interindividual variation in

PEPT1 transport activity in the intestine. Because of the vital role that PEPT1 plays in normal homeostasis, mutations that result in loss of activity likely have a high negative evolutionary selection pressure. This does not, however, preclude future discovery of polymorphs with variation in expression or activity. In the case of PEPT2, polymorphs have been identified that lack transport function and have differing affinity and pH sensitivity. Variable mRNA expression has also been observed, likely due to *cis* acting polymorphisms.[75] Thus there is a considerable variability in the PEPT2 gene, with a possible influence on the pharmacokinetics of drugs transported by PEPT2.

SLC19A1

SLC19A1, also known as reduced folate carrier-1 (RFC-1), is involved in the transport of folate and antifolate drugs into human cells. Resistance to folate anticancer drugs may be mediated by point mutations of this transporter. Since lack of nutritional folate is strongly associated with birth defects such as cleft palate, it would be expected that variants of the folate carrier might also be associated with these defects. While one study failed to show a strong correlation between genetic variants of RFC-1 and cleft palate, this same study did show modest evidence for an interaction between infant RFC-1 genotype and risk of certain congenital heart defects.[76] The specific variant examined was the SNP 80A>G, which results in the replacement of a histidine residue with an arginine in the protein.[77] The functional result of this replacement on the transport protein is unknown, but higher plasma folate levels were observed in individuals homozygous for A80 compared to individuals with a G80/G80 genotype.

Methotrexate is an example of a drug that is transported by the reduced folate carrier-1. The 80G>A polymorphism in RFC-1 has been associated with altered treatment efficacy in patients with rheumatoid arthritis treated with methotrexate. In one study, the probability of remission was 3.3-fold higher in patients with the 80AA genotype compared to those with the 80GG genotype. The frequency of the A allele was also found to be 14% higher in patients that responded to methotrexate compared to nonresponders. Additionally, aminotransferase activity was noted more frequently in carriers of the 80AA genotype.[78] All of this information suggests that evaluation of RFC-1 polymorphism could be useful for optimization of methotrexate therapy.

Another study examined the effect of the Gly80Ala polymorphism in RFC-1 in relation to risk for thrombosis.[79] Since folate lowers homocysteine, which is thrombogenic, reduction in the transport of folate might be expected to have an effect on the prevalence of thrombosis. This study did find a significant protective effect of the A allele against thrombosis. No effect on homocysteine plasma level was observed, but an increased extracellular to intracellular ratio of folate was seen. This is consistent with the biological role of RFC-1 and may explain the protective effect of the polymorph against thrombosis.

SLC28

There are three members of the *SLC28* gene family in humans: *SLC28A1, SLC28A2,* and *SLC28A3.* All of them encode nucleoside transporters coupled to ion gradients (i.e., concentrative nucleoside transporters CNT1, CNT2, and CNT3). CNT1 translocates pyrimidines, while CNT2 translocates purines. Both of them are coupled to sodium ion transport. The CNT3 transporter has broad selectivity and can transport nucleosides coupled to either sodium ions or protons. This coupling allows the transporters to move nucleosides against their concentration gradient. Besides transporting naturally occurring nucleosides such as adenosine, these transporters are vitally important in transporting anticancer/antiviral nucleosides into cells. Since nucleoside drugs are mostly hydrophilic molecules, cellular uptake is dependent on transport proteins. Along with the SLC29 family, SLC28 members are important for salvage processing of nucleosides. SNPs of the CNTs have been identified, but pharmacogenomic relevance is currently poorly defined.

SL29

The family *SLC29* genes code for equilibrative nucleoside transporter proteins (ENT). There are four members of this family in humans: SLC29A1 to SLC29A4 (ENT1 to ENT4). ENT1 is independent of sodium ion concentration, in contrast to concentrative nucleoside transporters. This transporter plays a role in cellular uptake of anticancer nucleoside analogs.[80] The clinical relevance of this finding is currently unclear, although a number of polymorphisms at this gene have been uncovered. In one study on a population of 256 Japanese cancer patients, 39 variations of the gene were found, with a highest frequency of 0.051.[81]

Summary

In summary, evidence is accumulating of the many ways in which genotype for individual transport proteins affects the response to a variety of medications. Additionally, the profound effect of racial/ethnic heritage on distribution of genotypic variation can no longer be ignored. This chapter has reviewed some of the transporters with accumulated evidence for pharmacogenomic relevance. Many other transporters have been identified that also may ultimately be found to be important for determining individual therapeutic response. Also, many more SNPs for transport proteins have been identified than have been studied in vivo. The advent of inexpensive broad genetic screening for transport protein polymorphisms will no doubt be instrumental in a new era of truly personalized therapy. For instance, DNA chips are now available that screen 100,000 SNPs in a matter of hours. In order to solidify treatment guidelines for genetically diverse populations, significant amounts of research continue to be needed in this area. Since few drugs are transported by just one carrier protein, other carriers may compensate for a deleterious SNP. Thus a single SNP is often not capable of altering the pharmacokinetics of a drug. For this reason, future studies that are more comprehensive in scope will offer more insight into the genetics of drug response.

References

1. Huang Y, Sadée W. Membrane transporters and channels in chemoresistance and -sensitivity of tumor cells. *Cancer Letters*. 2006;239:168.
2. Klein I, Sarkadi B, Varadi A. An inventory of the human ABC proteins. *Biochem Biophys Acta*. 1999;1461:237.
3. de Jong FA, de Jonge MJA, Verweij J, et al. Role of pharmacogenetics in irinotecan therapy. *Cancer Letters*. 2006;234:90.
4. Smith NF, Figg WD, Sparreboom A. Pharmacogenetics of irinotecan metabolism and transport: An update. *Toxicology in Vitro*. 2006;20:163.
5. Takane H, Kawamoto K, Sasaki T, et al. Life-threatening toxicities in a patient with UG-T1A1*6/*28 and SLCO1B1*15/*15 genotypes after irinotecan-based chemotherapy. *Cancer Chemother Pharmacol*. 2009;63:1165.
6. Takane H, Miyata M, Burioka N, et al. Severe toxicities after irinotecan-based chemotherapy in a patient with lung cancer: a homozygote for the SLCO1B1*15 allele. *Ther Drug Monit*. 2007;29:666.
7. Williams JA, Andersson T, Andersson TB, et al. PhRMA white paper on ADME pharmacogenomics. *J Clin Pharmacol*. 2008;48:849.

8. Oldham ML, Davidson AL, Chen J. Structural insights into ABC transporter mechanism. *Curr Opin Struct Biol.* 2008;18:726-733.

9. Davidson AL, Maloney PC. ABC transporters: how small machines do a big job. *Trends Microbiol.* 2007;15:448.

10. Rabow AA, Shoemaker RH, Sausville EA, et al. Mining the National Cancer Institute's tumor-screening database: identification of compounds with similar cellular activities. *J Med Chem.* 2002;45:818-840.

11. Martin F, Fromm ME. The pharmacogenomics of human P-glycoprotein. In: Licinio J, Wong ML, eds. *Pharmacogenomics: The Search for Individualized Therapies.* Weinheim, Germany: Wiley VCH; 2003:159-178.

12. Ambudkar SV, Kimchi-Sarfaty C, Sauna ZE, et al. P-glycoprotein: from genomics to mechanism. *Oncogene.* 2003;22:7468.

13. Leschziner GD, Andrew T, Pirmohamed M, et al. ABCB1 genotype and PGP expression, function and therapeutic drug response: a critical review and recommendations for future research [review]. *Pharmacogenomics J.* 2007;7:154-179.

14. Ameyaw MM, Regateiro F, Li T, et al. MDR1 pharmacogenetics: frequency of the C3435T mutation in exon 26 is significantly influenced by ethnicity. *Pharmacogenetics.* 2001;11:217.

15. Marzolini C, Paus E, Buclin T, et al. Polymorphisms in human MDR1 (P-glycoprotein): recent advances and clinical relevance. *Clin Pharmacol Ther.* 2004;75:13.

16. Pauli-Magnus C, Kroetz DL. Functional implications of genetic polymorphisms in the multidrug resistance gene MDR1 (ABCB1). *Pharm Res.* 2004;21:904.

17. Ieiri I, Takane H, Otsubo K. The MDR1 (ABCB1) gene polymorphism and its clinical implications. *Clin Pharmacokinet.* 2004;43:553.

18. Hoffmeyer S, Burk O, von Richter O, et al. Functional polymorphisms of the human multidrug-resistance gene: multiple sequence variations and correlation of one allele with P-glycoprotein expression and activity in vivo. *Proc Natl Acad Sci USA.* 2000;97:3473.

19. Eichelbaum M, Fromm MF, Schwab M. Clinical aspects of the MDR1 (ABCB1) gene polymorphism. *Ther Drug Monit.* 2004;26:180.

20. Pan JH, Han JX, Wu JM, et al. MDR1 single nucleotide polymorphism G2677T/A and haplotype are correlated with response to docetaxel-cisplatin chemotherapy in patients with non-small-cell lung cancer. *Respiration.* 2009;78:49-55.

21. Kim RB, Leake BF, Choo EF, et al. Identification of functionally variant MDR1 alleles among European Americans and African Americans. *Clin Pharmacol Ther.* 2001;70:189.

22. Schaeffeler E, Eichelbaum M, Brinkmann U, et al. Frequency of C3435T polymorphism of MDR1 gene in African people. *The Lancet.* 2001;358:383.

23. Min DI, Lee M, Ku YM, et al. Gender-dependent racial difference in disposition of cyclosporine among healthy African American and white volunteers. *Clin Pharmacol Ther.* 2000;68:478.

24. Elmore JG, Moceri VM, Carter D, et al. Breast carcinoma tumor characteristics in black and white women. *Cancer.* 1998;83:2509.

25. Cross CK, Harris J, Recht A. Race, socioeconomic status, and breast carcinoma in the US: what have we learned from clinical studies. *Cancer.* 2002;95:1988.

26. Aarnoudse AJ, Dieleman JP, Visser LE, et al. Common ATP-binding cassette B1 variants are associated with increased digoxin serum concentration. *Pharmacogenet Genomics.* 2008;18:299-305.

27. Verstuyft C, Schwab M, Schaeffeler E, et al. Digoxin pharmacokinetics and MDR1 genetic polymorphisms. *Eur J Clin Pharmacol.* 2003;58:809.

28. Sakaeda T, Nakamura T, Horinouchi M, et al. MDR1 genotype-related pharmacokinetics of digoxin after single oral administration in healthy Japanese subjects. *Pharm Res.* 2001;18:1400.

29. Hur EH, Lee JH, Lee MJ, et al. C3435T polymorphism of the MDR1 gene is not associated with P-glycoprotein function of leukemic blasts and clinical outcome in patients with acute myeloid leukemia. *Leuk Res.* 2008;32:1601.

30. Schuetz EG, Furuya KN, Schuetz JD. Interindividual variation in expression of P-glycoprotein in normal human liver and secondary hepatic neoplasms. *J Pharmacol Exp Ther.* 1995;275:1011-1018.

31. Davis M. Gender differences in p-glycoprotein: drug toxicity and response. *J Clin Oncol.* 2005;23:6439-6440.

32. Sai K, Kaniwa N, Itoda M, et al. Haplotype analysis of ABCB1/MDR1 blocks in a Japanese population reveals genotype-dependent renal clearance of irinotecan. *Pharmacogenetics.* 2003;13:741.

33. de Jong FA, Scott-Horton TJ, Kroetz DL, et al. Irinotecan-induced diarrhea: functional significance of the polymorphic ABCC2 transporter protein. *Clin Pharmacol Ther.* 2007;81:42.

34. Mathijssen RHJ, Marsh S, Karlsson MO, et al. Irinotecan pathway genotype analysis to predict pharmacokinetics. *Clin Cancer Res.* 2003;9:3246.

35. Mathijssen RHJ, de Jong FA, van Schaik RHN, et al. Prediction of irinotecan pharmacokinetics by use of cytochrome P450 3A4 phenotyping probes. *J Natl Cancer Inst.* 2004;96:1585.

36. Innocenti F, Kroetz DL, Schuetz E, et al. Comprehensive pharmacogenetic analysis of irinotecan neutropenia and pharmacokinetics. *J Clin Oncol.* 2009;27:2604-2614.

37. Han JY, Lim HS, Yoo YK, et al. Associations of ABCB1, ABCC2, and ABCG2 polymorphisms with irinotecan-pharmacokinetics and clinical outcome in patients with advanced non-small cell lung cancer. *Cancer.* 2007;110:138.

38. Balram C, Li J, Zhou QY, et al. Molecular mechanisms of interethnic differences in irinotecan disposition: impact of variants in ABCG2. *J Clin Oncol* (meeting abstracts.) 2005;23(16 suppl):2018.

39. Gradhand U, Kim RB. Pharmacogenomics of MRP transporters (ABCC1-5) and BCRP (ABCG2). *Drug Metab Rev.* 2008;40:317.

40. Conrad S, Kauffmann HM, Ito K, et al. A naturally occurring mutation in MRP1 results in a selective decrease in organic anion transport and in increased doxorubicin resistance. *Pharmacogenetics.* 2002;12:321-330.

41. Leslie EM, Letourneau IJ, Deeley RG, et al. Functional and structural consequences of cysteine substitutions in the NH2 proximal region of the human multidrug resistance protein 1 (MRP1/ABCC1). *Biochemistry.* 2003;42:5214.

42. Wang Z, Wang B, Tang K, et al. A functional polymorphism within the MRP1 gene locus identified through its genomic signature of positive selection. *Hum Mol Genet.* 2005;14:2075-2087.

43. Nakamura T, Yamamori M, Sakaeda T. Pharmacogenetics of intestinal absorption. *Curr Drug Deliv.* 2008;5:153.

44. Hulot JS, Villard E, Maguy A, et al. A mutation in the drug transporter gene ABCC2 associated with impaired methotrexate elimination. *Pharmacogenet Genomics.* 2005;15:277.

45. Noma B, Sasaki T, Fujimoto Y, et al. Expression of multidrug resistance-associated protein 2 is involved in chemotherapy resistance in human pancreatic cancer. *Int J Oncol.* 2008;33:1187.

46. Grant CE, Gao M, DeGorter MK, et al. Structural determinants of substrate specificity differences between human multidrug resistance protein (MRP) 1 (ABCC1) and MRP3 (ABCC3). *Drug Metab Dispos.* 2008;36:2571.

47. Lang T, Hitzl M, Burk O, et al. Genetic polymorphisms in the multidrug resistance-associated protein 3 (ABCC3, MRP3) gene and relationship to its mRNA and protein expression in human liver. *Pharmacogenetics.* 2004;14:155.

48. Müller P, Asher N, Heled M, et al. Polymorphisms in transporter and phase II metabolism genes as potential modifiers of the predisposition to and treatment outcome of de novo acute myeloid leukemia in Israeli ethnic groups. *Leukemia Research.* 2008;32:919.

49. Doerfel C, Rump A, Sauerbrey A, et al. In acute leukemia, the polymorphism -211C>T in the promoter region of the multidrug resistance-associated protein 3 (MRP3) does not determine the expression level of the gene. *Pharmacogenet Genomics.* 2006;16:149-150.

50. Krishnamurthy P, Schwab M, Takenaka K, et al. Transporter-mediated protection against thiopurine-induced hematopoietic toxicity. *Cancer Res.* 2008;68:4983.

51. Cusatis G, Sparreboom A. Pharmacogenomic importance of ABCG2. *Pharmacogenomics.* 2008;9:1005.

52. Mao Q, Unadkat JD. Role of the breast cancer resistance protein (ABCG2) in drug transport. *AAPS J.* 2005;7:118.

53. Krishnamurthy P, Schuetz JD. Role of ABCG2/BCRP in biology and medicine. *Annu Rev Pharmacol Toxicol.* 2006;46:381.

54. Adkison KK, Vaidya SS, Lee DY, et al. The ABCG2 C421A polymorphism does not affect oral nitrofurantoin pharmacokinetics in healthy Chinese male subjects. *Br J Clin Pharmacol.* 2008;66:233-239.

55. Kim HS, Sunwoo YE, Ryu JY, et al. The effect of ABCG2 V12M, Q141K and Q126X, known functional variants in vitro, on the disposition of lamivudine. *Br J Clin Pharmacol.* 2007;64:645-654.

56. Weiss J, Rose J, Storch CH, et al. Modulation of human BCRP (ABCG2) activity by anti-HIV drugs. *J Antimicrob Chemother.* 2007;59:238-245.

57. Cusatis G, Gregorc V, Li J, et al. Pharmacogenetics of ABCG2 and adverse reactions to gefitinib. *J Natl Cancer Inst.* 2006;98:1739-1742.

58. Dehghan A, Kottgen A, Yang Q, et al. Association of three genetic loci with uric acid concentration and risk of gout: a genome-wide association study. *Lancet.* 2008;372:1953-1961.

59. Mao Q. BCRP/ABCG2 in the placenta: expression, function and regulation. *Pharmaceutical Research.* 2008;25:1244-1255.

60. Kondo C, Suzuki H, Itoda M, et al. Functional analysis of SNPs variants of BCRP/ABCG2. *Pharmaceutical Research.* 2004;21:1895-1903.

61. SEARCH Collaborative Group, Link E, Parish S, Armitage J, et al. SLCO1B1 variants and statin-induced myopathy—a genomewide study. *N Engl J Med.* 2008;359:789-799.

62. Nishizato Y, Ieiri I, Suzuki H, et al. Polymorphisms of OATP-C (SLC21A6) and OAT3 (SLC22A8) genes: consequences for pravastatin pharmacokinetics. *Clin Pharmacol Ther.* 2003;73:554.

63. Rohrbacher M, Kirchhof A, Skarke C, et al. Rapid identification of three functionally relevant polymorphisms in the OATP1B1 transporter gene using pyrosequencing. *Pharmacogenomics.* 2006;7:167.

64. Murphy DL, Fox MA, Timpano KR, et al. How the serotonin story is being rewritten by new gene-based discoveries principally related to SLC6A4, the serotonin transporter gene, which functions to influence all cellular serotonin systems. *Neuropharmacology.* 2008;55:932.

65. Hu XZ, Rush AJ, Charney D, et al. Association between a functional serotonin transporter promoter polymorphism and citalopram treatment in adult outpatients with major depression. *Arch Gen Psychiatry.* 2007;64:783-792.

66. Franke B, Hoogman M, Arias Vasquez A, et al. Association of the dopamine transporter (SLC6A3/DAT1) gene 9-6 haplotype with adult ADHD. *Am J Med Genet B Neuropsychiatr Genet.* 2008;147B:1576-1579.

67. Purper-Ouakil D, Wohl M, Orejarena S, et al. Pharmacogenetics of methylphenidate response in attention deficit/hyperactivity disorder: association with the dopamine transporter gene (SLC6A3). *Am J Med Genet B Neuropsychiatr Genet.* 2008;147B:1425-1430

68. Yoshida K, Takahashi H, Higuchi H, et al. Prediction of antidepressant response to milnacipran by norepinephrine transporter gene polymorphisms. *Am J Psychiatry.* 2004;161:1575-1580.

69. Li F, Maag H, Alfredson T. Prodrugs of nucleoside analogues for improved oral absorption and tissue targeting. *J Pharm Sci.* 2008;97:1109-1134.

70. Phan DD, Chin-Hong P, Lin ET, et al. Intra- and interindividual variabilities of valacyclovir oral bioavailability and effect of coadministration of an hPEPT1 inhibitor. *Antimicrob Agents Chemother.* 2003;47:2351.

71. Knutter I, Wollesky C, Kottra G, et al. Transport of angiotensin-converting enzyme inhibitors by H+/peptide transporters revisited. *J Pharmacol Exp Ther.* 2008;327:432-441.

72. Brandsch M, Knutter I, Bosse-Doenecke E. Pharmaceutical and pharmacological importance of peptide transporters. *J Pharm Pharmacol.* 2008;60:543-585.

73. Zhang EY, Fu DJ, Pak YA, et al. Genetic polymorphisms in human proton-dependent dipeptide transporter PEPT1: implications for the functional role of Pro586. *J Pharmacol Exp Ther.* 2004;310:437-445.

74. Anderle P, Nielsen CU, Pinsonneault J, et al. Genetic variants of the human dipeptide transporter PEPT1. *J Pharmacol Exp Ther.* 2006;316:636-646.

75. Pinsonneault J, Nielsen CU, Sadee W. Genetic variants of the human H+/dipeptide transporter PEPT2: analysis of haplotype functions. *J Pharmacol Exp Ther.* 2004;311:1088.

76. Shaw GM, Zhu H, Lammer EJ, et al. Genetic variation of infant reduced folate carrier (A80G) and risk of orofacial and conotruncal heart defects. *Am J Epidemiol.* 2003;158:747-752.

77. Chango A, Emery-Fillon N, de Courcy GP, et al. A polymorphism (80G->A) in the reduced folate carrier gene and its associations with folate status and homocysteinemia. *Mol Genet Metab.* 2000;70:310.

78. Drozdzik M, Rudas T, Pawlik A, et al. Reduced folate carrier-1 80G>A polymorphism affects methotrexate treatment outcome in rheumatoid arthritis. *Pharmacogenomics J.* 2007;7:404.

79. Yates Z, Lucock M. G80A reduced folate carrier SNP modulates cellular uptake of folate and affords protection against thrombosis via a non homocysteine related mechanism. *Life Sciences.* 2005;77:2735.

80. Huang Y, Anderle P, Bussey KJ, et al. Membrane transporters and channels: role of the transportome in cancer chemosensitivity and chemoresistance. *Cancer Res.* 2004;64:4294-4301.

81. Kim SR, Saito Y, Maekawa K, et al. Thirty novel genetic variations in the SLC29A1 gene encoding human equilibrative nucleoside transporter 1 (hENT1). *Drug Metab Pharmacokinet.* 2006;21:248.

82. Lal S, Wong ZW, Sandanaraj E, et al. Influence of *ABCB1* and *ABCG2* polymorphisms on doxorubicin disposition in Asian breast cancer patients. *Cancer Sci.* 2008;99:816-823.

83. Toh S, Wada M, Uchiumi T, et al. Genomic structure of the canalicular multispecific organic anion-transporter gene (MRP2/cMOAT) and mutations in the ATP-binding-cassette region in Dubin-Johnson syndrome. *Am J Hum Genet.* 1999;64:739.

84. Hoblinger A, Grunhage F, Sauerbruch T, et al. Association of the c.3972C>T variant of the multidrug resistance-associated protein 2 gene (MRP2/ABCC2) with susceptibility to bile duct cancer. *Digestion.* 2009;80:36.

85. Zamek-Gliszczynski MJ, Nezasa K, Tian X, et al. Evaluation of the role of multidrug resistance-associated protein (Mrp) 3 and Mrp4 in hepatic basolateral excretion of sulfate and glucuronide metabolites of acetaminophen, 4-methylumbelliferone, and harmol in Abcc3-/- and Abcc4-/- mice. *J Pharmacol Exp Ther.* 2006;319:1485-1491.

86. Zelcer N, van de Wetering K, Hillebrand M, et al. Mice lacking multidrug resistance protein 3 show altered morphine pharmacokinetics and morphine-6-glucuronide antinociception. *Proc Natl Acad Sci USA.* 2005;102:7274.

87. Muller PJ, Dally H, Klappenecker CN, et al. Polymorphisms in ABCG2, ABCC3 and CNT1 genes and their possible impact on chemotherapy outcome of lung cancer patients. *Int J Cancer.* 2009;124:1669.

88. Kobayashi K, Ito K, Takada T, et al. Functional analysis of nonsynonymous single nucleotide polymorphism type ATP-binding cassette transmembrane transporter subfamily C member 3. *Pharmacogenet Genomics.* 2008;18:823.

89. Ho LL, Kench JG, Handelsman DJ, et al. Androgen regulation of multidrug resistance-associated protein 4 (MRP4/ABCC4) in prostate cancer. *Prostate.* 2008;68:1421.

90. El-Sheikh AA, van den Heuvel JJ, Koenderink JB, et al. Effect of hypouricaemic and hyperuricaemic drugs on the renal urate efflux transporter, multidrug resistance protein 4. *Br J Pharmacol.* 2008;155:1066-1075.

91. Torky A-RW, Stehfest E, Viehweger K, et al. Immuno-histochemical detection of MRPs in human lung cells in culture. *Toxicology.* 2005;207:437.

92. Nies AT, Jedlitschky G, Konig J, et al. Expression and immunolocalization of the multidrug resistance proteins, MRP1-MRP6 (ABCC1-ABCC6), in human brain. *Neuroscience.* 2004;129:349.

93. Konig J, Hartel M, Nies AT, et al. Expression and localization of human multidrug resistance protein (ABCC) family members in pancreatic carcinoma. *Int J Cancer.* 2005;115:359.

94. Schuetz JD, Connelly MC, Sun D, et al. MRP4: a previously unidentified factor in resistance to nucleoside-based antiviral drugs. *Nat Med.* 1999;5:1048.

95. Jedlitschky G, Tirschmann K, Lubenow LE, et al. The nucleotide transporter MRP4 (ABCC4) is highly expressed in human platelets and present in dense granules, indicating a role in mediator storage. *Blood.* 2004;104:3603.

96. Dazert P, Meissner K, Vogelgesang S, et al. Expression and localization of the multidrug resistance protein 5 (MRP5/ABCC5), a cellular export pump for cyclic nucleotides, in human heart. *Am J Pathol.* 2003;163:1567.

97. Abla N, Chinn LW, Nakamura T, et al. The human multidrug resistance protein 4 (MRP4, ABCC4): functional analysis of a highly polymorphic gene. *J Pharmacol Exp Ther.* 2008;325:859.

98. Kiser JJ, Aquilante CL, Anderson PL, et al. Clinical and genetic determinants of intracellular tenofovir diphosphate concentrations in HIV-infected patients. *J Acquir Immune Defic Syndr.* 2008;47:298.

99. Shi Y, Terry SF, Terry PF, et al. Development of a rapid, reliable genetic test for pseudoxanthoma elasticum. *J Mol Diagn.* 2007;9:105.

100. Kim IS, Kim HG, Kim DC, et al. ABCG2 Q141K polymorphism is associated with chemotherapy-induced diarrhea in patients with diffuse large B-cell lymphoma who received frontline rituximab plus cyclophosphamide/doxorubicin/vincristine/prednisone chemotherapy. *Cancer Sci.* 2008;99:2496.

101. Gill RK, Pant N, Saksena S, et al. Function, expression, and characterization of the serotonin transporter in the native human intestine. *Am J Physiol Gastrointest Liver Physiol.* 2008;294:254.

102. Goldberg TE, Kotov R, Lee AT, et al. The serotonin transporter gene and disease modification in psychosis: Evidence for systematic differences in allelic directionality at the 5-HTTLPR locus. *Schizophr Res.* 2009;111:103.

103. Dervieux T, Kremer J, Lein DO, et al. Contribution of common polymorphisms in reduced folate carrier and gamma-glutamylhydrolase to methotrexate polyglutamate levels in patients with rheumatoid arthritis. *Pharmacogenetics.* 2004;14:733.

104. Ho RH, Choi L, Lee W, et al. Effect of drug transporter genotypes on pravastatin disposition in European- and African-American participants. *Pharmacogenet Genomics.* 2007;17:647.

105. Miura M, Satoh S, Inoue K, et al. Influence of SLCO1B1, 1B3, 2B1 and ABCC2 genetic polymorphisms on mycophenolic acid pharmacokinetics in Japanese renal transplant recipients. *Eur J Clin Pharmacol.* 2007;63:1161.

106. Rubio-Aliaga I, Daniel H. Peptide transporters and their roles in physiological processes and drug disposition. *Xenobiotica.* 2008;38:1022-1042.

107. Terada T, Irie M, Okuda M, et al. Genetic variant Arg57His in human H+/peptide cotransporter 2 causes a complete loss of transport function. *Biochem Biophys Res Commun.* 2004;316:416.

108. Govindarajan R, Bakken AH, Hudkins KL, et al. In situ hybridization and immunolocalization of concentrative and equilibrative nucleoside transporters in the human intestine, liver, kidneys, and placenta. *Am J Physiol Regul Integr Comp Physiol.* 2007;293:R1809-R1822.

Chapter 6

Pharmacodynamics and Pharmacogenomics

Kathy D. Webster, Pharm.D., Ph.D.

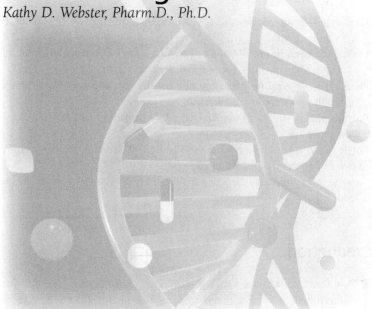

Learning Objectives

After completing this chapter, the reader should be able to

- Explain the key terms.
- List the common types of drug targets that are affected by genetic polymorphism.
- Describe the consequences of genetic variability on drug action.
- Describe the types of drug targets that have demonstrated or are associated with genetic variability and give examples of each type.
- Explain how genetic variability can indirectly modulate the overall drug response.
- Discuss the role of genetic variability on the incidence of adverse drug reactions.
- List common examples of genetic polymorphism and adverse drug reactions.
- Discuss the role of disease state biomarkers and drug response.

Key Definitions

Biomarker—An indicator of a particular disease state or a particular state of an organism.

Drug target—An enzyme or receptor protein that is a direct target of a drug, a signal transduction or downstream protein that mediates a drug response or a protein associated with a disease that is modified by a drug.

Epigenetics—Heritable changes in gene function that occurs without change in the sequence of nuclear DNA.

Genotype—Set of two alleles carried by an individual at a given polymorphic site.

Germline mutations—Genetic variation that is detectable and occurs in germ cells, a heritable mutation.

Haplotype—Group of alleles on a single chromosome that are closely linked such that they are inherited as a unit.

Linkage disequilibrium—Multiple SNPs that always appear together, the alleles are inherited as a unit, also known as a haplotype block.

Phenotype—Physical manifestation of a genetic trait or a general constitutional manifestation of health or disease in an individual.

Polymorphism—Genetic variation in the DNA sequence with a measurable frequency of detection above 1%.

Single nucleotide polymorphism (SNP)—Genetic variation at a single DNA base with a measurable frequency of detection above 1%.

Somatic cell mutations—Genetic variation that occurs only in an affected organ or disease locus (tumor), acquired mutation.

Introduction

The use of pharmacogenetic markers or biomarkers to identify patients who will most likely benefit from a given treatment is an important new tool for optimizing drug therapy. Pharmacogenetic studies associate a characteristic drug response (i.e., a phenotype), with a genetic polymorphism (i.e., a genotype). These polymorphisms may include single nucleotide polymorphisms (SNPs), nucleotide sequence repeats, insertions (I), deletions (D), or grouped mutations (haplotypes), which are characteristic of the genotype. A patient is considered homozygous if both copies of the gene, each allele, is the same and heterozygous if each of the alleles is different. Mutations can occur in both germline (inherited) DNA or somatic (tumor or tissue-specific) DNA.

Pharmacodynamic-based pharmacogenetic studies focus on drug targets. Altered drug response has been associated with allelic variants of genes encoding for molecular targets and their associated modifiers, or key proteins in the pathophysiology of systems affected by the drug. Over- or under-expression of normal proteins or production of variant proteins for receptors, enzymes, ion channels, transcription factors, and intracellular or extracellular signaling proteins can all modify drug response.

Clinical Pearl

Pharmacodynamic-based genetic variability is more complicated and less understood compared to pharmacokinetic-based genetic variability.

Our understanding of pharmacokinetic-based pharmacogenetics is more advanced than our understanding of pharmacodynamic-based pharmacogenetics. Unlike pharmacokinetic studies where a genetic variation in an enzyme or transporter might affect many drugs or disease states, pharmacodynamic studies generally focus on one drug, one drug class or one disease-specific target at a time. This more narrow focus slows the progress of pharmacodynamic-based pharmacogenetics. The correlation of pharmacogenetic variability in drug targets with clinical outcomes has shown inconsistent results, this may be due in part to attempts to relate single SNPs to pharmacodynamic variability whereas a more complex relationship may be present. Multiple SNPs or haplotypes may be better predictors of drug target response. In addition, the complexity of a drug response typically involves multiple components. For example a cell surface receptor typically utilizes a protein receptor which interfaces with a multi-component second messenger cascade; genetic variation in one or more of these components may affect the ultimate outcome of the drug response. Many physiological responses are likewise mediated by a balance between multiple receptor types, thus the complexity increases when trying to pinpoint the impact of a single genetic mutation. It is likely that a genetic profile of relevant genes would be more helpful than the genotyping of a single SNP or haplotypes in predicting therapeutic outcome.[1]

Variability in the drug response phenotype can also be due to more than one mutation which affects <u>both</u> the pharmacokinetic and the pharmacodynamic properties of the drug.[2] The pharmacokinetic characteristics will determine how much drug gets to the site of action while the pharmacodynamic characteristics will determine the responsiveness of the drug target. Two recently characterized examples, warfarin and beta blockers, illustrate this concept.

Warfarin, an anticoagulant drug with a narrow therapeutic index, shows significant variability in its dose response. Inappropriate dosing for an individual patient can lead to serious adverse outcomes; too much warfarin will result in excess bleeding while insufficient warfarin can result in blood-clot formation. Both of these conditions may be life-threatening. At least one pharmacokinetic and one pharmacodynamic polymorphism have been shown to affect the therapeutic response of warfarin (Figure 6-1). S-Warfarin, the most potent enantiomer of the racemic mixture is predominantly metabolized by CYP2C9. The cytochrome P450 enzyme, CYP2C9, has a well characterized genetic polymorphism (See Chapter 4 The Pharmacogenetics of Drug Metabolism). The CYP2C9*2 and *3 alleles are significantly less active than the wild-type allele, CYP2C9*1. An individual who carries one or more of the mutant alleles will have reduced metabolism of warfarin with a concomitant increase in drug levels and risk of hemorrhaging. The molecular target for warfarin is vitamin K epoxide reductase complex I (VKORCI). VKORCI converts vitamin K epoxide to the active reduced form of vitamin K which is required for synthesis of coagulation factors; warfarin inhibits this enzymatic conversion. A series of characterized haplotypes have been associated with high or low dose warfarin requirements (see the section in this chapter on enzymes as drug targets). The warfarin dose requirement is indicative of VKORCI enzymatic activity. A haplotype that requires low dose warfarin has a much lower intrinsic enzymatic activity compared to a haplotype that requires high dose warfarin. Thus, a patient with both decreased drug metabolism (CYP2C9 activity) and enhanced inhibition of the target (VKORCI) would require a much lower dose of warfarin compared to the "average patient" in order to achieve the desired therapeutic response. The combination of CYP2C9 and VKORCI genetic polymorphisms and other risk factors accounts for more than 50% of dosing variability seen with warfarin.[4]

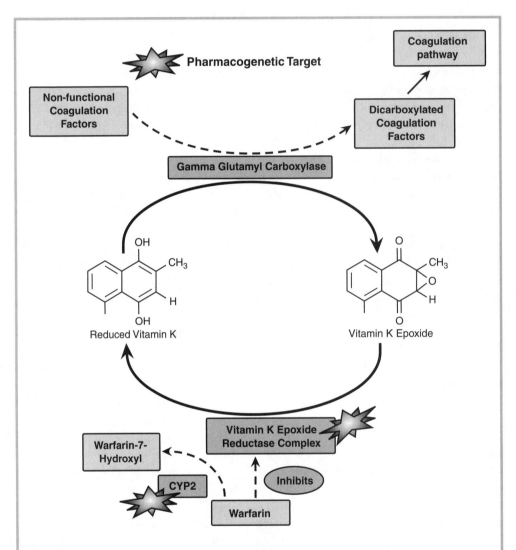

Figure 6.1 • Warfarin inhibits the vitamin K epoxide reductase complex (VKORC1), decreasing the availability of reduced vitamin K. Reduced vitamin K is required for synthesis of the coagulation factors, which must be activated to produce coagulation. Both pharmacokinetics and pharmacodynamics affect patient variability. The pharmacokinetic polymorphism is in cytochrome P450 2C9 (CYP2C9) and the pharmacodynamic polymorphisms are found in VKORC1. (Source: Figure modified from reference 3.)

The clinical outcomes of beta blockers or beta$_1$ adrenergic receptor antagonists are also affected by both pharmacokinetic and pharmacodynamic genetic variations. Many beta blockers are metabolized by another cytochrome P450 isoform, CYP2D6. Phenotypes for CYP2D6 metabolism can be classified as poor metabolizers (PM), intermediate metabolizers (IM), extensive metabolizers (EM) and ultra-rapid metabolizers (UM).[5] With chronic administration of an equivalent dose of the beta blocker metoprolol, PMs had approximately fivefold higher blood levels compared to non-PMs.[6] Metoprolol produced greater reductions in heart rate, diastolic blood pressure, and mean arterial pressure in the PMs. Several polymorphisms of the beta$_1$ adrenergic receptor have also been characterized (see the section in this chapter on cell surface receptors as drug targets). Some studies have shown increased response to beta blockers in patients homozygous for the *Arg389* allele.[7] Its seems likely that the variation in response to beta blockers is determined by the metabolism as well as the receptor response. However, no study has yet documented the clinical interaction between these genes.

Pharmacodynamic variability associated with germline or somatic DNA mutations may result in increased or decreased susceptibility to disease. A significant change in a drug-target protein that causes loss or excessive functional activity may result in a disease phenotype. Beta adrenergic receptor polymorphism has been associated with asthma,[8] genetic variation of serotonin receptors may predict the risk of developing depression,[9] and mutated K$^+$ channels can result in cardiac arrhythmias.[10] The gene for APOE4 has been associated with increased progression of both coronary heart disease and Alzheimer's disease.[11] Somatic mutations of growth factor receptors are associated with highly aggressive forms of cancer.[12] Natural selection favors emergence of genetic mutations that provide protections from specific diseases, thus Glucose -6-phosphate dehydrogenase (G6PD) polymorphisms were thought to have developed to provide protection against malaria.[13]

The goal of pharmacogenetics is to optimize drug efficacy and minimize toxicity based on an individual's genetic profile. Ideally the clinician will be able to predict the patient's drug response based on his DNA and use this information to pick the "right drug and the right dose." Genetic polymorphisms in proteins that are drug targets will obviously mediate variability in drug response. More subtle changes in proteins that affect the physiological context, provide secondary targets, or mediate the development or severity of a disease will indirectly cause variations in drug response.

 ## *Case Study*

- A 25-year-old Caucasian woman was recently diagnosed with a urinary tract infection (UTI).
- The physician prescribed trimethoprim-sulfamethoxazole combination.
- After several days, the patient developed QT-prolongation.
- Trimethoprim-sulfamethoxazole was discontinued and patient exhibited a normal electrocardiogram.
- The patient was then started on clarithromycin and developed QT prolongation with this antibiotic as well.
  1. What is the likely cause of QT-prolongation?
  2. What is the role of trimethoprim-sulfamethizole in this adverse affect?
  3. Why did clarithromycin also cause the same adverse affect?
  4. What is the best course of action for this patient?

Consequences of Genetic Variability and Drug Pharmacodynamics

Pharmacogenetics can profoundly affect the efficacy and safety of a drug. Functional variations in the coding sequence or expression level of a drug target protein can affect responses to a drug by altering drug–target interactions and/or subsequent signaling events, producing insufficient or excessive pharmacological activity. In some situations the genetic variant can result in a total lack of response to the drug entity. Mutations in somatic cells, tumors, can provide a unique target that is not found in normal tissues and thus provides a drug effect that is specific for the tumor tissue.

Changes in genes that affect the physiological environment (i.e., variations that produce an underlying disease state or more subtle changes in homeostasis) can result in variability in the therapeutic response or an increased or decreased incident of a particular adverse drug reaction (ADR). Genetic variation in nontarget receptors can also result in variable risk for ADRs.

A full understanding of the role that genetic variation can play in pharmacodynamics will optimize therapeutic decision making. Drugs that will not work or will precipitate an ADR can be avoided. Patients who need to start at a higher or lower dose can be identified and treated accordingly.

Genetic Variability of Drug Targets

A mutation in the gene of a protein that functions as a drug target can result in enhanced or reduced drug response. Typical drug targets include cell surface or cytosolic receptor proteins or enzymes. A list of drug targets associated with genetic variants that have resulted in a pharmacodynamic change are summarized in Table 6-1.

Table 6-1
Drug Targets Associated With Genetic Variability to Drug Response

Target	Type	Affected Drug/Class
Beta2 adrenergic receptor	Cell surface receptor	Beta-2 receptor agonists (8, 14–25)
Beta1 adrenergic receptor	Cell surface receptor 2nd messenger	Beta-1 receptor agonists and antagonists (7, 26–33)
Chemokine (C-C motif) Receptor 5(CCR5)	Cell surface receptor	CCR5 inhibitors (34–40)
Mu opioid receptor	Cell surface receptor	Opioids (41–44)
Serotonin transporter and receptor	Cell surface receptor	Selective serotonin reuptake inhibitors (45–50)
Estrogen receptors	Cytosolic receptor	Estrogen/tamoxifen (51–53)
Vitamin K Epoxide Reductase Complex 1	Enzyme	Warfarin (54)
5-Lipoxygenase	Enzyme	Zileuton (55–57)
Angiotensin Converting Enzyme	Enzyme	ACE inhibitors (58–62)
Cyclo-oxygenase 2	Enzyme	NSAIDs (63)

Cell Surface Receptors and Signal Transduction Systems

Beta Adrenergic Receptors

Variability in drug response can be related to changes in the cell surface receptor and/or its second messenger proteins. A classic example can be found with the G-protein-coupled beta adrenergic receptors. The effect of genetic polymorphism on the activity of these beta adrenergic receptors has been extensively studied and modified drug response has been documented for both Beta$_1$ and Beta$_2$ receptor subtypes.

Beta$_2$ adrenergic receptors (ADRB2) are important mediators of bronchodilation, venodilation, and lipid metabolism. Although there are many inconsistencies in studies on genetic polymorphism of ADRB2, mutants in the gene coding for ADRB2 have been associated with significant variability in the response of asthma patients to short acting beta $_2$ agonists (SABA). No consistent results have been seen with the long acting beta $_2$ agonists (LABA).[14] The ADRB2 has also shown variable response to the vascular affects of beta agonists.[15]

At least 13 SNPs have been documented; two important modified receptor proteins have been identified, Arg16Gly and the Gln27Glu.[6,16] There is some linkage disequilibrium with these two SNPs, in that the *Arg16* allele is usually linked to the *Glu27*allele, but the *Gly16* allele can be linked with either the *Glu27* or the *Gln27*allele.[17] Individuals with *GlyGly16* gene were found to have higher rates of drug response and increased down regulation with albuterol compared to patients with the *ArgArg16* gene.[18,19] Studies have documented a decline in peak expiratory flow rates and exacerbation of asthma with regular use of SABAs in patients with the

ArgArg16 receptor.[18,20,21] Limited studies on the long-term use of LABA in conjunction with inhaled corticosteroid use reported no difference with the *Arg16* allele.[22] Another low frequency variant allele, *Thr164Ile*, has been characterized both functionally and clinically.[23,24] The Ile164 receptor has a threefold reduction in affinity for beta agonists and a decrease in basal and agonist-stimulated adenylyl cyclase activity.[23] In the dorsal hand vein model, the Ile164 variant was associated with a fivefold reduction in sensitivity to ADBR2 agonist (isoproterenol)-mediated vasodilation while vasoconstrictor (epinephrine) sensitivity was increased.[24]

Some studies have supported the genetic associations described above, but other studies have shown no difference or have had opposing results. The effect of receptor mutations on beta$_2$ agonist response is variable in different ethnic groups and as a result it is likely that examination of haplotypes containing these SNPs might be more useful in predicting the clinical response to beta$_2$ agonist.[16,25]

Beta$_1$ adrenergic receptors (ADRB1) are important in regulating heart rate and contractility as well as renin release in the kidney. ADRB1 is coupled to the stimulatory G-protein, G$_s$, which activates adenylyl cyclase, and other non-cAMP pathways including various ion channels (Figure 6-2). The two most common ADRB1 genetic polymorphisms, Ser49Gly and Arg389Gly, modify resting heart rate and blood pressure, and enhance the response to beta agonists and antagonists.[26]

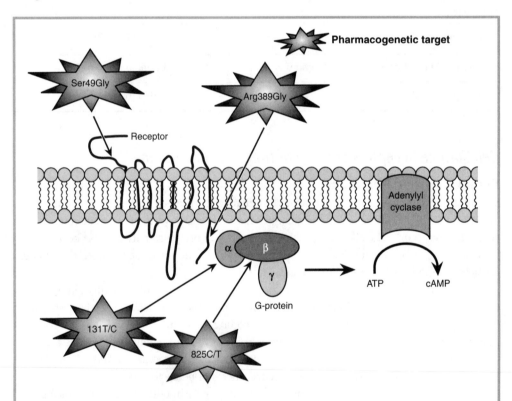

Figure 6.2 • The Ser49 and the Arg389 alleles in the receptor protein show enhanced receptor activity and increased response to metoprolol and other beta blockers. The 131C allele in the alpha subunit protein and the 825C allele in the beta subunit protein of the coupled Gs protein also show an increased response to beta blockers.

The Ser49Gly mutation showed variation in agonist-mediated down regulation as evidenced by increased receptor desensitization after exposure to isoproterenol compared to the wild type.[27] The Arg389Gly polymorphism is located in the intracellular cytoplasmic tail. The Arg389 receptor showed increased coupling to the G protein with enhanced adenylyl cyclase activity. As a result, second messenger activity increased under both basal and isoproterenol-stimulated conditions.[28] Patients homozygous for the *Arg389* allele had greater reduction in diastolic BP in response to metoprolol, a beta blocker, compared to patients who were carriers of the *Gly389* allele.[29] Hypertensive patients with the Ser49Arg389/Ser49Arg389 haplotypes were associated with the best systolic blood pressure response to metoprolol in both Caucasian and Chinese populations.[7,29] The pharmacodynamic variability of several cardiac parameters in response to beta blocker treatment has also been examined. Heart rate response to metoprolol was not affected by these polymorphisms but heart failure patients with the Arg389 variant or Ser49-Arg389 haplotype showed the greatest improvement in left ventricular ejection fraction after initiation of β-blocker therapy.[30,31]

A few studies have looked at mutations in the G_S protein associated with the ADRB1 receptor.[32,33] One study examined the response to atenolol in hypertensive patients with the 825C/T mutant in the beta subunit of the gene for the G_s protein (*GNB3*) of ADBR1.[32] The *T* allele has been associated with increased signal transduction. Females with the *CC* alleles showed a significant fall in blood pressure compared to the *T* carriers. An earlier study showed an enhanced response to beta blockers in Caucasian hypertensive patients with a SNP, 131T/C, in the gene for the alpha subunit of the G_s protein (GNAS) of ADBR1.[33] No specific beta blocker was used. The *131C* allele was associated with good responders however the functional basis of the variation in drug response is unclear. The ADBR1 receptor (Figure 6-2) is a model for altered drug response due to genetic variation in the cell surface receptor as well as the signal transduction system.

HIV Therapeutics

Drug response in human immunodeficiency virus type 1 (HIV-1) infections is dependent on both virus and host genetics.[34] To infect host cells HIV-1 must first bind to a CD4 antigen, a receptor on the cell surface of human helper T-cells, monocytes/macrophages, dendritic cells and glial cells. A co-receptor is also necessary for HIV-1 entry into the host cell. The human chemokine receptors CCR5 and CXCR4 are the main co-receptors used by the Macrophage-tropic (M- or CCR5-tropic) and the T-cell-tropic (T- or CXCR4-tropic) HIV-1 strains, respectively, for entering their CD4+ target cells. A protein on the surface of the HIV particle, glycoprotein 120, binds specifically to CD4 and the co-receptor forming a complex that allows the viral envelope to join with the host cell membrane and the virus to enter the host cell.

An allelic mutation of the CCR5 receptor has been identified that provides resistance against HIV-1 by blocking attachment to the receptor, thus denying entry of the virus in to the macrophage.[35] The mutation consists of a 32 nucleic acid deletion that prevents expression of the receptor on the cell surface. The homozygous variant provides almost complete resistance to HIV-1 infection while heterozygous alleles show partial resistance with slower disease progression. The CCR5-Delta32 deletion mutation has been found with a high frequency in Caucasian populations (10%), but has not been found in African, Asian, Middle Eastern, and American Indian populations.[36]

The observation that this genetic mutation can slow or delay the onset of AIDS in patient populations suggested that inhibitors of CCR5 might prohibit the entrance of the virus into the human cell and provide a novel form of antiretroviral therapy. Several CCR5 inhibitors have been developed, but only maraviroc/Selzentry® has been approved for treatment of AIDS.[34,37] In patients infected with the CCR5-tropic HIV-1 strain, maraviroc in combination with optimized antiretroviral therapy was shown to be effective and generally well-tolerated for at least 48 weeks.[38] Appropriate use of maraviroc requires that the virus is the CCR5-tropic HIV-1 strain.[37] The impact of host CCR5 polymorphisms on the efficacy of maraviroc is being evaluated.[39] Thus genetic variants of both the pharmacodynamic receptor and the infecting agent may be important for determining drug efficacy against HIV.

CNS Targets

The *OPRM1* gene encodes the protein for the mu opioid receptor; the mu receptor is responsible for mediation of the analgesic effects of most opioid drugs. A SNP in the intron region, A118G, results in an amino acid change from Asparagine to Aspartate at position 40. The *40Asp* allele occurs with a frequency of 10–19% in the Caucasian population.[40] The *40Asp* allele has been associated with decreased mRNA expression and receptor protein levels, as well as a decreased analgesic response to morphine.[41,42] The mu opioid receptor has also been implicated in the reward properties of several addictive substances including cocaine, alcohol, and opioids. Mu receptor antagonists like naltrexone have been used to treat alcohol and opioid dependence, variability in response to naltrexone for treatment of alcoholism has suggested a genetic component.[43] Alcohol-dependent patients with the 40Asp variant were shown to be more responsive to naltrexone and less likely to relapse into alcoholism.[44] Thus *OPRMI* genotyping might be useful in selecting treatment for alcoholism as well as pain management.

Another type of cell surface drug target is the serotonin transporter protein; this is a prime target for antidepressant drugs. Inhibition of the transporter results in increased synaptic levels of serotonin which modulates neuronal activity by allowing serotonin to bind other targets. Kirchheiner et al. have recently reviewed the impact of pharmacogenetics on antidepressants and antipsychotics.[45] Mutations in the serotonin transporter (SERT) and the 5-HT$_{2A}$ receptor were correlated with an increased response to selective serotonin reuptake inhibitors (SSRIs) in a European population.[46] SERT mutations resulted in variable expression of the transporter protein.[47] The 44 base pair insertion/deletion (*5HTTLPR*) in the promoter region of the gene results in a long (*l*) or short (*s*) allele. The (*l*) allele shows twofold higher expression and is associated with an increased response to the SSRIs compared to the (*s*) allele. Some studies in Asian populations have shown better response to fluoxetine with carriers of the (*s*) allele.[48] The frequency of the (*s*) allele is much higher in Asians (79%) than Caucasians (42%), thus ethnicity may explain the discrepancy in results.[45,49] A second SERT polymorphism was associated with antidepressant efficacy; the variable number tandem repeat (VNTR) polymorphism for SERT has three alleles with 9, 10, and 12 copies of the tandem repeat in the 2nd intron. The 12 copy tandem repeat allele had higher expression and was associated with better response to the SSRIs.[48] Although the serotonin receptor is not the direct pharmacological target for SSRIs, inhibition of SERT by the SSRIs will increase the levels of serotonin in the synapse and thus increase stimulation of serotonin receptors. Antidepressant activity is thought to result from the increase in serotonin activity at the receptors. Thus polymorphisms of the serotonin receptors could also affect the antidepressant activity of SSRIs. The 102T/C polymorphism in the 5-HT$_{2A}$ receptor showed better antidepressant response with one or two *102C* alleles compared to the *T/T* homozygote.[50] This is an example of how mutations in either a direct (SERT) or indirect (5-HT$_{2A}$) drug target can modify pharmacodynamic response.

Cytosolic Receptors

Cytosolic estrogen receptors (ER) are members of the nuclear steroid receptor superfamily. Two receptor types have been identified, ER-α and ER-β, these proteins are products of the *ER1* and *ER2* genes. Estrogen's positive effects on heart disease have been associated with its ability to raise plasma levels of high-density lipoprotein (HDL) cholesterol.[51] Herrington et al. evaluated 10 different variants of ER-α in postmenopausal women with coronary disease.[52] Women with the IVS1 (intervening sequence on intron 1) 401 C/C genotype and several other closely linked intron 1 polymorphisms had an increase in HDL cholesterol levels with hormone replacement therapy which was more than twice the increase observed in other women.

More recently, ER polymorphism and the lipid effects of tamoxifen were investigated in women being treated for breast cancer.[53] Tamoxifen is considered a selective estrogen receptor modifier (SERM) because it has both agonist and antagonist activity at various estrogen receptors. Genetic variants for both ER-α and ER-β were associated with differences in tamoxifen-mediated changes in HDL cholesterol, LDL cholesterol, and triglycerides. Tamoxifen effects differed in premenopausal and postmenopausal women. The mechanism for and the clinical significance of the ER mediated changes in lipids is unclear.

Enzyme Targets

Warfarin Response

There are numerous examples of genetic variation in enzymes that are used as drug targets. As previously discussed, warfarin's primary drug target is the enzyme VKORC1 (see Figure 6-1). Inhibition of VKORC1 interferes with vitamin K reduction and vitamin K-dependent carboxylation of clotting factors II, VII, IX and X, as well as protein C and S. Depletion of vitamin K results in the production of nonfunctional coagulation factors and loss of the coagulation. Genetic polymorphism in the *VKORC1* gene illustrates a clinically important example of variation in drug response associated with haplotypes rather than a single SNP.[54] Promoter and intronic *VKORC1* variants 1639G/A (3673), 1173C/T (6484), 1542G/C (6853), 2255C/T (7566) show strong linkage disequilibrium, they are inherited together. Haplotypes with the variant SNPs require low dose warfarin, are associated with lower gene expression and are called haplotype group A; the other haplotypes are considered group B. Haplotypes that contain variations in *VKORC1* generally result in patients who require high doses, BB (6.2 mg/d), moderate doses, AB (4.9 mg/d), or low doses, AA (2.7 mg/d), to achieve anticoagulation, depending on the level of enzyme expression.

Asthma Therapy

Variability in the gene *ALOX5* provides an example of a mutation in the promoter region that affects the expression of the normal enzyme protein, namely 5-lipoxygenase. 5-Lipoxygenase is the enzyme responsible for conversion of arachidonic acid to leukotrienes. Leukotrienes mediate inflammation, vasoconstriction, and bronchoconstriction and have been implicated in the pathophysiology of asthma.[55] Zileuton, an inhibitor of 5-lipoxygenase, can be used to decrease airway inflammation in patients with asthma. However, not all patients respond to this drug. The promoter region of the *ALOX5* gene shows variation in the number of tandem Sp1 binding motifs (5'GGGCGG3').[56] Transcription factors SP1 and Egr-1 bind to this sequence and up-regulate *ALOX5* transcription. Genetic variants in the promoter region may change the binding of these transcription factors and therefore the rate of 5-lipoxygenase transcription and the activation of leukotrienes under inflammatory conditions. The most common or wild type allele (frequency of 77%) has five repeats of the tandem Sp1 binding motif. Several mutant alleles contain three, four, or six tandem Sp1-binding motifs, these variants were associated with reduced transcription of the 5-lipoxygenase gene, as compared with the common allele.[57] Patients that had at least one copy of the wild type allele responded to therapy, but asthma patients who were homozygous for the mutant alleles had a decreased response to treatment with antileukotriene drugs thus indicating a pharmacogenetic effect of the promoter sequence on response to treatment.

ACE Inhibitors

The pharmacogenetics of angiotensin converting enzyme (ACE) and the antihypertensive effects of ACE inhibitors has been extensively studied.[58,59] The insertion (I)/deletion variant in intron 16 is characterized by the absence/or presence of 287 nucleotides.[60] The DD genotype has been associated with elevated levels of serum ACE.[60] Clinical effects associated with ACE inhibition polymorphism which have been studied include: blood pressure reduction, left ventricular hypertrophy, expression of angiotensin II type 1 receptor (AT_1R) messenger RNA, arteriole stiffness, heart rate, and renoprotection.[59] Carriers of the (I) allele treated with ACE inhibitors have been associated with a reduced regression of left ventricular hypertrophy, greater reduction of the glomerular filtration, and decreased expression of AT_1R messenger RNA as well as a greater reduction of diastolic blood pressure with AT_1R antagonists. Conflicting results have been seen regarding the influence of ACE inhibitors and the I/D polymorphism on reduction in blood pressure with some results showing no relationship, others showing an increased reduction in blood pressure with either the (I) or the allele. Ethnic diversity might explain the variable results, if an allele is more prevalent it may be easier to find a relationship between drug response and polymorphism. The (I) allele has a higher frequency in the Asian (62%) and the African American (60%) populations compared to the Caucasian population (50%).[59,61] A reduced response to ACE inhibitors and AT_1R antagonists among hypertensive African American patients is well documented.[62] However the relationship between the ACE I/D polymorphism, ethnicity, and response to ACE inhibitors remains unclear.

Inflammation

Cyclo-oxygenase (COX) 1 and 2 are important enzymes in the conversion of arachidonic acid to prostaglandins. Prostaglandins have an important role in mediation of inflammation and pain. Lee et al. examined the role of haplotypes of the COX1 (*PTGS1*) and COX2 (*PTGS2*) genes on enzyme expression and response to post-surgical pain relief of ibuprofen, a nonselective COX inhibitor, and rofecoxib, a selective COX-2 inhibitor.[63] A *PTGS2* haplotype block with four promoter and intron SNPs, -1290A/G,-765G/C, 3629G/A, 4068T/C, showed a differential response to the COX inhibitors. The homozygous major haplotype showed increased COX-2 expression in response to surgery and increased pain relief with rofecoxib, while the homozygous minor and the heterozygous haplotype showed decreased COX-2 expression and a better response to the nonselective inhibitor ibuprofen. This suggests that post-surgical pain was mediated by COX-2 in the patients homozygous for the major *PTGS2* haplotype and that post-surgical pain in other patient populations was predominantly mediated by COX-1. This provides an example of haplotype variants resulting in different enzyme activity and thus inhibitor drug response.

Polymorphisms That Indirectly Modulate Drug Response

Pharmacodynamic-based genetic variability can produce undesired or unexpected changes in drug response that are not directly due to changes in the drug target. Often these genetic mutations result in ADRs but can result in protection from ADRs or modification of drug efficacy. The polymorphism may result in a patient who is more susceptible to an adverse effect, because this mutation decreases their capacity to handle the stress of the drug therapy. This is illustrated by the decrease capacity to handle oxidative stress in individuals with decreased glucose-6-phosphate dehydrogenase activity. On the other hand, a genetic variant might provide added protection in some individuals who have an increased capacity to handle the drug-induced stress. Thus pharmacogenetics may offer an explanation for some "idiosyncratic reactions." Another type of indirect change in drug response can occur when genetic variation results in the increased sensitivity of a nontarget drug receptor, enzyme, or signaling pathway. Drug interactions with a nontarget protein can result in an increased side effect in genetically sensitive individuals as seen with the increased nausea associated with the SSRI, Paroxetine. Examples of pharmacodynamic polymorphisms that indirectly affect drug response are summarized in Table 6-2 and discussed in further detail below.

Table 6-2
Genetic Variability That Modify Drug Response

Mutation	Physiological Response	Affected Drug/Class
Glucose-6-phosphate dehydrogenase	Redox state of red blood cells	Drugs that cause oxidative stress (13)
Factor V and prothrombin	Coagulation	Oral contraceptives (67–71)
Human leukocytic antigen	Hypersensitivity reaction	Abacavir, carbamazepine, ximelagatran (72–76)
Cardiac potassium and sodium channels	QT-prolonging	Drugs that block the potassium channels (10, 78–84)
Serotonin receptor	Nausea	Selective serotonin reuptake inhibitors (87–88)
Dopamine receptor	Tardive dyskinesia	Antipsychotics (90)
Bradykinin receptor	Cough	ACE inhibitors (92)
Apolipoproteins, cholesterol transport proteins, mitochondrial proteins, resistin	Dyslipidemia, lipodystrophy	Anti-retroviral therapy (96–99)

Clinical Pearl

Idiosyncratic reactions may result from pharmacodynamic-based genetic variability.

Antineoplastic Response and Epigenetic Polymorphisms

Genetic differences may have indirect effects on drug response that are related to modification of the drug-target interactions. Epigenetics refers to changes in the phenotype or protein expression caused by mechanisms other than changes in the DNA sequence. Post-translational methylation variability has been seen in cancer cells. Increased or decreased methylation can modulate expression of enzymes and cell-cycle regulators. This in turn can impact prognosis or drug response. Improved antineoplastic response can be seen with mutations in enzymes involved in tumor DNA repair. Methylguanine methyltransferase (MGMT) is a DNA repair enzyme; increased activity of this enzyme can repair alkylated tumor DNA, resulting in poor response to chemotherapeutic alkylating agents. Methylation of the promoter region of the *MGMT* gene has been shown to decrease expression, decrease DNA repair and improve response of gliomas to treatment with alkylating agents carmustine or temozolomide.[64,65] A more recent study has examined the epigenetics of the response of gastric cancer to 5-fluorouracil-based drugs.[66] Methylation of the promoter region of *p16*, a cell cycle regulator gene, results in decreased expression of p16 and an increased response to the 5-fluorouracil analogs. The increased response to the 5-fluorouracil analogs is thought to be due to disruption of the cell cycle resulting in an increased numbers of cells in the S-phase, the phase most susceptible to antimetabolites. Profiling of aberrations in post-translational methylation of genes should allow better decision-making in antineoplastic choices.

Increased Incidence of Adverse Drug Reactions

Glucose-6-Phosphate Dehydrogenase and Oxidative Stress

One of the earliest and most common examples of a genetic polymorphism resulting in increased ADRs are the functional mutations of glucose-6-phosphate dehydrogenase (G6PD).[13] More than 400 million people carry mutant genes for this enzyme. Greater than 400 biochemical variants of this X-linked gene have been described, most of which result in defective enzyme activity. G6PD is an enzyme that catalyses the first step in the pentose phosphate pathway. The product of this reaction is NADPH (reduced form of nicotinamide adenine dinucleotide phosphate). NADPH is essential for the activity of enzymes that counterbalance oxidative stress. Defective G6PD results in decreased tolerance to oxidative stress and drugs that increase oxidative stress may precipitate hemolytic anemia in the presence of this defective enzyme. Individuals with the mutant G6PD have experienced increased incidence of hemolytic anemia when treated with drugs like anti-malarials, sulfonamides, sulfones, aspirin, ciprofloxacin, vitamin K analogs, chloramphenicol, and nitrofurantoin. The highest frequencies G6PD mutations are found in Africa, Asia, the Mediterranean, and the Middle East.

Thromboembolic Disorders

It has long been know that some women taking oral contraceptives are susceptible to thromboembolic disorders such as deep vein thrombosis (DVTs) or pulmonary embolism. Enhanced coagulation is thought to be related to elevation in prothrombin (factor II) levels.[67] Genetic variations in coagulation factors such as factor V and prothrombin may contribute to an increase in this risk.[68,69] Factor V is converted to the active form, factor Va, by thrombin. Activated factor V serves as an essential protein in the coagulation pathway and acts as a cofactor for the conversion of prothrombin to thrombin by factor Xa. Factor Va is inactivated by activated protein C (APC). APC resistance was associated with a variant allele identified as 1691G/A, a SNP found in exon 10 of the factor V(*F5*) gene, which results in a coding change Arg506Gln.[70] The 1691A allele is often referred to as factor V Leiden as it was characterized in a family in Belgium. Individuals with one or two alleles are more susceptible to clot formation. Another important mutation in the coagulation pathway is the SNP found in the 3' untranslated region of prothrombin, 20210G/A. Carriers of the 20210A allele have higher plasma prothrombin levels than controls with the normal 20210GG genotype and have a 2.8-fold increased risk of venous thrombosis.[71] The use of oral contraceptives in patients with either the 1691A allele or the 20210A allele results in a markedly higher incidence of DVTs since the combinations are synergistic rather than additive.[68,69]

Hypersensitivity Reactions

Hypersensitivity reactions are a common ADR, in some cases the allergic reaction can be related to a gene variant of the immune system. The human leukocyte antigen system (HLA) is the major histocompatibility complex (MHC) in humans. Hypersensitivity reactions have been associated with variant alleles of several HLA genes. About 5% of the patients taking the nucleoside reverse-transcriptase inhibitor (NRTI) abacavir experience a systemic hypersensitivity reaction which includes GI distress, rash fever and fatigue.[72] The *HLA-B*5701* and the *HLA-DR7* genes were associated with the abacavir-related hypersensitivity reaction.[73,74] A more serious hypersensitivity reaction, Stevens-Johnson syndrome, has occurred with the antiepileptic drug carbamazepine. This particular ADR has been associated with *HLA-B1502* in Han Chinese.[75] Recently a thrombin inhibitor, ximelagatran, was removed from the market because of hepatotoxicity, studies have revealed a strong association between this hepatotoxicity and the *HLA DRB1*0701* gene.[76]

QT-Interval Prolongation

Genetic variation in ion channel genes that are not drug targets can also have a role in predisposing patients to toxic effects of drugs. Individuals with variant alleles in ion channels may have substantial morbidity or mortality resulting from drugs that cause QT-interval prolongation and may also be inherently more susceptible to cardiac arrhythmias. QT- prolongation is a common life-threatening adverse effect which has resulted in removal of numerous drugs from the market.[77] Mutations in potassium or sodium channels can allow accumulation of excess intracellular positive ions in cardiac cells, leading to delayed repolarization or decrease in "repolarization reserve."[78] Drug induced or acquired QT-prolongation has been identified in individuals with the KCNQ1 and KCNE1 genes (IKS potassium channel), HERG and KCNE2 genes (I_{KR} potassium channel), and the SCN5A gene (sodium channel) variants.[79] Some antiarrhythmic drugs are expected to affect the QT-interval, but many noncardiovascular drugs also affect the QT-interval. The voltage-gated potassium channel involved in cardiac repolarization current I_{Kr} appears to be the main culprit in QT-prolongation based arrhythmias known as torsades de pointes.[10] Drugs which block this potassium channel can precipitate cardiac ar-rhythmias; several examples are listed in Table 6-3. The young woman in our case study was most likely experiencing an adverse drug reaction due to a potassium channel genetic polymor-phism. Her UTI would be handled more safely with antibiotics that do not bind and inhibit potassium channels. Understanding the genetic basis for QT-prolongation based arrhythmias could help improve drug development as well as patient safety.

Table 6-3
Noncardiac Drugs That Bind to Cardiac Potassium Channels

Drug	Class	Drug Target	Channel	Mutation	Reference
Clarithromycin	Antibiotic	I_{Kr} blocker	MiRP1(KCNE2)[a] Subunit of the I_{Kr} -Potassium Chan-nel	Q9E	(80)
Sulfamethox-azole	Antibiotic	I_{Kr} blocker	MiRP1(KCNE2)[a] Subunit of the I_{Kr} -Potassium Chan-nel	T8A	(81)
Cisapride	Prokinetic agent	I_{Kr} blocker	SCN5A Sodium Channel	L1825P	(82)
Terfenadine	Antihistamine	I_{Kr} blocker	KCNH2		(83)
Sibutramine	Serotonin and norepinephrine reuptake inhibitor	I_{Kr} blocker	KCNQ1	T265I	(84)

[a]MinK-related peptide 1-MiRP1 is also called KCNE2, subunit of IKr, inward rectifying potassium channel.

Serotonin Receptors and GI Side Effects

Drug side effects may be caused by the drug binding to ancillary receptors that are not the therapeutic target. A significant number of patients taking selective serotonin reuptake in-hibitors (SSRIs) like paroxetine (Paxil®) experience nausea as an undesired side effect. Even though paroxetine is believed to exert its anti-depressant effects by inhibiting the serotonin transporter, it is thought that activation of the 5-hydroxytryptamine 3B or 2A receptors (5-HT_{3B} or 5-HT_{2A}) mediates the SSRI-induced gastrointestinal side effects. The 5-HT_{3B} receptors located in the small intestinal mucosa and the chemotrigger zone in the CNS mediate the vomiting reflex and the 5-HT_{2A} receptor affects gut motility.[85] Studies using 5-HT_3 antagonists, cisapride and ondansetron, showed a reduction in SSRI-induced gastrointestinal side effects, a finding which suggests that 5-HT_3 receptors are involved in these GI effects.[86] The Tyr129Ser polymorphism of the *HTR3B* gene has been shown to significantly affect the incidence of nau-sea in a population of Japanese psychiatric patients treated with paroxetine. Patients with the Tyr/Tyr genotype had a fourfold higher risk of developing nausea compared to patients with the *Ser* allele. There was no correlation with the incidence of nausea and *HTR3A* gene or the *CYP2D6* gene polymorphisms.[87] Murphy et al. showed a strong correlation between genetic mutations in the 5-HT_{2A} receptor and side effect severity in patients treated with paroxetine.[88]

The *HTR2A 102T/C* SNP showed a frequency of 0.6:0.4, T:C, in a U.S. Caucasian population. Patients with the *CC* genotype showed a significantly higher incidence of GI complaints and discontinuation rate. The increased incidence of GI side effects associated with genetic variations in serotonin receptors provides an example of a shift in drug response due to a mutation in a secondary target.

Tardive Dyskinesia

Another example of the pharmacogenetics of a secondary target modifying drug response can be seen in the association of dopamine three (D_3) receptor mutations with an increased incidence of tardive dyskinesia (TD). TD is a serious, irreversible movement disorder that affects at least 20% of the patients taking traditional antipsychotic agents.[89] Many typical antipsychotics are thought to work through their antagonism of dopamine two (D_2) receptors; however, these drugs can also antagonize other dopamine receptors including the D_3 receptor. Numerous studies have identified a variant of the D_3 receptor (DRD3 ser9gly) in patients who develop TD. Patients homozygous for the *DRD3gly* allele show an increased incidence of TD and *in vitro* studies show higher affinity of dopamine for cells expressing the mutant gene product.[90]

Bradykinin-Mediated Cough

Although the primary therapeutic effect of ACE inhibitors results from blocking the conversion of angiotensin I to angiotensin II, ACE inhibitors also block the breakdown of bradykinin. Bradykinin is thought to mediate some of the adverse effects of the ACE inhibitors including the dry persistent cough seen in about 10% of the patients taking ACE inhibitors.[91] Variants in the bradykinin B_2 receptor have been implicated in a predisposition for this ADR. Mukae et al. looked at the incidence of cough and genetic polymorphism of genes for ACE, angiotensin II type I and type II receptor, and the bradykinin B_2 receptor in a hypertensive Japanese population.[92] Patients with one or two copies of the *-58T* allele of the bradykinin B_2 receptor had a higher incidence of cough compared to patients with the *-58CC* genotype. This promoter region variant resulted in higher expression of the bradykinin B_2 receptor protein.

Anti-Retroviral Therapy and Dyslipidemia

Anti-retroviral therapy (ART) can cause elevation in serum triglycerides, decrease in high-density lipoprotein, insulin resistance, and lipodystrophy which is the loss of peripheral adipose tissue with a concomitant an increase in abdominal adiposity.[93] These affects on lipids are independent of the drug target used to suppress HIV proliferation. Protease inhibitors and nucleotide reverse transcriptase inhibitors (NRTIs) have been shown to alter the expression of adipogenic transcription factors, genes involved in lipid metabolism and cell cycle control.[94] NRTIs deplete adipocyte mitochondrial DNA (mtDNA) with an associated decrease in mtDNA copy number, and stimulate mitochondrial proliferation, fat wasting and adipocyte loss.[95] Not all patients experience the same degree of dyslipidemia and lipodystrophy with ART suggesting a genetic component. Susceptibility to ART lipid and mitochondrial disturbances shows a complex relationship with a number of genetic polymorphisms; patient populations with compromised lipid metabolism and adipocyte mitochondrial function may be more sensitive to these adverse effects.[96] Variants of apolipoproteins APOA5 and APOC3, interacting with *APOE* genotypes, have been associated with an increase in severity of ART-induced dyslipidemia and lipodystrophy. Genetic polymorphisms of the nuclear transcription-factor sterol response element binding proteins (*SREBP1c*) and of tumor necrosis factor-a (*TNFa*), which can also affect lipid metabolism, have yielded contrasting results in patients treated with ART. In addition to supporting the role of *APOA5*, *APOC3*, and *APOE* polymorphisms, Arnedo et al. demonstrated that variant alleles of the genes for ATP-binding cassette (ABC) protein cholesterol transporter (ABCA1) and cholesteryl ester transfer protein (CETP) also contributed to elevation of plasma triglyceride and decreased high-density lipoprotein-cholesterol levels related to ART exposure.[97] More recently other allele variants have been associated with ART-induced lipidemias. The hemochromatosis gene (*HFE*) is known to impact mitochondrial function, Hulgen et al. found that a specific mutation in the HFE gene, *HFE 187C/G*—was protective against fat loss in patient's treats with ART.[98] An extensive evaluation of genes in patients treated with ART showed a strong association of ART-induced metabolic complications with a genetic variation in *resistin*, a gene previously implicated in obesity and insulin resistance.[99] Although the genetic variability associated with ART-induced adverse lipid metabolism remains unclear, identification of all predisposing factors remains an important goal in optimizing therapy.

Disease States and Biomarkers

Certain disease states have been associated with a genetic mutation and often this same genetic mutation has also been associated with altered efficacy to a particular drug therapy. A genetic mutation that is associated with a disease or a particular subpopulation of that disease is termed a biomarker. The relationship of the biomarker to therapeutic outcome may be directly related to a genetic mutation in the drug target, indirectly through changes in the ability of the drug to reach the drug target or due to the linkage of this mutation to other pathological changes. Below are several examples that can be used to illustrate the direct association between the disease biomarker and the therapeutic outcome based on a specific drug target.

Alzheimer's Disease

Alzheimer's disease has been associated with a genetic polymorphism of APOE, a protein involved in the expression of Choline acetyltransferase.[100] Choline acetyltransferase is required for synthesis of acetylcholine. The *APOE4* allele (Cys112Arg) is associated with a poor prognosis and a decreased response to tacrine, Cognex®, an acetylcholinesterase inhibitor that is used to increase endogenous acetylcholine levels.[11] A beneficial response to tacrine and a better prognosis is seen individuals with the *APOE2* and *APOE3* alleles. This differential response seems to be more important in women compared to men.[101] Two other acetylcholinesterase inhibitors, rivastigmine, Aricept® and galanthamine (galantamine), Razadyne® also show increased response rates in *APOE2/3* compared to patients with the *APOE4* allele.[102,103] It is thought that the number of functional presynaptic cholinergic fibers in the brains of AD patients carrying the *APOE4* allele may be too low to benefit from the neurochemical and therapeutic action of acetylcholinesterase inhibitors.[104]

Cancer

Somatic or acquired mutations in tumor cell DNA can produce individual variability in response to cancer treatment. Growth factor biomarkers have been used to predict therapeutic outcomes and design specific drug entities. Activation of the EGFR (epidermal growth factor receptor) or other ErbB family members promotes cell growth and survival, and these receptors are often overexpressed in solid tumors. Pharmacogenetics of cancer treatment based on targeting growth factor receptors has recently been reviewed.[12] A diagram of the ErbB type receptor is presented in Figure 6-3. Dimerization of ErbB receptors or EGFR containing tyrosine kinase results in phosphorylation of an intracellular tyrosine residue on the dimerized receptor. This phosphorylation initiates the enrollment of other cytosolic proteins that ultimately affect gene expression and various biological outcomes. Numerous cancers including: chronic myelogenous leukemia, breast, ovarian, glioma, colon, bladder and non small-cell lung cancer and squamous-cell carcinomas of the head and neck, have been associated with excess activity due to overexpression or mutation of these receptors.[105] Not only is the development of cancer and its prognosis associated with these genetic mutations but these mutations provide a prime target for drugs directed specifically at the tumor cells. Several small molecule tyrosine kinase inhibitors and monoclonal antibodies to the receptor have found clinical application. A summary of these types of drugs can be found in Table 6-4. Inhibition of growth factor-mediated gene expression by these drugs results in decreased tumor cell growth and angiogenesis which may result in tumor cell death. Cancer cells that do not contain these somatic mutations will not respond to these drugs. Normal cells that do not contain these receptors will likewise not be affected thus avoiding many of the typical cytotoxic side effects associated with cancer chemotherapy. Testing for the overexpressed growth factor receptors is crucial for identifying the patient population that may benefit from a specific treatment. Herceptin is an example of a drug that was approved by the FDA with a required test to identify overexpression of HER2 protein, a member of the ErbB family.[106] Growth factor receptor inhibitors may not work if additional mutations are present downstream from the receptor in the signaling cascade. For example, mutations that result in overexpression of *K-ras,* a small G-protein downstream of EGFR, can overcome the positive effects of cetuximab (an EGFR antibody) in treatment of advanced colorectal cancer.[107]

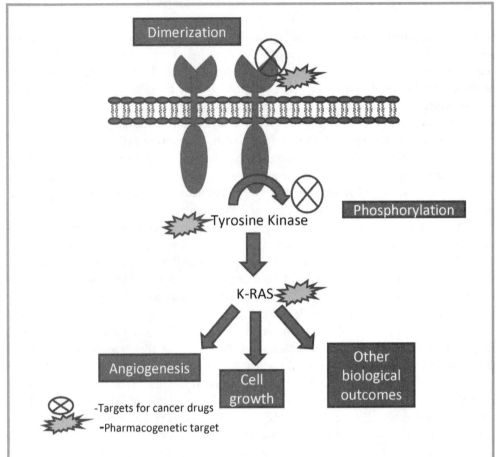

Figure 6.3 • Figure 6-3. Somatic mutations in tumor cells can result in excess activity of the ErbB receptors. These receptor mutations have provided unique targets for cancer drugs, antibodies to the receptor or protein kinase inhibitors. Conversely mutations in other genes (i.e., the downstream RAS gene have resulted in insensitivity to these cancer drugs).

Table 6-4
Growth Factor Inhibitors in Cancer

Drug	Type	Target	Cancer	Reference
Trastuzumab *Herceptin*	Monoclonal antibody	ErbB2 or HER2	Breast	(106)
Cetuximab *Erbitux*	Monoclonal antibody	ErbB1 or EDGFR	Colorectal, SCCHN	(107)
Bevacizumab *Arastin*	Monoclonal antibody	VEGF	Colorectal, NSCLC, breast	(108)
Panitumumab *Vectibix*	Monoclonal antibody	ErbB1 or EDGFR	Colorectal	(12)
Imatinib *Glivec*	Tyrosine kinase inhibitor	BCR-ABL, multiple kinases	Chronic and acute myelogenous leukemia, GIST, glioblastoma	(109)
Gefitinib *Iressa* Erlotinib *Tarceva*	Tyrosine kinase inhibitor	ErbB1 or EDGFR	NSCLC	(110,111)
Sorafenib *Nexvar*	Tyrosine kinase inhibitor	VEGFR, multiple kinases	Renal cell carcinoma	(108)
Sunitinib *Sutent*	Tyrosine kinase inhibitor	VEGFR, multiple kinases	Renal cell and hepatocellular carcinoma, GIST	(108,111)

ErbB2 = erythroblastic leukemia viral oncogene homolog 2; HER2 = human epidermal growth factor receptor 2; ErbB1 = erythroblastic leukemia viral oncogene homolog 1; EDGFR = epidermal growth factor receptor; SCCHN = squamous-cell carcinoma of the head and neck; VEGF(R) = vascular endothelial growth factor (receptor); NSCLC = nonsmall cell lung cancer; BCR-ABL = breakpoint cluster region-Abelson; GIST = gastrointestinal stromal tumor.

Summary

Our understanding of pharmacodynamic-based genetic variation is still in its early stages. Haplotype and genome wide studies have provided better indicators of the importance of specific polymorphisms variations in drug response. The complexity of drug targets and their interactions with other proteins have made it difficult to translate the information regarding individual genetic variants into useful therapeutic strategies. On the other hand, pharmacodynamic genetic polymorphisms can provide a better explanation for "idiosyncratic" adverse drug reactions. Better designed studies and more extensive genetic mapping should allow better prediction of optimal drug response and avoidance of adverse drug reactions.

References

1. Evans WE, Johnson JA. Pharmacogenomics: the inherited basis for interindividual differences in drug response. *Annu Rev Genomics Hum Genet.* 2001;2:9-39.
2. Evans WE, McLeod HL. Pharm.D. Pharmacogenomics: drug disposition, drug targets, and side effects. *N Engl. J Med.* 2003;348:538-549.
3. Hall AM, Wilkins MR. Warfarin: a case history in pharmacogenetics. *Heart.* 2005;91:563-564.
4. Michaud V, Vanier MC, Brouillette D, et al. Combination of phenotypic assessments and CYP2C9-VKORC1 polymorphisms in the determination of warfarin dose requirements in heavily medicated patients. *Clin Pharmacol Ther.* 2007;83:740-748.
5. Sachse C, Brockmöller J, Bauer S, et al. Cytochrome P450 2D6 variants in a Caucasian population: allele frequencies and phenotypic consequences. *Am J Hum Genet.* 1997;60:284-295.
6. Rau T, Wuttke H, Michels LM, et al. Impact of the CYP2D6 genotype on the clinical effects of metoprolol: a prospective longitudinal study. *Clin Pharmacol Ther.* 2009;85:269-272.
7. Liu J, Liu ZQ, Tan ZR, et al. Beta1-adrenergic receptor polymorphisms influence the response to metoprolol monotherapy in patients with essential hypertension. *Clin. Pharmacol Ther.* 2006;80:23-32.
8. Reihsaus E, Innis M, MacIntyre N, et al. Mutations in the gene encoding for the beta(2)-adrenergic receptor in normal and asthmatic subjects. *Am J Resp Cell Molec Biol.* 1993;8:334-339.
9. Wong M-L, Licinio J. From monoamines to genomic targets: a paradigm shift for drug discovery in depression. *Nat Rev Drug Discov.* 2004;3:136-151.
10. Roepke TK, Abbott GW. Pharmacogenetics and cardiac ion channels. *Vasc Pharmacol.* 2006;44:990-106.
11. Poirier J, Delisle MC, Quirion R, et al. Apolipoprotein E4 allele as a predictor of cholinergic deficits and treatment outcome in Alzheimer disease. *Proc Natl Acad Sci USA.* 1995;92:12260-12264.
12. Krejsa C, Rogge M, Sadee W. Protein therapeutics: new applications for pharmacogenetics. *Nat Rev Drug Discov.* 2006;5:507-521.
13. Cappellini MD, Fiorelli G. Glucose-6-phosphate dehydrogenase deficiency. *Lancet.* 2008;371:64–74.
14. Contopoulos-Ioannidis DG, Kouri I, Ioannidis JP. Pharmacogenetics of the response to beta 2 agonist drugs: a systematic overview of the field. *Pharmacogenomics.* 2007;8:933-958.
15. Dishy V, Gbenga MD, Sofowora, G. The effect of common polymorphisms of the β–adrenergic receptor on agonist-mediated vascular desensitization. *N Engl J Med.* 2001;345:1030-1035.
16. Drysdale C, McGraw DW, Stack C, et al. Complex promoter and coding region β 2-adrenergic receptor haplotypes alter receptor expression and predict in vivo responsiveness. *Proc Natl Acad Sci USA.* 2000;97:10483-10488.
17. Dewar JC, Wheatley AP, Venn A, et al. β2-adrenoceptor polymorphisms are in linkage disequilibrium but are not associated with asthma in an adult population. *Clin Exp Allergy.* 1998;28:442-448.
18. Israel E, Chinchilli VM, Ford JG, et al. Use of regularly scheduled albuterol treatment in asthma: genotype-stratified, randomised, placebo-controlled cross-over trial. *Lancet.* 2004;364:1505-1512.
19. Green SA, Turki J, Innis M, et al. Amino-terminal polymorphisms of the human β2-adrenergic receptor imparts distinct agonist-promoted regulatory properties. *Biochemistry.* 1994;33:9414-9419.
20. Israel E, Drazen JM, Liggett SB, et al. The effect of polymorphisms of the β(2)-adrenergic receptor on the response to regular use of albuterol in asthma. *Am J Respir Crit Care Med.* 2000;162:75-80.
21. Taylor DR, Drazen JM, Herbison GP, et al. Asthma exacerbations during long term β agonist use: influence of β(2)-adrenoceptor polymorphism. *Thorax.* 2000;55:762-767.
22. Bleecker ER, Postma DS, Lawrance RM, et al. Effect of ADRB2 polymorphisms on response to long acting β2-agonist therapy: a pharmacogenetic analysis of two randomised studies. *Lancet.* 2007;370:2118-2125.
23. Green SA, Cole G, Jacinto M, et al. A polymorphism of the human β2-adrenergic receptor within the fourth transmembrane domain alters ligand binding and functional properties of the receptor. *J Biol Chem.* 1993;268:23116-23121.
24. Dishy V, Landau R, Sofowora GG, et al. Beta-2-adrenoceptor thr164ile polymorphism is associated with markedly decreased vasodilator and increased vasoconstrictor sensitivity in vivo. *Pharmacogenetics.* 2004;14:517-522.

25. Liggett, SB. β-Adrenergic receptor pharmacogenetics. *Am J Respir Crit Care Med.* 2000;161:S1-97-S201.

26. Johnson JA, Shin J. Pharmacogenetics of β-Blockers. *Pharmacotherapy.* 2007;27:874-887.

27. Rathz DA, Brown KM, Kramer LA, et al. Amino acid 49 polymorphisms of the human beta1-adrenergic receptor affect agonist promoted trafficking. *J Cardiovasc Pharmacol.* 2002;39:155-160.

28. Mason DA, Moore JD, Green SA, et al. A gain-of-function polymorphism in a G-protein coupling domain of the human beta1-adrenergic receptor. *J Biol Chem.* 1999;274:12670-12674.

29. Johnson JA, Zineh I, Puckett BJ, et al. β1-Adrenergic receptor polymorphisms and antihypertensive response to metoprolol. *Clin Pharmacol Ther.* 2003;74:44-52.

30. Beitelshees AL, Zineh I, Yarandi HN, et al. Influence of phenotype and pharmacokinetics on beta-blocker drug target pharmacogenetics. *Pharmacogenomics J.* 2006;6:174-178.

31. Mialet-Perez, J. Rathz DA, Petrashevskaya NN, et al. Beta 1-adrenergic receptor polymorphisms confer differential function and predisposition to heart failure. *Nat Med.* 2003;9:1300-1305.

32. Filigheddu F, Reid JE, Troffa C, et al. Genetic polymorphisms of the β-adrenergic system: association with essential hypertension and response to β-blockade. *Pharmacogenomics J.* 2004;4:154-160.

33. Jia, H. Hingorani AD, Sharma P, et al. Association of the G(s) alpha gene with essential hypertension and response to beta-blockade. *Hypertension.* 1999;34:8-14.

34. Reiche EMV, Bonametti AM, Voltarelli JC, et al. Genetic polymorphisms in the chemokine and chemokine receptors: impact on clinical course and therapy of the human immunodeficiency virus type 1 infection (HIV-1). *Curr Med Chem.* 2007;14:1325-1334.

35. Samson M, Libert F, Doranz BJ, et al. Resistance to HIV-1 infection in Caucasian individuals bearing mutant alleles of the CCR-5 chemokine receptor gene. *Nature.* 1996;382:722-725.

36. Martinson JJ, Chapman NH, Rees DC, et al. Global distribution of the CCR5 gene 32-basepair deletion. *Nat Genet.*1997;16:100-103.

37. Raphael D. A new class of anti-HIV therapy and new challenges. *N Engl J Med.* 2008;359:1510-1511.

38. Gulick RM, Lalezari J, Goodrich J, et al. Maraviroc for previously treated patients with R5 HIV-1 infection. *N Engl J Med.* 2008;359:1429-1441.

39. Ketas TJ, Kuhmann SE, Palmer A, et al. Cell surface expression of CCR5 and other host factors influence the inhibition of HIV-1 infection of human lymphocytes by CCR5 ligands. *Virology.* 2007;364:281-290.

40. Lotsch J, Geisslinger G. Are mu-opioid receptor polymorphisms important for clinical opioid therapy? *Trends Mol Med.* 2005;11:82-89.

41. Zhang Y, Wang D, Johnson AD, et al. Allelic expression imbalance of human mu receptor (*OPRM1*) caused by variant A118G. *J Biol Chem.* 2006;280:326118-32624.

42. Campa D, Gioia A, Tomei A, et al. Association of *ABCB1/MDR1* and *OPRM1* gene polymorphisms with morphine pain relief. *Clin Pharmacol Ther.* 2008;83:559-566.

43. Anton RF, Drobes DJ, Voronin K, et al. Naltrexone effects on alcohol consumption in a clinical laboratory paradigm: temporal effects of drinking. *Psychopharmacology.* 2004;173:32-40.

44. Oslin DW, Berrettini W, Kranzler HR, et al. A functional polymorphism on the μ-opioid receptor gene is associated with naltrexone response in alcohol-independent patients. *Neuropsychopharmacology.* 2003;28:1546-1552.

45. Kirchheiner J, Nickchen K, Bauer M, et al. Pharmacogenetics of antidepressants and antipsychotics: the contribution of allelic variations to the phenotype of drug response. *Mol Psychiatry.* 2004;9:442-473.

46. Smeraldi E, Zanardi R, Benedetti F, et al. Polymorphism within the promoter of the serotonin transporter gene and antidepressant efficacy of fluvoxamine. *Mol Psychiatry.*1998;3:508-511.

47. Lesch KP, Bengel D, Heils A, et al. Association of anxiety-related traits with a polymorphism in the serotonin transporter gene regulatory region. *Science.* 1996;274:1527-1531.

48. Kim DK, Lim SW, Lee S, et al. Serotonin transporter gene polymorphism and antidepressant response. *Neuroreport.* 2000;11:215-219.

49. Kunugi H, Hattori M, Kato T, et al. Serotonin transporter gene polymorphisms: ethnic difference and possible association with bipolar affective disorder. *Mol Psychiatry.*1997;2:457-462.

50. Minov C, Baghai TC, Schule C, et al. Serotonin-2A-receptor and -transporter polymorphisms: lack of association in patients with major depression. *Neurosci Lett.* 2001;303:119-122.

51. Gerhard M, Ganz P. How do we explain the clinical benefits of estrogen? From bedside to bench. *Circulation.*1995;92:5-8.

52. Herrington DM, Howard TD, Hawkins GA, et al. Estrogen-receptor polymorphisms and effects of estrogen replacement on high-density lipoprotein cholesterol in women with coronary disease. *N Engl J Med.* 2002;346:967-974.

53. Ntukidem NI, Nguyen AT, Stearns V, et al. Estrogen receptor genotypes, menopausal status, and the lipid effects of tamoxifen. *Clin Pharmacol Ther.* 2008;83:702-710.

54. Rieder MJ, Reiner AP, Gage BF, et al. Effect of VKORC1 haplotypes on transcriptional regulation and warfarin dose. *N Engl J Med.* 2005;52:2285-2293.

55. Drazen JM, Israel E, O'Byrne PM. Treatment of asthma with drugs modifying the leukotriene pathway. *N Engl J Med.* 1999;340:197-206.

56. In KH, Asano K, Beier D, et al. Naturally occurring mutations in the human 5-lipoxygenase gene promoter that modify transcription factor binding and reporter gene transcription. *J Clin Invest.* 1997;99:1130-1137.

57. Drazen JM, Yandava CN, Dube L, et al. Pharmacogenetic association between ALOX5 promoter genotype and the response to anti-asthma treatment. *Nat Genet.* 1999;22:168-170.

58. Schelleman H, Klungel OH, van Duijn CM, et al. Drug-gene interaction between the insertion/deletion polymorphism of the angiotensin-converting enzyme gene and antihypertensive therapy. *Ann Pharmacother.* 2006;40:212-218.

59. Schelleman H, Stickler BHC, de Boer A, et al. Drug-gene interaction between genetic polymorphisms antihypertensive therapy. *Drugs.* 2004;64:1801-1816.

60. Rigat B, Hubert C, Alhenc-Gelas F, et al. An insertion/deletion polymorphism in the angiotensin I-converting enzyme gene accounting for half the variance of serum enzyme levels. *J Clin Invest.* 1990;86:1343-1346.

61. Wu J, Kraja AT, Oberman A, et al. A summary of the effects of antihypertensive medications on measured blood pressure. *Am J Hypertens.* 2005;18:935-942.

62. Frazier L, Turner ST, Schwartz GL, et al. Multilocus effects of the renin-angiotensin- aldosterone system genes on blood pressure response to a thiazide diuretic. *Pharmacogenomics J.* 2004;4:17-23.

63. Lee Y-S, Kim H, Wu T-X, et al. Genetically mediated interindividual variation in analgesic responses to cyclooxygenase inhibitory drugs. *Clin Pharmacol Ther.* 2006;79:407-418.

64. Esteller M, Garcia-Foncillas J, Andion E, et al. Inactivation of the DNA-repair gene MGMT and the clinical response of gliomas to alkylating agents. *N Engl J Med.* 2000;343:1350-1354.

65. Hegi ME, Diserens A-C, Godard S, et al. Clinical trial substantiates the predicative value of MGMT-methylation in glioblastoma patients treated with temozolomide. *Clin Cancer Res.* 2004;10:1871-1874.

66. Mitsuno M, Kitajima Y, Ide T, et al. Aberrant methylation of *p16* predicts candidates for 5-fluorouracil-based adjuvant therapy in gastric cancer patients. *J Gastroenterol.* 2007;42:866-873.

67. Kluft C, Lansik M. Effect of oral contraceptives on haemostasis variables. *Thromb Haemost.* 1997;78:315-326.

68. Van Hylckama Vlieg A, Rosendaal FR. Interaction between oral contraceptive use and coagulation factor levels in deep venous thrombosis. *J Thromb Haemostasis.* 2003;1:2186-2190.

69. Martinelli I, Taioli E, Cetin I, et al. Interaction between the *G20210A* mutation of the prothrombin gene and oral contraceptive use in deep vein thrombosis. *Arterioscler Thromb Vasc Biol.* 1999;19:700-703.

70. Bertina RM, Koeleman BPC, Koster T, et al. Mutation in blood coagulation factor V associated with resistance to activated protein C. *Nature.* 1994;369:64-67.

71. Poort SR, Rosendaal FR, Reitsma PH, et al. A common genetic variation in the 3'-untranslated region of the prothrombin gene is associated with elevated plasma prothrombin levels and an increase in venous thrombosis. *Blood.* 1996;88:3698-3703.

72. Hetherington S, McGuirk S, Powell G, et al. Hypersensitivity reactions during therapy with the nucleoside reverse transcriptase inhibitor abacavir. *Clin Ther.* 2001;23:1603-1614.

73. Mallal S, Nolan D, Witt C, et al. Association between presence of *HLA-B*5701*, *HLA-DR7*, and *HLA-DQ3* and hypersensitivity to HIV-1 reverse-transcriptase inhibitor abacavir. *Lancet.* 2002;359:727-732.

74. Hetherington S, Hughes AR, Mosteller M, et al. Genetic variations in HLA-B region and hypersensitivity reactions to abacavir. *Lancet.* 2002;359:1121-1122.

75. Chung WH, Hung SI, Hong HS, et al. Medical genetics: a marker for Stevens-Johnson syndrome. *Nature.* 2004;428:486.

76. Kindmark A, Jawaid A, Harbron CG, et al. Genome-wide pharmacogenetic investigation of a hepatic adverse event without clinical signs of immunopathology suggests an underlying immune pathogenesis. *Pharmacogenomics J.* 2008;8:186-195.

77. Wilke RA, Lin DW, Roden D, et al. Identifying genetic risk factors for serious adverse drug reactions: current progress and challenges. *Nat Rev Drug Discov.* 2007;6:904-916.

78. Roden DM. Taking the idio out of idiosyncratic: predicting torsades de pointes. *Pacing Clin Electrophysiol.* 1998;21:1029-1034.

79. Mank-Seymour AR, Richmond JL, Wood LS, et al. Association of torsades de pointes with novel and known single nucleotide polymorphisms in long QT syndrome genes. *Am Heart J.* 2006;152:1116-1222.

80. Abbott GW, Sesti F, Spawski I, et al. MiRP1 forms I_{Kr} potassium channels with HERG and is associated with cardiac arrhythmia. *Cell.*1999;97:175-187.

81. Sesti F, Abbott GW, Wei J, et al. A common polymorphism associated with antibiotic-induced cardiac arrhythmia. *Proc Natl Acad Sci USA.* 2000;97:10613-10618.

82. Makita N, Horie M, Nakamura T, et al. Drug-Induced Long-QT Syndrome Associated With a Subclinical SCN5A Mutation. *Circulation.* 2002;106:1269-1274.

83. Fitzgerald PT, Ackerman MJ. Drug-induced torsades de pointes: the evolving role of pharmacogenetics. *Heart Rhythm* 2005;2:S30–S37.

84. Harrison-Woolrych M, Clark DW, Hill GR, et al. QT interval prolongation associated with sibutramine treatment. *Br J Clin Pharmacol.* 2006;6:464-469.

85. Gershon MD. Review article: serotonin receptors and transporters: roles in normal and abnormal gastrointestinal motility. *Aliment Pharmacol Ther.* 2004;20:S3-S14.

86. Bergeron R, Blier P. Cisapride for the treatment of nausea produced by selective serotonin reuptake inhibitors. *Am J Psychiatry.* 1994;151:1084-1086.

87. Sugai T, Suzuki Y, Sawamura K, et al. The effect of 5-hydroxytryptamine 3A and 3B receptor genes on nausea induced by paroxetine. *Pharmacogenomics J.* 2006;6:351-356.

88. Murphy GM, Kremer C, Rodrigues HE, et al. Pharmacogenetics of antidepressant medication intolerance. *Am J Psychiatry.* 2003;160:1830-1835.

89. Janno S, Holi M, Tuisku K, et al. Prevalence of neuroleptic-induced movement disorders in chronic schizophrenia inpatients. *Am J Psychiatry.* 2004;161:160-163.

90. Lerer B, Segman RH, Fangerau H, et al. Pharmacogenetics of tardive dyskinesia: combined analysis of 780 patients supports association with dopamine D3 receptor gene Ser9Gly polymorphism. *Neuropsychopharmacology.* 2002;27:105-119.

91. Karpman I. Cough from ACE inhibitors. *Am Heart J.* 1988;116:1658.

92. Mukae S, Itoh S, Aoki S, et al. Association of polymorphisms of the renin-angiotensin system and bradykinin B2 receptor with ACE-inhibitor-related cough. *J Human Hypertens.* 2002;16:857-863.

93. Behrens G, Dejam A, Schmidt H, et al. Impaired glucose tolerance, beta cell function and lipid metabolism in HIV patients under treatment with protease inhibitors. *AIDS.* 1999;13:63-70.

94. Pacenti M, Barzon L, Favaretto F, et al. Microarray analysis during adipogenesis identifies new genes altered by antiretroviral drugs. *AIDS.* 2006;20:1691-1705.

95. Nolan D, Hammond E, Martin A, et al. Mitochondrial DNA depletion and morphologic changes in adipocytes associated with nucleoside reverse transcriptase inhibitor therapy. *AIDS.* 2003;17:1329-1338.

96. Bonnet E, Genoux A, Bernard J, et al. Impact of genetic polymorphisms on the risk of lipid disorders in patients on anti-HIV therapy. *Clin Chem Lab Med.* 2007;45:815-821.

97. Arnedo M, Taffe P, Sahli R, et al. Contribution of 20 single nucleotide polymorphisms of 13 genes to dyslipidemia associated with antiretroviral therapy. *Pharmacogenet Genomics.* 2007;17:755-764.

98. Hulgan T, Tebas P, Canter JA, et al. Hemochromatosis gene polymorphisms, mitochondrial haplogroups, and peripheral lipoatrophy during antiretroviral therapy. *J Infect Dis.* 2008;197:858-866.

99. Ranade K, Geese WJ, Noor M, et al. Genetic analysis implicates resistin in HIV lipodystrophy. *AIDS.* 2008;22:1561-1568.

100. Poirier J. Apolipoprotein E in animal models of CNS injury and in Alzheimer's disease. *Trends Neurosci.* 1994;17:525-530.

101. Farlow MR, Lahiri DK, Poirier J, et al. Treatment outcome of tacrine therapy depends on apolipoprotein genotype and gender of the subjects with Alzheimer's disease. *Neurology.* 1998;50:669-677.

102. MacGowan SH, Wilcock GK, Scott M. Effect of gender and apolipoprotein E genotype on response to anticholinesterase therapy in Alzheimer's disease. *Int J Geriatr Psychiatry.* 1998;13:625-630.

103. Farlow M, Lane R, Kudaravalli S, et al. Differential qualitative responses to rivastigmine in APOE epsilon 4 carriers and noncarriers. *Pharmacogenomics J.* 2004;4:332-335.

104. Soininen H, Kosunen O, Helisalmi S, et al. A severe loss of choline acetyltransferase in the frontal cortex of Alzheimer patients carrying apolipoprotein E4 allele. *Neurosci Lett.* 1995;187:79-82.

105. Holbro T, Hynes NE. ErbB receptors: directing key signaling networks throughout life. *Annu Rev Pharmacol Toxicol.* 2004;44:195-217.

106. Pegram MD, Konecny G, Slamon DJ. The molecular and cellular biology of HER2/neu gene amplification/overexpression and the clinical development of herceptin (trastuzumab) therapy for breast cancer. *Cancer Treat Res.* 2000;103:57-75.

107. Karapetis CS, Khambata-Ford S, Jonker DJ, et al. K-ras mutations and benefit from cetuximab in advanced colorectal cancer. *N Engl J Med.* 2008;350:1757-1765.

108. Ellis LM, Hicklin DJ. VEGF-targeted therapy: mechanisms of anti-tumour activity. *Nat Rev Cancer.* 2008;8:579-591.

109. Capdeville R, Buchdunger E, Zimmermann J, et al. *Glivec* (STI571, imatinib), a rationally developed, targeted anticancer drug. *Nat Rev Drug Discov.* 2002;1:493-502.

110. Lynch TJ, Bell DW, Sordella R, et al. Activating mutations in the epidermal growth factor receptor underlying responsiveness of non–small-cell lung cancer to gefitinib. *N Engl J Med.* 2004;350:2129-2139.

111. Ikediobi ON. Somatic pharmacogenomics in cancer. *Pharmacogenomics J.* 2008;8:305-314.

Part II

Applications of Pharmacogenomics in Therapeutics

Chapter 7

Cardiovascular Disease

Kathryn M. Momary, Pharm.D., BCPS; Michael A. Crouch, Pharm.D., FASHP, BCPS

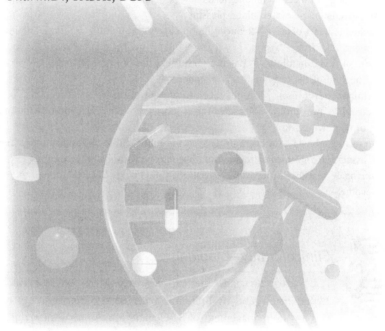

Learning Objectives

After completing this chapter, the reader should be able to

- Identify genetic variants that have been associated with drug therapy response in cardiovascular disease.
- Translate data from genetic studies in cardiovascular disease to clinical practice.
- Distinguish between polymorphisms that have demonstrated clinical utility from those that are still under investigation.
- Design a therapeutic management plan based on genetic information for warfarin and clopidogrel therapy.
- Theorize which polymorphisms are likely to be used in future cardiovascular practice.

Key Definitions

Arrhythmia—Abnormal electrical activity within the heart.

Dosing algorithm—A flow diagram that considers clinical, laboratory, and/or genetic characteristics to predict dosing requirements.

Dual antiplatelet therapy—Usually refers to aspirin in combination with clopidogrel or another antiplatelet agent.

Dyslipidemia—Altered blood lipid concentrations.

Heart failure—A condition where the heart is incapable of providing sufficient blood flow to the body to meet metabolic needs.

Hypertension—Elevated blood pressure.

Ischemic heart disease—Reduced blood supply through the coronary arteries that supply the heart muscle.

Loss of function allele—A polymorphism that has been associated with impaired metabolic function of the enzyme that it encodes.

Primary prevention—Measures taken to prevent disease.

Secondary prevention—Measures taken to prevent recurrence and/or additional manifestations of a known disease.

Stent thrombosis—An acute or delayed thrombus within an intracoronary stent, which may be associated with a catastrophic outcome (e.g., myocardial infarction).

Surrogate marker—A measurable change in physiology believed to lead to an eventual outcome.

Clinical Study—Clopidogrel

A 64-year-old Asian-American woman with a past medical history of diabetes, hypertension, and dyslipidemia received two drug-eluting stents (DES) 10 days ago for the management of ST-elevation myocardial infarction. Before undergoing primary percutaneous coronary intervention, she received a single dose of aspirin (325 mg) and clopidogrel (600 mg). Her current drug regimen includes atorvastatin 20 mg daily, EC aspirin 325 mg daily, clopidogrel 75 mg daily, fosinopril 10 mg daily, metoprolol XL 50 mg daily, esomeprazole 20 mg daily, and metformin 1 gm daily. As part of a clinical trial, platelet function testing was performed today with light transmission aggregometry (20 micromole/ADP). The residual platelet aggregation was found to be 60%, which supports she is a nonresponder to clopidogrel and is at increased risk of ischemic events.

1. What genetic polymorphism may explain why this patient is a nonresponder to clopidogrel?
2. What drug-drug interactions must be considered, along with genetic testing, in this clopidogrel nonresponder?
3. What are potential therapeutic options that can be used to overcome nonresponsiveness to clopidogrel?

Introduction

Despite many advances in the treatment of cardiovascular disease (CVD), it remains the leading killer of both men and women in the United States (U.S.). On average, one death occurs every 38 seconds because of CVD. In addition, it is estimated that direct and indirect cost of care for CVD will exceed 503.2 billion dollars in 2010.[1]

Given the large burden CVD has on society, efforts have been made to improve treatment and outcomes associated with cardiovascular disease. Many large scale trials have assessed treatment modalities for CVD resulting in the publication of numerous consensus guidelines. These guidelines drive the management of cardiovascular diseases, including hypertension, dyslipidemia, ischemic heart disease, and heart failure to name a few.[2-4] Drug therapy recommendations make up the majority of these guidelines.

A shortcoming of guideline driven therapy is that it may lead to empiric therapeutic choices that do not consider patient specific factors. However, there is significant interpatient variability in response to many drugs used to treat cardiovascular diseases. This variability is due to numerous factors, such as age, race, sex, concomitant medications and concomitant disease states. However, even after these patient specific factors are considered, there remains a significant amount of interpatient variability in response. This has led many to assess the role of genetic variability as a potential contributor.

Anticoagulant and Antiplatelet Agents

An area of active research is pharmacogenomic variation related to agents that affect coagulation or platelet activity. Many of these agents have promising lines of research, including warfarin, aspirin, dipyridamole, clopidogrel, and the glycoprotein IIb/IIIa receptor inhibitors. In fact, warfarin is the best current example of the utilization of pharmacogenomics to alter drug dosing in direct patient care.

Warfarin

Warfarin pharmacogenomic research shows great promise. Clinically, this is extremely relevant since warfarin has a narrow therapeutic range, multiple drug-drug and drug-food interactions, and it remains the only available oral anticoagulant with over 30 million prescriptions written in the U.S. annually.[5] There are numerous clinical and demographic variables that influence warfarin dosing, including age, nutritional status, and hepatic function, among others. Even when one considers the known clinical variables that alter warfarin dosing, the precision of dosing remains low. Polymorphisms in the genes encoding two enzymes, CYP2C9 and vitamin K epoxide reductase complex subunit 1 (VKORC1), contribute significantly to warfarin dose requirements (Figure 7-1).

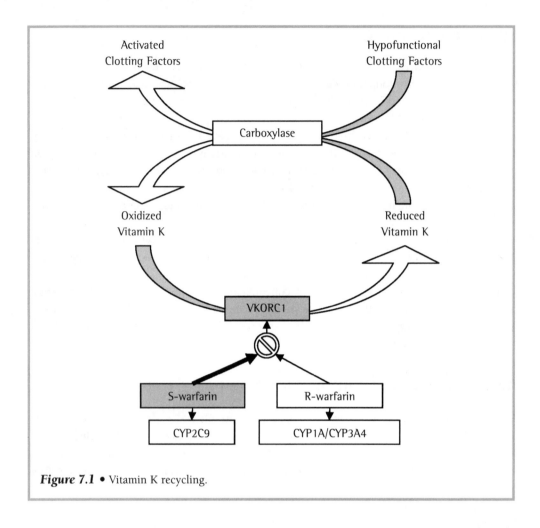

Figure 7.1 • Vitamin K recycling.

Warfarin is highly metabolized and hence its effects can be altered by genetic variation that modifies drug metabolism. Warfarin is a racemic mixture (R and S isomers) with the S-isomer being about five times more potent. Warfarin is cleared by multiple CYP isoenzymes, but the more potent S-isomer undergoes metabolism via the CYP2C9 isoenzyme.

The initial research regarding genetic variation with warfarin focused on altered metabolism via CYP2C9. *CYP2C9*1* encodes for the wild-type enzyme that is consistent with normal extensive metabolism of warfarin. Two common single nucleotide polymorphisms (SNPs) have been discovered, *CYP2C9*2* and *CYP2C9*3*. The *CYP2C9*2* variant has an arginine replaced with a cysteine at position 144 in exon 3, which occurs in about 10% to 20% of Caucasians and rarely in African Americans and Asians (Table 7-1). In the *CYP2C9*3* variant, isoleucine is replaced with leucine at exon 7. This occurs in about 7% to 9% of the population.[6] Patients can be homozygous for each allele (e.g., CYP2C9*1/*1, CYP2C9*2/*2) or heterozygous (e.g., CYP2C9*1/*2). Overall, CYP2C9*2 variants have about a 30% reduction in enzymatic activity corresponding to a 17% reduction in dose if one variant is present. CYP2C9*3 has an 80% reduction in activity equivalent to a 37% reduction in dose if at least one variant is present.[7] Other *CYP2C9* alleles (*CYP2C9*5*, *6, and *11) have also been reported, with *CYP2C9*6* having little effect on metabolic activity but reduced activity has been reported with *CYP2C9*5* and *11.[8] However, these polymorphisms have not been consistently or independently associated with warfarin dose requirements. When considering warfarin dose requirements, there is a gene-dose relationship, where *1/*1, *1/*2, and *1/*3 subjects require average dosages of 5.63, 4.88, and 3.32 mg of warfarin daily, respectively.[9] Posession of multiple variant alleles is associated with even lower daily dosages.

Table 7–1

Racial Differences in Estimated Allele Frequencies Relevant to Warfarin Pharmacokinetics and Pharmacodynamics[8]

		Allele Frequencies %		
		European Americans	African American	Hong Kong Chines
CYP2C9				
CYP2C9*1	–	80.9	95.9	97
CYP2C9*2	rs1799853	12.8	1.3	3
CYP2C9*3	rs1057910	6.3	1.9	–
CYP2C9*5	rs28371686	–	0.9	
VKORC1				
–1639G	–	63.9	89.1	13
–1639A	rs992321	36.1	10.9	87

Another key point of warfarin research is that altered metabolism also changes time to steady-state, requiring longer periods before dose adjustment.[9] Thus, genetic variability in the pharmacokinetics of warfarin leads not only to decreased dose requirements, but alterations in other pharmacokinetic parameters which may effect timing of dose adjustment. This change in pharmacokinetic properties may be why patients possessing a CYP2C9*2 or *3 allele are at increased risk of both time above goal INR range and serious or life-threatening bleeding.[10-13] In fact, even taking CYP2C9 genotype into account prior to warfarin dosing does not decrease this risk.[13]

Recently, the gene encoding the active site for warfarin (VKORC1) was identified. Vitamin K epoxide reductase mediates the conversion from oxidized to reduced vitamin K, which is necessary for the activation of clotting factors II, VII, IX, X and proteins C, and S (Figure 7-1). Binding of warfarin to this enzyme blocks vitamin K recycling and prevents the activation of clotting factors. Thus, warfarin leads to hypofunctional clotting factors and an anticoagulated state. Altered response to warfarin at VKORC1 changes how patients respond to warfarin therapy. Various VKORC1 polymorphisms have been identified but the two most widely studied include C1173T and G-1639A.[8] These two polymorphisms along with several others often occur together in Caucasians and are thus said to be in linkage disequilibrium. Therefore, looking at only one of these polymorphisms (often the G-1639A SNP) is sufficient to characterize the genetic variability in the Caucasian population. However, less is known about the linkage disequilibrium patterns in non-Caucasian populations, such as African Americans. The frequencies of the variant VKORC1 1173T or -1639A alleles are well characterized in several racial groups, and these variant alleles are most common in the Asian population compared to those of European-American decent and are uncommon in African Americans (Table 7-1).

In Caucasians, these variant alleles have been associated with decreased vitamin K epoxide reductase messenger RNA levels.[9] Therefore, possession of either variant allele is associated with increased warfarin sensitivity that is likely due to decreased available vitamin K epoxide reductase to block. *VKORC1* -1639AA genotype corresponds with patients that are more sensitive to warfarin, whereas GG corresponds to patients that are less sensitive to therapy. Mean warfarin dose requirements for patients with AA, GA, and GG genotypes are 2.7, 4.9, and 6.2 mg daily, respectively.[14] Prior to the genetic characterization of *VKORC1*, warfarin dosing nomograms had used race as a predictor of warfarin dose requirements. We now know that African Americans and Asians require higher and lower warfarin doses respectively, compared to Caucasians, because of the difference in *VKORC1* allele frequencies in these populations.

Based on the previously described results, warfarin became the first cardiovascular drug to have a change in its package insert adding pharmacogenetic information, specifically stating "…lower initiation doses should be considered for patients with certain genetic variations in *CYP2C9* and *VKORC1* enzymes…"[15] The potential benefits of pharmacogenetic guided dosing are to achieve the correct INR sooner, maintain the INR within range better, and to prevent complications. Two studies suggest possible benefit of pharmacogenomic based warfarin dosing.[7,16] In one study, there was a nonsignificant reduction in serious clinical events in those who received pharmacogenomic dosing.[17] A more recent investigation, found a lower rate of minor hemorrhage in subjects with *CYP2C9* genotype-guided warfarin dosing.[16]

Various dosing algorithms have been developed based on the available pharmacogenomic data and other clinical variables (e.g., age, weight, height, gender, race, etc.).[13,18,19] A recent study provides guidance regarding estimation of the warfarin dose with clinical and pharmacogenetic data.[20] The authors created a dosing algorithm in 4,043 racially diverse subjects and validated it in a cohort of 1,009 subjects. The pharmacogenetic algorithm, which took into account both genotype and clinical information (drug interactions, body size, race, and smoking status), accurately identified individuals that required markedly lower dosing (<21 mg/week) and those requiring higher dosing (>49 mg/week), which was necessary in 46.2% of the population. Overall, the pharmacogenetic algorithm, as compared to the clinical algorithm, better predicted the stable dose of warfarin required to achieve the target INR. This dosing algorithm can be found at warfarindosing.org.

Although dosing algorithms are available, there are numerous questions that need to be answered before routine pharmacogenetic testing for warfarin (or any other medication) will occur in a clinical setting. First, is the safety of warfarin enhanced with pharmacogenetic testing? As previously mentioned, only slight, and often nonsignificant, reductions in adverse events have been found when genotyping is used prospectively to predict warfarin dose requirements.[16,17] It is important to remember that even the best dosing algorithms to date only predict 40% to 60% of the variability in warfarin dose requirements.[13,18-20] However, larger studies assessing prospective genotyping of warfarin are currently under way. These results should shed light on the clinical utility of pharmacogenetic guided warfarin therapy. Also, is it cost effective to routinely screen all warfarin patients before initiating warfarin therapy? This last question has been assessed in a paper by the AEI-Brookings Joint Center for Regulatory Studies and a publication by Eckman et al. with conflicting results.[21,22] While the AEI-Brookings paper found that universally utilized genotype guided therapy would be cost effective, these results have been criticized. In addition, the paper by Eckman et al. found that prospective warfarin genotyping was unlikely to be cost effective.[22] However, as genotyping methods become less expensive, these results may change.

Aspirin

Aspirin is a standard therapy in patients with or at high-risk of ischemic heart disease or stroke. It has been shown to reduce the risk of death, myocardial infarction, and nonfatal stroke in this patient population.[23] Moreover, aspirin in addition to clopidogrel plays an important role in duel antiplatelet therapy after percutaneous coronary intervention.

Aspirin exhibits its antiplatelet effect by inhibiting cyclooxygenase-1 (COX-1), which is responsible for production of thromboxane A_2 (TXA_2). TXA_2 is one of many factors that promote platelet activation that subsequently leads to platelet aggregation. Aspirin is not effective in all patients and numerous variables may be responsible for this phenomenon, including platelet agonists beyond TXA_2 (e.g., adenosine diphosphate), gender differences, and patient adherence. The term *aspirin resistance* has been coined to represent this phenomenon. This term can be defined further as clinical resistance, where there is the occurrence of an atherothrombotic event despite aspirin therapy, and biologic/pharmacodynamic resistance, where aspirin fails to inhibit platelet function as determined by assay.[24]

Polymorphisms of the gene encoding COX-1 (*PTGS1*) have been evaluated as a potential cause of decreased response to aspirin. The promoter region, specifically the A-842G polymorphism, has been the focus of research associated with aspirin resistance. Studies in coronary artery disease, using laboratory assays, suggest the -842G allele is associated with a reduced response to aspirin, although contradictory data have been published in subjects with recurrent ischemic stroke.[25-28]

The gene (*ITGB3*) that encodes the glycoprotein IIIA (GPIIIA) receptor has also been evaluated as a second potential cause of aspirin resistance. The Leu33Pro SNP occurs in exon 2 of *ITGB3* and defines the P1[A1] and P1[A2] variants.[29] In vitro, the P1[A2] allele, which occurs at a frequency of 15%, has been associated with increased platelet activation and aggregation.[30,31] In addition, possession of the variant P1[A2] allele has been associated with an increased risk of stent thrombosis after percutaneous coronary intervention and other adverse cardiovascular outocmes.[32] However, these data have been inconsistent.[33] Similarly, studies investigating the role of this polymorphism in aspirin resistance are unclear. In fact, The *ITGB3* variant P1[A2] allele has been associated with both increased and decreased response to aspirin; while still other studies have found no association.[26,34,35] Of note, all of these studies used different methods to determine aspirin resistance. This highlights the importance of phenotype choice in pharmacogenomics studies. Due to the inconsistency of the data currently available, clinical genotyping for aspirin response cannot be recommended.

Clopidogrel

Clopidogrel is another important antiplatelet agent commonly used in clinical practice. In addition to being a viable option in patients that cannot take aspirin, clopidogrel is a standard of care in patients after percutaneous coronary intervention with stent placement. Dual antiplatelet therapy (clopidogrel in addition to aspirin) is necessary after stent placement to prevent in-stent thrombosis. However, not all patients respond similarly to treatment.

There is significant variability in the pharmacokinetics of clopidogrel, beginning with its absorption in the gastrointestinal tract via p-glycoprotein. Additionally, clopidogrel is a prodrug and requires conversion to its active form via numerous CYP450 isoenzymes. The active metabolite then exerts its effects by inhibiting adenosine diphosphate activity via the $P2Y_{12}$ receptor. There are various ways in which polymorphisms can lead to altered drug effect at the receptor site. In fact, up to 30% of natural variation in platelet reactivity is related to genetic inheritance.[36] Specifically, genetic variability in the CYP450 system and in $P2Y_{12}$ have been studied for their role in clopidogrel response. Much like aspirin, clopidogrel response can also be characterized through clinical outcomes or via platelet aggregation tests.

Genetic variability in the gene encoding the $P2Y_{12}$ receptor (*P2RY12*) has been well studied. Several SNPs in *P2RY12* have been assessed for their association with clopidogrel response. The majority of the SNPs studied were in linkage disequilibrium and occurred together. The largest study to date assessed the role of the T744C polymorphism in clopidogrel efficacy as assessed by both biologic and clinical response.[37] They found no association between this SNP and response to clopidogrel. Other studies have found similar results.[38] Therefore, genotyping of *P2RY12* polymorphisms is not used to predict clopidogrel response.

Genetic variation in pathways involved in drug absorption and metabolism can also lead to reduced response to clopidogrel. P-glycoprotein is involved in clopidogrel absorption and the role of three *ABCB1* SNPs (C3435T, G2677T, and C1236T) have been evaluated. Lower clopidogrel concentration (both Cmax and AUC) after a single dose of 300 and 600 mg were noted in subjects that were homozygous for the variant 3435T.[39] Of interest, a larger loading dose of 900 mg overcame this difference. However, this change in pharmacokinetic parameters has not been consistently associated with clinical response to clopidogrel.[40,41] Until further studies are completed, genotyping of *ABCB1* in patients receiving clopidogrel cannot be recommended.

Other studies have evaluated the role of altered metabolism with clopidogrel. Various isoenzymes of the CYP450 system have been evaluated including CYP3A4, CYP3A5, and CYP2C19. *CYP3A4* polymorphisms (*CYP3A4*1B*, *CYP3A4*3*, intervening sequence [IVS] 7+258A>G, IVS7+849C>T, and IVS10+12G>A) have been assessed and only the IVS10+12A was associated with increased response to clopidogrel therapy, but with conflicting results.[42,43] Contradictory results have been found with polymorphisms of *CYP3A5*.[41,42,44,45]

Several well characterized polymorphisms in the gene encoding CYP2C19 have been studied for their role in clopidogrel response. The *CYP2C19*2* and *3* variant alleles are associated with decreased CYP2C19 function compared to *CYP2C19*1*. Approximately 30% of Caucasians, 40% of African Americans, and more than 55% of East Asians carry one of these variant alleles. Three studies recently documented that possession of two loss of function *CYP2C19* alleles was associated with an increased risk of cardiovascular events with clopidogrel therapy.[40,42,46] These studies are conflicting however on the response of subjects possessing only one loss of function allele. Two studies, a genetic analysis of the Trial to Assess Improvement in Therapeutic Outcomes by Optimizing Platelet Inhibition with Prasugrel-Thrombolysis in Myocardial Infarction (TRITON-TIMI) 38 and a registry study of young subjects status post myocardial infarction, found that possession of at least one loss of function *CYP2C19* allele was associated with increased risk of cardiovascular events.[42] However, the other study, which genotyped subjects in the French Registry of Acute ST-Elevation and Non-ST-Elevation Myocardial Infarction, demonstrated that subjects possessing two loss of function *CYP2C19* alleles had worse outcomes.[40] These studies demonstrate clearly that possessing at least two loss of function alleles is associated with increased risk of adverse cardiovascular events in patients receiving clopidogrel. In fact, these data have led to pharmacogenetic information being added to the clopidogrel package insert. The updated package insert states "CYP2C19 poor metabolizer status is associated with diminished response to clopidogrel. The optimal dose regimen for poor metabolizers has yet to be determined."[47] It is currently unclear; however, whether patients with just one loss of function allele will have worse outcomes with clopidogrel therapy. In addition, no studies have documented how patients with loss of function *CYP2C19* alleles should be managed. However, a novel thienopyridine (prasugrel) recently received FDA approval for patients with unstable angina or myocardial infarction who undergo PCI. Prasugrel does not undergo the same extensive metabolism as clopidogrel and is less likely to be susceptible to genetic variation in the CYP450 system. Patients who possess loss of function *CYP2C19* alleles would be good candidates for prasugrel therapy. Additionally, ticlopidine may be considered in clopidogrel nonresponders. Nonresponse to both clopidogrel and ticlopidine has been found to occur only in 3.5% of patients.[48]

Abciximab/GPIIbIIIas

GP IIb/IIIa receptor inhibitors are potent antiplatelet agents used in select situations, such as acute coronary syndromes and percutaneous coronary intervention. All of these agents block the GP IIb/IIIa receptors, but abciximab also has activity on receptors involved in platelet adhesion (e.g., vitronectin). One investigation found that platelets with the *ITGB3* Pl$^{A1/A2}$ genotype were more sensitive to inhibition by abciximab.[35] Conversely, another study found that platelets with the Pl$^{A1/A2}$ genotype are less completely inhibited with abciximab.[49] While a third study found that this polymorphism had no effect on the interindividual variability in the platelet inhibitory effects of the three GPIIb/IIIa inhibitors.[50] Therefore, no genotyping can currently be recommended to predict response to these medications.

Agents for Hypertension, Heart Failure, and Ischemic Heart Disease

Agents for the management of hypertension, heart failure, and ischemic heart disease have various pharmacogenomic considerations that may guide therapy. Interpatient variability has been noted with the beta-blockers, angiotensin-converting-enzyme (ACE) inhibitors, angiotensin receptor blockers (ARBs), diuretics, and hydralazine. This section addresses the pharmacogenomic basis for these alterations as well as relevant clinical data.

Beta-blockers

The primary site of action for beta-blockers is the adrenergic system, specifically the beta-1 (β1) and beta-2 (β2) receptors. These receptors are polymorphic and genetic variation may result in an altered treatment response. The effect of pharmacogenomics on β-blocker response may also differ based on the pharmacologic characteristics of the agent. For instance, some β-blockers are relatively selective for the β1 receptor (e.g., metoprolol) whereas others are nonselective (e.g., propranolol). Moreover, certain agents may have α-adrenergic receptor blockade (e.g., carvedilol) or intrinsic sympathomimetic activity (e.g., pindolol).

The gene encoding the β1 receptor (*ADRB1*) has two well studied polymorphisms (Arg-389Gly and Ser49Gly) (Table 7-2). Of note, frequencies of these polymorphisms appear to vary based on ethnic background. For the *ADRB1* gene, both the variant 389Gly and 49Gly alleles occur more frequently in African Americans than Causasians.[51] In vitro, these polymorphisms have been shown to affect the function of the receptor as well as its cell signaling.[52,53] Specifically, data demonstrate that the wild-type 389Arg and 49Ser alleles have been associated with increased in-vitro activity. This increased activity suggests that patients possessing an *ADRB1* 389Arg or 49Gly allele for *ADRB1* would have better response to β-blockade. Polymorphisms of *ADRB1* have been well studied in patients with hypertension and heart failure.

Table 7-2
Relevant Genes Related to Cardiovascular Drugs

Drug	Gene (name)	Polymorphisms Studied	Type of Alteration
Beta blockers	*ADRB1*	Arg389Gly, Ser49Gly	Pharmacodynamic
	ADRB2	Arg16Gly, Glu27Gln	Pharmacodynamic
	CYP2D6		Pharmacokinetic
	(e.g., metoprolol, carveidolol)		
ACE inhibitors and ARBs	AGT	Met325Thr	Pharmacodynamic
	ACE	I/D	Pharmacodynamic
	AGTR1	A1166C	Pharmacodynamic
Statins	HMGCR		Pharmacodynamic
	APOE	ε2, ε3, ε4	Pharmacodynamic
	MTHFR	C677T	Pharmacodynamic
	CBS	Insertion/deletion	Pharmacodynamic
	ADAMTS1	Asp227Pro	Pharmacodynamic
	FCAR	Asp92Asn	Pharmacodynamic
	KIF6	Trp719Arg	Pharmacodynamic
	CYP3A5	CYP3A5*3	Pharmacokinetic
	SLCO1B1	rs4149056 T/C	Pharmacokinetic
Ezetimibe	NPC1L1	C1735G, A25342C, T27677C, A-133G, C-18A, C1679G	Pharmacodynamic
Digoxin	ABCB1	C3435T	Pharmacokinetic
Propafenone	CYP2D6	Genotype and Phenotype	Pharmacokinetic
Flecainide	CYP2D6	Genotype and Phenotype	Pharmacokinetic
Procainamide	NAT2	Genotype and Phenotype	Pharmacokinetic

Response to β-blockers in hypertension is highly variable, with up to 60% of patients on treatment not achieving adequate control with monotherapy.[54,55] Genetic variation may be a contributing factor. Clinical trials have validated in-vitro hypotheses and subjects with the 389Arg genotype have been shown to exhibit a greater reduction of blood pressure with β-blocker therapy.[56-60] Many of these investigations, however, have focused on response to metoprolol, and the results may not be applicable to other β-blockers given the pharmacodynamic variability of the agents mentioned previously. Discordant data regarding blood pressure response based on genetic variation have been published for other β-blockers, specifically atenolol and bisoprolol.[56,57,61] Genotyping for *ADRB1* polymorphisms maybe useful in patients receiving metoprolol, although it is unclear if the difference in blood pressure lowering correlates with improved clinical outcomes. Therefore, currently genotyping for *ADRB1* polymorphisms cannot be recommended for patients receiving β-blockers for hypertension.

In heart failure, several studies have evaluated polymorphisms of *ADRB1* and response to β-blocker therapy. Similar to the data in hypertension, it is subjects with the 389Arg genotype that showed improved response, including a greater reduction in left ventricular diameter and improvement in left ventricular ejection fraction.[62,63] In addition, heart failure subjects with the 49Ser genotype had a higher mortality rate as compared to the 49Gly genotype; however, the use of β-blockers therapy mitigated this difference.[64] Contrary data, however, have been published. A substudy of the MERIT-HF trial found no association between heart failure outcomes or response to β-blocker therapy (metoprolol) and the Arg389 genotype.[65] This study is difficult to interpret though, because statistical analysis of the interaction between *ADRB1* genotype and treatment and their association with outcome was not presented. Another study of 637 heart failure subjects enrolled in registries found no association between β-receptor genotypes and survival in heart failure with metoprolol or carvedilol.[66]

Additional data with bucindolol substantiates a potential association between response to β-blocker therapy in heart failure and genetic variation in *ADRB1*. In the Beta-blocker Evaluation of Survival (BEST) study, bucindolol was evaluated in subjects with NYHA class III and IV heart failure. When compared to standard of care, bucindolol showed no overall survival benefit.[67] When considering the hazard ratios for death in prespecified subgroups, it was suggested that there was a difference in response based on race. African-American subjects did not receive any benefit from bucindolol therapy while non–African-American subjects had a significant reduction in mortality with bucindolol. Given the differing frequency of polymorphisms in the β-adrenergic receptor genes by race, genetic variation may have played a role in the differing response.

A genetic substudy of BEST (n=1040) evaluated the association between the *ADRB1* Arg-389Gly and α2c 322-325 WT/Del polymorphisms and mortality with bucindolol therapy.[68] Subjects who were 389Arg homozygotes had a statistically higher rate of overall survival with bucindolol therapy compared to placebo. The subjects in the favorable genotype group also had reduced heart failure hospitalization and cardiovascular hospitalization. In contrast, subjects possessing the 389Gly allele had no response to bucindolol therapy. No association was seen with the α2c 322-325 WT/Del polymorphism. Although this study is remarkable because it identified those who may respond to bucindolol based on genetic testing, numerous questions must be resolved. For example, why is *ADRB1* genotype associated with response to bucindolol therapy in heart failure, but not metoprolol or carvedilol response? What are the incentives for genetic testing and who will pay for it? Does a genetically identified bucindolol responder do better than standard metoprolol or carvedilol treated patients? Bucindolol attempted to earn FDA approval based on the results of the BEST substudy. The FDA, however, deemed that additional data were needed. Only when or if bucindolol receives FDA approval, can *ADRB1* genotyping be recommended for bucindolol therapy in this patient population.

The gene encoding the β2 receptor (*ADRB2*) has two polymorphisms of interest (Gly16Arg and Gln27Glu) (Table 7-2). The *ADRB2* 16Gly and 27Gln alleles have been associated with reduced sensitivity to isoproterenol (a β1 and β2 receptor agonist) in vitro.[69] Similar to the *ADRB1* gene, the frequency of polymorphisms in *ADRB2* differ based on race. The *ADRB2* 16Arg allele frequency is 0.39 among Caucasians, 0.49 among African Americans, and 0.51 among Chinese. The *ADRB2* 27Gln is more frequent in African Americans (0.81) and Chinese (0.91) compared to Caucasians (0.754). Genetic variation in *ADRB2* has been assessed in ischemic heart disease, specifically in patients with acute coronary syndrome. One investigation considered the effect of the *ADRB1* Arg389Gly and Ser49Gly and the *ADRB2* Gly16Arg and Glu27Gln polymorphisms on survival in subjects receiving β-blocker therapy after an acute coronary syndrome.[70] This prospective cohort study found that subjects prescribed β-blocker therapy after ACS had different survival based on *ADRB2* genotype. Subjects homozygous for both the 27Gln and 16Arg alleles who received β-blocker therapy, had increased 3-year mortality compared to other genotypes. No association between mortality and *ADRB2* genotype was seen in non–β-blocker treated subjects; however, the population of non–β-blocker treated subjects was small. This suggests that the polymorphisms are associated specifically with β-blocker response and not ACS mortality in general. However without confirmatory studies, assessing *ADRB2* genotype for β-blocker therapy in ACS cannot be recommended.

It has also been hypothesized that β-blocker response is related to genetic variability in drug metabolizing enzymes. Because carvedilol, metoprolol, propranolol, labetalol, and timolol are metabolized by CYP2D6, and well known polymorphisms in the gene encoding CYP2D6 lead to variable CYP2D6 activity, there is the potential for altered metabolism.[51] Altered metabolism could then lead to changes in the efficacy or safety of the β-blocker, which is extensively discussed in Chapter 4. Studies have shown that patients classified as poor metabolizers based on *CYP2D6* genotype do have increased β-blocker concentrations. However, β-blockers have a wide therapeutic window and the majority of studies have found no association between variance in *CYP2D6* genotype and response to β-blocker therapy.[63,71]

Angiotensin-Converting Enzyme Inhibitors and Angiotensin II Receptor Blocker

Angiotensin-converting enzyme (ACE) inhibitors and angiotensin II receptor blockers (ARBs) are common agents used in the management of hypertension, heart failure, and ischemic heart disease. Both agents mitigate the renin-angiotensin-aldosterone system, albeit by different mechanisms. ACE inhibitors block the step that prevents the conversion of angiotensin I to angiotensin II. Angiotensin II, through its interaction with the angiotensin type 1(AT1) receptor, is responsible for the detrimental effects in cardiac disease, such as vasoconstriction, excess aldosterone release, and water retention. ARBs exert their effects by blocking angiotensin II at the AT1 receptor.

There are polymorphisms in three genes that are relevant to ACE inhibitor and ARB therapy (Table 7-2). The gene encoding angiotensinogen has a common polymorphism, Met235Thr, which has been associated with higher angiotensin concentrations and elevated blood pressure.[72] The angiotensin converting enzyme, which converts angiotensin I to angiotensin II, also has a common insertion/deletion polymorphism, which occurs in approximately 27% of the population.[73] The *ACE* I/D polymorphism has been associated with ACE plasma levels. Finally, the gene encoding the AT1 receptor also has the A1166C single nucleotide polymorphism (SNP).

The *ACE* I/D polymorphism is one of the most frequently studied polymorphisms in pharmacogenetics and hypertension. Two large studies have evaluated the association between this polymorphism and blood pressure response or other outcomes related to ACE inhibitor therapy, specifically lisinopril and perindopril.[74,75] Both of these studies found no association between response to ACE inhibitor therapy and *ACE* I/D genotype. Data from these two very large, randomized, controlled trials provide strong evidence that the *ACE* I/D polymorphism is not associated with treatment outcomes in hypertension.

Despite results with the I/D polymorphism, *ACE* continues to be considered a good candidate gene for explaining some of the variability seen with ACE inhibitor therapy. In fact, subjects from the African American Study of Kidney Disease and Hypertension (AASK) trial who were randomized to ramipril therapy were genotyped for three polymorphisms down stream from the *ACE* I/D polymorphism (G12269A, C17888T, G20037A).[76] These polymorphisms had previously been linked to ACE plasma levels. The AASK investigators specifically assessed whether these polymorphisms or haplotypes were associated with time required to reach blood pressure goal in 347 of the AASK study subjects who received ramipril. They found that subjects who were heterozygous at *ACE* position 12269 reached their blood pressure goal slower than either homozygote genotype at the same position. The small sample size and limited racial population make the results of this study difficult to apply; however, future studies will likely assess genetic variation in *ACE* beyond the I/D polymorphism.

The angiotensinogen polymorphism, Met235Thr, has also been evaluated in hypertension. Possession of the 235Thr allele has been associated with increased angiotensinogen levels and blood pressure response to ACE inhibitor therapy.[73,77] However, differing results have been found in other studies. One study found an association between the *AGT* 235Thr allele and an increased risk of myocardial infarction in subjects receiving ACE inhibitor therapy, whereas another study suggested that possession of this same allele was associated with a lower risk of stroke.[78,79] These discordant data make it difficult to draw a firm conclusion related to the *AGT* Met235Thr polymorphisms. Other related polymorphisms have also been evaluated with variable results.

The final gene directly related to ARB therapy is the gene encoding the AT1 receptor (*AGTR1*). The A1166C SNP has been evaluated for its role in response to losartan therapy. Studies have shown that the 1166C allele is associated with a greater reduction in blood pressure, while other studies have shown that the 1166A allele was associated with a decrease in myocardial stiffness.[80,81] In addition, no association has been seen between blood pressure reduction with ARB therapy and this SNP.[82] Small studies have also assessed the role of this polymorphism in the response to ARB therapy in heart failure. This will likely be an expanding area of interest, but currently genotyping for this polymorphism in patients with hypertension or heart failure cannot be recommended.

Diuretics

The use of thiazide diuretics is a standard of care for individuals with uncomplicated hypertension. Thiazide diuretics exert their effect by blocking sodium and chloride reabsorption in the distal tubule. Adducin, an α/β heterodimeric protein, is a cytoskeletal protein that plays a role in cell signal transduction and is associated with renal sodium reabsorption. Polymorphisms in the gene encoding the α-adducin sub-unit (*ADD1*) may be associated with response to thiazides in hypertensive individuals. The *ADD1* Gly460Trp SNP has been well studied. Possession of the 460Trp allele has been associated with an increased risk of hypertension and specifically salt sensitive hypertension.[83] In addition, the 460Trp allele has been linked to greater reductions in blood pressure and decreased risk of MI or stroke with thiazide diuretic treatment.[83-86] However, results related to this *ADD1* polymorphism have been inconsistent.[87] In fact, two large, randomized studies have further assessed the association between the *ADD1* Gly460Trp SNP and CHD outcomes in hypertensives receiving thiazide diuretics.[88,89] No association was found with *ADD1* genotype and CHD risk or response to thiazide diuretic therapy in either study. These conflicting results limit the clinical utility of *ADD1* genotyping to predict response to diuretic therapy.

In addition, polymorphisms in the genes encoding the β3 subunit of the G protein gene (*GNB3*), endothelial nitric oxide synthase (*NOS3*), *ACE*, WNK lysine deficient protein kinase 1 (*WNK1*), *ADRB2*, the γ subunit of the nonvoltage-gated sodium channel (*SCNNIG*) have been found to make small contributions to thiazide induced changes in blood pressure.[86,87,90-92] However, without multiple studies replicating the results listed above genotyping for these polymorphisms cannot currently be recommended for patients receiving diuretic therapy.

Hydralazine/Isosorbide Dinitrate

The combination of hydralazine and isosorbide dinitrate has shown benefit for patients with heart failure, with early data demonstrating a lower mortality compared to placebo.[93] It is believed that the combination of hydralazine and nitrates is effective in heart failure because nitrates serve as a nitric oxide donor that leads to venodilation while hydralazine vasodilates arterial smooth muscle. In addition, hydralazine may have antioxidant properties which decrease tolerance to nitrates in heart failure patients.[94] However, when compared to ACE inhibitor therapy, specifically enalapril, the ACE inhibitor was superior in reducing mortality.[95] A subsequent subgroup analysis, however, demonstrated that African-American subjects did not show the improved benefit with enalapril.[96] This finding led to the A-HeFT trial, which evaluated the use of hydralazine and isosorbide dinitrate in self-identified African-American subjects with heart failure.[97] A-HeFT demonstrated a substantial reduction in mortality in African-American subjects treated with the hydralazine-nitrate combination when added to standard therapy (ACE inhibitors and β-blockers).

Genetic variation is one of the possible underlying reasons for this difference in response to hydralazine and nitrates between Caucasians and African Americans. The Genetic Risk of Heart Failure in African Americans (GRAHF) study, a genetic substudy of A-HeFT, was initiated in order to assess the genetic differences between these two racial groups with respect to the development of heart failure and response to hydralazine and nitrates.[98] Subjects were genotyped for a promoter region polymorphism (T-344C) in the gene encoding aldosterone synthase (*CYP11B2*). Possession of the -344C allele has been associated with increased aldosterone synthase activity, increased risk of hypertension, and left ventricular remodeling. In addition, the -344C allele is significantly more prevalent in Caucasian heart failure patients. In this study of African-American subjects, the -344C allele was associated with poorer hospitalization-free survival and increased mortality. African-American subjects possessing a -344C allele did not receive the same benefit from the hydralazine and nitrate treatment as those with -344TT genotype did (which is the most prevalent genotype in African Americans).

Based on the mechanism of action of the hydralazine/nitrate combination and the difference in prevalence of variants in *NOS3* (the gene encoding endothelial nitric oxide synthase) in African Americans compared to Caucasians, it was hypothesized that *NOS3* genotype may predict those that would benefit from this combination.[99] Three *NOS3* polymorphisms (T-786C, intron 4a/4b, and Glu298Asp) have been studied. The -786T, 4a, and 298Glu alleles are found more frequently in African Americans than in Caucasians. However, only the Glu298Asp polymorphism influenced treatment outcomes, with the fixed dosed combination of hydralazine-isosorbide dinitrate improving the composite score and quality of life in the Glu298Glu subset only. These studies suggest that the *CYP11B2* T-344C or the *NOS3* Glu298Asp polymorphisms maybe associated with response to hydralazine and nitrates in African Americans, but until confirmatory evidence is published from a separate cohort, genotyping for these SNPs cannot be recommended. In addition, these genetic studies have only been completed in African Americans. Therefore, it is unclear if SNPs in *CYP11B2* or *NOS3* are associated with response to hydralazine and nitrate combination therapy in Caucasians.

Agents for Dyslipidemia

Interpatient variability has been noted with agents used in the treatment of dyslipidemia. Several studies have sought to characterize the source of this variation. This section addresses the pharmacogenomic basis for these alterations as well as the relevant clinical data.

Statins

3-hydroxy-3-methylglutaryl coenzyme A reductase (HMG-CoA) reductase inhibitors (statins) are used primarily for lowering low density lipoprotein concentrations (LDL-C). In addition, statins have been demonstrated to decrease morbidity and mortality in patients with elevated LDL-C. However, there is substantial variability in LDL lowering with statin therapy. Genes associated with both the pharmacokinetics and pharmacodynamics of statins have been studied for their contribution to this variability.

While the metabolic pathways for statins vary, they all share a uniform mechanism of action. All statins are competitive inhibitors of HMG-CoA reductase, which is the rate limiting enzyme involved in cholesterol synthesis. Therefore, several studies have assessed the role of variation in the gene encoding HMG-CoA reductase (*HMGCR*) in statin response.

Single gene-association studies have documented an association between *HMGCR* genotype and lipid response to statin therapy.[100,101] However, when multiple genes associated with statin response have been assessed, the results have been inconsistent.[102-104] Moreover, while *HMGCR* genotype has been associated with LDL response to pravastatin therapy in one study, it was not found to be associated with LDL response to other statins in additional studies.[102,103] Polymorphisms in this gene have also never been linked to the morbidity and mortality improvements seen with statin therapy.

Genes encoding proteins involved in lipid homeostasis and inflammation have also been studied for their association with statin response. Apolipoproteins are found on lipoprotein particles and facilitate cellular uptake of these lipoproteins. Apolipoprotein E (ApoE) has been well studied for its association with statin response. There are three common apoE isoforms: ε2, ε3, and ε4. The ε2 allele has been associated with greater LDL-C reduction with statin therapy.[105] This was confirmed in a large study assessing multiple genes involved in statin response in subjects receiving atorvastatin, lovastatin, fluvastatin, pravastatin, and simvastatin.[103] Specifically, subjects carrying the ε2 rare variant allele had a 3.5% greater reduction in LDL; but this association with LDL lowering was weaker than that found with age and gender. However, even these results have been inconsistent.[102] An association has also been demonstrated between *APOE* genotype and risk of MI or death. This was done in a 966 subject subset of the Scandinavian Simvastatin Survival Study (4S).[106] They found that risk of death was increased in *APOE* ε4 carriers; however, this excess risk was abolished with simvastatin treatment. This is in contrast to the previous study in which possession of the *APOE* ε2, not the ε4, allele was associated with improved LDL lowering with statins.[103] In other words, while those who carry the *APOE* ε2 allele have better LDL lowering with statins, carriers of the *APOE* ε4 allele may actually derive the most life-saving benefits from simvastatin therapy. Therefore, *APOE* genotype may provide information, beyond LDL lowering, on event reduction with statins. The two studies highlight the importance of studying not only the surrogate marker (LDL lowering) but also important clinical outcomes (MI or death) in cardiovascular pharmacogenomic studies. *APOE* genotype appears to be associated both with LDL response and clinical outcomes with statin therapy. However, without confirmation from additional studies clinical use of *APOE* genotype cannot be recommended.

Genetic variation in enzymes involved in the regulation of homocysteine levels have also been studied for their role in statin response. Homocysteine has been shown to play a role in oxidative stress and endothelial damage and is considered to be a risk factor for CAD. Subjects in the GenHAT subset of ALLHAT were genotyped for two polymorphisms in the gene encoding methylenetetrahydrofolate reductase (*MTHRF*) and one in the gene encoding cystathionine-β-synthase (*CBS*); both of which are involved in the regulation of homocysteine levels.[107] Subjects in ALLHAT were randomized in an open label fashion to treatment with pravastatin 40 mg/day or usual care and were followed for 6 years to assess CHD death, nonfatal MI, and all cause mortality. The *MTHFR* C677T and *CBS* insertion variants were found to be associated with pravastatin response. Specifically, subjects with the *MTHFR* 677CC genotype had a protective effect from pravastatin where as T allele carriers did not. Subjects carrying a *CBS* insertion allele had an increased risk of CHD and all cause mortality compared to subjects without an insertion allele. In addition, the deleterious effects of the CBS insertion allele were alleviated with the use of pravastatin. These data suggest that polymorphisms in genes involved in homocysteine regulation and homeostasis may play a role in pravastatin response. However, the data from this study are difficult to interpret as pravastatin did not demonstrate a beneficial effect in the overall ALLHAT study.[108]

The Cholesterol and Recurrent Events (CARE) study and West of Scotland Coronary Prevention Study (WOSCOPS) populations have been used to assess the role of genetics in pravastatin response. CARE was a secondary prevention study primarily in male subjects with average cholesterol levels, which randomized subjects to pravastatin 40 mg/day or placebo.[109] WOSCOPS was a double-blind, placebo controlled primary prevention trial in men with hypercholesterolemia randomized to pravastatin 40mg/day or placebo.[110] The primary outcome in CARE was coronary event or nonfatal MI and in WOSCOPS it was the combined incidence of nonfatal MI and death from CHD. The gene encoding ADAMTS1 a matrix metalloproteinase, theoretically involved in the stability of the fibrous cap of atherosclerotic lesions, has been studied in both populations.[111] Specifically, the *ADAMTS1* Ala227Pro polymorphism was associated with coronary event risk and pravastatin response in the Caucasian male population of both studies. In CARE, 227 pro/pro homozygotes had an increased risk of CHD and nonfatal MI compared to 227Ala allele carriers. *ADAMTS1* 227pro/pro homozygotes also received greater benefit from pravastatin therapy. This association was confirmed in WOSCOPS. The Asp92Asn polymorphism in the gene encoding the myeloid IgA Fc receptor (*FCAR*), which is involved in the activation of monocytes and macrophages and thus inflammation, was assessed in the same manor.[112] The *FCAR* 92Asn allele was associated with increased risk of CHD and nonfatal MI in both CARE and WOSCOPS. In CARE, the risk of MI was reduced in carriers of the 92Asn allele but not in noncarriers. In WOSCOPS however, both carriers and noncarriers of the 92Asn allele received benefit from pravastatin. The differing results from CARE and WOSCOPS maybe due to the difference in the primary and secondary prevention populations. It is important to note, however, that the *FCAR* Asp92Asn and the *ADAMTS1* Ala227Pro polymorphisms have only been studied in Caucasian males receiving pravastatin. The results of these genetic studies cannot be extrapolated to other patient groups or other statins. Before considering genotyping for either of these polymorphisms, additional studies in a broader range of patients will be necessary.

The role of the Trp719Arg polymorphism in the gene encoding KIF6, a kinesin involved in intracellular transport, has also been found to be associated with risk of MI and CHD in both CARE and WOSCOPS.[113] Specifically, possession of the 719Arg allele was associated with an increased risk of CHD in both studies. In addition, 719Arg allele carriers had greater risk reduction with pravastatin compared to non carriers in both studies. The role of this polymorphism was also assessed in subjects from the Pravastatin or Atorvastatin Evaluation and Infection Therapy –Thrombolysis in MI 22 study (PROVE IT-TIMI 22). PROVE IT-TIMI 22 enrolled subjects recently hospitalized for ACS, in stable condition after any planned revascularization, and randomized them to atorvastatin 80mg/day or pravastatin 40mg/day and to gatifloxacin or placebo in a 2 x 2 factorial design.[114] Only Caucasian subjects were utilized in this genetic analysis.[115] Subjects possessing the 719Arg variant allele had a significantly reduced risk of death or major adverse cardiovascular event with atorvastatin compared to pravastatin. However, there was no difference in atorvastatin or pravastatin response in noncarriers. This is in contrast to the data from CARE and WOSCOPS where pravastatin ameliorated the increased risk of CHD associated with the 719Arg allele; atorvastatin 80 mg/day actually decreased the risk of CHD in carriers compared to noncarriers. While, the *KIF6* Trp719Arg polymorphism has been studied in three separate populations, it has still only been studied in Caucasians and only with simvastatin and atorvastatin. While these results are strong, they cannot be extrapolated to other patient groups or other medications in the statin class. In addition, the functional consequence of this polymorphism is unknown, as is the role of this specific kinesin protein in CHD. Without knowledge of the functional role of this protein and this polymorphism, regular genotyping cannot be recommended.

While statins all share the same mechanism of action, each has different pharmacokinetic properties. CYP3A4 plays an important role in the metabolism of lovastatin, simvastatin, and atorvastatin, while fluvastatin is metabolized primarily by CYP2C9.[116] Pravastatin and rosuvastatin are primarily eliminated as unchanged parent compound in the feces and the urine (Table 7-3). Thus, variability in the genes encoding CYP450 enzymes does not uniformly affect statins as a class. In addition, while studies have linked polymorphisms in genes encoding CYP450 enzymes with changes in statin pharmacokinetic parameters, the clinical meaning of these pharmacokinetic changes is unknown.[105] Studies assessing the effect of CYP450 polymorphisms on statin lipid lowering effects have been inconsistent. Currently, there does not appear to be a role for genotyping CYP450 enzymes in patients receiving statin therapy. However, knowledge of the genetic variability in a patient's drug metabolizing enzymes could possibly allow clinicians to better predict the effect of drug interactions on statin therapy. Theoretically, patients who do not express certain CYP450 enzymes or express deficient enzymes maybe more susceptible to enzyme inhibition drug interactions with statin therapy. These drug interactions can lead to increased statin concentrations and perhaps adverse events. Little data exists related to the role of CYP450 genetic variability and statin drug interactions currently. Nevertheless, pharmacists could play in a role in utilizing genetic information related to drug metabolizing enzymes to prevent clinically significant consequences associated with statin drug interactions.

Table 7–3

Role of Metabolic Enzymes and Transporter Proteins in the Pharmacokinetics of the Different Statin[116]

	Metabolizing CYP450 Enzymes	Active Metabolite	Transporter Proteins
Atorvastatin	3A4, 3A5	Yes	OATP1B1, MDR1
Fluvastatin	2C9	No	OATP1B1, MDR1
Lovastatin	3A4, 3A5	Yes	OATP1B1, MDR1
Pravastatin	None	No	OATP1B1, MDR1
Rosuvastatin	None[a]	Yes	OATP1B1
Simvastatin	3A4, 3A5, 2C8	Yes	OATP1B1, MDR1

[a]Approximately 10% of rosuvastatin is metabolized by CYP2C.

Polymorphisms in genes encoding CYP450 enzymes have also been assessed for their role in statin adverse effects; however, these data are inconsistent as well. A retrospective case-control study of atorvastatin-induced muscle damage found no association between the incidence of muscle damage and genotype; however, they did find an association between genotype and the severity of muscle damage.[117] Specifically, *CYP3A5* genotype was associated with the degree of serum creatine kinase elevation in those subjects on single lipid lowering therapy with atorvastatin. While there may be an association with atorvastatin induced muscle damage and *CYP3A5* genotype, each statin has its own metabolic pathway; therefore, CYP3A5 genotype is not likely to be associated with all statin-induced muscle damage. However, in the future *CYP3A5* genotype may be determined prior to initiation of statin therapy so that those patients at high risk for atorvastatin-induced muscle damage may be monitored more closely or initiated on a different statin. Assessing polymorphisms in other CYP450 enzymes to predict statin adverse events cannot be recommended at this time.

All statins appear to undergo active transport during their absorption, distribution, or elimination. Transport of statins into hepatic cells is particularly important as this is the site of statin effect. In addition, transport into hepatic cells is necessary for the clearance of statins. Transporters studied for their role in statin response (Table 7-3) include organic anion transporting polypeptide (OATP) 1B1, OATP2B1, OATP2A8, multidrug resistant protein (MDR) 1, and multidrug resistance associated protein (MRP) 2.[116] Polymorphisms in the gene encoding MDR1 (*ABCB1*) have been associated with lipid lowering response to statins, but these results have been inconsistent.[105] OATP1B1 facilitates the hepatic uptake of most statins and has been well studied with the most consistent results. Variants in the gene encoding OATP1B1 (*SLCO1B1*) have been associated with simvastatin, pravastatin, and fluvastatin pharmacokinetics and efficacy. However, the strongest association demonstrated with *SLCO1B1* is with statin-induced myopathy. Each additional copy of the variant rs4149056 C allele in *SLCO1B1* has been associated with an increased risk of myopathy induced by simvastatin 80 mg.[118] Importantly, this association was replicated in a study of myopathy induced by simvastatin 40 mg/day. While the majority of myopathy cases occurred in subjects carrying the rs4149056 C allele, this polymorphism was not associated with all cases of myopathy. Thus, it is likely that other genetic variants and clinical factors play a role in statin-induced myopathy. In addition, this study only assessed simvastatin induced myopathy. Theoretically, as all statins undergo transport via OATP1B1, this may be a class effect. However, these data currently cannot be extrapolated to predict risk with other statins. In the future, genotyping for the *SLCO1B1*rs4149056 C allele may allow for the prediction of those patients who require more frequent monitoring for myopathy or lower initial statin doses.

The pharmacogenetic data assessing statin response is complicated for several reasons. Statins differ in both their pharmacokinetic properties and pharmacodynamic potency and thus data from a study on one statin cannot be extrapolated to the class. In addition, much of the data available on statin pharmacogenomics comes from genotyping subjects from completed statin clinical trials. Each trial has unique inclusion criteria and study end-points. Therefore, it is difficult to replicate the pharmacogenetic interactions that have been seen. The role of statins in lipid lowering is likely mediated by numerous genes as well. In addition, CHD is a complex disease state likely involving multiple genetic pathways. In the future, a pharmacogenetic method of predicting statin response will likely involve genotyping multiple polymorphisms in multiple genes. Until there are data available for this technique, utilizing genotype to predict statin response cannot be recommended.

Ezetimibe

Ezetimibe is also utilized for lowering LDL-C. Ezetimibe lowers serum LDL-C levels by blocking the Niemann-Pick C1-like 1 (NPC1L1) intestinal cholesterol transporter. The first genetic association report for ezetimibe was in a resistant patient who was found to have rare non-synonymous *NPC1L1* gene mutations.[119] The gene was then further sequenced in additional patients and approximately 140 SNPs and 5 insertion/deletion polymorphisms have been identified.

Two studies have assessed the association between *NPC1L1* genotype and LDL response to ezetimibe. The first study found a haplotype, made up of 3 SNPs, to be associated with percent LDL reduction from baseline.[120] In fact those subjects possessing at least one copy of the *NPC1L1* haplotype alleles studied (1735C, 25342A, 27677T) had smaller LDL reduction from baseline with ezetimibe. The second study also used three *NPC1L1* SNPs to create haplotype groups; however, they utilized different SNPs from the previous study.[121] They found that possession of the haplotype -133A, -18A, 1679G was associated with increased LDL lowering. However, because each study found different *NPC1L1* SNPs and haplotypes to be associated with ezetimibe response, it is as yet unclear which polymorphism or haplotype may actually be leading to the altered LDL lowering response. In addition, there were impressive racial differences in the allele frequencies for the SNPs studied. At this time, regular genotyping for *NPC1L1* polymorphisms to predict ezetimibe response cannot be recommended. In addition, as discussed with statins, lipid homeostasis involves several pathways with many different genes. Therefore, a polygenetic approach will likely be necessary to assess ezetimibe response.

It is also possible that genetic variability could affect the pharmacokinetics of ezetimibe. Ezetimibe is primarily metabolized by UDP glucuronosyltransferase 1 family, polypeptide A1 (UGT1A1).[122] Both ezetimibe and ezetimibe glucuronide are substrates for the efflux pumps ABCB1 and ABCC2. These efflux pumps and UGT1A1 are susceptible to drug interactions and these interactions have been shown to modulate the effects of ezetimibe. When subjects were given the ABCB1, ABCC2, and UGT1A1 inducer rifampin, clearance of ezetimibe and ezetimibe glucuronide was significantly increased and the sterol-lowering effects of ezetimibe were abolished.[123] *UGT1A1*, *ABCB1*, and *ABCC2* also have functionally characterized genetic variation. The role of this genetic variation in ezetimibe response is unknown, however theoretically patients with variants associated with decreased functionality could have increased response to ezetimibe while patients with increased functionality could have decreased response. Genotyping for polymorphisms associated with ezetimibe pharmacokinetics cannot be recommended at this time. However, pharmacists should consider the implications of drug interactions on ezetimibe response.

Antiarrhythmic Agents

Antiarrhythmic agents in general have narrow therapeutic windows and are often highly susceptible to drug-drug interactions. In addition, some arrhythmias can lead to death, especially if they are not used appropriately. All of this has led to significant study of the pharmacogenomics of antiarrhythmic therapy in order to improve response and decrease adverse events.

Procainamide

Procainamide is a class Ia antiarrhythmic used for the treatment of several different arrhythmias. It is metabolized by n-acetyltransferases (NAT) to n-acetylprocainamide (NAPA), an active metabolite, which also possesses antiarrhythmic properties. NAT1 is consistently expressed in most patients; however, NAT2 is variably expressed and plays a major role in the production of NAPA. The majority of patients receiving procainamide therapy will develop autoantibodies over time and possibly drug induced lupus. An early study showed that subjects who had a slow-acetylator phenotype developed antinuclear antibodies earlier than rapid acetylators.[124] This was confirmed in a later study of subjects who received long term procainamide therapy.[125] However, these authors found that acetylator status was not associated with the risk of developing drug related lupus, only with increased antibody formation. Also, theoretically patients with *NAT2* genotypes associated with rapid-acetylation may have increased NAPA concentrations and thus increased anti-arrhythmic effects and possible excessive QT prolongation. However, this has not been documented in the literature. While *NAT2* genotyping may predict the rate at which patients will develop autoantibodies with procainamide therapy, the clinical utility of this is unclear.

Propafenone

Propafenone is a class Ic antiarrhythmic medication used for the treatment of supraventricular arrhythmias. Propafenone exerts its effects by blocking fast inward sodium current and has some β-receptor blocking properties at higher concentrations. Propafenone is primarily metabolized by CYP2D6 while CYP1A2 and CYP3A4 also contribute to its metabolism. Genetic classification of CYP2D6 activity is complex; however, patients are generally classified as poor metabolizers, extensive metabolizers, and ultrarapid metabolizers. CYP2D6 functional status can be determined via genotyping or phenotyping. Approximately 5% to 10% of Caucasians and African Americans are considered to be poor metabolizers and essentially make no active CYP2D6.[126] Patients who are classified as CYP2D6 poor metabolizers have decreased propafenone clearance. This decrease in clearance leads to an increase in propafenone serum concentrations, which has more β-blocking properties then its active metabolites. The additional β-blockade seen in CYP2D6 poor metabolizers can lead to clinically significant adverse events in asthmatic patients due to effects on β2-receptors. Also, subjects with paroxysmal atrial fibrillation classified as CYP2D6 poor metabolizers have been found to be more likely to maintain normal sinus rhythm with propafenone than extensive metabolizers. However, the data are inconsistent. Another more recent study assessed the role of propafenone in the prevention of tachyarrhythmias after cardiac surgery.[127] These authors did find a significant association between propafenone pharmacokinetics and CYP2D6 metabolizer status based on genotype. However, CYP2D6 metabolizer status was not associated with arrhythmia risk in subjects receiving propafenone. While it is well documented that *CYP2D6* genotype, and thus metabolizer status, does effect the pharmacokinetics of propafenone, it is unclear if this translates into differences in clinical outcomes. For this reason, routine CYP2D6 genotyping cannot be recommended for patients receiving propafenone therapy.

Flecainide

Flecainide is also a class Ic antiarrhythmic primarily used for supraventricular arrhythmias. Flecainide undergoes both hepatic and renal clearance. Like propafenone, CYP2D6 is the primary enzyme responsible for the metabolism of flecainide. Therapy with flecainide is challenging because there is substantial interpatient variability in its pharmacokinetics and increased concentrations can lead to excessive widening of the QRS interval. While therapeutic drug monitoring can be done for flecainide, it is possible that assessing metabolizer status for CYP2D6 may help to predict a patient's dose response to flecainide. Pharmacokinetic studies with flecainide have used both genotyping and phenotyping methods to classify CYP2D6 metabolizer status. Two of the studies, which used genotyping to assess CYP2D6 metabolizer status, demonstrated an association between *CYP2D6* genotype and flecainide pharmacokinetics, with poor metabolizers having decreased flecainide clearance.[128,129] Inclusion of CYP2D6 genotype, body weight, age, sex, and serum creatinine explained approximately 50% of the variability in flecainide pharmacokinetics. However, another study utilized phenotyping to classify CYP2D6 status did not find an association between CYP2D6 metabolizer status and flecainide pharmacokinetics.[130] It is possible that CYP2D6 contributes to some of the variability seen in flecainide dose response; however, the data are inconsistent. At this time CYP2D6 genotyping or phenotyping cannot be recommended to predict flecainide dosing.

Amiodarone

Amiodarone is a class III antiarrhythmic, which is effective for both supraventricular and ventricular arrhythmias. Amiodarone metabolism is extensive with involvement of both phase I and phase II drug metabolizing enzymes. CYP3A4 and CYP2C8 are known to play a key role in amiodarone metabolism. In addition, amiodarone is a potent inhibitor of CYP3A4, CYP1A2, CYP2C9, and CYP2D6 leading to multiple drug interactions. While genetic variation in any of these metabolic enzymes may lead to alterations in amiodarone clearance or its propensity for drug interactions, there is little data to support this. At this time, genotyping for alterations in CYP450 isoenzymes to predict amiodarone response cannot be recommended.

Digoxin

Digoxin exerts its effects by inhibiting sodium-potassium adenosine triphosphatase and is used in both atrial fibrillation and heart failure. Digoxin is an ABCB1 substrate and the role of *ABCB1* polymorphisms in digoxin pharmacokinetics has been well studied. In fact, digoxin was the first drug documented to be effected by *ABCB1* polymorphisms. The most studied polymorphism is the C3435T SNP.[131,132] Several studies have demonstrated an association between digoxin pharmacokinetics and *ABCB1* polymorphisms; however, the results have been very inconsistent. While ABCB1 is an important consideration for drug interactions with digoxin; at this time, genotyping for *ABCB1* polymorphisms to predict digoxin pharmacokinetics cannot be recommended. It is also possible that polymorphisms related to digoxin's pharmacodynamics (i.e., sodium-potassium ATPase, which is digoxin's site of action) may affect digoxin response.[126] However, there is currently no data to support this.

Pro-arrhythmic Effects of Medications

The pro-arrhythmic effects of medications (both those used to treat arrhythmias and those used for other indications) have been well studied. Interest in these rare adverse events is due to the fact that they can be life threatening and require a significant amount of patient monitoring. Proarrhythmia is generally defined as the worsening of the arrhythmia being treated or generation of a new arrhythmia with medication therapy.[133] Genetic studies have focused on drug induced increases in the QT interval and drug induced torsades de pointes. The focus on genetic factors associated with drug induced prolonged QT intervals is due to the knowledge gained from many years of studying and evaluating congenital long QT syndromes. In addition, the association between prolonged QT interval and torsades de pointes has been well documented.

The QT interval on an electrocardiogram represents the action potentials of ventricular myocytes. The ventricular action potential is made up of several currents produced by different ion channels. The action potential is prolonged when either there is increased inward current or decreased outward current. The heart has significant built in redundancy as several ion channels participate in the ventricular action potential. This redundancy is termed *repolarization reserve*. Thus, variation in one ion channel will not necessarily lead to an increase in the QT interval. A combination of factors is generally necessary for patients to exhibit both congenital and drug induced long QT syndromes. Several clinical factors, beyond genetic variation in ion channels, have been associated with an increased risk of drug induced long QT syndromes and it is thought that these factors affect the heart's *repolarization reserve*.[133] These factors include but are not limited to hypokalemia, recent conversion of atrial fibrillation, advanced heart disease, and female gender.

Factors influencing the pharmacokinetics of medications may also affect the risk of drug induced long QT syndrome. The risk of drug induced long QT syndrome maybe increased if the clearance of a drug is decreased via either a drug interaction or genetic variants in hepatic enzyme systems. Pharmacists should be particularly vigilant in monitoring for drug interactions with medications known to prolong the QT interval. In addition, if genetic variability in hepatic enzyme systems for a patient is known this should be considered as well.

Polymorphisms in several of the genes encoding ion channels associated with ventricular action potential have been studied for their role in congenital long QT syndromes because of their possible effect on *repolarization reserve*.[134] Mutations found in genes encoding potassium voltage-gated channels (KCNQ1, KCNH2, KCNE1, KCNE2) and in a sodium voltage gated channel (SCN5A) have been associated with risk for congenital long QT syndrome. Because the ion channels have been associated with congenital long QT syndrome they are a logical starting place for assessing drug induced long QT syndrome. Medications can prolong the QT interval by blocking the ion channel pore, inducing conformational changes in the ion channel pore, and/or decreasing production of the proteins encoding the ion channels. The amino acid structure of KCNH2 appears to make this ion channel pore particularly susceptible to drug blockade. Polymorphisms in the gene encoding KCNH2 may affect its susceptibility to drug binding. Polymorphisms in *SCN5A* may also contribute to the risk of drug induced long QT syndrome. However, while polymorphisms in several genes encoding ion channels have been found to be associated with risk of drug induced long QT syndrome, none of these results have been replicated in other studies. Prior to utilizing pharmacogenetic information to predict proarrhythmic risk with medications a genetic variant must be validated in separate, distinct populations. In addition, an understanding of the biology and physiology of the polymorphism is necessary.

Currently using genetic information to predict pro-arrhythmia risk cannot be recommended. The volume of knowledge on this topic is growing and with validated genetic markers, genotyping may in the future be clinically useful. However, utilizing genetic information to predict risk of drug induced long QT syndrome will likely be complex due to the redundancy in the system. It is unlikely that polymorphisms in a single gene or a single clinical risk factor will be sufficient to predict risk. Therefore a pharmacogenomic approach to predicting risk for drug induced long QT syndrome will be necessary where multiple genes are assessed along with clinical factors.

Summary

The study of pharmacogenomics in the area of cardiology is growing exponentially. Data are currently available to support prospective genotyping for warfarin therapy. In addition, well characterized genetic data is available for clopidogrel and bucindolol. It is likely only a matter of time before this information is used clinically. Furthermore, with the continuing growth of literature in this area, our clinical use of genetics in cardiovascular drug therapy is likely to expand.

References

1. American Heart Association, ed. *Heart Disease and Stroke Statistics — 2010 Update.* Dallas, TX: American Heart Association; 2010.
2. Chobanian AV, Bakris GL, Black HR, et al. The seventh report of the joint national committee on prevention, detection, evaluation, and treatment of high blood pressure: The JNC 7 report. *JAMA.* 2003;289:2560-2572.
3. Expert Panel on Detection, Evaluation, and Treatment of High Blood Cholesterol in Adults. Executive summary of the third report of the national cholesterol education program (NCEP) expert panel on detection, evaluation, and treatment of high blood cholesterol in adults (adult treatment panel III). *JAMA.* 2001;285:2486-2497.
4. Heart Failure Society of America. HFSA 2006 comprehensive heart failure practice guideline. *J Card Fail.* 2006;12:e1-e122.
5. Wysowski DK, Nourjah P, Swartz L. Bleeding complications with warfarin use: A prevalent adverse effect resulting in regulatory action. *Arch Intern Med.* 2007;167:1414-1419.
6. Herman D, Locatelli I, Grabnar I, et al. Influence of CYP2C9 polymorphisms, demographic factors and concomitant drug therapy on warfarin metabolism and maintenance dose. *Pharmacogenomics J.* 2005;5:193-202.
7. Sanderson S, Emery J, Higgins J. CYP2C9 gene variants, drug dose, and bleeding risk in warfarin-treated patients: a HuGEnet systematic review and meta-analysis. *Genet Med.* 2005;7:97-104.
8. Limdi NA, Veenstra DL. Warfarin pharmacogenetics. *Pharmacotherapy.* 2008;28:1084-1097.
9. Higashi MK, Veenstra DL, Kondo LM, et al. Association between CYP2C9 genetic variants and anticoagulation-related outcomes during warfarin therapy. *JAMA.* 2002;287:1690-1698.
10. Schalekamp T, vanGeest-Daalderop JH, deVries-Goldschmeding H, et al. Acenocoumarol stabilization is delayed in CYP2C93 carriers. *Clin Pharmacol Ther.* 2004;75:394-402.

11. Freeman BD, Zehnbauer BA, McGrath S, et al. Cytochrome P450 polymorphisms are associated with reduced warfarin dose. *Surgery.* 2000;128:281-285.
12. Kamali F, Khan TI, King BP, et al. Contribution of age, body size, and CYP2C9 genotype to anticoagulant response to warfarin. *Clin Pharmacol Ther.* 2004;75:204-212.
13. Voora D, Eby C, Linder MW, et al. Prospective dosing of warfarin based on cytochrome P-450 2C9 genotype. *Thromb Haemost.* 2005;93:700-705.
14. Rieder MJ, Reiner AP, Gage BF, et al. Effect of VKORC1 haplotypes on transcriptional regulation and warfarin dose. *N Engl J Med.* 2005;352:2285-2293.
15. Warfarin (Coumadin®) [package insert]. Princeton, NJ: Bristol-Myers Squibb; August 2007.
16. Caraco Y, Blotnick S, Muszkat M. CYP2C9 genotype-guided warfarin prescribing enhances the efficacy and safety of anticoagulation: A prospective randomized controlled study. *Clin Pharmacol Ther.* 2008;83:460-470.
17. Anderson JL, Horne BD, Stevens SM, et al. Randomized trial of genotype-guided versus standard warfarin dosing in patients initiating oral anticoagulation. *Circulation.* 2007;116:2563-2570.
18. Aquilante CL, Langaee TY, Lopez LM, et al. Influence of coagulation factor, vitamin K epoxide reductase complex subunit 1, and cytochrome P450 2C9 gene polymorphisms on warfarin dose requirements. *Clin Pharmacol Ther.* 2006;79:291-302.
19. Sconce EA, Khan TI, Wynne HA, et al. The impact of CYP2C9 and VKORC1 genetic polymorphism and patient characteristics upon warfarin dose requirements: Proposal for a new dosing regimen. *Blood.* 2005;106:2329-2333.
20. International Warfarin Pharmacogenetics Consortium, Klein TE, Altman RB, et al. Estimation of the warfarin dose with clinical and pharmacogenetic data. *N Engl J Med.* 2009;360:753-764.
21. McWilliam A, Lutter R, Nardinelli C. Health care savings from personalizing medicine using genetic testing: the case of warfarin. 2006;Working Paper 06-23.
22. Eckman MH, Rosand J, Greenberg SM, et al. Cost-effectiveness of using pharmacogenetic information in warfarin dosing for patients with nonvalvular atrial fibrillation. *Ann Intern Med.* 2009;150:73-83.
23. Antithrombotic Trialists' Collaboration. Collaborative meta-analysis of randomised trials of antiplatelet therapy for prevention of death, myocardial infarction, and stroke in high risk patients. *BMJ.* 2002;324:71-86.
24. Dorsch MP, Lee JS, Lynch DR, et al. Aspirin resistance in patients with stable coronary artery disease with and without a history of myocardial infarction. *Ann Pharmacother.* 2007;41:737-741.
25. Maree AO, Curtin RJ, Chubb A, et al. Cyclooxygenase-1 haplotype modulates platelet response to aspirin. *J Thromb Haemost.* 2005;3:2340-2345.
26. Lepantalo A, Mikkelsson J, Resendiz JC, et al. Polymorphisms of COX-1 and GPVI associate with the antiplatelet effect of aspirin in coronary artery disease patients. *Thromb Haemost.* 2006;95:253-259.
27. Hillarp A, Palmqvist B, Lethagen S, et al. Mutations within the cyclooxygenase-1 gene in aspirin non-responders with recurrence of stroke. *Thromb Res.* 2003;112:275-283.
28. Clappers N, van Oijen MG, Sundaresan S, et al. The C50T polymorphism of the cyclooxygenase-1 gene and the risk of thrombotic events during low-dose therapy with acetyl salicylic acid. *Thromb Haemost.* 2008;100:70-75.
29. Faraday N, Becker DM, Becker LC. Pharmacogenomics of platelet responsiveness to aspirin. *Pharmacogenomics.* 2007;8:1413-1425.
30. Feng D, Lindpaintner K, Larson MG, et al. Increased platelet aggregability associated with platelet GPIIIa PlA2 polymorphism: The Framingham offspring study. *Arterioscler Thromb Vasc Biol.* 1999;19:1142-1147.
31. Goodall AH, Curzen N, Panesar M, et al. Increased binding of fibrinogen to glycoprotein IIIa-proline33 (HPA-1b, PlA2, zwb) positive platelets in patients with cardiovascular disease. *Eur Heart J.* 1999;20:742-747.
32. Walter DH, Schachinger V, Elsner M, et al. Platelet glycoprotein IIIa polymorphisms and risk of coronary stent thrombosis. *Lancet.* 1997;350:1217-1219.
33. Ridker PM, Hennekens CH, Schmitz C, et al. PIA1/A2 polymorphism of platelet glycoprotein IIIa and risks of myocardial infarction, stroke, and venous thrombosis. *Lancet.* 1997;349:385-388.

34. Macchi L, Christiaens L, Brabant S, et al. Resistance in vitro to low-dose aspirin is associated with platelet PlA1 (GP IIIa) polymorphism but not with C807T(GP Ia/IIa) and C-5T kozak (GP ibalpha) polymorphisms. *J Am Coll Cardiol.* 2003;42:1115-1119.

35. Michelson AD, Furman MI, Goldschmidt-Clermont P, et al. Platelet GP IIIa pl(A) polymorphisms display different sensitivities to agonists. *Circulation.* 2000;101:1013-1018.

36. Quinn MJ, Topol EJ. Common variations in platelet glycoproteins: Pharmacogenomic implications. *Pharmacogenomics.* 2001;2:341-352.

37. Cuisset T, Frere C, Quilici J, et al. Role of the T744C polymorphism of the P2Y12 gene on platelet response to a 600-mg loading dose of clopidogrel in 597 patients with non-ST-segment elevation acute coronary syndrome. *Thromb Res.* 2007;120:893-899.

38. Bura A, Bachelot-Loza C, Ali FD, et al. Role of the P2Y12 gene polymorphism in platelet responsiveness to clopidogrel in healthy subjects. *J Thromb Haemost.* 2006;4:2096-2097.

39. Taubert D, vonBeckerath N, Grimberg G, et al. Impact of P-glycoprotein on clopidogrel absorption. *Clin Pharmacol Ther.* 2006;80:486-501.

40. Simon T, Verstuyft C, Mary-Krause M, et al. Genetic determinants of response to clopidogrel and cardiovascular events. *N Engl J Med.* 2009;360:363-375.

41. Shuldiner AR, O'Connell JR, Bliden KP, et al. Association of cytochrome P450 2C19 genotype with the antiplatelet effect and clinical efficacy of clopidogrel therapy. *JAMA.* 2009;302:849-857.

42. Mega JL, Close SL, Wiviott SD, et al. Cytochrome p-450 polymorphisms and response to clopidogrel. *N Engl J Med.* 2009;360:354-362.

43. Angiolillo DJ, Fernandez-Ortiz A, Bernardo E, et al. Contribution of gene sequence variations of the hepatic cytochrome P450 3A4 enzyme to variability in individual responsiveness to clopidogrel. *Arterioscler Thromb Vasc Biol.* 2006;26:1895-1900.

44. Smith SM, Judge HM, Peters G, et al. Common sequence variations in the P2Y12 and CYP3A5 genes do not explain the variability in the inhibitory effects of clopidogrel therapy. *Platelets.* 2006;17:250-258.

45. Suh JW, Koo BK, Zhang SY, et al. Increased risk of atherothrombotic events associated with cytochrome P450 3A5 polymorphism in patients taking clopidogrel. *CMAJ.* 2006;174:1715-1722.

46. Collet JP, Hulot JS, Pena A, et al. Cytochrome P450 2C19 polymorphism in young patients treated with clopidogrel after myocardial infarction: A cohort study. *Lancet.* 2009;373:309-317.

47. Clopidogrel (Plavix®) [package insert]. Bridgewater, NJ: Sanofi-Aventis and Bristol Meyers Squibb; May 2009.

48. Campo G, Valgimigli M, Gemmati D, et al. Poor responsiveness to clopidogrel: Drug-specific or class-effect mechanism? evidence from a clopidogrel-to-ticlopidine crossover study. *J Am Coll Cardiol.* 2007;50:1132-1137.

49. Wheeler GL, Braden GA, Bray PF, et al. Reduced inhibition by abciximab in platelets with the PlA2 polymorphism. *Am Heart J.* 2002;143:76-82.

50. Weber AA, Jacobs C, Meila D, et al. No evidence for an influence of the human platelet antigen-1 polymorphism on the antiplatelet effects of glycoprotein IIb/IIIa inhibitors. *Pharmacogenetics.* 2002;12:581-583.

51. Shin J, Johnson JA. Pharmacogenetics of beta-blockers. *Pharmacotherapy.* 2007;27:874-887.

52. Mason DA, Moore JD, Green SA, et al. A gain-of-function polymorphism in a G-protein coupling domain of the human beta1-adrenergic receptor. *J Biol Chem.* 1999;274:12670-12674.

53. Levin MC, Marullo S, Muntaner O, et al. The myocardium-protective gly-49 variant of the beta 1-adrenergic receptor exhibits constitutive activity and increased desensitization and down-regulation. *J Biol Chem.* 2002;277:30429-30435.

54. Comparison of propranolol and hydrochlorothiazide for the initial treatment of hypertension. II. results of long-term therapy. Veterans Administration Cooperative Study Group on Antihypertensive Agents. *JAMA.* 1982;248:2004-2011.

55. Materson BJ, Reda DJ, Cushman WC, et al. Single-drug therapy for hypertension in men: a comparison of six antihypertensive agents with placebo. *N Engl J Med.* 1993;328:914-921.

56. Karlsson J, Lind L, Hallberg P, et al. Beta1-adrenergic receptor gene polymorphisms and response to beta 1-adrenergic receptor blockade in patients with essential hypertension. *Clin Cardiol.* 2004;27:347-350.

57. Sofowora GG, Dishy V, Muszkat M, et al. A common beta 1-adrenergic receptor polymorphism (Arg389Gly) affects blood pressure response to beta-blockade. *Clin Pharmacol Ther*. 2003;73:366-371.

58. Johnson JA, Zineh I, Puckett BJ, et al. Beta 1-adrenergic receptor polymorphisms and antihypertensive response to metoprolol. *Clin Pharmacol Ther*. 2003;74:44-52.

59. Liu J, Liu ZQ, Yu BN, et al. Beta 1-adrenergic receptor polymorphisms influence the response to metoprolol monotherapy in patients with essential hypertension. *Clin Pharmacol Ther*. 2006;80:23-32.

60. Liu J, Liu ZQ, Tan ZR, et al. Gly389Arg polymorphism of beta1-adrenergic receptor is associated with the cardiovascular response to metoprolol. *Clin Pharmacol Ther*. 2003;74:372-379.

61. O'Shaughnessy KM, Fu B, Dickerson C, et al. The gain-of-function G389R variant of the beta 1-adrenoceptor does not influence blood pressure or heart rate response to beta-blockade in hypertensive subjects. *Clin Sci (Lond)*. 2000;99:233-238.

62. Mialet Perez J, Rathz DA, Petrashevskaya NN, et al. Beta 1-adrenergic receptor polymorphisms confer differential function and predisposition to heart failure. *Nat Med*. 2003;9:1300-1305.

63. Terra SG, Hamilton KK, Pauly DF, et al. Beta 1-adrenergic receptor polymorphisms and left ventricular remodeling changes in response to beta-blocker therapy. *Pharmacogenet Genomics*. 2005;15:227-234.

64. Magnusson Y, Levin MC, Eggertsen R, et al. Ser49Gly of beta 1-adrenergic receptor is associated with effective beta-blocker dose in dilated cardiomyopathy. *Clin Pharmacol Ther*. 2005;78:221-231.

65. White HL, deBoer RA, Maqbool A, et al. An evaluation of the beta-1 adrenergic receptor Arg-389Gly polymorphism in individuals with heart failure: A MERIT-HF sub-study. *Eur J Heart Fail*. 2003;5:463-468.

66. Sehnert AJ, Daniels SE, Elashoff M, et al. Lack of association between adrenergic receptor genotypes and survival in heart failure patients treated with carvedilol or metoprolol. *J Am Coll Cardiol*. 2008;52:644-651.

67. Beta-Blocker Evaluation of Survival Trial Investigators. A trial of the beta-blocker bucindolol in patients with advanced chronic heart failure. *N Engl J Med*. 2001;344:1659-1667.

68. Liggett SB, Mialet-Perez J, Thaneemit-Chen S, et al. A polymorphism within a conserved beta(1)-adrenergic receptor motif alters cardiac function and beta-blocker response in human heart failure. *Proc Natl Acad Sci U S A*. 2006;103:11288-11293.

69. Khalaila JM, Elami A, Caraco Y. Interaction between beta 2 adrenergic receptor polymorphisms determines the extent of isoproterenol-induced vasodilatation ex vivo. *Pharmacogenet Genomics*. 2007;17:803-811.

70. Lanfear DE, Jones PG, Marsh S, et al. Beta 2-adrenergic receptor genotype and survival among patients receiving beta-blocker therapy after an acute coronary syndrome. *JAMA*. 2005;294:1526-1533.

71. Rau T, Wuttke H, Michels LM, et al. Impact of the CYP2D6 genotype on the clinical effects of metoprolol: A prospective longitudinal study. *Clin Pharmacol Ther*. 2009;85:269-272.

72. Winkelmann BR, Russ AP, Nauck M, et al. Angiotensinogen M235T polymorphism is associated with plasma angiotensinogen and cardiovascular disease. *Am Heart J*. 1999;137:698-705.

73. Momary KM. Cardiovascular pharmacogenomics. *J Pharm Pract*. 2007;20:265-276.

74. Arnett DK, Davis BR, Ford CE, et al. Pharmacogenetic association of the angiotensin-converting enzyme insertion/deletion polymorphism on blood pressure and cardiovascular risk in relation to antihypertensive treatment: The genetics of hypertension-associated treatment (GenHAT) study. *Circulation*. 2005;111:3374-3383.

75. Harrap SB, Tzourio C, Cambien F, et al. The ACE gene I/D polymorphism is not associated with the blood pressure and cardiovascular benefits of ACE inhibition. *Hypertension*. 2003;42:297-303.

76. Bhatnagar V, O'Connor DT, Schork NJ, et al. Angiotensin-converting enzyme gene polymorphism predicts the time-course of blood pressure response to angiotensin converting enzyme inhibition in the AASK trial. *J Hypertens*. 2007;25:2082-2092.

77. Hingorani AD, Jia H, Stevens PA, et al. Renin-angiotensin system gene polymorphisms influence blood pressure and the response to angiotensin converting enzyme inhibition. *J Hypertens*. 1995;13:1602-1609.

78. Schelleman H, Klungel OH, Witteman JC, et al. Angiotensinogen M235T polymorphism and the risk of myocardial infarction and stroke among hypertensive patients on ACE-inhibitors or beta-blockers. *Eur J Hum Genet*. 2007;15:478-484.

79. Bis JC, Smith NL, Psaty BM, et al. Angiotensinogen Met235Thr polymorphism, angiotensin-converting enzyme inhibitor therapy, and the risk of nonfatal stroke or myocardial infarction in hypertensive patients. *Am J Hypertens*. 2003;16:1011-1017.

80. Miller JA, Thai K, Scholey JW. Angiotensin II type 1 receptor gene polymorphism predicts response to losartan and angiotensin II. *Kidney Int*. 1999;56:2173-2180.

81. Diez J, Laviades C, Orbe J, et al. The A1166C polymorphism of the AT1 receptor gene is associated with collagen type I synthesis and myocardial stiffness in hypertensives. *J Hypertens*. 2003;21:2085-2092.

82. Kurland L, Melhus H, Karlsson J, et al. Angiotensin converting enzyme gene polymorphism predicts blood pressure response to angiotensin II receptor type 1 antagonist treatment in hypertensive patients. *J Hypertens*. 2001;19:1783-1787.

83. Cusi D, Barlassina C, Azzani T, et al. Polymorphisms of alpha-adducin and salt sensitivity in patients with essential hypertension. *Lancet*. 1997;349:1353-1357.

84. Glorioso N, Manunta P, Filigheddu F, et al. The role of alpha-adducin polymorphism in blood pressure and sodium handling regulation may not be excluded by a negative association study. *Hypertension*. 1999;34:649-654.

85. Psaty BM, Smith NL, Heckbert SR, et al. Diuretic therapy, the alpha-adducin gene variant, and the risk of myocardial infarction or stroke in persons with treated hypertension. *JAMA*. 2002;287:1680-1689.

86. Sciarrone MT, Stella P, Barlassina C, et al. ACE and alpha-adducin polymorphism as markers of individual response to diuretic therapy. *Hypertension*. 2003;41:398-403.

87. Turner ST, Chapman AB, Schwartz GL, et al. Effects of endothelial nitric oxide synthase, alpha-adducin, and other candidate gene polymorphisms on blood pressure response to hydrochlorothiazide. *Am J Hypertens*. 2003;16:834-839.

88. Gerhard T, Gong Y, Beitelshees AL, et al. Alpha-adducin polymorphism associated with increased risk of adverse cardiovascular outcomes: Results from GENEtic Substudy of the International Verapamil SR-trandolapril Study (INVEST-GENES). *Am Heart J*. 2008;156:397-404.

89. Davis BR, Arnett DK, Boerwinkle E, et al. Antihypertensive therapy, the alpha-adducin polymorphism, and cardiovascular disease in high-risk hypertensive persons: The genetics of hypertension-associated treatment study. *Pharmacogenomics J*. 2007;7:112-122. Epub 2006 May 16.

90. Turner ST, Schwartz GL, Chapman AB, et al. C825T polymorphism of the G protein beta(3)-subunit and antihypertensive response to a thiazide diuretic. *Hypertension*. 2001;37:739-743.

91. Turner ST, Schwartz GL, Chapman AB, et al. WNK1 kinase polymorphism and blood pressure response to a thiazide diuretic. *Hypertension*. 2005;46:758-765.

92. Maitland-van der Zee AH, Turner ST, Schwartz GL, et al. A multifocus approach to the antihypertensive pharmacogenetics of hydrochlorothiazide. *Pharmacogenet Genomics*. 2005;15:287-293.

93. Cohn JN, Archibald DG, Ziesche S, et al. Effect of vasodilator therapy on mortality in chronic congestive heart failure: results of a Veterans Administration cooperative study. *N Engl J Med*. 1986;314:1547-1552.

94. Gogia H, Mehra A, Parikh S, et al. Prevention of tolerance to hemodynamic effects of nitrates with concomitant use of hydralazine in patients with chronic heart failure. *J Am Coll Cardiol*. 1995;26:1575-1580.

95. Cohn JN, Johnson G, Ziesche S, et al. A comparison of enalapril with hydralazine-isosorbide dinitrate in the treatment of chronic congestive heart failure. *N Engl J Med*. 1991;325:303-310.

96. Carson P, Ziesche S, Johnson G, et al. Racial differences in response to therapy for heart failure: Analysis of the vasodilator-heart failure trials. vasodilator-heart failure trial study group. *J Card Fail*. 1999;5:178-187.

97. Taylor AL, Ziesche S, Yancy C, et al. Combination of isosorbide dinitrate and hydralazine in blacks with heart failure. *N Engl J Med*. 2004;351:2049-2057.

98. McNamara DM, Tam SW, Sabolinski ML, et al. Aldosterone synthase promoter polymorphism predicts outcome in African Americans with heart failure: Results from the A-HeFT trial. *J Am Coll Cardiol*. 2006;48:1277-1282.

99. McNamara DM, Tam SW, Sabolinski ML, et al. Endothelial nitric oxide synthase (NOS3) polymorphisms in African Americans with heart failure: Results from the A-HeFT trial. *J Card Fail.* 2009;15:191-198.

100. Krauss RM, Mangravite LM, Smith JD, et al. Variation in the 3-hydroxyl-3-methylglutaryl coenzyme a reductase gene is associated with racial differences in low-density lipoprotein cholesterol response to simvastatin treatment. *Circulation.* 2008;117:1537-1544.

101. Donnelly LA, Doney AS, Dannfald J, et al. A paucimorphic variant in the HMG-CoA reductase gene is associated with lipid-lowering response to statin treatment in diabetes: A GoDARTS study. *Pharmacogenet Genomics.* 2008;18:1021-1026.

102. Chasman DI, Posada D, Subrahmanyan L, et al. Pharmacogenetic study of statin therapy and cholesterol reduction. *JAMA.* 2004;291:2821-2827.

103. Thompson JF, Man M, Johnson KJ, et al. An association study of 43 SNPs in 16 candidate genes with atorvastatin response. *Pharmacogenomics J.* 2005;5:352-358.

104. Polisecki E, Muallem H, Maeda N, et al. Genetic variation at the LDL receptor and HMG-CoA reductase gene loci, lipid levels, statin response, and cardiovascular disease incidence in PROSPER. *Atherosclerosis.* 2008;200:109-114.

105. Mangravite LM, Thorn CF, Krauss RM. Clinical implications of pharmacogenomics of statin treatment. *Pharmacogenomics J.* 2006;6:360-374.

106. Gerdes LU, Gerdes C, Kervinen K, et al. The apolipoprotein epsilon4 allele determines prognosis and the effect on prognosis of simvastatin in survivors of myocardial infarction: a substudy of the Scandinavian simvastatin survival study. *Circulation.* 2000;101:1366-1371.

107. Maitland-van der Zee AH, Lynch A, Boerwinkle E, et al. Interactions between the single nucleotide polymorphisms in the homocysteine pathway (MTHFR 677C>T, MTHFR 1298 A>C, and CBSins) and the efficacy of HMG-CoA reductase inhibitors in preventing cardiovascular disease in high-risk patients of hypertension: The GenHAT study. *Pharmacogenet Genomics.* 2008;18:651-656.

108. The ALLHAT Officers and Coordinators for the ALLHAT Collaborative Research Group. Major outcomes in high-risk hypertensive patients randomized to angiotensin-converting enzyme inhibitor or calcium channel blocker vs diuretic: the antihypertensive and lipid-lowering treatment to prevent heart attack trial (ALLHAT). *JAMA.* 2002;288:2981-2997.

109. Sacks FM, Pfeffer MA, Moye LA, et al. The effect of pravastatin on coronary events after myocardial infarction in patients with average cholesterol levels. cholesterol and recurrent events trial investigators. *N Engl J Med.* 1996;335:1001-1009.

110. Shepherd J, Cobbe SM, Ford I, et al. Prevention of coronary heart disease with pravastatin in men with hypercholesterolemia. west of Scotland coronary prevention study group. *N Engl J Med.* 1995;333:1301-1307.

111. Sabatine MS, Ploughman L, Simonsen KL, et al. Association between ADAMTS1 matrix metalloproteinase gene variation, coronary heart disease, and benefit of statin therapy. *Arterioscler Thromb Vasc Biol.* 2008;28:562-567.

112. Iakoubova OA, Tong CH, Chokkalingam AP, et al. Asp92Asn polymorphism in the myeloid IgA fc receptor is associated with myocardial infarction in two disparate populations: CARE and WOSCOPS. *Arterioscler Thromb Vasc Biol.* 2006;26:2763-2768.

113. Iakoubova OA, Tong CH, Rowland CM, et al. Association of the Trp719Arg polymorphism in kinesin-like protein 6 with myocardial infarction and coronary heart disease in 2 prospective trials: The CARE and WOSCOPS trials. *J Am Coll Cardiol.* 2008;51:435-443.

114. Cannon CP, Braunwald E, McCabe CH, et al. Intensive versus moderate lipid lowering with statins after acute coronary syndromes. *N Engl J Med.* 2004;350:1495-1504.

115. Iakoubova OA, Sabatine MS, Rowland CM, et al. Polymorphism in KIF6 gene and benefit from statins after acute coronary syndromes: Results from the PROVE IT-TIMI 22 study. *J Am Coll Cardiol.* 2008;51:449-455.

116. Neuvonen PJ, Niemi M, Backman JT. Drug interactions with lipid-lowering drugs: Mechanisms and clinical relevance. *Clin Pharmacol Ther.* 2006;80:565-581.

117. Wilke RA, Moore JH, Burmester JK. Relative impact of CYP3A genotype and concomitant medication on the severity of atorvastatin-induced muscle damage. *Pharmacogenet Genomics.* 2005;15:415-421.

118. SEARCH Collaborative Group, Link E, Parish S, et al. SLCO1B1 variants and statin-induced myopathy—a genomewide study. *N Engl J Med*. 2008;359:789-799.

119. Wang J, Williams CM, Hegele RA. Compound heterozygosity for two non-synonymous polymorphisms in NPC1L1 in a non-responder to ezetimibe. *Clin Genet*. 2005;67:175-177.

120. Hegele RA, Guy J, Ban MR, et al. NPC1L1 haplotype is associated with inter-individual variation in plasma low-density lipoprotein response to ezetimibe. *Lipids Health Dis*. 2005;4:16.

121. Simon JS, Karnoub MC, Devlin DJ, et al. Sequence variation in NPC1L1 and association with improved LDL-cholesterol lowering in response to ezetimibe treatment. *Genomics*. 2005;86:648-656.

122. Schmitz G, Schmitz-Madry A, Ugocsai P. Pharmacogenetics and pharmacogenomics of cholesterol-lowering therapy. *Curr Opin Lipidol*. 2007;18:164-173.

123. Oswald S, Haenisch S, Fricke C, et al. Intestinal expression of P-glycoprotein (ABCB1), multidrug resistance associated protein 2 (ABCC2), and uridine diphosphate-glucuronosyltransferase 1A1 predicts the disposition and modulates the effects of the cholesterol absorption inhibitor ezetimibe in humans. *Clin Pharmacol Ther*. 2006;79:206-217.

124. Woosley RL, Drayer DE, Reidenberg MM, et al. Effect of acetylator phenotype on the rate at which procainamide induces antinuclear antibodies and the lupus syndrome. *N Engl J Med*. 1978;298:1157-1159.

125. Mongey AB, Sim E, Risch A, et al. Acetylation status is associated with serological changes but not clinically significant disease in patients receiving procainamide. *J Rheumatol*. 1999;26:1721-1726.

126. Darbar D, Roden DM. Pharmacogenetics of antiarrhythmic therapy. *Expert Opin Pharmacother*. 2006;7:1583-1590.

127. Morike K, Kivisto KT, Schaeffeler E, et al. Propafenone for the prevention of atrial tachyarrhythmias after cardiac surgery: A randomized, double-blind placebo-controlled trial. *Clin Pharmacol Ther*. 2008;84:104-110.

128. Lim KS, Cho JY, Jang IJ, et al. Pharmacokinetic interaction of flecainide and paroxetine in relation to the CYP2D6*10 allele in healthy Korean subjects. *Br J Clin Pharmacol*. 2008;66:660-666.

129. Doki K, Homma M, Kuga K, et al. Effect of CYP2D6 genotype on flecainide pharmacokinetics in Japanese patients with supraventricular tachyarrhythmia. *Eur J Clin Pharmacol*. 2006;62:919-926.

130. Tenneze L, Tarral E, Ducloux N, et al. Pharmacokinetics and electrocardiographic effects of a new controlled-release form of flecainide acetate: comparison with the standard form and influence of the CYP2D6 polymorphism. *Clin Pharmacol Ther*. 2002;72:112-122.

131. Chowbay B, Li H, David M, et al. Meta-analysis of the influence of MDR1 C3435T polymorphism on digoxin pharmacokinetics and MDR1 gene expression. *Br J Clin Pharmacol*. 2005;60:159-171.

132. Leschziner GD, Andrew T, Pirmohamed M, et al. ABCB1 genotype and PGP expression, function and therapeutic drug response: a critical review and recommendations for future research. *Pharmacogenomics J*. 2007;7:154-179.

133. Roden DM. Proarrhythmia as a pharmacogenomic entity: A critical review and formulation of a unifying hypothesis. *Cardiovasc Res*. 2005;67:419-425.

134. Kannankeril PJ. Understanding drug-induced torsades de pointes: a genetic stance. *Expert Opin Drug Saf*. 2008;7:231-239.

Chapter 8

Hematology/Oncology Pharmacogenomics

Todd A. Thompson, Ph.D.

Learning Objectives

After completing this chapter, the reader should be able to

- Define terms necessary for understanding concepts relevant to cancer pharmacogenomics.
- Describe the three areas that define cancer pharmacogenomics.
- Distinguish between pharmacodynamic and pharmacokinetic considerations in cancer pharmacogenomics.
- Identify specific genetic variants that impact the use of cancer chemotherapeutic agents including alkylating agents, purine analogs, pyrimidine analogs, topoisomerase I inhibitors, antimetabolites, and selective estrogen receptor modulators.
- Describe the three distinct areas of cancer prevention that may be targeted by cancer chemopreventive measures.
- Describe the difference between variant forms of cancers (e.g., sarcomas versus carcinomas; leukemia versus solid tumors) and pharmacogenomics relevant to different forms of cancer.

- Describe how differences between hereditary (i.e., germline) variants and somatic mutations that develop during cancer progression are determined.
- Give examples of how differences between hereditary (i.e., germline) variants and somatic mutations that develop during cancer progression can be used to optimize cancer therapy.
- Explain a critical difference between technologies used to analyze mRNA expression and genetic variants found in DNA (e.g., SNPs).
- Describe key differences between genome-wide association studies and candidate gene studies.

Key Definitions

Cancer—A disease of abnormal cellular proliferation in which cells have invaded tissue locally or at locations distant from their site of origin.

Cancer chemoprevention—Drug-based interventions for individuals at increased risk for cancer development that may be useful in preventing cancer onset. These risk factors may include environmental factors, hereditary factors, or both.

Cancer chemotherapy—Upon cancer diagnosis, drug-based therapeutics that may be used to treat specific types of cancer. In many cases, cancer chemotherapy is used in conjunction with surgical and radiological cancer treatments.

Candidate gene study—Genetic association study performed to assess the association of specific gene variants (e.g., in a candidate gene) with a phenotype of interest such as an adverse drug response.

Carcinoma—Cancers of epithelial tissue origin. Glandular tissues, such as the breast and prostate, lead to the formation of adenocarcinomas.

Copy number variation (CNV)—Regions of DNA or genes that can vary in the number of copies present (e.g., *CYP2D6*).

Differentiation—In most tissues, the process that involves the progression from a progenitor cell to cells with distinct characteristics associated with the functional role of the tissue. For many tissues, cancer is believed to arise from tissue progenitor cells and thus the cancer may exhibit differentiated characteristics associated with the tissue of origin.

Epigenetics—Modifications of genetic material that are associated with changes in gene expression, but do not alter the basepair sequence of DNA. These include changes in DNA methylation state and alterations of histones, such as acetylation.

Genome-wide association studies—Studies performed to comprehensively examine genetic variations present in DNA (i.e., a person's whole genome) for association with a specific phenotype such as a specific response to drug treatment. Such a study does not *a priori* assume that a particular gene or genes is associated with individual drug response.

Indel—Insertion/deletion of a segment of DNA (i.e., greater than or equal to two basepairs).

Leukemia—A group of cancers derived from blood forming cells.

Messenger RNA (mRNA)—The ribonucleic acid polymer derived from DNA through the process of transcription providing the code for protein production through translation.

Microarray—A nucleotide hybridization-based technology used either to measure characteristics of nucleic acids such as the specific presence of thousands of distinct cellular mRNAs or to measure specific variants of DNA.

Multidrug resistance—Resistance to drug action usually in reference to the action of cell membrane transport proteins that export drugs from the intracellular compartment to outside the cell preventing the drug from acting on its intracellular target (e.g., ATP binding cassette proteins; see p-glycoprotein).

Oligonucleotide—A stretch of nucleotides ranging up to approximately 50 basepairs.

Oncogenes—Genes associated with cancer development that have normal cellular counterparts or proto-oncogenes. The activation of oncogenes involves a genetic event such as a mutation, which may alter the activity of the gene product or a translocation of the oncogene resulting in altered regulation of gene expression. Compare oncogenes to tumor suppressor genes.

Oncology (cancer biology)—The study of cancer often with an emphasis on cancer development and therapy.

P-glycoprotein—(ABCB1; multiple drug resistance 1) an efflux pump present in many cell types. In some cancers, p-glycoprotein is over-expressed and is responsible for cancer chemotherapeutic drug resistance due to the actions of p-glycoprotein pumping the drug out of the cancer cell precluding interactions with the intracellular therapeutic target.

Polymerase chain reaction—A technique used to amplify segments of DNA that most commonly use special thermal stable DNA polymerases. The segment of DNA amplified is determined by DNA primers specific to the region of interest.

Polymorphic variants—Differences in the DNA between two individuals that may account for the genetic basis of phenotype. Such variations may include SNPs, indels, and CNVs. The terms *polymorphic variants, genetic variants, variants,* and *alleles* are used interchangeably throughout this chapter.

Sarcomas—A group of cancers originating from cells of mesodermal origin, such as bone and other connective tissues.

Single nucleotide polymorphism (SNP)—Genetic variants between individuals present at a single, distinct basepair location in DNA.

Splice site variants—Variants of mRNA due to differential processing of introns and exons from the immature mRNA transcript. These variants may result in multiple transcripts present from a single gene, which may in turn result in multiple proteins with variable activities.

Thiopurine methyltransferase deficiency—A deficiency in thiopurine methyltransferase activity due to genetic variants in the thiopurine methyltransferase gene with reduced ability to metabolize the purine analogs such as mercaptopurine and thioguanine.

Tumor suppressor genes—Genes coding for proteins that deter cancer development through regulation of cell growth and division. During cancer development, genetic events may occur that inactivate tumor suppressor genes (e.g., *TP53, RB1*). Because tumor suppressor genes are often inactivated in cancer, the consequence of genetic changes to these genes is difficult to rectify therapeutically. Compare the term *tumor suppressor genes* to *oncogenes*.

Case Study—Pharmacogenomic Considerations for Tamoxifen Therapy

Beatrice is a 45-year-old nulliparous, premenopausal Caucasian female. Her mother died of breast cancer shortly after immigrating to the United States from Israel. Beatrice's older sister, Gertrude, was diagnosed with breast cancer while in her 50s, which was estrogen receptor positive, supporting her as a strong candidate for tamoxifen therapy. However, Gertrude's cancer did not respond to tamoxifen therapy. Additional chemotherapeutic measures to treat Gertrude's cancer were not successful and eventually she died from her breast cancer.

During self-examination, Beatrice palpated a small mass present in her right breast, which, on mammography was found to present as a radio-dense mass. The cancer was biopsied and evaluated to identify a stage IIa infiltrating lobular carcinoma. A lumpectomy was performed to remove the cancerous mass from Beatrice's right breast. In addition, all axillary lymph nodes were removed for analyses.

A metastatic workup was negative. In addition, the cancer was found to be estrogen and progesterone receptor positive without amplification of ErbB2. Performance of an Oncotype DX© Breast Cancer Assay on a histological sample of Beatrice's breast cancer resulted in a low recurrence score (less than 18). Based on these findings, standard therapeutic practice would consider Beatrice to be a good candidate for tamoxifen therapy. However, her physician felt more information was necessary to be confident that Beatrice did not have other factors that would affect the success of tamoxifen therapy.

1. What hereditary gene variants are known that may be contributing factors to the development of Beatrice's breast cancer? Which of these may be consistent with Beatrice's family history and ethnic background?
2. Name a possible pharmacokinetic pharmacogenomic consideration that may affect the efficacy of tamoxifen therapy. How could screening for variants be used to optimize therapeutic strategies for the chemotherapy of Beatrice's breast cancer?

Introduction

Pharmacogenomics has the potential to significantly enhance optimization of cancer therapeutics. Because cancer is frequently a terminal disease, it is critical to utilize the most effective therapeutic regimen to treat the disease and under the best circumstances enact a cure. Many different classes of cancer chemotherapeutic agents have been developed, largely over the past seven decades. These include alkylating agents, purine and pyrimidine analogs, folic acid antimetabolites, topoisomerase inhibitors, taxanes, and hormonal modulators. Specific protocols that utilize these agents are continually being optimized to provide the most effective treatments for the many different types of cancers ranging from hematological cancers to solid cancers, including sarcomas and carcinomas. Therapeutics for all cancer chemotherapeutic classes has been heavily influenced by the advent of cancer pharmacogenomics. Additionally, our increasing understanding of molecular lesions associated with cancers, a key area of cancer pharmaco-genomics, is greatly assisting the development of novel targeted cancer therapeutics.

Understanding of the role that heredity plays in both the recognition of cancer syndromes and the biology of drug action is increasing. Cancer is a disease known to involve numerous changes to the cellular genome. These changes include modifications to both DNA and mRNA expression. Thus, cancer pharmacogenomics incorporates an understanding of hereditary factors that alter genes associated with cancer predisposition, as well as genetic changes that occur in the multistage process of carcinogenesis including alterations in the expression of genes, which affect drug metabolism (Figure 8-1). Methods have been developed for research and clinical use (e.g., microarrays) to examine genetic variants from a patient's DNA. Microarrays have also been developed that allow the assessment of changes that occur in mRNA expression present in cancer cells. Information combined from each of these different types of genetic assays can now be utilized to provide personalized cancer therapy for individual patients.

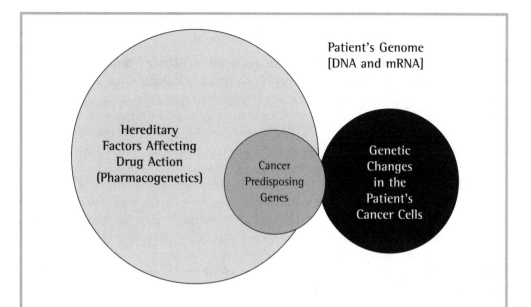

Patient's Genome
[DNA and mRNA]

Hereditary
Factors Affecting
Drug Action
(Pharmacogenetics)

Cancer
Predisposing
Genes

Genetic
Changes
in the
Patient's
Cancer Cells

Figure 8.1 • Areas of genomics contributing to cancer pharmacogenomics include analyses of both DNA and mRNA expression. As in traditional pharmacogenetics, hereditary factors have a significant role in determining both the effectiveness and toxicities associated with cancer chemotherapy. Currently, studies are evaluating the role of cancer predisposing genes associated with cancer syndromes and their impact on cancer chemotherapy as a subset of hereditary factors. In addition, genetic changes, such as mutations and alterations in gene expression, that occur in the patient's cancer cells during the progression of the cancer may have a significant impact in both determining the effectiveness of drug therapy as well as in providing information useful for targeting drug therapy.

Because genetic considerations in cancer therapy include both hereditary factors as well as genetic contributions that occur during cancer progression, individualized drug therapy for cancer is a quintessential example of the increasing impact of the field of pharmacogenomics on cancer therapy. Additionally, a growing area of cancer pharmacogenomics addresses cancer prevention. Individuals with a recognized genetic predisposition to cancer or that engage in high-risk activities for cancer may be strong candidates for cancer prevention approaches. These measures may include drug-based strategies that define the emerging field of chemo-prevention. The field of pharmacogenomics offers exceptional promise for the future of cancer therapy, in both optimizing therapeutic strategies as well as reducing the side-effects associated with cancer chemotherapeutics, which are often based on the hereditary genetics of the patient as well as genetic considerations of the cancer. The ability to correlate pharmacogenomic characteristics of a cancer and an individual's specific DNA profile with responsiveness to a specific drug provides an "individualized" approach to pharmacotherapy that is having a significant impact on pharmacy practice. This chapter provides an overview of pharmacogenomics used in pharmacy that is of key relevance to cancer chemoprevention and therapy.

General Considerations in Cancer Pharmacogenomics

Pharmacokinetics in Cancer Pharmacogenomics—Drug Metabolism

As with other areas of pharmacogenomics, important considerations for the pharmaco-genomics of cancer therapeutic agents can generally be divided into two broad classifications: pharmacokinetics, or the disposition of the drug in the body (especially in relationship to drug transport and metabolic activity in the body that may alter drug action), and pharmacodynam-ics, or the action of the drug on the body (e.g., the action of a drug on a specific drug receptor). Pharmacodynamic considerations important to cancer pharmacogenomics will be discussed in the following section. Pharmacokinetic considerations in pharmacogenomics were critical in the early observations of adverse drug reactions that led to an understanding of genetic contri-butions to drug activity. Pharmacokinetic considerations primarily relate to metabolic actions that facilitate drug inactivation and excretion. However, drug metabolism may also have an im-portant impact on the activation of prodrugs (e.g., the metabolism of codeine to morphine).

There are many different enzymes involved in the metabolism of drugs used in cancer che-motherapy. One of the most pervasive families of metabolic enzymes is the cytochrome P450's (CYPs).[1] In humans, 57 different *CYP* genes have been identified. Substrates for different CYP members vary and almost all drugs are metabolized by more than a single CYP. Polymorphic variants of the CYPs are extensive and involve virtually all possible forms of genetic variants in-cluding SNPs, indels, and CNVs. Because numerous variants of CYPs have been identified, they have been organized into the more succinct designations of poor, intermediate, extensive, and ultrarapid metabolizers. For example, numerous variants of CYP2D6 have been identified such that the metabolic profile for different CYP2D6 variants themselves have been classified into groups of poor, intermediate, extensive, and ultrarapid metabolizers.[2] Many other classes of drug metabolizing enzymes have highly significant roles in cancer pharmacogenomics. These include UDP glucuronosyl transferases, thiopurine methyltransferases, N-acetyl transferases, and cytidine deaminase to name a few. A complete listing of metabolic enzymes important in drug metabolism is beyond the scope of this chapter (see Chapter 4), though many important examples are featured throughout. It is important to recognize that numerous polymorphic variants of drug metabolizing enzymes exist and many have been identified that have a vital role in cancer pharmacogenomics.

Pharmacodynamics in Cancer Pharmacogenomics—Drug Targets

Pharmacological considerations for most drugs address the action of the drug on the drug target. Many drug targets are proteins (i.e., gene products) with specialized cellular activity. The genes associated with the drug target may exist in variant forms, which may result in the production of different amino acid sequences in the gene product. Such differences in amino acid sequences of these gene products can have pronounced functional consequences that impact the efficacy of drug action. This paradigm of drug action regarding pharmacodynamics applies to cancer chemotherapeutic agents. Importantly, our understanding of drug targets is a key consideration in the design of candidate gene studies, where polymorphic variants in the accepted drug target gene are logical candidates for investigating associations for differences in drug action between individuals.

An example of pharmacodynamic considerations in cancer pharmacogenomics includes the target of 5-fluorouracil (5-FU), thymidylate synthase (*TYMS*). As will be discussed, *TYMS* possesses a number of well-established polymorphic variants.[3] Although it seems reasonable to consider that variants of *TYMS* might affect the actions of 5-FU, this has not proven to be decisive from a clinical standpoint. However, the action of folic acid inhibitors, such as methotrexate, which indirectly affect TYMS, may be affected by *TYMS* variants.[4] In many instances, candidate gene analysis comparing target gene variants with drug action have failed to show meaningful associations to explain differences in drug action. More recently, due to a more thorough knowledge of genetic variants, genome-wide association studies (GWAS) are being performed to identify variants that may account for differences in drug action among individuals. In these studies, genetic variants are tested without choosing a candidate gene or genes. Interestingly, GWAS have resulted in many meaningful and unexpected variants accounting for individual differences in drug action. Thus, association studies for determining genetic variants affecting drug action do not necessarily follow the sensibility of pharmacodynamic considerations in cancer pharmacogenomics studies. Because of the unexpected success of GWAS findings in all areas of pharmacogenomics, including cancer pharmacogenomics, they will be discussed in greater detail in later sections.

Drug Efflux Pumps

Drug transport pumps represent a special case with potential relevance to either the pharmacokinetics or pharmacodynamics of cancer pharmacogenomics, depending on the context of drug action. The plasma cell membrane contains pumps that allow the transfer of small molecules into (i.e., uptake pumps) and out of (i.e., efflux pumps) the cell. These pumps control the transfer of a vast array of molecules, from small ions such as sodium to relative large cancer therapeutic agents (e.g., docetaxel). There are numerous pumps (or transporters) that may be selectively expressed in different cell types; however, the large array of pumps is categorized into families based on activity and similarity of the encoded proteins. Of particular importance to cancer therapy are efflux pumps that remove cancer therapeutic agents from the inside of the cancer cell, preventing the drug from reaching their therapeutic target. Therefore, drug efflux pumps present a special case regarding pharmacodynamic and pharmacokinetic considerations in pharmacogenomics. Because efflux pumps actively remove drugs from cells, an activity important to drug disposition, these proteins may have a critical role in the pharmacokinetics of drug action. However, these proteins may also be the target of drug action, whereby pharmacodynamic considerations are relevant. Examples of efflux pumps with activity important to cancer therapy include the mitoxantrone resistance protein and P-glycoprotein.

Mitoxantrone Resistance Protein

The mitoxantrone resistance protein (MXR or ABCG2) is also referred to as the breast cancer resistance protein. It is an efflux transporter that confers resistance to important classes of cancer chemotherapeutic agents that include the anthracyclines, anthracenediones (e.g., mitoxantrone), and camptothecins, such as topotecan and irinotecan.[5] MXR has been implicated in therapeutic resistance for acute myelogenous leukemia and breast cancer.[6] Although many variants of MXR have been identified, further studies are necessary to determine what therapeutic consequence these variants have on the outcome of cancer therapy.

Multiple Drug Resistance 1 (P-glycoprotein)

Among the most extensively investigated efflux pumps associated with resistance to cancer therapy is P-glycoprotein (MDR1 or ABCB1). P-glycoprotein was first identified in cancer cells as an over-expressed protein that is believed to be important in the resistance of many cancers to chemotherapeutic agents. Drugs that may be pumped from cells by P-glycoprotein include anthracyclines, calcium channel blockers, digoxin, paclitaxel, and vinca alkaloids.[7] Many variants of P-glycoprotein have been identified, and a few may have important effects on the activity of this protein. Hoffmeyer et al. examined the DNA sequence from 21 individuals to identify 15 polymorphic variants.[8] Of these variants, one designated C3435T was found to have a significant impact on the expression of P-glycoprotein. Individuals homozygous (i.e., two copies of the same allele) for the T form of P-glycoprotein were found to have reduced duodenal protein expression levels of P-glycoprotein, which was believed to be responsible for increased drug plasma protein levels. In this case, P-glycoprotein variants could have an important impact on pharmacokinetic properties related to drug administration. However, to date, modification of cancer therapy based on the presence of specific genetic variants of P-glycoprotein has yet to be successfully translated into contemporary pharmacotherapy.

Pharmacogenomics of Cancer Chemotherapeutic Agents

Many different classes of cancer chemotherapies are available with a broad scope of therapeutic applications for the many different forms of cancer. As found throughout pharmacogenomics, many different genetic polymorphisms are known that affect the action of cancer chemotherapies. Classes of cancer chemotherapeutic agents that are known to be affected by genetic variants include purine and pyrimidine analogs, folic acid antimetabolites, topoisomerase I inhibitors, and selective hormone receptor modulators. Some key examples of cancer therapies associated with relevant genetic variants are listed in Table 8-1.

Table 8-1
Pharmacogenomics of Cancer Chemotherapeutic Agents

Drug Class	Cancer Chemotherapeutic Agent	Gene(s)
Alkylating agents	Cyclophosphamide	CYP2B6, CYP2C9, CYP2C19, CYP3A4
Folic acid antimetabolites	Methotrexate	DHFR, TYMS
Hormone modulators	Tamoxifen	CYP2D6
Purine antimetabolites	Mercaptopurine	TPMT
	Thioguanine	TPMT
Pyrimidine antimetabolites	Gemcitabine	Cytidine deaminase
	5-Fluorouracil	DYPD, TYMS
Topoisomerase inhibitors	Irinotecan	UGT1A1

Purine Analogs (e.g., 6-mercaptopurine and 6-thioguanine)

Purine analogs such as mercaptopurine and thioguanine are used in the treatment of acute lymphoblastic leukemia. Mercaptopurine and thioguanine are activated to form thioguanine nucleotides that are incorporated into DNA and RNA causing DNA damage and cytotoxicity. A major metabolic pathway involved in the inactivation of these drugs is S-methylation catalyzed by thiopurine S-methyltransferase (TPMT) using S-adenosyl-L-methionine as the S-methyl donor. Interestingly, although metabolism of mercaptopurine and thioguanine by TPMT is a major route of their inactivation, the physiologic function of TPMT is uncertain.

Multiple genetic variations of the *TPMT* gene have been identified.[9] However, only three variants are present with sufficient prevalence to have a clinical impact. These are designated TPMT *2, *3A, and *3C. The *2 variant is due to a G238C variant that results in the substitution of an alanine with a proline at amino acid 80 and a 100-fold decrease in enzyme activity. The *3A variant has been ascribed to multiple differences in a single gene that include G460A and A719G variants resulting in the substitution of an alanine with a threonine and a tyrosine with a cysteine at amino acids 154 and 240, respectively. The *3C variant is representative of the A719G variant only of *3A. As with the *2 variant, *3A and *3C variants have greatly reduced TPMT activity. Because of the severe toxicity associated with reduced mercaptopurine or thioguanine clearance in individuals harboring these TPMT variants, screening for these variants prior to treatment with these purine analogs is now becoming commonplace.

An important pharmacogenomic consideration in the use of purine analogs is that reduced dosing levels due to the presence of TPMT variants does not reduce therapeutic efficacy, but greatly reduces toxicity associated with the use of purine analogs (reviewed in Chapter 10. At least 15 other variants of TPMT have been identified but at lower frequencies than TPMT *2, *3A, and *3C. Variations among ethnic groups are extensive and may necessitate further characterization of additional TPMT variants for therapeutic considerations among specific ethnic groups.[9]

Clinical Pearl

Due to the potentially severe toxicities associated with thiopurine treatment and the limited opportunities to achieve therapeutic efficacy, factors affecting therapy are critical and impact thiopurine dosing. For example, reductions in 6-mercaptopurine dosing levels are instituted for both the presence of a single TPMT variant form (i.e., individuals heterozygous for TPMT variants with reduced activity). More extreme dosage reductions are instituted for those individuals with two TPMT variants having reduced activity (i.e., homozygous for reduced activity TPMT variants). In these individuals, dose reductions of up to 90% the standard dosing levels may be warranted.[10]

Pyrimidine Analogs (e.g., 5-fluorouracil and gemcitibine)

Pyrimidine analogs are used in the treatment of tumors such as colorectal and gastric cancers. The drug 5-fluorouracil (5-FU) is a pyrimidine analog that acts as a uracil analog and functions, in part, by inhibiting thymidylate synthase (TYMS), which results in decreased thymidine production and inhibition of DNA synthesis. 5-FU itself is not active but requires metabolism through pyrimidine salvage pathways to produce the active forms.

TYMS is expressed both in normal cells and cancer cells and is a key enzyme involved in the synthesis of thymidylate. Because TYMS is the key target of 5-FU activity, genetic variants of the *TYMS* gene have been investigated at length.[3] Polymorphic variants affecting *TYMS* expression have been identified with variations in the 5′ and 3′ untranslated regions of the *TYMS* gene.[11] For the 5′ untranslated region, three copies of a 28 basepair tandem repeat have been described. For the 3′ untranslated region, a 6 basepair deletion has been described that results in reduced *TYMS* gene expression. However, to date, the impact of these variants on *TYMS* gene expression and patient response to 5-FU at present is unclear.[12] In contrast, *TYMS* variants may affect response to folic acid antimetabolite therapies (see below).

A key enzyme involved in pyrimidine catabolism is dihydropyrimidine dehydrogenase (DPYD), which is important in the breakdown of 5-fluorouracil. It is estimated that approximately 5% to 10% of the population possess a deficiency in DPYD enzyme activity. *DPYD* is a complex gene in which many genetic variants have been identified. A splice site variant, designated IVS14+1G>A, results in a deficiency of DPYD with resultant 5-FU associated toxicity, as reported by Van Kuilenburg et al. In this study, 28% of patients were found to harbor the IVS14+1G>A variant.[13] Because of its high prevalence, screening for the IVS14+1G>A *DPYD* variant in patients before 5-FU administration was recommended.[13]

Gemcitabine is a deoxycytidine analog with a broad spectrum of antitumor activity including hard-to-treat cancers such as pancreatic and nonsmall-cell lung cancer. Inactivation of gemcitabine occurs by metabolism to 2′, 2′-difluorodeoxyuridine through the actions of cytidine deaminase. Sugiyama et al. examined the pharmacokinetics of gemcitabine in a study of 256 Japanese patients receiving a 30-minute intravenous infusion of 800 or 1,000 mg/m^2 gemcitabine.[14] It was found that individuals with a G208A variant of cytidine deaminase (designated CDA*3), which has a threonine in place of an alanine at amino acid 70, had decreased clearance of gemcitabine and an increased incidence of neutropenia when coadministered with 5-FU. In fact, a patient homozygous for the CDA*3 variant suffered life-threatening toxicity after gemcitabine treatment.[15]

Folic Acid Antimetabolites (e.g., methotrexate)

Folic acid antimetabolites were among the first cancer chemotherapies with broad use in cancer treatment including breast, head and neck, GI, and lung cancers, as well as osteosarcomas and acute lymphoblastic leukemia (ALL). A primary action of these agents is the blockade of dihydrofolate reductase (DHFR). Inhibiting the conversion of folic acid to tetrahydrofolate results in cell cycle arrest due to inhibition of DNA, RNA, and protein synthesis. Variants in thymidylate synthase (TYMS) have also been suggested to affect the efficacy of folic acid antimetabolites. Both pharmacodynamic and pharmacokinetic considerations are believed to contribute to the pharmacogenomics of folic acid antimetabolites.

Few variants of the DHFR gene have been identified. In a laboratory setting, cells exposed to methotrexate have been shown to develop mutations in the DHFR gene that confer resistance to methotrexate.[16] However, these mutations have not been linked to the use of methotrexate in a clinical setting. Similarly, genetic amplifications of the DHFR gene have been produced in cell lines cultured to develop methotrexate resistance.[17,18] Currently, it is unclear whether or not variants of DHFR affecting enzyme activity or levels of DHFR have a significant impact on the action of folic acid antimetabolites in cancer treatment.

As presented for pyrimidines analogs, variants in *TYMS* are of importance in the pharmacogenomics of folic acid antimetabolites. Anticancer drugs such as methotrexate inhibit this enzyme in cancer cells in order to interfere with cancer cell nucleic acid metabolism. As discussed previously, an indel of two or three 28 basepair repeats has been identified in the promoter of the *TYMS* gene. The presence of a triplet of the 28 basepair repeat is associated with higher levels of *TYMS* expression.[3] Krajinovic et al. examined the variability in response to methotrexate in children treated for acute lymphoblastic leukemia based on the presence of these variants.[4] Among 205 children treated with methotrexate, those homozygous for the triple 28 basepair repeat were found to have a worse outcome than children with other *TYMS* gene variants.[4] Based on this observation, the investigators concluded that, "Genotyping of thymidylate synthase might make it possible to individualize treatment for patients with acute lymphoblastic leukemia."[4]

Topoisomerase I Inhibitors (e.g., irinotecan)

Irinotecan is used for the treatment of metastatic colorectal and lung cancers. It is a semisynthetic derivative of camptothecin that exhibits anticancer activity through inhibition of topoisomerase I, which is necessary for DNA replication. Biotransformation of irinotecan to SN-38 by carboxylesterases is required for the potent antitumor activity of irinotecan. From a pharmacogenomic standpoint, polymorphic variants of carboxylesterases would be expected to affect the efficacy of irinotecan. However, variants affecting SN-38 production have not been described. Instead, the inactivation of SN-38 by glucuronidation has pharmacogenomic consequences.

UDP glucuronosyltransferases are a family of enzymes that are responsible for the glucuronidation of drugs, steroids, bilirubin, and other fat soluble molecules to form excretable metabolites. SN-38 is a substrate for UDP glucuronosyltransferase 1A1 (UGT1A1). Variants of this gene are associated with Crigler-Najjar syndrome. In addition, variants are associated with decreased SN-38 excretion. Ratain's group first reported the altered metabolism of SN-38 in liver cells from individuals with a variant in the promoter region of the *UGT1A1* gene.[19] This variant, designated UGT1A1*28, has an additional TA repeat in the promoter region of the *UGT1A1* gene (i.e., seven TAs compared to six) that result in decreased UGT1A1 liver expression. The reduced levels of UGT1A1 results in decreased SN-38 hepatic excretion and toxicity due to elevated SN-38 levels. Interestingly, this variant is also commonly associated with Gilbert syndrome, which is manifested as a mild form of hyperbilirubinemia.[20,21]

Selective Estrogen Receptor Modulators (e.g., tamoxifen and raloxifene)

Tamoxifen and raloxifene are selective estrogen receptor modulators (SERMs) that act as estrogen antagonists in estrogen receptor positive breast cancers.[22] Many breast cancers express estrogen receptor alpha, which, in the presence of estrogen, acts to promote breast cancer cell growth. Inhibition of estrogen receptor activation reduces the proliferative activity of breast cancer cells. In this regard, SERMs block the interaction of estrogens with the estrogen receptor, thereby reducing breast cancer cell proliferation. Tamoxifen is prescribed for breast cancer treatment of estrogen receptor positive breast cancer in premenopausal women, whereas raloxifene may be prescribed for treatment in postmenopausal patients.[22]

As pointed out previously, the CYPs are a large family of enzymes responsible for the oxidative metabolism of many xenobiotics, including many cancer chemotherapeutic agents.[1] One of the most polymorphic forms of the CYPs is *CYP2D6*, which is also one of the most important in the metabolism of tamoxifen to one of its most active forms 4-hydroxytamoxifen. However, polymorphic variants of *CYP2D6* exist that code for proteins that do not efficiently metabolize tamoxifen to 4-hydroxytamoxifen.[23] One of the more prevalent variants with reduced activity is designated CYP2D6*4, present in 17% to 21% of the Caucasian population. CYP2D6*4 occurs from a G to A variation present in the first basepairs of exon 4 of the *CYP2D6* gene, resulting in a splice site shift and the generation of a premature termination codon. Individuals homozygous for CYP2D6*4 lack CYP2D6 activity and individuals either heterozygous or homozygous for CYP2D6*4 are deemed poor metabolizers. Although conflicting results are observed when comparing clinical studies on the efficacy of tamoxifen and *CYP2D6* variants, in 2006 the Food and Drug Administration recommended an update on the tamoxifen label to reflect an increased recurrence in breast cancer patients who are CYP2D6 poor metabolizers.[24]

Clinical Pearl

Metabolism of drugs by metabolic enzymes, such as CYPs, is often associated with drug excretion and impairment of activity may be associated with increased levels of parent drug and increased toxicity. As discussed, CYP variants can have a pronounced effect on drug excretion. Alternatively, as in the case of tamoxifen, therapeutic efficacy of a drug may be dictated by metabolism to the active form by metabolic enzymes, which may also be affected by the presence of specific polymorphic variants. Therefore, drug action resulting from genetic variants is not always predictable and requires a careful pharmacological assessment before the full physiologic effects of these variants are accurately understood.

Taxanes (paclitaxel and docetaxel)

Taxanes are novel cancer therapeutic agents that act through promoting and stabilizing the assembly of microtubule formation by preventing depolymerization. Taxanes include paclitaxel, which is a dipertene plant derivative from the needles and bark of the western yew tree, and docetaxel, a semisynthetic analog of paclitaxel that is derived from the European yew tree. Taxanes have found to have broad efficacy for the treatment of many forms of cancer. Pharmacokinetic considerations have been the focus of pharmacogenomic studies evaluating the cancer chemotherapeutic efficacy of the taxanes.

Metabolism of docetaxel by CYPs is considered a major route of elimination.[1] For example, CYP3A4 is known to metabolize docetaxel to its inactive hydroxylated forms. Thus, high CYP3A4 activity would be expected to result in reduced therapeutic efficacy of docetaxel. In support of this concept, Engels et al. found that inhibition of CYP3A4 using ketoconazole decreased the clearance of docetaxel.[25] Clinically, although many CYP3A4 variants have been recognized, there is currently limited support that these variants affect docetaxel activity in cancer treatment. Because of interindividual diversity in paclitaxel pharmacokinetics and the identification of a CYP3A4 haplotype associated with paclitaxel pharmacokinetics, applications of pharmacogenomics to optimizing paclitaxel therapy are anticipated.[26]

Alkylating Agents (e.g., cyclophosphamide)

Cyclophosphamide is an alkylating agent that is used primarily for the treatment of lymphomas and breast cancer. As with tamoxifen, cyclophosphamide is a prodrug that requires metabolism by CYPs to produce the active form of the drug.[1] Multiple CYP forms are able to activate cyclophosphamide including CYP 2B6, 2C9, 2C19, and 3A4/5. Studies are ongoing to determine the effect of variants in these *CYP* genes on the efficacy of cyclophosphamide therapy.

Pharmacogenomics of Cancer Chemoprevention

As discussed later, genetic variants exist that are associated with a predisposition to cancer. Development of multiple cancers, an early age of onset, and the development of cancers among relatives may all be suggestive of hereditary factors contributing to cancer predisposition.[27] A goal of pharmacogenomics includes the institution of preventive measures to reduce the likelihood of developing cancers, which may be greatly improved by performing genetic screens for variants associated with cancer predisposition. In addition, cancer chemopreventive measures may be prudent among individuals that engage in high-risk activities for cancer development. Strategies for cancer prevention can be divided in three distinct areas: primary, secondary, and tertiary prevention.

Primary cancer prevention involves preventive measures among individuals not currently diagnosed with cancer, but who may be involved in high risk activities (e.g., working with radiation) or that have a genetic predisposition to cancer development. An example of a promising cancer primary chemopreventive intervention includes the use of nonsteroidal anti-inflammatory drugs for the prevention of colorectal cancer development.[28] Colorectal cancer is the third leading cause of cancer cases and deaths in the U.S.[29] Results from epidemiologic studies support that regular aspirin intake is associated with a reduced risk of colorectal cancer development.[30] Other nonsteroidal anti-inflammatory drugs have also shown efficacy in prevention of colorectal cancer.[31] Although not firmly established, it is anticipated that genetic factors will have a significant role in the efficacy of colorectal cancer preventive measures, which will open the field of chemopreventive pharmacogenomics in the primary prevention setting.[31] Secondary prevention involves measures among individuals diagnosed with premalignant lesions to reduce the chance that these lesions progress to more advanced stages of disease. An example of secondary prevention may include the institution of chemopreventive measures upon the identification of preneoplastic lesions in colon cancer (e.g., polyps).[32]

Tertiary prevention measures are taken by individuals that have been treated for cancer to prevent further cancer development. An example of tertiary prevention is the use of tamoxifen to prevent tumor development in a contralateral breast in high-risk individuals. Pharmacogenomic considerations that apply to tamoxifen therapy for breast cancer are also relevant to tamoxifen chemoprevention of breast cancer. The breast cancer preventive potential of tamoxifen in women with breast cancer predisposing genetic variants in *BRCA1* or *BRCA2* was studied for contralateral breast cancer development.[33] In this study, tamoxifen treatment was found to reduce the risk of contralateral breast cancer by 50%.[33] In addition to colon and breast cancer, chemoprevention of cancer is being investigated for head and neck, lung, bladder, prostate, skin, and cervical cancer.[34] With an increased understanding of cancer genetics, the ability to estimate a risk to cancer development will become an increasingly important element of healthcare. In the future of pharmacy practice, it is likely that cancer pharmacogenomics will include greater considerations for cancer chemopreventive measures.

Cancer Genetics and Pharmacogenomics

Cancer is a genomic disease. During cancer progression, genetic modifications (i.e., mutations) develop within the disease. In the early stages of cancer, mutations occur in a select subpopulation of cells (i.e., the nascent cancer cell) that may facilitate the progression of the disease. In many instances, the molecular abnormalities caused by the cytogenetic changes can be targeted therapeutically (Table 8-2). Key examples include the treatment of breast cancers over-expressing an amplified *Her-2/neu* gene (i.e., treated with trastuzumab) and chronic myelogenous leukemia associated with translocations resulting in a novel fusion gene Bcr-Abl (i.e., treated with imatinib).[35,36] Mutations found in cancer cells are not inherited as they would likely be detrimental to the development of the organism. However, there are cancer syndromes that involve genetic factors that may predispose an individual to cancer development as will be described later. Because, in an increasing number of cases, drug therapy for a specific cancer targets the proteins that are associated with gene mutations, genetic considerations in cancer pharmacogenomics is to a large degree distinct from pharmacogenomic considerations associated with inborn genetic variants.

Table 8-2
Examples of Genetic Modifications in Cancers and Targeted Therapies

Cancer Types	Genetic Modification	Targeted Therapy
Hematologic cancers		
Acute myeloid leukemia	*FLT3* mutations	Tyrosine kinase inhibitors
Acute promyelocytic leukemia	*PML:RARα* - t(15;27)	All-trans retinoic acid
Chronic myelogenous leukemia	*BCR:ABL* fusion	Imatinib
Carcinomas		
Breast cancer	*ErbB2* amplification	Trastuzumab
Colorectal	*EGFR* and *KRAS* mutations	Cetuximab
Prostate cancer	*TMPRSS2:ETS* fusion	(In development)

Genetic Changes Occurring During Cancer Progression

Hematologic Malignancies

Hematologic cancers are those malignancies that affect the blood forming cells and are distinct from solid cancers in many respects, including the therapeutic regimens used to treat these diseases. Examples of hematologic malignancies include acute lymphoblastic leukemia, acute myeloid leukemia (and the subtype acute promyelocytic leukemia), chronic lymphocytic leukemia, and chronic myelogenous leukemia. Many hematologic malignancies are associated with gene translocations that have critical roles in the development and maintenance of the cancerous phenotype and have been associated with high-risk disease. In some instances, the gene product associated with these translocations has been exploited as a therapeutic target.

Acute Lymphoblastic Leukemia (ALL)

Acute lymphoblastic leukemia (ALL) is the most common childhood cancer.[37] Multiple genetic lesions that are associated with ALL have proven useful in determining disease prognosis. Historically, these genetic lesions have been determined cytogenetically. For example, a chromosomal translocation that occurs in ALL is t(12;21), which is associated with good prognosis. However, not all genetic changes in ALL are easily identifiable and some patients experience treatment failure or disease relapse after therapy, or may experience severe treatment-related toxicities.[38]

Significant progress has occurred in the treatment of ALL over the past four decades. As discussed previously, antimetabolites such as 6-mercaptopurine and methotrexate may be used in ALL treatment. Thus, the pharmacogenomic considerations that apply to these drugs must be considered in the treatment of ALL. For example, variants in TPMT as discussed should be assessed to avoid severe toxicity associated with 6-mercaptopurine among individuals carrying less active variants of this gene.

Acute Myeloid Leukemia (AML)

Acute myeloid leukemia (AML) is more common than ALL and occurs primarily in adults. AML is a heterogeneous group of leukemia that result from clonal transformation of hematopoietic precursors through the acquisition of chromosomal rearrangements and multiple gene mutations.[39] In addition to cytogenetic considerations, dysplastic features, the patient's preceding history, and age are important prognostic factors for AML.

As with most leukemia, AML can be characterized by genetic modifications present in the disease. An example of a genetic change present in approximately a third of AML patients are mutations in the *FLT3* gene.[40] FLT3 (fms-like tyrosine kinase 3) is a receptor tyrosine kinase found to be expressed in hematopoietic stem/progenitor cells. Mutations found in *FLT3* in AML patients include internal tandem duplications and point mutations that lead to a constitutively active receptor. Presence of these mutations in AML patients has been associated with a higher relapse rate to conventional therapies. Tyrosine kinase inhibitors targeting FLT3 have been designed and are in clinical trials for AML treatment. In addition, anti-FLT3 antibodies are being developed to therapeutically target the FLT3 protein in AML.[40]

Acute promyelocytic leukemia (APL) is a subtype of AML that is cytogenetically classified by a balanced reciprocal translocation between chromosomes 15 and 17, resulting in the fusion between the promyelocytic leukemia gene and the retinoic acid receptor alpha gene.[41] The complete remission rate for APL has greatly increased since the use of all-trans retinoic acid (ATRA) was introduced for the treatment of APL because it works as a differentiating agent. However, relapse following ATRA treatment still occurs such that it must be combined with other chemotherapies to optimize response. Interestingly, altered expression of CYP2D6, which is important in retinoid metabolism, may have an impact in relapse to ATRA treatment.[42]

Clinical Pearl

Prior to the use of ATRA, the long-term response rate for APL treatment was lower than 10%. Although relapse can occur with ATRA, the addition of ATRA to APL treatment regimens has increased the number of long-term survivors to nearly 80%.[43] ATRA therapy for APL represents a strategy based on rational drug design, resulting from a heightened understanding of molecular lesions associated with specific cancers.

Chronic Lymphocytic Leukemia (CLL)

Chronic lymphocytic leukemia (CLL) is a blood cancer of B-lymphocyte origin that occurs primarily in adults. Prognostic groups of CLL are based on genetic changes.[44] One of the more common genetic modifications associated with CLL is a deletion located in the long arm of chromosome 13. The specific genetic elements contributing to CLL from chromosome 13 deletion are not known. However, because this likely represents a deletion of a tumor suppressor gene and the absence of a target, therapeutic interventions based on this molecular lesion may not lend themselves to targeted therapeutics.

Chronic Myelogenous Leukemia (CML)

As with other leukemias, chronic myelogenous leukemia (CML) is cytogenetically classified by a reciprocal translocation. In the case of CML, this translocation occurs between chromosomes 9 and 22 involving a fusion of the ABL proto-oncogene from chromosome 9 with the breakpoint cluster region (BCR) of chromosome 22. This chromosomal fusion is referred to as the Philadelphia chromosome. Upon translocation, the regulation of *ABL* expression is altered resulting in oncogenic character. More specifically, the ABL protein has tyrosine kinase activity that alters cell cycle regulation. A breakthrough in CML treatment occurred with the discovery of imatinib, a comparatively selective ABL tyrosine kinase inhibitor.[45] The success of imatinib in CML treatment has prompted the discovery of other tyrosine kinase inhibitors for cancer therapy, including advanced agents for the treatment of CML, and has served as a paradigm for rational drug design.[36,46]

Carcinomas

Early models of carcinoma development illustrated that cancer proceeds in multiple stages contributing to the progression of the disease.[47] In these models, cancer development begins with the *initiating lesion,* representing the first stage in cancer development, which is genetic in origin. That is, the initiation stage necessarily involves the production of mutations that can facilitate cancer development. The subsequent *promotion stage* of cancer development may also involve carcinogenic mutations. However, promotion is primarily associated with changes in gene expression that further facilitate cancer development. The *progression stage* of cancer development is associated with the production of the key genetic changes that lead to malignancy. Note that genetic lesions associated with sarcoma progression have also been identified and have important therapeutic implications. Because sarcomas are relatively rare forms of cancer compared to carcinomas, they are not covered in this chapter. The numbers of genetic lesions identified that are associated with the stages of carcinoma development are growing rapidly, facilitating the discovery of novel therapeutic targets. A few key examples are provided here.

Breast Cancer

The identification of *BRCA1* and *BRCA2* gene variants associated with familial breast cancer represents a historical breakthrough in medical genetics. Breast cancer is the most prominent form of cancer to develop among women in the U.S.[29] Among these cancers, approximately 10% are associated with mutations in *BRCA1* or *BRCA2*.[48] As noted in the pharmacogenomics of cancer chemoprevention, tamoxifen use was found to reduce the risk of contralateral breast cancer in women with predisposing variants in the *BRCA1* or *BRCA2* genes.[49]

Clinical Pearl

Ethnic heritage may provide useful information regarding inherited genetic variants. For example, women of Ashkenazi Jewish descent have a 21% to 30% presence of founder mutations in *BRCA1* or *BRCA2* among those diagnosed with breast cancer before 50 years of age compared to an approximately 6.1% rate among non-Jewish women.[50] Thus, medical genetics related to ethnicity may assist the identification of inherited variants that can impact therapeutic decisions.

Gene amplifications observed in cancers may result in the over-expression of proteins that contribute to disease pathology. An example is the ErbB2 protein (also referred to as Her2/neu) in breast cancer. The *ErbB2* gene codes for a protein that belongs to the same family of proteins as the epidermal growth factor receptor (i.e., ErbB1). Over-expression of ErbB2 is associated with a poorer prognosis in breast cancer. Monoclonal antibody therapies (e.g., trastuzumab) targeted at the ErbB2 protein have been developed that can be effective in the treatment of breast cancers over-expressing ErbB2. Analysis of breast cancers for ErbB2 over-expression has become a standard of practice to optimize therapies for breast cancer using monoclonal antibody therapies, such as trastuzumab.

Colorectal Cancer

Genomic changes associated with the progression of colorectal cancer have been extensively investigated.[51] Among the lesions identified, activating mutations in the *KRAS* gene are present in approximately 40% of these cancers and likely represent an early event (i.e., initiating lesion) in colorectal cancer progression. The presence of activating mutations in the *KRAS* oncogene of colorectal cancers has been found to influence the efficacy of EGFR-targeted therapies.[52] For example, cetuximab, an anti-EGFR antibody, has been used effectively in the treatment of advanced colorectal cancer. Lievre et al. reported a zero percent response to cetuximab among 24 patients with *KRAS* mutations in their cancer compared to a 40% response among 65 patients without these mutations ($P<0.001$).[53] These results, combined with results from previous studies, strongly suggest that *KRAS* mutations be considered in cetuximab treatment for advanced colorectal cancers.[53]

Prostate Cancer

Gene fusions and chromosomal rearrangements, as associated with hematologic malignancies, have not been as extensively investigated in carcinomas. The identification of molecular lesions found with frequency in prostate cancer has occurred only recently. An example is the TM-PRSS2/ETS family gene fusions.[54] These gene fusions involve the androgen-regulated *TMPRSS2* gene located on chromosome 21, which codes for a transmembrane serine protease. The ETS (erythroblastosis virus E26 transformation sequence) family members that are found fused with *TMPRSS2* include *ERG*, *ETV1*, or *ETV4*, which are transcription factors with transforming potential (i.e., change cells to possess cancer-associated characteristics). Because the *TMPRSS2* gene is androgen-sensitive, current hormonal ablation therapies may act in part through down-regulation of the fusion product activity. Targeted therapies for TMPRSS2/ETS are currently in development.[54]

Genetics of Cancer Syndromes

Familial connections to cancer were recognized long before precise genetic variants were identified as contributing factors to these hereditary diseases. Of particular importance are cancer preventive measures for individuals predisposed to cancer syndromes. With regard to pharmacy practice, this will likely lead to the dispensing of drugs important as cancer chemopreventative agents. An example is the recognition that COX inhibitors are preventive for colorectal cancer. As presented, daily aspirin supplementation is recognized as reducing colorectal cancer development. Importantly, the influence of these genetic contributors in cancer development is now being incorporated therapeutically. Examples of cancers with known familial contributing factors are listed in Table 8-3.

Table 8-3
Cancer Syndromes and Associated Predisposing Genes

Cancer Syndrome	Genes Associated with Syndrome
Familial breast and ovarian cancer	*BRCA1, BRCA2*
Hereditary nonpolyposis colorectal cancer	*MLH1, MSH2, MSH6, PMS1, PMS2*
Multiple endocrine neoplasia	*MEN 1, MEN 2A/B*
Li-Fraumeni syndrome	*TP53*
Retinoblastoma	*RB1*

Genetic Screening Methods Used in Cancer Pharmacogenomics

The base sequence of DNA refers to the consecutive order of guanine (G), adenine (A), thymine (T), and cytosine (C) bases, which defines DNA as the genetic code. Under ideal conditions, the complete DNA sequence for each person would be available for pharmacogenomic studies as this is the most comprehensive information for assessing polymorphic variants. For example, DNA sequence information allows the assessment of all forms of genetic variants including SNPs, indels, and CNVs. Thus, for pharmacogenomic studies, DNA sequence information would be utilized as it necessarily contains all genetic contributors relevant for assessing pharmacogenomic endpoints. However, the technological complexity, time, and cost of a comprehensive sequencing of each patient's DNA are currently prohibitive for routine clinical performance. Thus, the less comprehensive, but technically more feasible use of microarray-based nucleic acid analysis is rapidly becoming the standard of practice.

Because microarray-based technologies are advancing for nucleic acid analysis in the clinical setting, a basic understanding of the use of these methods is desirable. Different types of microarrays are available for the analyses of nucleic acids. These technologies can be used to analyze either DNA or mRNA. DNA microarray technology relies on the hybridization of complementary pieces of DNA present in relatively short stretches of DNA (e.g., approximately 25 base pairs = oligonucleotide). Over this stretch of DNA sequence, hybridization can be optimized so that only regions of DNA that match perfectly will hybridize. It is this precise hybridization of complementary segments of nucleic acids present as part of the microarray system with DNA or mRNA derived from a patient sample that forms the basis of microarray analysis. Thousands to hundreds of thousands of different oligonucleotides representing different genetic variants can be assayed in a single microarray run. Microarrays may also be used to determine cellular levels of mRNA being expressed, which is referred to as gene expression profiling.

Gene Expression Profiling

Gene expression profiling is used to assess the aberrant expression of genes associated with a person's cancer. Determination of mRNA expression in cancers is an increasingly important means of profiling cancers and can be effective in identifying subgroups of cancers. For the microarray analysis of mRNA, samples are typically required from both normal and diseased tissue. This allows the identification of mRNA expression differences that facilitate an understanding of abnormal mRNA expression occurring in cancer cells. This information may guide an understanding of the pathological basis of the disease as well as facilitate the identification of novel therapeutic targets. The ability to use gene expression profiling to optimize cancer therapy, in part, distinguishes cancer pharmacogenomics from pharmacogenomics applied to many other disease states. The profiling of genes abnormally expressed in breast cancer is a key example of the clinical use of gene expression profiling.

The Oncotype DX assay can be performed to help determine therapeutic strategies for breast cancer. This assay is a gene expression-based test of 21 genes that are used to quantify the likelihood of breast cancer recurrence in women with early stage disease. The genes analyzed include 16 breast cancer-related genes (e.g., *Her2/neu*, *estrogen receptor*, *progesterone receptor*) and five reference genes.[55] Currently, this test is recommended for women with node-negative, estrogen-receptor positive invasive breast cancer and post-menopausal women with node-positive, hormone-receptor positive invasive breast cancer. Results from the assay are provided in the form of a recurrence score. From clinical studies performed using the Oncotype DX assay it was determined that, "The likelihood of distant recurrence at 10 years increases continuously with an increase in the assay recurrence score result." These results can be used to make more informed treatment decisions based on pharmacogenomic information.

Clinical Pearl

Breast cancer samples used for the Oncotype DX Breast Cancer Assay are provided as paraffin blocks derived from histological samples. A multigene expression assay is performed resulting in the assignment of a recurrence score. A key question addressed is whether or not chemotherapy in addition to tamoxifen treatment may be beneficial. The likelihood of distant recurrence at 10 years increases with the recurrence score value. A 6.8% rate of distant recurrence at 10 years is associated with a recurrence score less than 18, suggesting these patients derive minimal benefit from additional chemotherapy. In contrast, a 30.5% rate is associated with a score of greater than or equal to 31, where substantial benefit may be gained from additional chemotherapy.

Gene expression profiling is also being used to estimate the response of patients to therapy. For example, these methods are being developed to assess the characteristics and to optimize the treatment of hematological malignancies.[56] To date, treatments for leukemia are largely based on genotypic characteristics of the leukemic blast, clinical features of the patient, and the initial therapeutic response.[57] In one example, a study was carried out to assess the utility of gene expression profiling to identify at initial diagnosis children that may have a poor therapeutic response.[58] It was concluded that altered expression of early blast regression genes may be helpful in identifying patients that may be at risk for inferior responses to treatment.[58] Examples from breast cancer and acute leukemia illustrate the increasing utility of gene expression profiling in cancer pharmacogenomics to improve cancer therapy.

Screening for Genetic Variation in Cancer Susceptibility and Drug Response

Microarrays can be used to determine inherited genetic variations in a person's DNA (e.g., DNA obtained from a cheek swab). Such an analysis could be performed to assess the many variants as described in the section on pharmacogenomics of cancer chemotherapeutic agents. The majority of these microarray assays examine the presence of known SNPs. Alternatively, DNA from a tumor sample can be analyzed by microarrays to determine mutations that have arisen in a specific cancer. In fact, genome-wide profiling may be used to identify genetic changes in specific types of cancer to determine consistency of genetic changes in these cancers. For example, using microarray-based techniques to exam genetic alterations in ALL, genetic changes in key cellular pathways, including lymphoid differentiation, cell cycle regulation, and drug responsiveness have been identified.[59] The analysis of variations in DNA may greatly facilitate the identification of strategies to individualize cancer therapy. Key examples include the treatment of breast cancers over-expressing an amplified *Her-2/neu* gene.[35] A genotyping panel for assessing response to cancer chemotherapy is in clinical trials.[60] An advantage of microarray analyses of DNA is the ability to analyze may thousands of genetic changes from a single sample.

Genome-Wide Association Studies (GWAS)

Genome-wide association studies (GWAS) are performed to comprehensively examine genetic variations present in DNA (i.e., a person's whole genome) among individuals with an identifiable condition, such as a specific response to drug treatment. GWAS are performed using high-resolution, microarray-based DNA screening technologies, most commonly analyzing for known SNPs (i.e., SNPs identified in previous studies of genetic variants). Using GWAS, significant progress is being made in the identification of genes associated with adverse drug reactions.[61] As long as groups of individuals with a specific phenotype can be identified, such as an adverse response to a drug, GWAS can be performed to assess the genetic variants that may be shared among a specific group.[61]

GWAS are a hypothesis generating means of determining genetic variants that may have an impact on cancer therapy. Such a study does not *a priori* assume that a particular gene or genes is associated with individual drug response, as is true for a candidate gene study (i.e., those studies where specific genes are picked for variant analyses based on an understanding of the disease state and genes associated with the drug's actions). Thus, the gene or genes identified that may be associated with the identified genetic variant(s) in a GWAS may be unexpected and often require further examination to determine how these variants relate to the drug's action.

Summary

Cancer pharmacogenomics includes both distinct and traditional elements of pharmacogenomics. From a traditional standpoint, polymorphic variants are known that affect both pharmacokinetic and pharmacodynamic aspects of pharmacogenomics in cancer chemotherapy. Unique to cancer pharmacogenomics is the determination of specific mutations associated with an individual's cancer. In addition, through the use of gene expression analyses, characteristics of each independent cancer can be determined, which will allow for highly personalized cancer therapeutics. An emerging area of cancer pharmacogenomics is the identification of genetic variants associated with cancer development that may be modulated by chemopreventive agents. These agents hold strong potential as preventive measures for specific cancers. The field of chemoprevention is poised to become a major component of pharmacy practice. These unique areas of pharmacogenomics combine with traditional pharmacogenomics to illustrate the enormous potential of cancer pharmacogenomics in pharmacy practice.

Acknowledgments

The author is grateful for the insightful advice provided by Drs. Mark Holdsworth, Pharm.D., Debra MacKenzie, Ph.D., and Ian Rabinowitz, MD in the preparation of this chapter.

References

1. Rodriguez-Antona C, Ingelman-Sundberg M. Cytochrome P450 pharmacogenetics and cancer. *Oncogene*. 2006;25:1679-1691.
2. Cascorbi I. Pharmacogenetics of cytochrome P4502D6: genetic background and clinical implications. *Eur J Clin Invest*. 2003;33S2:17-22.
3. Marsh S. Thymidylate synthase pharmacogenetics. *Invest New Drugs*. 2005;23:533-537.
4. Krajinovic M, Costea I, Chiasson S. Polymorphism of the thymidylate synthase gene and outcome of acute lymphoblastic leukemia. *Lancet*. 2002;359:1033-1034.
5. Lepper ER, Nooter K, Verweij J, et al. Mechanisms of resistance to anticancer drugs: the role of the polymorphic ABC transporters ABCB1 and ABCG2. *Pharmacogenomics*. 2005;6:115-138.
6. Hardwick LJ, Velamakanni S, van Veen HW. The emerging pharmacotherapeutic significance of the breast cancer resistance protein (ABCG2). *Br J Pharmacol*. 2007;151:163-174.
7. Zhou SF. Structure, function, and regulation of P-glycoprotein and its clinical relevance in drug disposition. *Xenobiotica*. 2008;38:802-832.

8. Hoffmeyer S, Burk O, von Richter O, et al. Functional polymorphisms of the human multidrug resistance gene: multiple sequence variations and correlation of one allele with P-glycoprotein expression and activity in vivo. *Proc Natl Acad Sci, USA.* 2000;97:3473-3478.

9. Zhou S. Clinical pharmacogenomics of thiopurine S-methyltransferase. *Curr Clin Pharmacol.* 2006;1:119-128.

10. Eichelbaum M, Ingelman-Sundberg M, et al. Pharmacogenomics and individualized drug therapy. *Annu Rev Med.* 2006;57:119-137.

11. Nief N, Le Morvan V, Robert J. Involvement of gene polymorphisms of thymidylate synthase in gene expression, protein activity, and anticancer drug cytotoxicity using the NCI-60 panel. *Eur J Cancer.* 2007;43:955-962.

12. Showalter SL, Showalter TN, Witkiewicz A, et al. Evaluating the drug-target relationship between thymidylate synthase expression and tumor response to 5-fluorouracil. Is it time to move forward? *Cancer Biol Ther.* 2008;7:986-994.

13. Van Kuilenburg AB, Meinsma R, Zoetekouw L, et al. High prevalence of the IVS14+1G>A mutation in the dihydropyrimidine dehydrogenase gene of patients with severe 5-fluorouracil-associated toxicity. *Pharmacogenetics.* 2002;12:555-558.

14. Sugiyama E, Kaniwa N, Kim S-R, et al. Pharmacokinetics of gemcitabine in Japanese cancer patients: the impact of a cytidine deaminase polymorphism. *J Clin Oncol.* 2007;25:32-42.

15. Ueno H, Kaniwa N, Okusaka T, et al. Homozygous CDA*3 is a major cause of life-threatening toxicities in gemcitibine-treated Japanese cancer patients. *Br J Cancer.* 2009;100:870-873.

16. Blakley RL, Sorrentino BP. In vitro mutations in dihydrofolate reductase that confer resistance to methotrexate: potential for clinical application. *Hum Mutat.* 1998;11:259-263.

17. Singer MJ, Mesner LD, Friedman CL, et al. Amplification of the human dihydrofolate reductase gene via double minutes is initiated by chromosome breaks. *Proc Nat Acad Sci, USA.* 2000;97:7921-7926.

18. Banerjee D, Mayer-Kuchuk P, Capiaux G, et al. Novel aspects of resistance to drugs targeted to dihydrofolate reductase and thymidylate synthase. *Biochim Biophys Acta.* 2002;1587:164-173.

19. Iyer L, King CD, Whitington PF, et al. Genetic predisposition to the metabolism of irinotecan (CPT-11). Role of uridine diphosphate glucuronosyltransferase isoform 1A1 in the glucuronidation of its active metabolite (SN-38) in human liver microsomes. *J Clin Invest.* 1998;101:847-854.

20. Bosma PJ, Chowdhury JR, Bakker C, et al. The genetic basis of the reduced expression of bilirubin UDP-glucuronosyltransferase 1 in Gilbert's syndrome. *N Engl J Med.* 1995;333:1171-1175.

21. Strassburg CP. Pharmacogenetics of Gilbert's syndrome. *Pharmacogenomics.* 2008;9:703-715.

22. Swaby RF, Sharma CGN, Jordan VC. SERMs for the treatment and prevention of breast cancer. *Rev Endocr Metab Disord.* 2007;8:229-239.

23. Goetz MP, Kamal A, Ames MM. Tamoxifen pharmacogenomics: the role of CYP2D6 as a predictor of drug response. *Clin Pharmacol Ther.* 2008;83:160-166.

24. Dezentje VO, Guchelaar H-J, Nortier JWR, et al. Clinical implications of CYP2D6 genotyping in tamoxifen treatment for breast cancer. *Clin Cancer Res* 2009;15:15-21.

25. Engels FK, Ten Tije AJ, Baker SD, et al. Effect of cytochrome P450 3A4 inhibition on the pharmacokinetics of docetaxel. *Clin Pharmacol Ther.* 2004;75:448-454.

26. Mielke S. Individualized pharmacotherapy with paclitaxel. *Curr Opin Oncol.* 2007;19:586-589.

27. Foulkes WD. Inherited susceptibility to common cancers. *New Engl J Med.* 2008;359:2143-2153.

28. Ulrich CM, Bigler J, Potter JD. Non-steroidal anti-inflammatory drugs for cancer prevention: promise, perils, and pharmacogenetics. *Nat Rev Cancer.* 2006;6:130-140.

29. Jemal A, Siegel R, Ward E, et al. Cancer statistics, 2008. *CA Cancer J Clin.* 2008;58:71-96.

30. Chan AT, Giovannucci EL, Meyerhardt JA, et al. Aspirin dose and duration of use and risk of colorectal cancer in men. *Gastroenterology.* 2008;134:21-28.

31. Cross IT, Poole EM, Ulrich CM. A review of gene-drug interactions for nonsteroidal anti-inflammatory drug use in preventing colorectal neoplasia. *Pharmacogenomics J.* 2008;8:237-247.

32. Sinicrope FA, Gill S. Role of cyclooxygenase-2 in colorectal cancer. *Cancer Metastasis Rev.* 2004;23:63-75.

33. Metcalfe K, Lynch HT, Ghadirian P, et al. Contralateral breast cancer in BRCA1 and BRCA2 mutation carriers. *J Clin Oncol.* 2004;22:2328-2335.

34. Tsao AS, Kim ES, Hong WK. Chemoprevention of cancer. *CA Cancer J Clin.* 2004;54:150-180.

35. Pegram MD, Konecny G, Slamon DJ. The molecular and cellular biology of HER2/neu gene amplification/overexpression and the clinical development of herceptin (trastuzumab) therapy for breast cancer. *Cancer Treat Res.* 2000;103:57-75.

36. Druker BJ. Perspectives on the development of a molecularly targeted agent. *Cancer Cell.* 2002;1:31-36.

37. Ansari M, Krajinovic M. Pharmacogenomics in cancer treatment defining genetic bases for interindividual differences in responses to chemotherapy. *Curr Opin Pediatr.* 2007;19:15-22.59.

38. Cunningham L, Aplenc R. Pharmacogenetics of acute lymphoblastic leukemia treatment response. *Exper Opin Pharmacother.* 2007;8:2519-2531.

39. Rubnitz JE, Gibson B, Smith FO. Acute myeloid leukemia. *Pediatr Clin North Am.* 2008;55:21-51.

40. Small D. Targeting FLT3 for treatment of leukemia. *Semin Hematol.* 2008;45:S17-S21.

41. Wang ZY, Chen Z. Acute promyelocytic leukemia: from highly fatal to highly curable. *Blood.* 2008;111:2505-2515.

42. Quere R, Baudet A, Cassinat B, et al. Pharmacogenomic analysis of acute promyelocytic leukemia cells highlights CYP26 cytochrome metabolism in differential all-trans retinoic acid sensitivity. *Blood.* 2007;109:4450-4460.

43. Lengfelder E, Saussele S, Weisser A, et al. Treatment concepts of acute promyelocytic leukemia. *Crit Rev Oncol Hematol.* 2005;56:261-274.

44. Döhner H, Stilgenbauer S, Benner A, et al. Genomic aberrations and survival in chronic lymphocytic leukemia. *N Engl J Med.* 2000:343;1910-1916.

45. Druker BJ, Lydon NB. Lessons learned from the development of an abl tyrosine kinase inhibitor for chronic myelogenous leukemia. *J Clin Invest.* 2000;105:3-7.

46. Eck MJ, Manley PW. The interplay of structural information and functional studies in kinase drug design: insights from BCR-ABL. *Curr Opin Cell Biol.* 2009;21:288-295.

47. Kemp CJ. Multistep skin cancer in mice as a model to study the evolution of cancer cells. *Semin Cancer Biol.* 2005;15:460-473.

48. Olopade OI, Grushko TA, Nanda R, et al. Advances in breast cancer: pathways to personalized medicine. *Clin Cancer Res.* 2008;14:7988-7999.

49. Narod SA, Brunet JS, Ghadirian P, et al. Tamoxifen and risk of contralateral breast cancer in BRCA1 and BRCA2 mutation carriers: a case-control study. Hereditary Breast Cancer Clinical Study Group. *Lancet.* 2000;356:1876-1881.

50. Rubenstein W. Hereditary breast cancer in Jews. *Familial Cancer.* 2004;3:249-257.

51. Kinzler KW, Vogelstein B. Lessons from hereditary colorectal cancer. *Cell* 1996;87:159-170.

52. Balko JM, Black EP. A gene expression predictor of response to EGFR-targeted therapy stratifies progression-free survival to cetuximab in KRAS wild-type metastatic colorectal cancer. *BMC Cancer.* 2009;9:145.

53. Lievre A, Bachet J-B, Boige V, et al. KRAS mutations as an independent prognostic factor in patients with advanced colorectal cancer treated with cetuximab. *J Clin Oncol.* 2008;26:374-379.

54. Shah RB, Chinnaiyan AM. The discovery of common recurrent transmembrane protease serine 2(TMPRSS2)-erythroblastosis virus E26 transforming sequence (ETS) gene fusions in prostate cancer: significance and clinical implications. *Adv Anat Pathol.* 2009;16:145-153.

55. Paik S, Tang G, Shak S, et al. Gene expression and benefit of chemotherapy in women with node-negative, estrogen receptor-positive breast cancer. *J Clin Oncol.* 2006;24:3726-3734.

56. Bacher U, Kohlmann A, Haferlach T. Perspectives of gene expression profiling for diagnosis and therapy in haematological malignancies. *Brief Funct Genomic Proteomic.* 2009;8:184-193.

57. Bhojwani, Moskowitz N, Raetz EA, Carroll WL. Potential of gene expression profiling in the management of childhood acute lymphoblastic leukemia. *Pediatric Drugs.* 2007;9:149-156.

58. Bhojwani D, Kang H, Menezes RX, et al. Gene expression signatures predictive of early response and outcome in high risk childhood acute lymphoblastic leukemia: a Children's Oncology Group Study. *J Clin Oncol.* 2008;26:4376-4384.

59. Mullighan CG, Dowing JR. Genome-wide profiling of genetic alterations in acute lymphoblastic leukemia: recent insights and future directions. *Leukemia.* 2009;23:1209-1218.

60. Dai Z, Papp AC, Wang D, et al. Genotyping panel for assessing response to cancer chemotherapy. *BMC Med Genomics.* 2008;1:24.

61. Nelson MR, Bacanu S-A, Li L, et al. Genome-wide approaches to identify pharmacogenetic contributions to adverse drug reactions. *Pharmacogenomics J.* 2009;9:23-33.

Chapter 9

Central Nervous System

Megan Jo Ehret, Pharm.D., BCPP

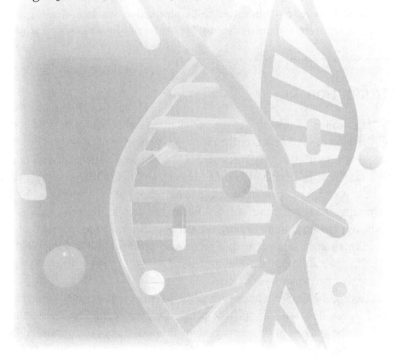

Learning Objectives

After completing this chapter, the reader should be able to

- Describe the utility of pharmacogenomics in the treatment of various psychiatric disorders including: major depressive disorder, schizophrenia, bipolar disorder, and attention deficit hyperactivity disorder.
- Describe the utility of pharmacogenomics in the treatment of various neurological disorders including: multiple sclerosis, migraine, Alzheimer's disease, Parkinson's disease, pain, and epilepsy.
- Discuss potential barriers to the use of pharmacogenomics in the treatment of psychiatric and neurological disorders.

Key Definitions

Response—Treatment of depression that results in at least 50% improvement in symptoms.

Remission—Treatment of depression that results in removal of essentially all symptoms.

Typical antipsychotic—First generation antipsychotics, primary pharmacological property of dopamine 2 antagonism, this is responsible for their antipsychotic efficacy but also for many of their side effects.

Atypical antipsychotic—Second generation antipsychotics, primary pharmacological property is coupling of dopamine 2 antagonism with serotonin 2A antagonism.

Opioids—Compounds, both natural and synthetic that have morphine-like actions, that are mu-opioid receptor agonists used for the treatment of mild to severe, acute, and chronic pain.

Introduction

The human brain is one of the body's most complex organs. This complexity makes the treatment of disorders of the central nervous system (CNS) very challenging. A patient's response to the many medications used to treat various disorders of the brain can be highly variable. The Human Genome Project identified >30,000 genes that are polymorphic, and the expression of many of these gene's have been found to occur in the brain or play a role in enhancing the brain's function.[1,2] Although research in the area of CNS disorders is growing quickly, our understanding of why certain populations either respond or do not respond or experience an adverse effect with a given medication is still lacking. Pharmacogenomics can potentially play an important role in determining the genetic differences that alter a patient's response to a particular medication.

Currently, the CNS is a highly researched system with regards to medication response, adverse drug reactions, and genetic risk factors. Diseases of the CNS are the third largest area with regards to the amount of pharmacogenomic information in the published literature.[3] Approximately 15 package inserts for psychotropic medications currently contain pharmacogenomic-prescribing information.[4] Given the importance of predicting drug response and adverse drug reactions, the applications of pharmacogenomics in CNS therapeutics will likely continue to grow.

Case Study—Bipolar Disorder, Most Recent Episode Depression

CT is a 40-year-old male who is experiencing his second episode of bipolar disorder. He presents with a lack of energy and loss of hope for the future. He feels that he is worthless to society and would like to hurt himself. He complains of a loss of appetite, decreased concentration, an inability to sleep, and a lack of motivation. He has had one previous hospitalization for mania where he was prescribed lithium and risperidone. He felt that the medication never truly helped him.

Questions:

1. What genes or drug targets are currently being researched for drug response in bipolar disorder in regards to mood stabilizers?

2. Discuss the current literature regarding the association of treatment response with risperidone and known genetic differences.
3. How can pharmacogenomics affect a patient's response to antidepressants?

Psychiatric Disorders

Major Depressive Disorder

According to the National Comorbidity Survey Replication, 16.2% of the population studied had a history of major depressive disorder, and only 65% to 70% of patients with this diagnosis improved with drug therapy.[5] In double-blind efficacy trials, initial treatment with antidepressants appears to lead to remission in only 35% to 47% of patients.[6,7] A meta-analysis of 315 studies compared the efficacy of the tri-cyclic antidepressants (TCAs) to the selective serotonin reuptake inhibitors (SSRIs) and found similar response rates in the treatment of depression and dysthymia.[8] With the discovery of the newer antidepressants, higher response and remission rates may be expected.

The mechanism of action of the antidepressants varies by class, but most increase the neurotransmitters norepinephrine (NE) and serotonin (5HT). See Table 9-1 for detailed information regarding mechanism of action of the various antidepressant medications.[9] All of these pathways can be sources of genetic variability in a patient's response to the antidepressants.

Table 9-1
Mechanism of Action of Antidepressant Medications[9]

Medication	Mechanism of Action
Monoamine Oxidase Inhibitors Phenelzine (Nardil®) Selegiline (Emsam®) Tranylcypromine (Parnate®)	Increases endogenous concentrations of norepinephrine, dopamine, and serotonin by inhibition of monoamine oxidase, which is the enzyme responsible for their breakdown
Tricyclics Amitriptyline (Elavil®) Amoxapine (Asendin®) Clomipramine (Anafranil®) Desipramine (Norpramin®) Doxepin (Sinequan®) Imipramine (Tofranil®) Maprotiline (Ludiomil®) Nortriptyline (Pamelor®) Protriptyline (Vivactil®) Trimipramine (Surmontil®)	Increases the synaptic concentration of serotonin and norepinephrine by inhibition of their reuptake by the presynaptic neuronal membrane

Continued on next page

Table 9-1 *(Continued)*

Medication	Mechanism of Action
Selective Serotonin Reuptake Inhibitors Citalopram (Celexa®) Escitalopram (Lexapro®) Paroxetine (Paxil®) Fluoxetine (Prozac®) Fluvoxamine (Luvox®) Sertraline (Zoloft®)	Inhibits the reuptake of serotonin in the presynaptic neurons
Serotonin Norepinephrine Reuptake Inhibitors Desvenlafaxine (Pristiq®) Duloxetine (Cymbalta®) Venlafaxine (Effexor®)	Potently inhibits neuronal reuptake of serotonin and norepinephrine; weakly inhibits dopamine reuptake
Bupropion (Wellbutrin®)	Weakly inhibits the neuronal uptake of norepinephrine and dopamine
Nefazodone (Serzone®)	Inhibits neuronal reuptake of serotonin and norepinephrine; blocks 5HT2 and alpha1 receptors
Trazodone (Desyrel®)	Inhibits the reuptake of serotonin; causes adrenoreceptor subsensitivity; induces significant changes in 5HT presynaptic receptor adrenoreceptors
Mirtazapine (Remeron®)	Increases release of serotonin and norepinephrine by antagonizing central presynaptic alpha2-adrenergic receptors; potently antagonizing the 5HT2 and 5HT3 receptors; antagonizes the H1 histamine and moderately antagonizes the peripheral alpha1-adrenergic and muscarinic receptors

One of the most studied genes affecting the treatment of depression is the serotonin transporter gene (SLC6A4), which is located on chromosome 17q.[10,11] SLC6A4 is a protein structure made up of 12 transmembrane helices with an extracellular loop between helices three and four. This transporter is responsible for the reuptake of 5HT into the presynaptic neurons.

A well-characterized variant of this gene is a functional polymorphism located in the 5' promoter region, 5HT transporter gene-linked polymorphic region (5-HTTLPR).[12,13] The polymorphism consists of a repetitive region containing 16 imperfect repeat units of 22 base pairs (bp) located ~1,000bp upstream of the transcriptional start site. It is polymorphic because of an insertion/deletion of units six-eight, which produces a short (s) allele that is 44bp shorter than the long (l) allele.[12,13] Although originally thought to be bi-allelic, very long and extra-long alleles have been identified in a small percentage of Japanese and African Americans (<<5%).[14]

More than 20 studies have investigated this particular polymorphism with regards to antidepressant treatment. SSRIs have been the focus for the majority of these studies. In all of the Caucasian studies of unipolar or bipolar depressed patients, at least nominally significant associations could be found between the long variant and antidepressant response.[15-25] This was different with an Asian population, in which several studies found an association with the s-allele and better outcomes with SSRI antidepressants.[26-32] The s-allele is present in 50% of Caucasians and 75% of Asians.[14] This ultimately leads to very few Asians who would present with a homozygous l-allele, a finding that could explain the difference in associations with response and 5-HTTLPR. Larger population based studies need to be completed to determine the role of this polymorphic gene and the response to antidepressants.

Clinical Pearl

The serotonin transporter gene is an important and highly studied gene in terms of antidepressant response. Statistically significant associations have been found between variations in this gene and antidepressant response. Currently, point of care testing is not being completed for this polymorphism.

Additional polymorphisms within the SLC6A4 gene could also account for some of the variation in drug response that is observed. An association of a single nucleotide polymorphism (SNP), rs25531, which is located upstream of the 5-HTTLPR, has been reported with response to fluoxetine treatment.[24] It has been proposed that rs25531 and 5-HTTLPR are in linkage disequilibrium with each other (r^2=0.75).[24] In the presence of the G-allele of rs25531, the l-allele of 5-HTTLPR seems to be associated with reduced drug response. Likewise in the presence of the A-allele of rs25531, the s-allele of the 5-HTTLPR seems to be associated with reduced drug response.[24] The influences of this and other SNPS in the serotonin transporter protein gene need to be considered when utilizing this information to determine drug response.

Polymorphisms in the genes that code for the various serotonin receptors have also been studied with regards to their role in altering the efficacy of various antidepressants. The 5-HT 1A receptor has one SNP located in the promoter region, C-1019G, which has shown a trend association between the G allele and various antidepressant response (p=0.049).[33] An additional study did demonstrate a combined effect when measuring the C-1019G SNP with a variation on the SLC6A4 (5-HTTLPR) gene in 130 patients treated with an SSRI over 12 weeks. It was determined that patients with the "risk genotype" (s/s-G/G) were more likely to not achieve remission (p=0.009).[34] The SNP within the 5-HT 2A receptor gene, rs7997910, demonstrated an 18% absolute risk of having no response to treatment compared to those homozygous for the other allele in a study of 1,953 patients treated with citalopram. The A allele of rs7997910 was six times more frequent in white than black participants, with treatment being less effective in the black participants.[35] Although additional studies regarding other serotonin receptors have been completed, they failed to demonstrate an association between genetic variation and the effectiveness of antidepressants.[36]

Additional areas of interest, which have been studied to a lesser extent to determine an association between efficacy and the antidepressants, include the g-protein coupled receptors, tryptophan hydroxylase I, monoamine oxidase, dopamine receptor genes, noradrenergic receptor gene, nitric oxide, angiotensin-converting enzyme, interleukin-1 beta, stress hormone system, and phosphodiesterase. Information on each of these genes can be found in Table 9-2. Routine use of these polymorphic genes in practice will require larger studies to be completed.

Table 9-2
Pharmacogenomic Studies of Various Antidepressants in Unipolar Depression

Polymorphism	Number of Patients Studied	Medication	Association with Response
G-protein coupled receptor C825T			
	N=169 (ref. 21)	Fluoxetine or nortriptyline	None
	N=106 (ref. 37)	Various antidepressants	T-allele reduced response to nortriptyline only (p<0.05)
Tryptophan Hydroxylase A218C			
	N=121 (ref. 38)	Paroxetine	C-allele associated with response (p=0.001)
	N=66 (ref. 39)	Fluvoxamine	None
	N=96 (ref. 40)	Fluoxetine	C-allele associated with response (p<0.05)
Monoamine Oxidase A VNTR			
	N=64 (ref. 39)	Moclobemide	None
	N=66 (ref. 41)	Fluvoxamine	None
Dopamine 2 receptor S311C			
	N=364 (ref. 42)	Fluvoxamine or paroxetine	None

Continued on next page

Table 9–2 *(Continued)*

Polymorphism	Number of Patients Studied	Medication	Association with Response
Dopamine 4 receptor VNTR			
	N=364 (ref. 42)	Fluvoxamine or paroxetine	None
Noradrenergic G1165C			
	N=259 (ref. 43)	Various antidepressants	C-allele associated with improved response (p=0.05)
Norepinephrine G1287A			
	N=96 (ref. 44)	Milnacipran	T-allele associated with response (p=0.03)
	N=241 (ref. 45)	Nortriptyline	G-allele associated with response (p<0.001)
Nitric Oxide C267T			
	N=114 (ref. 46)	Fluoxetine	None
Angiotensin-converting enzyme insertion/ deletion			
	N=99 (ref. 47)	Various antidepressants	D-allele associated with response (p<0.0001)
	N=313 (ref. 48)	Various antidepressants	None
	N=100 (ref. 49)	Venlafaxine or fluoxetine	None
Interleukin 1 Beta -511C/T			
	N=157 (ref. 50)	Fluoxetine	T-allele trended for an association with response (p=0.05)

Continued on next page

Table 9-2 (*Continued*)

Polymorphism	Number of Patients Studied	Medication	Association with Response
Stress Hormone System CRHR1			
	N=80 (ref. 51)	Desipramine or fluoxetine	GAG haplotype associated with response (p=0.03)
Glucocorticoid Receptor			
	N=367 (ref. 52)	Various antidepressants	ER22/EK23 genotype associated with response (p=0.008)
Phosphodiesterase			
	N=284 (ref. 53)	Desipramine or fluoxetine	Response associated with the rs1549870 in PDE1A (p=0.005) and rs18880916 in PDE11A (p=0.04)
		Fluoxetine	Response associated with rs2544934 in PDE6A (p=0.03), rs884162 in PDE8B (p=0.02), and rs3770018 in PDE11A (p=0.007)

To help determine the utility of the plethora of information evolving with antidepressant responsiveness and pharmacokinetic pharmacogenomics, a review was undertaken by the Evaluation of Genomic Applications in Practice and Prevention (EGAPP) Working Group to investigate the evidence for genetic testing for CYP450 polymorphisms in the management of patients with nonpsychotic depression treated with SSRIs.[54] The group determined that there was a paucity of evidence regarding the use of CYP450 genotyping as a guide to the management of SSRIs for patients with nonpsychotic depression. No prospective studies of CYP450 genotyping, to guide treatment and measure subsequent clinical outcomes, have been completed. The investigators concluded that there is a lack of sufficient evidence for incorporation of any of the CYP450 genotyping tests into guidelines for clinical practice. Realizing that CYP450 genotyping may only be one of several genetic variants affecting response to antidepressant treatment, the group recommended that more research is needed in this area combining pharmacokinetics and pharmacodynamics. The investigators called for extreme caution in interpreting any CYP genotyping results until prospective evidence-based research provides data to prove an unequivocal association between variations in CYP450 genotypes and SSRI treatment outcomes in the treatment of major depressive disorder.[55] Additional studies have also shown similar results to the finding of the EGAPP group.[56]

Clinical Pearl

The utility of CYP450 genotyping in the treatment of depression is currently undergoing further evaluation.

Schizophrenia

The Epidemiologic Catchment Area Study estimated that 0.6% to 1.9% of the population suffers from schizophrenia.[57] Efficacy studies have demonstrated a response rate to antipsychotics of 60-70% for patients with schizophrenia, although the Clinical Antipsychotic Trials of Intervention Effectiveness (CATIE) demonstrated a much poorer clinical outcome with the atypical antipsychotics when they were used in general clinical practice.[58,59] Given these statistics, researchers have focused on investigating the various genetic components to the response to these medications. Pharmacogenomic studies have focused on atypical antipsychotic agents with emphasis on identifying candidate genes coding for receptors or metabolizing enzymes that have been identified in preclinical and clinical studies. Recent pharmacogenomic studies have also investigated neurotransmitter disposition, second messenger systems, and peripheral neurotransmitters.[60]

The primary treatment model for schizophrenia is the antipsychotics, although there is considerable variation in the treatment response with these medications.[61] The typical antipsychotics work by blockade of the dopamine 2 (D2) receptors, while the atypical antipsychotics are also antagonists at 5-HT2A and 2C receptors in addition to D2 receptors.[62,63] Many researchers have studied the D2, 5-HT2A and 2C receptors in hopes of finding an association with antipsychotic efficacy. These studies have utilized various ethnic races, medications, and definitions of response. Table 9-3 summarizes the various studies, which have been completed in efforts to determine genetic differences in relationship to antipsychotic efficacy.

Table 9–3
Pharmacogenomic Studies of Response in Schizophrenia

Target	Polymorphism	Number of Patients Race or Ethnicity	Medication	Association with Response
Serotonin 1A (ref. 64)	C-1019G	68 German-Caucasian	Risperidone, haloperidol	C-allele associated with improvement in negative symptoms
Serotonin 2A (ref. 65)	102T/C	99 Chinese	Clozapine	102C associated with poor response
(ref. 66)	102T/C, His452Try	733 Caucasian	Clozapine	102C associated with poor response

Continued on next page

Table 9-3 (*Continued*)

Target	Polymorphism	Number of Patients Race or Ethnicity	Medication	Association with Response
(ref. 67)	His452Try, 1438A/G, 102T/C	185 Mixed races	Clozapine	452His allele associated with improved response
(ref. 68)	1438A/G	42 Caucasian	Olanzapine	-1438A/A genotype associated with negative symptom improvement
(ref. 69)	102T/C, 1438G/A	63 Turkish	Risperidone	102 T/T and -1438 A/A genotypes associated with improvement
(ref. 70)	102T/C	100 Chinese	Risperidone	102 C/C genotype associated with improvement
(ref. 71)	102T/C, 516C/T, Thr25Asn, His45Tyr	42 Caucasian	Olanzapine	None
(ref. 72)	-1438G>A, 102 T>C, H452Y	73 Japanese	Risperidone	None
Serotonin 2C (ref. 67)	Cys23Ser	185 Mixed races	Clozapine	None
(ref. 71)	Cys23Ser	42 Caucasian	Olanzapine	None
(ref. 73)	759C/T	177 Chinese	Risperidone, clozapine	-759C associated with symptom improvement
Serotonin 6 (ref. 74)	C267T	99 Chinese	Clozapine	267 T/T genotype associated with better response
Brain derived neurotrophic factor (ref. 75)	Val66Met	93 Chinese	Clozapine	Val66Val genotype associated with clinical response
Catechol-o-methyltransferase (ref. 72)	Val158Met	73 Japanese	Risperidone	None

Continued on next page

Table 9-3 *(Continued)*

Target	Polymorphism	Number of Patients Race or Ethnicity	Medication	Association with Response
(ref. 76)	Val108/158Met	86 Mixed races	Clozapine	158Met allele associated with improvement
(ref. 77)	Val108/158Met	Not described	Olanzapine	158Met allele predicted working memory performance
Dopamine receptor 1 (ref. 78)	2,2 genotype	15 Mixed races	Clozapine	2,2 genotype associated with response
Dopamine receptor 2 (ref. 79)	-141C Ins/Del Taq 1 polymorphism	135 Chinese	Chlorpromazine	-141C Ins/Del: no Del greater improvement
(ref. 80)	Taq 1 polymorphism	57 Caucasian	Haloperidol	Heterozygous better improvement in positive symptoms
(ref. 72)	-141C Ins/Del Taq 1A	73 Japanese	Risperidone	DRD2 haplotype associated with improvement
(ref. 73)	Taq 1A	177 Chinese	Risperidone, clozapine	None
(ref. 81)	12 SNPs spanning the DRD2 gene	232 Mixed races	Clozapine	Taq 1A, Taq 1B, and rs1125394 haplotype associated with response
(ref. 82)	Ser311Cys	123 Chinese	Risperidone	311Cys allele associated with improvement
(ref. 83)	6 SNPs spanning the DRD2 gene	125 Chinese	Risperidone	-241A allele associated with improvement
(ref. 84)	A-241G, -141C ins/del	61 Mixed races	Risperidone, olanzapine	214G allele associated with faster response; -141C Del allele carriers had delayed response

Continued on next page

Table 9-3 (*Continued*)

Target	Polymorphism	Number of Patients Race or Ethnicity	Medication	Association with Response
Dopamine receptor 3 (ref. 73)	Ser9Gly	177 Chinese	Risperidone, clozapine	Ser9 associated with symptom improvement
(ref. 85)	Ser9Gly	32 Pakistani	Clozapine	9Gly allele associated with response
(ref. 86)	Ser9Gly	123 Chinese	Risperidone	9Ser allele associated with negative symptom improvement
(ref. 87)	5 SNPs scanning the DRD3 gene	130 Chinese	Risperidone	None
Dopamine receptor 4 (ref. 88)	VNTR in exon 3	81 Chinese	Clozapine	5 repeat allele of exon 3 associated with response
Norepinephrine transporter (ref. 89)	G1287A, T-182C	75 Caucasians	Olanzapine, risperidone	A1287 allele associated with improvement
G-protein beta 3 subunit (ref. 90)	C825T	145 Mixed races	Clozapine	825C/C genotype associated with clinical improvement
(ref. 91)		42 Caucasian	Olanzapine	None
Regulator of G-protein signaling 4 (ref. 92)	4 SNPs	120 Chinese	Risperidone	A/A genotype at rs10917670: greater improvement in social function A/A at rs2661319 associated with greater improvement
NMDA receptor subunit 2B (ref. 93)	Genetic variants	Chinese	Clozapine	2664 C/C genotype required higher doses for stabilization
Type 3 metabotropic glutamate receptor (ref. 94)	rs274622, rs724226, rs917071, rs1468412, rs1989796, and rs1476455	42 Caucasian	Olanzapine	Significant predicators of negative symptom improvement ($p<0.001$)

Continued on next page

Table 9-3 (*Continued*)

Target	Polymorphism	Number of Patients Race or Ethnicity	Medication	Association with Response
Multiple drug resistance gene (ref. 95)	C1236T, G2677TA, C3435T	42 Caucasian	Olanzapine	3453T carriers had greater response at higher olanzapine plasma levels
(ref. 96)		130 Chinese	Risperidone	1236T allele associated with improvement
Interleukin 1 receptor antagonist (ref. 97)	VNTR	154 Caucasians	Haloperidol, risperidone, olanzapine	IL-1Rn *2 had greater improvement
Synaptosomal associated protein of 25K Da gene (ref. 98)		59 Mixed races	Mixed	Mn/I polymorphism associated with clinical improvement
DAT (dopamine transporter) (ref. 99)	Ser8Gly, VNTR	75 Caucasians	Olanzapine, quetiapine, risperidone	DRD3 S/S genotype associated with response
(ref. 100)	6 SNPs	130 Chinese	Risperidone	None

Clinical Pearl

The D2 and 5HT-2A and 2C receptors are currently being investigated for an association between genetic variability and treatment response in schizophrenia.

A pharmacogenomic test for clozapine had previously been on the market but is currently undergoing redevelopment. The Pgxpredict: CLOZAPINE Test (Prediction of clozapine induced aganulocytosis) was developed by Genaissance Pharmaceuticals Inc. The test focused on two genes associated with clozapine-induced agranulocytosis. Three genes, which the company has yet to name publicly, may be examples of leads for future proof of mechanism studies to understand the pathophysiology of clozapine-induced agranulocytosis. The company has stopped offering the first generation of this test, but is continuing to focus their resources on developing a second-generation test. The first test may not have eliminated the need for blood monitoring in those with negative results, and patients with positive results may not have had options besides clozapine.[101]

Adverse Effects: Weight Gain, Tardive Dyskinesia

Antipsychotics can induce substantial weight gain causing diabetes, lipid abnormalities, and psychological distress.[102] Treatment emergent weight gain varies within the class of antipsychotics, with several agents causing severe weight gain and others limited weight gain. An individual's propensity to develop weight gain not only encompasses the medication he or she is taking, but also genetic factors.[102] Candidate genes that have demonstrated significant findings related to weight gain include the 5HT2C and adrenergic α2a (ADRα2a) receptor genes, as well as those for leptin and guanine nucleotide binding protein (GNB3).[102] Refer to Table 9-4 for information on studies regarding those genes.

Table 9-4
Significant Studies Regarding Weight Gain and Antipsychotics

Gene	Polymorphism	Population	Association	Response
CYP2D6 (ref. 103)	Allele *1, *3, *4	Caucasians	*3 and *4	Associated with weight gain (p=0.009)
Serotonin 2C (ref. 104)	–759C/T	Han Chinese	–759T allele	Less weight gain after 6 wk (p<0.0001) and after 10 wk (p=0.0003)
(ref. 105)	–759C/T	Caucasians and African Americans	–759T	Trend for men to gain more weight (p=0.047)
(ref. 106)	–759C/T	Han Chinese	–759T allele	Gained significantly less weight (p=0.02)
(ref. 107)	–759C/T	Spanish Caucasians	–759T	Less weight gain after 6 wk (p=0.003), 3 months (p=0.01), and 9 months (p=0.03)
(ref. 108)	759C/T	Caucasians	–759T	No carriers gained 10% or more compared with 40.7% of carriers with the C allele (p=0.003)
(ref. 109)	759C/T	Caucasians, African Americans, Hispanic	-759T allele	Experienced less BMI changes (p=0.002)

Continued on next page

Table 9-4 *(Continued)*

Gene	Polymorphism	Population	Association	Response
Alpha-adrenergic 2a (ref. 110)	−1291 C/G	Chinese	GG genotype	Significantly associated with increased weight gain (p=0.02); weight gain >7% significantly associated with G-alleles (p<0.01)
(ref. 111)	−1291 C/G	Koreans	GG genotypes and G-alleles	Significantly higher in subjects with severe weight gain >10% (p=0.03)
G-protein beta 3 subunit (ref. 112)	C825T	Chinese	T/T genotype	Experienced more weight gain (p=0.003)
Leptin (ref. 113)	−2548A/G	Han Chinese	Carriers of A/A genotype	Gained more weight (p=0.003)
(ref. 107)	−2548A/G	Spanish Caucasians	G/G genotype	Gained more weight after 9 months (p=0.03)
(ref. 114)	−2548A/G	Han Chinese	3 G/A genotypes	Increased BMI (p=0.039), strong effect on BMI gain in males (p=0.004), not females (P>0.05)
Dopamine receptor 4 (ref. 115)	VNTR	Caucasians	Homozygous for the shorter alleles	Increase in BMI was significantly less (p=0.003)

Genomas, a personalized medicine company, has developed a patented system called the PhyzioType system which is an ensemble of DNA markers from several genes coupled with a biostatistical algorithm to predict an individual's risk of developing adverse drug reactions (ADRs), including antipsychotic-induced metabolic syndrome.[116] The current prototype DNA microarray includes 384 SNPs from 222 genes representing insulin resistance, glucose metabolism, energy homeostasis, adiposity, apolipoproteins and receptors, fatty acids and cholesterol metabolism, lipases and receptors, cell signaling and transcriptional regulation, growth factors, drug metabolism, blood pressure, vascular signaling, endothelial dysfunction, coagulation and fibrinolysis, vascular inflammation, cytokines, various neurotransmitter systems, and behavior (satiety).[117] In addition to these genes, the system also uses biostatistical algorithms that are based on physiogenomics, the medical application of sensitivity analysis and systems engineering.[118]

Thus far, studies have demonstrated three associations using the PhzioType system. Patients taking olanzapine, quetiapine, or chlorpromazine were found to have the acetyl coenzyme A carboxylase a-SNP (rs4072032) in the hypertriglyceridemia model and a neuropeptide Y (rs1468271) and ACCb (rs2241220) polymorphism in the hypercholesterolemia model.[117,119] Larger population-based studies are needed to further determine the utility of this system in mainstream practice.

Tardive Dyskinesia

Tardive dyskinesia (TD) is a debilitating motor disorder, characterized by hyperkinetic involuntary, repetitive and purposeless movements predominantly of the orofacial region. The movements can include chewing, tongue protrusion, lip smacking, puckering, and pursing of the lips and rapid eye blinking. Choreoathetotic movements of the limb and trunk region have also been observed.[120] TD develops in 20% to 30% of chronic schizophrenic patients on long-term treatment with typical antipsychotic drugs.[121] Genetic factors (i.e., drug metabolizing enzymes, neurotransmitters, and oxidative stress pathway genes) and nongenetic factors (i.e., advanced age, presence of early extrapyramidal symptoms (EPS), female gender, African American ethnicity, organic brain dysfunction, smoking, and duration of exposure to typical antipsychotic drugs) are both thought to play a role in TD pathogenesis.[122]

Pharmacogenomic studies have determined the following candidate genes have polymorphisms significantly associated with the development of tardive dyskinesia: CYP2D6, CYP1A2, CYP17-α, DRD2, dopamine receptor 3 (DRD3), dopamine receptor 4 (DRD4), catechol-o-methyltransferase (COMT), 5-HT2A, 5-HT2C, opioid receptor, estrogen receptor α, manganese superoxide dismutase, glutathione-S-transferase M1, NAD (P) H dehydrogenase, quinone 1, and nitric oxide synthase 3.[123-136] These studies, like many similar pharmacogenomic studies, were carried out in a wide range of ethnic populations. However, associations of CYP2D6 (*10), CYP1A2 (*1F), DRD2 (rs1800497/Taq 1A) and DRD3 (Ser9Gly) with TD have been the most widely replicated. Table 9-5 provides a more detailed summary of these studies. Again, larger, more diverse studies need to be completed prior to the implementation of these tests in mainstream healthcare.

Table 9-5
Significant Studies Regarding Tardive Dyskinesia and Antipsychotics

Gene	Polymorphism	Population	Association	Response
CYP2D6 (ref. 137)	Alleles *3, *4, *10	Japanese	*10	Associated with total AIMS scores and with TD presence/absence
(ref. 138)	Allele *10	Chinese	*10/*10 genotype	Females significantly associated with TD (p=0.004)
(ref. 139)	Alleles *2, *3, *4, *10, *12	Japanese	*2 and *10	Associated with the development of EPS
(ref. 140)	C188T	Chinese	*10	Significant association in males (p=0.001)
CYP1A2 (ref. 141)	734C/A (CYP1A2 *1F), −163C>A	Caucasians and African American	C/C genotype	Associated with higher AIMS scores particularly in smokers (p=0.008)

Continued on next page

Table 9-5 (*Continued*)

Gene	Polymorphism	Population	Association	Response
(ref. 142)	*1F, *1C	North Indian	Carriers of the A allele of *1C	Increased severity (p=0.016)
Dopamine receptor 2 (ref. 124)	−141C Ins/Del, Taq1 B, Taq1 D, S311C, Taq1 A	Chinese	B2 homozygotes of Taq1 B and A2 homozygotes of Taq1 A confer predisposition	Protective haplotype combination
(ref. 125)	Meta-analysis of pooled data from 20 genetic studies of TD	Mixed	A2 variant of Taq1 A SNP	Associated with increased risk (p=0.026)
Dopamine receptor 3 (ref. 126)	Ser9Gly	Scottish	Gly/Gly	Susceptibility (p=0.02)
(ref. 123)	Ser9Gly	Jewish	Gly/-	Susceptibility (p=0.02)
(ref. 128)	Ser9Gly	Chinese	Gly/-	Predisposing genotype (p=0.009)
(ref. 129)	Ser9Gly	Korean	Gly/Gly	Associated with TD (p=0.028)
(ref. 130)	Ser9Gly	Mixed races	Gly/Gly genotype score	Associated with higher AIMS (p<0.0001)
(ref. 131)	Ser9Gly, MnSOD Ala9Val	Chinese Han	MnSOD -9Val and DRD 9Ser	Synergistic effects (p=0.04)
(ref. 132)	Ser9Gly	Chinese	Ser/Ser	Associated with TD (p=0.012)
(ref. 133)	Ser9Gly	Mixed races	Gly/-	Associated with severe TD (p=0.02)
(ref. 134)	Ser9Gly (meta-analysis)	Mixed races	Gly allele	Susceptibility (p=0.04)
Serotonin 2C and Dopamine Receptor 3 (ref. 123)	Cys23Ser and Ser9Gly	Jewish	Ser allele associated with TD	Cys/Ser and Ser/Ser genotypes associated with TD in females (p=0.02); Cys/Ser and Ser/Ser genotypes associated with orofacial dyskinesias

Continued on next page

Table 9-5 *(Continued)*

Gene	Polymorphism	Population	Association	Response
CYP17-α, Dopamine Receptor 3 (ref. 123)	T-C polymorphism in the promoter region and DRD3 Ser9Gly	Jewish	Homozygosity for A2 allele	Significantly associated with orofacial (p<0.04), distal (p<0.05), and incapacitation (p<0.04) scores of AIMS in presence of the dopamine DRD3 gene Gly allele

Bipolar Disorder

Bipolar disorder (BD) is a chronic and often severe psychiatric disorder that is characterized by alternating manic and depressive episodes. It affects approximately 1% of the general population.[143] The gold standard of treatment for BD is lithium. The response to lithium is variable, with about 30% of subjects being excellent responders, and 25% being non-responders.[144] More recently, there has been a greater use of other anticonvulsants such as valproic acid (VPA) and carbamazepine as primary prophylactic agents. Response rates with these agents are similar to that of lithium.[145]

Studies attempting to identify genes that may predict lithium response have recently begun to emerge. A number of studies have demonstrated an association with lithium response and variability in a gene/target, such as the MN blood group, a blood group antigen caused by mutations in the Glycophorin A gene, phospholipase C-gamma 1, inositol polyphosphate 1-polyphosphatase, mitochondrial DNA (polymorphisms 5178 and 10398), glycogen synthase kinase-3β, X-box binding protein cyclic-AMP responsive element binding proteins, and the tryptophan hydroxylase (TPH) gene.[146-153]

Studies, which have resulted in a lack of association between lithium response and specific genes/targets, include the following genes/targets: 5-HT1A, 5-HT2A and 5-HT2C, brain-derived neurotrophic factor (BDNF), INPPI, serotonin transporter gene, activator protein 2β (AP-2β), breakpoint cluster region gene, glycogen synthase kinase-3β (GSK-3β).[154-162] Although many different studies have been completed, a predictive gene or target site with clinical significance has yet to be identified and replicated. The results obtained so far, however, provide hope for additional investigation in this area.[163]

In addition to the use of mood stabilizers in treatment of bipolar disorder, antidepressants can also be used in the depressive episode. Similar studies to those discussed in the depression section, have been conducted with depressed bipolar patients. The only gene that has demonstrated a positive association with antidepressant response is the Gβ3 gene.[164] Those genes demonstrating a negative response, i.e., an association with decreased response to an antidepressant, include TPH and 5HTT.[165-167] Further studies are required to determine the difference in response to antidepressants in unipolar depression versus bipolar disorder depression.

ADHD

Attention deficit hyperactivity disorder (ADHD) is one of the most common neurobehavioral disorders of childhood that can persist through adolescence and into adulthood. Chronic levels of inattention, impulsive hyperactivity, or both characterize it such that daily functioning is compromised.[168] There are few predictors of medication response that exist in the treatment of ADHD. Without this type of information, treatment is often determined empirically, similar to many other central nervous system disorders.[169]

Preliminary studies have suggested that candidate genes involved in the catecholamine pathway could influence individual responses to ADHD treatment. Results from several studies are contradictory, and the nature, magnitude, and direction of the genetic effects remains unclear. Also, although most studies focus on the use of methylphenidate, there are many other medications currently used in the treatment of ADHD. Table 9-6 describes the studies to date reviewing an association with methylphenidate response and genetic polymorphisms.

Table 9-6
Methylphenidate Response Association Studies in ADHD

Gene	Location	Outcome	Reference
Dopamine transporter	New York	Decreased response with homozygous 10-repeat	170
	Brazil	Decreased response with homozygous 10-repeat	171
	Ireland	Increased response with number of 10-repeat	172
	New York	No effect	173
	Korea	Decreased response with homozygous 10-repeat	174
	Washington, DC	Different dose-response curves by DAT1 genotype, decreased response with homozygous nine-repeat	175
	Montreal	Worsening with homozygous nine-repeat on parent ratings	176
	Netherlands	No effect	177
	United States	No effect	178
	Boston (adults)	No effect	179
	Brazil	No effect	180
	Paris	Decreased response with homozygous 10-repeat	180
Dopamine receptor 2	New York	No effect	170
Dopamine receptor 4	New York	No effect	170

Continued on next page

Table 9-6 *(Continued)*

Gene	Location	Outcome	Reference
	New York	Higher doses for normalization needed for seven-repeat	173
	United States	No effect on symptoms; increased picking, irritability, social withdrawal	178
	Korea	Decreased response with seven-repeat allele	182
	Brazil	No effect	180
Synaptosomal-associated protein	United States	Increased irritability and abnormal movements	178
Norepinephrine transporter protein 1	China	Decreased response for homozygous A-allele	183
Adrenergic α2A receptor	Brazil	Improved response on inattention symptoms with g-allele	184
	Brazil	Improved inattentive symptoms with g-allele	185
Serotonin receptors (1B, 2A)	Brazil	No effect	180
Serotonin transporter	Brazil	No effect	180

Clinical Pearl

The majority of ADHD treatment response association studies in pharmacogenomics have focused on methylphenidate. The results have been contradictory.

In addition to the various stimulants used to treat ADHD, a nonstimulant medication, atomoxetine, is also approved for the treatment of ADHD. Clinical development trials demonstrated that CYP2D6 metabolizer status influenced dosing titration and ultimately approved dosing limits. A recent meta-analysis describes the outcome data from several atomoxetine trials.[186] Subjects who were CYP2D6 poor metabolizers had greater symptom improvement than extensive metabolizers. This was likely due to the higher drug concentrations in the blood and CNS. Higher rates of appetite suppression and insomnia were also reported more often in the poor metabolizer group. This group also experienced greater increases in medication-related pulse and blood pressure changes.

Neurologic Disorders

Multiple Sclerosis

Multiple sclerosis (MS) is a demyelinating disease of the central nervous system with inflammatory and degenerative components.[187] To date, few reports have addressed pharmacogenetic issues in MS.[188] Two negative studies on polymorphisms in the interferon beta (INF-β) receptor genes (IFNAR1 and IFNAR2) and the promoter region of the IL-10 gene demonstrated no significant differences between responders and non-responders to IFN-β therapy.[189,190]

Despite these negative results, researchers using Mini-Lymphochip (MLC) cDNA microarrays demonstrated that responder and non-responder phenotypes to IFN-β differ in their gene expression profile in peripheral blood mononuclear cells.[191] This study found that the IL-8 gene in these cells was down regulated in responders compared to the non-responders.

Migraine

Migraines are a complex disorder caused by a combination of genetic and environmental factors.[192] The disorder can be described as a complex spectrum including the following features: craniofacial pain, autonomic dysfunctions, mood disregulations, and spreading cortical disturbance represented by both positive and negative aura phenomena.[193-197] The current gold standard for the acute treatment of migraines is the triptans. The triptans act selectively as agonists on 5-HT1B/1D receptors producing vasoconstriction of meningial vessels as well as direct action on central pathways of trigeminal transmission.[198,199] One study has investigated the relationship between polymorphisms of the 5-HT1B receptor and clinical response to sumatriptan. The study concluded that there was no difference in drug response or cardiovascular side effects associated with genotype.[200] Additional studies in this area are warranted.

Alzheimer's Disease

Alzheimer's disease (AD) is a non-reversible, progressive dementia manifested by gradual deterioration in cognition and behavior. Approximately 10% to 15% of the direct costs for treating dementia can be attributed to pharmacological treatment, while only 10% to 20% of the patients are moderate responders to conventional anti-dementia drugs, with questionable cost-effectiveness.[201-203] The exact etiology of AD is unknown. Genetic factors have been linked to errors in protein synthesis, which result in the formation of abnormal proteins involved in the pathogenesis of AD.[204] Mutations in the presenilin 1, amyloid precursor protein (APP), and presenilin 2 lead to an increase in the accumulation of amyloid beta (Aβ) in the brain. An increase in Aβ results in oxidative stress, neuronal destruction, and the clinical syndrome of AD.[205] Apolipoprotein (apo) E has also been identified as a strong risk factor for late-onset AD. Individuals who are carriers of two or more apo E4 alleles have an earlier onset of AD (approximately six years) compared with non-carriers.[204]

Numerous studies have been conducted to determine the influence of the apoE genotype on drug response in AD. In the monogenic-related studies, the apoE-4/4 carriers are the poorest responders to medication.[206-217] In trigenic-related studies, involving apoE, presenilin 1 and 2, the best responders are those patients carrying the 331222-, 341122-, 341222-, and 441112- genomic profiles. The worst responders in all genomic clusters were those patients with the 441122+ genotype.[218-226] These results demonstrate the deleterious effect of the apoE-4/4 genotype on AD therapeutics in combination with the other AD-related genes.[227]

The current treatment for AD, the cholinesterase inhibitors, are metabolized via the CYP450 pathway. Studies have demonstrated that poor metabolizers and ultra-rapid metabolizers are the poorest responders to pharmacological treatment, while the extensive and intermediate metabolizers are the best responders.[222,223,226,228] In light of the emerging data, it seems very plausible that the determination of response to pharmacological treatment for AD could depend on the interaction of genes involved in the drug metabolism and those genes associated with AD pathogenesis.[228]

Parkinson's Disease

Parkinson's disease is a progressive neurodegenerative disease, which is characterized by continuous cell loss in the nigrostriatal system, approximately 10% per year by positron-emission tomography.[229] Recently, evidence highlighting the importance of environmental factors and the interaction with genetics has prompted a number of association studies on the role of gene polymorphisms in the risk of Parkinson's disease.[230] Although many studies have attempted to discover an association for the risk of developing Parkinson's disease, little has been done in terms of an association between drug response and a particular genotype. One study done in a Caucasian population demonstrated that patients with higher erythrocyte COMT activity had less favorable clinical response to levodopa.[231] With new emerging data on the genetic links to development of Parkinson's disease, the potential for more studies on the genetics of drug response is high.

Epilepsy

Many different types of seizures, which vary in severity, appearance, cause, consequence, and management, characterize epilepsy. Each year, approximately 125,000 new epilepsy cases occur in the United States.[232] The treatment goal for epilepsy is complete elimination of seizures, no side effects, and an optimal quality of life.[233] The majority of literature regarding pharmacogenetics data in the field of epilepsy currently deals with the pharmacokinetics of antiepileptic drugs (AEDs).[234]

The AED, phenytoin, is metabolized via CYP2C9, which is known to have several genetic polymorphisms.[235] Two of the known SNPs, CYP2C9*2^1 (Arg144Cys) and CYP2C9*3 (Ile359Leu), have been shown to increase the risk of intoxication by medium range doses of phenytoin in homozygous and heterozygous carriers.[236-243] Phenytoin is also metabolized via CYP2C19. Two mutant CYP2C19$_{m1}$ and/or CYP2C19$_{m2}$ alleles have been found to be associated with reduced metabolism.[244] Several other studies have shown that mutant CYP2C19 is associated with moderately diminished metabolism of phenytoin.[240,245]

Unlike phenytoin, phenobarbital has conflicting data on the influence of genetic polymorphisms in CYP isoenzymes.[246] Phenobarbital is metabolized via CYP2C19. A group of researchers demonstrated a moderate decrease in clearance of phenobarbital in CYP2C19*2/*2 and *2/*3 genotypes relative to those with CYP2C19 *1/ *1; however, this report was not confirmed in a subsequent study.[247,248]

A third AED, valproic acid (VPA), was the focus of one study examining the role of CYP2C9 polymorphisms in the biotransformation of VPA into its hepatotoxic and inactive metabolites. The homozygous and heterozygous genotypes of alleles CYP2C9*2 and CYP2C9*3 were associated with a decrease in the formation of both these metabolites. The consequences for the hepatotoxicity and teratogenicity of the drug have not been determined so far.[249,250]

In addition to the CYP isoenzyme genotypes, P-glycoprotein (PGP) variations can alter the intracerebral penetration of several AEDs, such as carbamazepine, phenytoin, phenobarbital, valproic acid, gabapentin, topiramate, lamotrigine, and felbamate.[250,251] PGP is encoded in humans by the multi-drug resistance MDR1 gene (designated ABCB1).[252,253] The ABCB1 gene is polymorphic, and seven retrospective case-control studies have been published on the issue of genetic risk factors for pharmacoresistance in epilepsy associated with the multi-drug resistance transporter.[254-260] Four of the case reports demonstrated a positive response,[254-257] finding an association of genetic polymorphisms with AED pharmacoresistance, while three showed negative results. [258-260] A more recent study found no association of several polymorphisms within ABCB1 and any of the outcome measures (time to first seizure after starting drug therapy, time to 12-month remission, or time to drug withdrawal due to unacceptable adverse effects or to lack of seizure control).[261] More studies are needed in this area with stratification for epilepsy syndromes and the use of a unified definition of pharmacoresistance.[262,263]

Polymorphisms in drug targets of AEDs are another area where association studies with pharmacoresistance have begun. Currently there is a published study, which has demonstrated an association between variants in the α-subunit of a voltage-gated sodium channel with differing response to carbamazepine and phenytoin.[264] Further studies are needed in this area for each AED before this information can be utilized prior to prescribing these medications.

Few studies have been completed with determination of an association between adverse drug reactions and polymorphisms in regards to AEDs. Cutaneous adverse effects of drugs are rare, but there have been isolated case reports of familial observations of Stevens-Johnson syndrome (SJS) and the Drug Reaction with Eosinophilia and Systemic Symptoms (DRESS) syndrome with the AEDs.[265-267] Human leukocyte antigen (HLA) genotyping in a recent study of a Han Chinese population who developed SJS after exposure to carbamazepine revealed HLA-B*1502 alleles in all patients.[268] A replication study showed that only 33% of patients had the HLA*1502 allele with SJS and carbamazepine, although this study was done in Asian ancestry patients.[269] The HLA region may contain important genes for SJS, but it is not a universal marker since it is most likely linked to a specific ethnic background.[267]

Pain

Opioids, compounds both natural and synthetic that have morphine-like actions, are mu opioid receptor agonists used for the treatment of mild to severe, acute, and chronic pain.[270] They are characterized as having a narrow therapeutic index, with the most serious toxicity being respiratory depression.[270] Many factors may play a role in balancing pain control without causing respiratory depression/sedation: the patient characteristics; the patient's perception, severity, and likely duration of pain; the opioid drug and dosing regimen; and the genetic make-up of the patient. The determination of the role of pharmacogenomics in opioid pain control is difficult as the various experimental pain stimuli are different from the numerous clinical pain responses, and the identification of the genes involved in pain control are only now being elucidated.

The mu opioid receptor (OPRM1) is the primary binding site target for the opioid drugs. There are 100 variants in the OPRM1 identified, with greater than 20 producing amino-acid changes with a frequency of greater than one percent.[271,272] The most commonly identified SNP is A118G (frequency of 2% to 48%, ethnicity dependent), which leads to a loss of putative N-glycosylation site in the extracellular receptor region.[272] Several studies have been completed to determine the role of this polymorphism on the efficacy and/or dosage requirements of opioids.

The results have demonstrated the polymorphism is thought to cause a decrease opioid effect and an increase in opioid dosage requirement in patients needing pain control. These results are thought to be opioid drug and response specific, though, owing to the contribution of environmental factors and other genes affecting opioid responses.[273-277]

The metabolism of opioid medications through the CYP450 system has been more extensively studied. A significant correlation between CYP2D6 phenotype and the ability to metabolize weaker opioids (codeine, dihydrocodeine, oxycodone, hydrocodone, and tramadol) to their more potent hydroxyl metabolites (morphine, dihydromorphine, oxymorphone, and hydromorphone) has been established.[278-306] The importance of pharmacogenomics in opioid pain control is currently at the state of explaining variability in drug response and toxicity. Large ethnically diverse studies with standardized protocols are needed before this knowledge can be translated into clinical practice.[307]

Summary

With the increasing number of medications used to treat all of the varying disorders of the CNS, prescribing the correct one for each patient will become increasing more difficult. There are numerous genetic factors that cause the CNS disorders and many more, which may ultimately lead to response or failure of a medication. In addition, the amount of adverse drug reactions that these types of medications can cause is staggering.

Currently research is focusing on almost every aspect of treatment with disorders of the CNS, with the most pronounced data in the treatment of depression. Current remission rates with depression are low even with the numerous medications available to treat the disorder. Pharmacogenomics could play a very important role in the future treatment of depression. With increasing research into varying genetic differences between ethnic groups, responders and nonresponders to medications, and those that experience adverse reactions, the future may hold promise for an improved method of prescribing an effective medication for each patient the first time.

References

1. Sutcliffe JG. mRNA in the mammalian central nervous system. *Annu Rev Neurosci.* 1998;11:157-198.
2. Colantuoni C, Purcell AE, Bouton CM, et al. High throughput analysis of gene expression in the human brain. *J Neurosci Res.* 2000;59:1-10.
3. Zineh I, Pebanco GD, Aquilante C, et al. Discordance between availability of pharmacogenetics studies and pharmacogenetics-based prescribing information for the top 200 drugs. *Ann Pharmacother.* 2006;40:639-644.
4. Zineh I, Gerhard T, Aquilante CL, et al. Availability of pharmacogenomics-based prescribing information in drug package inserts for currently approved drugs. *Pharmacogenomics J.* 2004;4:354-358.
5. Kessler RC, Berglund P, Demler O. The epidemiology of major depressive disorders: results from the National Comorbidity Survey replication (NCS-R). *JAMA.* 2003;289:3095-3105.
6. Thase ME, Entsuah AR, Rudolph RL. Remission rates during treatment with venlafaxine or selective serotonin reuptake inhibitors. *Br J Psychiatry.* 2001;178:234-241.
7. Mulrow CP, Williams JW Jr, Trivedi M, et al. Treatment of depression-newer pharmacotherapies. *Evid Rep Technol.* 1999;7:1-4.
8. Thase ME, Haight BR, Richard N, et al. Remission rates following antidepressant therapy with bupropion or selective serotonin reuptake inhibitors: a meta-analysis of original data from seven randomized controlled trials. *J Clin Psychiatry.* 2005;66:974-981.

9. Mann JJ. The medical management of depression. *N Engl J Med.* 2005;353:1819-1834.

10. Ramamoorthy S, Leibach FH, Mahesh VB, et al. Partial purification and characterization of the human placental serotonin transporter. *Placenta.* 1993;14:449-461.

11. Lesch KP, Wolozin BL, Estler HC, et al. Isolation of a cDNA encoding the human brain serotonin transporter. *J Neural Transm Gen Sect.* 1993;91:67-72.

12. Lesch KP, Bengel D, Heils A, et al. Association of anxiety-related traits with a polymorphism in the serotonin transporter gene regulatory region. *Science.* 1996;274:1527-1531.

13. Heils A, Teufel A, Petri S, et al. Allelic variation of human serotonin transporter gene expression. *J Neurochem.* 1996;66:2621-2624.

14. Gelernter J, Cubells JF, Kidd JR, et al. Population studies of polymorphisms of the serotonin transporter protein gene. *Am J Med Genet.* 1999;88:61-66.

15. Smeraldi E, Zanardi R, Benedetti F, et al. Polymorphism within the promoter of the serotonin transporter gene and antidepressant efficacy of fluoxamine. *Mol Psychiatry.* 1998;3:508-511.

16. Zanardi R, Benedetti F, Di Bella D, et al. Efficacy of paroxetine in depression is influenced by a functional polymorphism within the promoter of the serotonin transporter gene. *J Clin Psychopharmacol.* 2000;20:105-107.

17. Pollock BG, Ferrell RE, Mulsant BH, et al. Allelic variation in the serotonin transporter promoter affects onset of paroxetine treatment response in late-life depression. *Neuropsychopharmacology.* 2000;35:587-590.

18. Arias B, Catalan R, Gastro C, et al. 5-HTTLPR polymorphism of the serotonin transporter gene predicts nonremission in major depression patients treated with citalopram in a 12-week follow up study. *J Clin Psychopharmacol.* 2003;23:563-567.

19. Zanardi R, Serretti A, Rossini D, et al. Factors affecting fluvoxamine antidepressant activity; influence of pindolol and 5-HTTLPR in delusional and nondelusional depression. *Biol Psychiatry.* 2001;50:323-330.

20. Rausch JL, Johnson ME, Fei YJ, et al. Initial conditions of serotonin transporter kinetics and genotype: influence on SSRI treatment trial outcome. *Biol Psychiatry.* 2001;51:723-732.

21. Joyce PR, Mulder RT, Luty SE, et al. Age-dependent antidepressant pharmacogenomics: polymorphisms of the serotonin transporter and G protein beta3 subunit as predictors of response to fluoxetine and nortriptyline. *Int J Neuropsychopharmacol.* 2003;6:339-346.

22. Durham LK, Webb SM, Milos PM, et al. The serotonin transporter polymorphism, 5HTTLPR, is associated with a faster response time to sertraline in an elderly population with major depressive disorder. *Psychopharmacology.* 2004;174:525-529.

23. Murphy GM Jr, Hollander SB, Rodrigues HE, et al. Effects of the serotonin transporter gene promoter polymorphism on mirtazapine and paroxetine efficacy and adverse events in geriatric major depression. *Arch Gen Psychiatry.* 2004;61:1163-1169.

24. Serretti A, Cusin C, Rossini D, et al. Further evidence of a combined effect of SERTPR and TPH on SSRIs response in mood disorders. *Am J Med Genet B Neuropsychiatr Genet.* 2004;129:36-40.

25. Kraft JB, Slager SL, McGrath PJ, et al. Sequence analysis of the serotonin transporter and associations with antidepressant response. *Biol Psychiatry.* 2005;58:374-381.

26. Kim DK, Lim SW, Lee S, et al. Serotonin transporter gene polymorphism and antidepressant response. *Neuroreport.* 2002;11:215-219.

27. Ito K, Yoshida K, Sato K, et al. A variable number of tandem repeats in the serotonin transporter gene does not affect the antidepressant response to fluvoxamine. *Psychiatry Res.* 2002;111:235-239.

28. Yoshida K, Ito K, Sato K, et al. Influence of the serotonin transporter gene-linked polymorphic region on the antidepressant response to fluvoxamine in Japanese depressed patients. *Prog Neuropsychopharmacol Biol Psychiatry.* 2002;26:383-386.

29. Yu YW, Tsai SJ, Chen TJ, et al. Association study of the serotonin transporter promoter polymorphism and symptomatology and antidepressant response in major depressive disorders. *Mol Psychiatry.* 2002;7:1115-1119.

30. Lee MS, Lee HY, Lee HJ, et al. Serotonin transporter promoter gene polymorphism and long-term outcome of antidepressant treatment. *Psychiatr Genet.* 2004;14:111-115.

31. Kato M, Ikenaga Y, Wakeno M, et al. Controlled clinical comparison of paroxetine and fluvoxamine considering the serotonin transporter promoter polymorphism. *Int Clin Psychopharmacol.* 2005;20:151-156.

32. Kim H, Lim SW, Seonwoo K, et al. Monoamine transporter gene polymorphisms and antidepressant responses in Koreans with late-life depression. *JAMA*. 2006;296:1609-1618.

33. Lemonde S, Du L, Bakish D, et al. Association of the C(-1019)G 5-HT 1A functional promoter polymorphism with antidepressant response. *Int J Neuropsychopharmacology*. 2004;7:501-506.

34. Arias B, Catalan R, Gastro C, et al. Evidence for a combined genetic effect of the 5-HT (1A) receptor and serotonin transporter genes in the clinical outcome of major depressive patients treated with citalopram. *J Psychopharmacol*. 2005;19:166-172.

35. McMahon FJ, Buervenich S, Charney D, et al. Variation in the gene encoding the serotonin 2A receptor is associated with outcome of antidepressant treatment. *Am J Hum Genet*. 2006;78:804-814.

36. Wu WH, Huo SJ, Cheng CY, et al. Association study of the 5-HT (6) receptor polymorphism (C267T) and symptomatology and antidepressant response in major depressive disorders. *Neuropsychobiology*. 2001;44:172-175.

37. Lee HJ, Cha JH, Ham BJ, et al. Association between a G-protein beta 3 subunit gene polymorphism and the symptomology and treatment responses of major depressive disorders. *Pharmacogenomics J*. 2004;4:29-33.

38. Serretti A, Zanardi R, Rossini D, et al. Influence of tryptophan hydroxylase and serotonin transporter genes on fluvoxamine antidepressant activity. *Mol Psychiatry*. 2001;6:586-592.

39. Yoshida K, Naito S, Takahashi H, et al. Monoamine oxidase: a gene polymorphism, tryptophan hydroxylase gene polymorphism and antidepressant response to fluoxamine in Japanese patients with major depressive disorder. *Prog Neuropsychopharmacol Biol Psychiatry*. 2002;26:1279-1283.

40. Peters EJ, Slager SL, McGrath PJ, et al. Investigation on serotonin-related genes in antidepressant response. *Mol Psychiatry*. 2004;9:879-889.

41. Muller DJ, Schulze TG, Macciardi F, et al. Moclobemide response in depressed patients: association study with a functional polymorphism in the monoamine oxidase A promoter. *Pharmacopsychiatry*. 2002;35:157-158.

42. Serretti A, Zanardi R, Cusin C, et al. No association between dopamine D2 and D4 receptor gene variants and antidepressant activity of two selective reuptake inhibitors. *Psychiatry Res*. 2001;104:195-203.

43. Zill P, Baghai TC, Engel R, et al. Beta-1-adrenergic receptor gene in major depression: influence on antidepressant treatment response. *Am J Med Genet*. 2003;120B:85-89.

44. Yoshida K, Takahashi H, Higuchi H, et al. Prediction of antidepressant response to milnacipran by norepinephrine transporter gene polymorphisms. *Am J Psychiatry*. 2004;161:1575-1580.

45. Kim H, Lim SW, Kim S, et al. Monoamine transporter gene polymorphisms and antidepressant response in Koreans with late-life depression. *JAMA*. 2006;296:1609-1618.

46. Yu YW, Chen TJ, Wang YC, et al. Association analysis for neuronal nitric oxide synthase gene polymorphism with major depression and fluoxetine response. *Neuropsychobiology*. 2003;47:137-140.

47. Baghai TC, Schule C, Zwanzger P, et al. Possible influence of the insertion/deletion polymorphism in the angiotensin 1-converting enzyme gene on therapeutic outcome in affective disorders. *Mol Psychiatry*. 2001;6:258-259.

48. Hong CJ, Wang YC, Tsai SJ. Association study of angiotensin 1-converting enzyme polymorphism and symptomatology and antidepressant response in major depressive disorders. *J Neural Transm*. 2002;109:1209-1214.

49. Baghai TC, Schule C, Zill P, et al. The angiotensin I converting enzyme insertion/deletion polymorphism influences therapeutic outcome in major depressed women, but not in men. *Neurosci Lett*. 2004;363:38-42.

50. Yu YW, Chen TJ, Hong CJ, et al. Association study of the interleukin-1 beta (c-511T) genetic polymorphism with major depressive disorder, associated symptomatology, and antidepressant response. *Neuropsychopharmacology*. 2003;28:1182-1185.

51. Licinio J, O'Kirwan F, Irizarry K, et al. Association of a corticotropin-releasing hormone receptor 1 haplotype and antidepressant treatment response in Mexican-Americans. *Mol Psychiatry*. 2004;9:1075-1082.

52. van Rossum ECF, Binder EB, Mayer M, et al. Polymorphisms of the glucocorticoid receptor gene and major depression. *Biol Psychiatry*. 2006;59:681-688.

53. Wong ML, Whelan F, Deloukas P, et al. Phosphodiesterase genes are associated with susceptibility to major depression and antidepressant treatment response. *Proc Natl Acad Sci.* 2006;103:15124-15129.

54. Evaluation of Genomic Applications in Practice and Prevention (EGAPP) Working Group. Recommendations from the EGAPP Working Group: testing for cytochrome P450 polymorphisms in adults with nonpsychotic depression treated with selective serotonin reuptake inhibitors. *Genetics Medicine.* 2007;9:819-825.

55. Thakur M, Grossman I, McCrory DC, et al. Review of evidence for genetic testing for CYP450 polymorphisms in management of patients with nonpsychotic depression with selective serotonin reuptake inhibitors. *Genetics Medicine.* 2007;9:826-835.

56. Peters EJ, Slager SL, Kraft JB, et al. Pharmacokinetic genes do no influence response or tolerance to citalopram in the STAR*D sample. *PLOS ONE.* 2008;3:e1872.

57. Jones P, Buckley P. *Schizophrenia.* London: Mosby; 2006.

58. Bishop JR, Ellingrod VL. Neuropsychiatric pharmacogenomics: moving toward a comprehensive understanding of predicting risks and response. *Pharmacogenomics.* 2004;5:463-477.

59. Lieberman JA, Stroup TS, McEvoy JP, et al. Effectiveness of antipsychotic drugs in patients with chronic schizophrenia. *N Engl J Med.* 2005;353:1209-1223.

60. Leckband SG, Bishop JR, Ellingrod V. Pharmacogenomics in psychiatry. *J Pharm Prac.* 2007;20:252-264.

61. Moore TA, Buchanan RW, Buckley PF, et al. The Texas Medication Algorithm Project antipsychotic algorithm for schizophrenia: 2006 update. *J Clin Psychiatry.* 2007;68:1751-1762.

62. Kapur S, Mamo D. Half a century of antipsychotics and still a central role for dopamine D2 receptors. *Prog Neuropsychopharmacol Biol Psychiatry.* 2003;27:1081-1090.

63. Meltzer HY, Li Z, Kaneda Y, et al. Serotonin receptors: their key role in drugs to treat schizophrenia. *Prog Neuropsychopharmacol Biol Psychiatry.* 2003;27:1159-1172.

64. Mossner R, Schuhmacher A, Kuhn K, et al. Functional serotonin 1A receptor variant influences treatment response to atypical antipsychotics in schizophrenia. *Pharmacogenet Genomics.* 2009;19:91-94.

65. Yu YW, Tsai SJ, Yang KH, et al. Evidence for an association between polymorphism in the serotonin-2a receptor variant (102T/C) and increment of N100 amplitude in schizophrenics treated with clozapine. *Neuropsychobiology.* 2001;43:79-82.

66. Arranz MJ, Munro J, Sham P, et al. Meta-analysis of studies on genetic variation in 5-HT2A receptors and clozapine response. *Schizophr Res.* 1998;32:93-99.

67. Masellis M, Basile V, Meltzer HY, et al. Serotonin subtype 2 receptor genes and clinical response to clozapine in schizophrenia patients. *Neuropsychopharmacology.* 1998;19:123-132.

68. Ellingrod VL, Lund BC, Miller D, et al. 5-HT2A receptor promoter polymorphism, -1438G/A and negative symptom response to olanzapine in schizophrenia. *Psychopharmacol Bull.* 2003;37:109-112.

69. Herken H, Erdel ME, Esgi K, et al. The relationship between the response to risperidone treatment and 5-HT2A receptor gene (T102C and -1438G/A) polymorphism in schizophrenia. *Bull Clin Psychopharmacol.* 2003;13:161-166.

70. Lane HY, Chang YC, Chiu CC, et al. Association of risperidone treatment response with a polymorphism in the 5-HT(2A) receptor gene. *Am J Psychiatry.* 2002;159:1593-1595.

71. Ellingrod VL, Perry PJ, Lund BC, et al. 5HT2A and 5HT2C receptor polymorphisms and predicting clinical response to olanzapine in schizophrenia. *J Clin Psychopharmacol.* 2002;22:622-624.

72. Yamanouchi Y, Iwata N, Suzuki T, et al. Effect of DRD2, 5-HT2A, and COMT genes on antipsychotic response to risperidone. *Pharmacogenomics J.* 2003;3:356-361.

73. Reynolds GP, Yao Z, Zhang X, et al. Pharmacogenetics of treatment in first-episode schizophrenia: D3 and 5-HT2C receptor polymorphisms separately associate with positive and negative symptom response. *Eur Neuropsychopharmacol.* 2005;15:143-51.

74. Yu YW, Tsai SJ, Lin CH, et al. Serotonin-6 receptor variant (C267T) and clinical response to clozapine. *Neuroreport.* 1999;10:1231-1233.

75. Hong CJ, Yu YW, Lin CH, et al. An association study of a brain-derived neurotrophic factor Val66Met polymorphism and clozapine response of schizophrenic patients. *Neurosci Lett.* 2003;349:206-208.

76. Woodward ND, Jayathilake K, Meltzer HY. COMT val108/158met genotype, cognitive function, and cognitive improvement with clozapine in schizophrenia. *Schizophr Res.* 2007;90:86-96.

77. Bertolino A, Caforio G, Blasi G, et al. Interaction of COMT (Val(108/158)Met) genotype and olanzapine treatment on prefrontal cortical function in patients with schizophrenia. *Am J Psychiatry.* 2004;161:1798-1805.

78. Potkin SG, Basile VS, Jin Y, et al. D1 receptor alleles predict PET metabolic correlates of clinical response to clozapine. *Mol Psychiatry.* 2003;8:109-113.

79. Wu S, Xing Q, Gao R, et al. Response to chlorpromazine treatment may be associated with polymorphisms of the DRD2 gene in Chinese schizophrenic patients. *Neuroscience Lett.* 2005;376:1-4.

80. Schafer M, Rujescu D, Ina G, et al. Association of short-term response to haloperidol treatment with a polymorphism in the dopamine D_2 receptor gene. *Am J Psychiatry.* 2001;158:802-804.

81. Hwang R, Shinkai T, De Luca V, et al. Association study of 12 polymorphisms spanning the dopamine D receptor gene and clozapine treatment response in two treatment refractory/intolerant populations. *J Psychopharmacology.* 2005;181:179-187.

82. Lane HY, Lee CC, Chang YC, et al. Effects of dopamine D2 receptor Ser311Cys polymorphism and clinical factors on risperidone efficacy for positive and negative symptoms and social function. *Int J Neuropsychopharmacol.* 2004;7:461-470.

83. Xing Q, Qian X, Li H, et al. The relationship between the therapeutic response to risperidone and the dopamine D2 receptor polymorphism in Chinese schizophrenia patients. *Int J Neuropsychopharmacol.* 2006;1-7.

84. Lencz T, Robinson DG, Xu K, et al. DRD2 promoter region variation as a predictor of sustained response to antipsychotic medication in first-episode schizophrenia patients. *Am J Psychiatry.* 2006;163:529-531.

85. Scharfetter J, Chaudhry HR, Hornik K, et al. Dopamine D3 receptor gene polymorphism and response to clozapine in schizophrenic Pakistani patients. *Eur Neuropsychopharmacol.* 1999;10:17-20.

86. Lane HY, Hsu SK, Liu YC, et al. Dopamine D3 receptor Ser9Gly polymorphism and risperidone response. *J Clin Psychopharmacol.* 2005;25:6-11.

87. Xuan J, Zhao C, He G, et al. Effects of the dopamine D_3 receptor (DRD3) gene polymorphisms on risperidone response: a pharmacogenetic study. *Neuropsychopharmacology.* 2008;33:305-311.

88. Zhao AL, Zhao JP, Zhang YH, et al. Dopamine D4 receptor gene exon III polymorphism and interindividual variation in response to clozapine. *Int J Neurosci.* 2005;115:1539-1547.

89. Meary A, Brousee G, Jamain S, et al. Pharmacogenetic study of atypical antipsychotic drug response: involvement of the norepinephrine transporter gene. *Am J Med Genet Part B.* 2008;147B:491-494.

90. Muller DJ, De L V, Sicard T, et al. Suggestive association between the C825T polymorphism of the G-protein beta3 subunit gene (GNB3) and clinical improvement with antipsychotics in schizophrenia. *Eur Neuropsychopharmacol.* 2005;15:525-531.

91. Bishop JR, Ellingrod VL, Moline J, et al. Pilot study of G-protein beta3 subunit (C825T) polymorphism and clinical response to olanzapine or olanzapine-related weight gain in persons with schizophrenia. *Med Sci Monit.* 2006;12:BR47-50.

92. Lane HY, Liu YC, Huang CL, et al. RGS4 polymorphisms predict clinical manifestations and responses to risperidone treatment in patients with schizophrenia. *J Clin Psychopharmacol.* 2008;28:64-68.

93. Hong CJ, Yu YW, Lin CH, et al. Association analysis for NMDA receptor subunit 2B (GRIN2B) genetic variants and psychopathology and clozapine response in schizophrenia. *Psychiatr Genet.* 2001;11:219-222.

94. Bishop JR, Ellingrod VL, Moline J, et al. Association between the polymorphic GRM3 gene and negative symptom improvement during olanzapine treatment. *Schizophr Res.* 2005;77:253-260.

95. Lin YC, Ellingrod VL, Bishop JR, et al. The relationship between P-glycoprotein (PGP) polymorphisms and response to olanzapine treatment in schizophrenia. *Ther Drug Monit.* 2006;28:668-672.

96. Xing Q, Gao R, Li H, et al. Polymorphisms of the ABCB1 gene are associated with the therapeutic response to risperidone in Chinese schizophrenia patients. *Pharmacogenomics.* 2006;7:987-993.

97. Mata I, Crespo-Facorro B, Perez-Iglesias R, et al. Association between the interleukin-1 receptor antagonist gene and negative symptom improvement during antipsychotic treatment. *Am J Med Genet B Neuropsychiatr Genet.* 2006;141:939-943.

98. Muller DJ, Klempan TA, De Luca V, et al. The SNAP-25 gene may be associated with clinical response and weight gain in antipsychotic treatment of schizophrenia. *Neurosci Lett.* 2005;379:81-89.

99. Szekeres G, Keri S, Juhasz A, et al. Role of dopamine D3 receptor (DRD3) and dopamine transporter (DAT) polymorphism in cognitive dysfunctions and therapeutic response to atypical antipsychotics in patients with schizophrenia. *Am J Med Genet B Neuropsychiatr Genet.* 2004;124:1-5.

100. Zhang A, Xing Q, Wang L, et al. Dopamine transporter polymorphisms and risperidone response in Chinese schizophrenia patients: an association study. *Pharmacogenomics.* 2007;8:1337-1345.

101. de Leon J. Pharmacogenomics: the promise of personalized medicine for CNS disorders. *Neuropsychopharmacology.* 2009;34:159-172.

102. Muller DJ, Kennedy JL. Genetics of antipsychotic treatment emergent weight gain in schizophrenia. *Pharmacogenomics.* 2006;7:863-887.

103. Ellingrod VL, Miller D, Schultz SK, et al. CYP2D6 polymorphisms and atypical antipsychotic weight gain. *Psychiatr Genet.* 2002;12:55-58.

104. Reynolds GP, Zhang ZJ, Zhang XB. Association of antipsychotic drug-induced weight gain with a 5-HT2C receptor gene polymorphism. *Lancet.* 2002;359:2086-2087.

105. Basile VS, Masellis M, De Luca V, et al. 759T/C genetic variation of 5HT(2C) receptor and clozapine-induced weight gain. *Lancet.* 2002;360:1790-1791.

106. Reynolds GP, Zhang Z, Zhang X. Polymorphism of the promoter region of the serotonin 5-HT(2C) receptor gene and clozapine-induced weight gain. *Am J Psychiatry.* 2003;160:677-679.

107. Templeman LA, Reynolds GP, Arranz B, et al. Polymorphisms of the 5HT2C receptor and leptin genes are associated with antipsychotic drug-induced weight gain in Caucasian subjects with a first-episode psychosis. *Pharmacogenet Genomics.* 2005;15:195-200.

108. Ellingrod VL, Perry PJ, Ringold JC, et al. Weight gain associated with the -795C/T polymorphism of the 5HT2C receptor and olanzapine. *Am J Med Genet B NeuroPsychiatr Genet.* 2005;134:76-78.

109. Miller del D, Ellingrod VL, Holman TL, et al. Clozapine-induced weight gain associated with the 5HT2C receptor -795C/T polymorphism. *Am J Med Genet B NeuroPsychiatr Genet.* 2005;133:97-100.

110. Wang YC, Bai YM, Chen JY, et al. Polymorphism of the adrenergic receptor α 2a-1291C>G genetic variation and clozapine-induced weight gain. *J Neural Transm.* 2005;112:1463-8.

111. Park YM, Chung YC, Lee SH, et al. Weight gain associated with the α(2a)-adrenergic receptor -1291 C/G polymorphism and olanzapine treatment. *Am J Med Genet B NeuroPsychiatr Genet.* 2006;141:394-397.

112. Wang YC, Bai YM, Chen JY, et al. C825T polymorphism in the human G protein β3 subunit gene is associated with long-term clozapine treatment-induced body weight change in the Chinese population. *Pharmacogenet Genomics.* 2005;15:743-748.

113. Zhang ZJ, Yao ZJ, Mou XD, et al. Association of -2548G/A functional polymorphism in the promoter region of leptin gene with antipsychotic agent-induced weight gain. *Zhonghua Yi Xue Za Zhi.* 2003;83:2119-2123.

114. Zhang XY, Tan YL, Zhou DF, et al. Association of clozapine-induced weight gain with a polymorphism in the leptin promoter region in patients with chronic schizophrenia in a Chinese population. *J Clin Psychopharmacol.* 2007;27:246-251.

115. Popp J, Leucht S, Heres S, et al. DRD4 48bp VNTR but not 5-HT$_{2C}$ Cys23Ser receptor polymorphism is related to antipsychotic-induced weight gain. *Pharmacogenomics J.* 2009;9:71-77.

116. Genomas. Available at: www.genomas.net. Accessed October 10, 2008.

117. de Leon J, Correa JC, Ruano G, et al. Exploring genetic variations that may be associated with direct effects of some antipsychotics on lipid levels. *Schizophr Res.* 2008;98:40-46.

118. Ruano G, Goethe JW, Caley C, et al. Physiogenomic comparison of weight profiles of olanzapine- and risperidone-treated patients. *Mol Psychiatry.* 2007;12:474-482.

119. de Leon J, Susce MT, Johnson M, et al. A clinical study of the association of antipsychotics with hyperlipidemia. *Schizophr Res.* 2007;92:95-102.

120. Casey DE. Tardive dyskinesia. *West J Med.* 1990;153:535-541.

121. Yassa R, Jeste DV. Gender differences in tardive dyskinesia: a critical review of the literature. *Schizophr Bull.* 1992;18:701-715.

122. Thelma BK, Srivastava V, Tiwari AK. Genetic underpinnings of tardive dyskinesia: passing the baton to pharmacogenetics. *Pharmacogenomics.* 2008;9:1285-1306.

123. Segman RH, Heresco-Levy U, Yakir A, et al. Interactive effect of cytochrome P450 17α-hydroxylase and dopamine D3 receptor gene polymorphisms on abnormal involuntary movements in chronic schizophrenia. *Biol Psychiatry.* 2002;51:261-263.

124. Liou YJ, Lai IC, Liao DL, et al. The human dopamine receptor D2 (DRD2) gene is associated with tardive dyskinesia in patients with schizophrenia. *Mol Psychiatry.* 2007;12:794-795.

125. Bakker PR, van Harten PN, van Os J. Antipsychotic-induced tardive dyskinesia and polymorphic variations in COMT, DRD2, CYP1A2, and MnSOD genes: a meta-analysis of pharmacogenetic interactions. *Mol Psychiatry.* 2008;13:544-556.

126. Steen VM, Lovlie R, MacEwan T, et al. Dopamine D3-receptor gene variant and susceptibility to tardive dyskinesia in schizophrenic patients. *Mol Psychiatry.* 1997;2:139-145.

127. Segman RH, Neeman T, Heresco-Levy U, et al. Genotypic association between the dopamine D3 receptor gene and tardive dyskinesia in chronic schizophrenia. *Mol Psychiatry.* 1999;4:247-253.

128. Liao DL, Yeh YC, Chen HM, et al. Association between the Ser9Gly polymorphism of the dopamine D3 receptor gene and tardive dyskinesia in Chinese schizophrenic patients. *Neuropsychobiology.* 2001;44:95-98.

129. Woo SI, Kim JW, Rha E, et al. Association of the Ser9Gly polymorphism in the dopamine D3 receptor gene with tardive dyskinesia in Korean schizophrenics. *Psychiatry Clin Neurosci.* 2002;56:469-474.

130. Lerer B, Segman RH, Fangerau H, et al. Pharmacogenetics of tardive dyskinesia: combined analysis of 780 patients supports association with dopamine D3 receptor gene Ser9Gly polymorphism. *Neuropsychopharmacology.* 2002;27:105-119.

131. Zhang ZJ, Zhang XB, Hou G, et al. Interaction between polymorphisms of the dopamine D3 receptor and manganese superoxide dismutase genes in susceptibility to tardive dyskinesia. *Psychiatr Genet.* 2003;13:187-192.

132. Chong SA, Tan EC, Tan CH, et al. Polymorphisms of dopamine receptors and tardive dyskinesia among Chinese patients with schizophrenia. *Am J Med Genet B Neuropsychiatr Genet.* 2003;116:51-54.

133. de Leon J, Susce MT, Pan RM, et al. Polymorphic variations in GSTM1, GSTT1, PgP, CYP2D6, CYP3A5, and dopamine D2 and D3 receptors and their association with tardive dyskinesia in severe mental illness. *J Clin Psychopharmacol.* 2005;25:448-456.

134. Bakker PR, van Harten PN, van Os J. Antipsychotic-induced tardive dyskinesia and the Ser9Gly polymorphism in the DRD3 gene: a meta analysis. *Schizophr Res.* 2006;83:185-192.

135. Segman RH, heresco-Levy U, Finkel B, et al. Association between the serotonin 2C receptor gene and tardive dyskinesia in chronic schizophrenia: additive contribution of 5-HT2Cser and DRD3gly alleles to susceptibility. *Psychopharmacology (Berlin).* 2000;152:408-413.

136. Chen CH, Wei FC, Koong FJ, et al. Association of Taq1 A polymorphism of dopamine D2 receptor gene and tardive dyskinesia in schizophrenia. *Biol Psychiatry.* 1997;41:827-829.

137. Ohmori O, Suzuki T, Kojima H, et al. Tardive dyskinesia and debrisoquine 4- hydroxylase (CYP2D6) genotype in Japanese schizophrenics. *Schizophr Res.* 1998;32:107-113.

138. Lam LC, Garcia-Barcelo MM, Ungvari GS, et al. Cytochrome P450 2D6 genotyping and association with tardive dyskinesia in Chinese schizophrenic patients. *Pharmacopsychiatry.* 2001;34:238-241.

139. Inada T, Senoo H, Iijima Y, et al. Cytochrome P450 II D6 gene polymorphisms and the neuroleptic-induced extrapyramidal symptoms in Japanese schizophrenic patients. *Psychiatr Genet.* 2003;13:163-168.

140. Liou YJ, Wang YC, Bai YM, et al. Cytochrome P-450 2D6*10 C188T polymorphism is associated with antipsychotic-induced persistent tardive dyskinesia in Chinese schizophrenic patients. *Neuropsychobiology.* 2004;49:167-173.

141. Basile VS, Ozdemir V, Masellis M. A functional polymorphism of the cytochrome P450 1A2 (CYP1A2) gene: association with tardive dyskinesia in schizophrenia. *Mol Psychiatry.* 2000;5:410-417.

142. Tiwari AK, Deshpande SN, Rao AR, et al. Genetic susceptibility to tardive dyskinesia in chronic schizophrenia subjects: I. Association of CP1A3 gene polymorphism. *Pharmacogenomics J.* 2005;5:60-69.

143. Akiskal HS, Bougeois ML, Angst J, et al. Reevaluating the prevalence of and diagnostic composition within the broad clinical spectrum of bipolar disorders. *J Affect Disord.* 2000;59:5-30.

144. Rybakowski JK, Chlopocka-Wozniak M, et al. The prophylactic effect of long-term lithium administration in bipolar patients entering treatment in the 1970s and 1980s. *Bipolar Disord.* 2001;3:63-67.

145. Kasper S, Stamenkovic M, Letmaier M, et al. Atypical antipsychotics in mood disorders. *Int Clin Psychopharmacol.* 2002;3:1-10.

146. Alda M, Grof P, Grof E. MN blood groups and bipolar disorder: evidence of genotypic association and Hardy-Weinberg disequilibrium. *Biol Psychiatry.* 1998;44:361-363.

147. Turecki G, Grof P, Cavazzoni P, et al. Evidence for a role of phospholipase C-gamma1 in the pathogenesis of bipolar disorder. *Mol Psychiatry.* 1998;3:534-538.

148. Steen VM, Lovlie R, Osher Y, et al. The polymorphic inositol polyphosphate 1-phosphatase gene as a candidate for pharmacogenetic prediction of lithium-responsive manic-depressive illness. *Pharmacogenetics.* 1998;8:259-268.

149. Del Zompo M, Ardau R, Palmas MA, et al. Lithium response: association study with two candidate genes. *Mol Psychiatry.* 1999;4:566.

150. Serretti A, Lilli R, Lorenzi C, et al. Tryptophan hydroxylase gene and response to lithium prophylaxis in mood disorders. *J Psychiatr Res.* 1999b;33:371-377.

151. Wahizuka S, Ikeda A, Kato N, et al. Possible relationship between mitochondrial DNA polymorphisms and lithium response in bipolar disorder. *Int J Neuropsychopharmacol.* 2003;6:421-424.

152. Masui T, Hashimota R, Kusumi I, et al. A possible association between the -116C/G single nucleotide polymorphism of the XBP1 gene and lithium prophylaxis in bipolar disorder. *Int J Neuropsychopharmacol.* 2006;9:83-88.

153. Mamdani F, Alda M, Grof P, et al. Lithium response and genetic variation in the CREB family of genes. *Am J Med Genet B Neuropsych Genet.* 2008;147B:500-504.

154. Michelon L, Meira-Lima I, Cordeiro Q, et al. Association study of the INPP1, 5HTT, BDNF, AP-2β and GSK-3β GENE variants and retrospectively scored response to lithium prophylaxis in bipolar disorder. *NeuroSci Lett.* 2006;403:288-293.

155. Masui T, Hashimoto R, Kusumi I, et al. Lithium response and Val66Met polymorphism of the brain-derived neurotrophic factor gene in Japanese patients with bipolar disorder. *Psychiatr Genet.* 2006;16:49-50.

156. Serretti A, Lorenzi C, Lilli R, et al. Serotonin receptor 2A, 2C, 1A genes and response to lithium prophylaxis in mood disorders. *J Psychiatric Res.* 2000;34:89-98.

157. Dmitrzak-Weglarz M, Rybakowski JK, Suwalska A, et al. Association of 5-HT_{2A} and 5-HT_{2C} serotonin receptor gene polymorphisms with prophylactic lithium response in bipolar patients. *Pharmacol Rep.* 2005;57:761-765.

158. Szczepankiewicz A, Rybakowski JK, Suwalska A, et al. Association study of the glycogen synthase kinse-3β gene polymorphism with prophylactic lithium response in bipolar patients. *World J Biol Psychiatry.* 2006;3:158-161.

159. Lovlie R, Berle JO, Stordal E, et al. The phospholipase C-gamma gene (PLCG1) and lithium-responsive bipolar disorder: re-examination of an intronic dinucleotide repeat polymorphism. *Psychiatr Genet.* 2001;11:41-43.

160. Masui T, Hashimoto R, Kusumi I, et al. A possible association between missense polymorphism of the breakpoint cluster region gene and lithium prophylaxis in bipolar disorder. *Prog Neuropsychopharmacol Biol Psychiatry.* 2008;32:204-208.

161. Serretti A, Lorenzi C, Cusin C, et al. SSRIs antidepressant activity is influenced by Gbeta3 variants. *Eur Neuropsychopharmacol.* 2003;13:117-122.

162. Benedetti F, Serretti A, Poniggia A, et al. Long-term response to lithium salts in bipolar illness is influenced by the glycogen synthase kinase 3-beta -50T/C SNP. *Neurosic Lett.* 2005;376:51-55.

163. Mamdani F, Jaitovich Groisman I, Alda M, et al. Pharmacogenetics and bipolar disorder. *Pharmacogenomics J.* 2004;4:161-170.

164. Zill P, Baghi TC, Zwanzger P, et al. Evidence for an association between a G-protein beta3-gene variant with depression and response to antidepressant treatment. *Neuroreport.* 2000;11:1893-1897.

165. Serretti A, Zanardi R, Cusin C, et al. Influence of tryptophan hydroxylase and serotonin transporter genes on fluvoxamine antidepressant activity. *Mol Psychiatry.* 2001;6:586-592.

166. Serretti A, Zandardi R, Cusin C, et al. Tryptophan hydroxylase gene associated with paroxetine antidepressant activity. *Eur Neuropsychopharmacol.* 2001;11:375-380.

167. Mundo E, Walker M, Cate T, et al. The role of serotonin transporter protein gene in antidepressant-induced mania in bipolar disorder: preliminary findings. *Arch Gen Psychiatry.* 2001;58:539-544.

168. Centers for Disease Control and Prevention: What is Attention-Deficit/Hyperactivity Disorder? Available at: http://www.cdc.gov/ncbddd/adhd/what.htm Accessed October 30, 2008.

169. Stein MA, McGough JJ. The pharmacogenomic era: promise for personalizing attention deficit hyperactivity disorder therapy. *Child Adolesc Psychiatric Clin N Am.* 2008;17:475-490.

170. Winsberg BG, Comings DE. Association of the dopamine transporter gene (DAT1) with poor methylphenidate response. *J Am Acad Child Adolesc Psychiatry.* 1999;38:1474-1477.

171. Roman T, Szobot C, Martine S, et al. Dopamine transporter gene and response to methylphenidate in attention-deficit/hyperactivity disorder. *Pharmacogenomics.* 2002;12:497-499.

172. Kirley A, Lowe N, Hawi A, et al. Association of the 480bp DAT1 allele with methylphenidate response in a sample of Irish children with ADHD. *Am J Med Genet.* 2003;121B:50-54.

173. Hamarman S, Fossella J, Ulger C, et al. Dopamine receptor 4 (DRD4)7-repeat allele predicts methylphenidate dose response in children with attention deficit hyperactivity disorder. *J Child Adolesc Psychopharmacol.* 2004;14:564-574.

174. Cheon KA, Ryu YH, Kim JW, et al. The homozygosity for the 10-repeat allele at dopamine transporter gene and dopamine transporter density in Korean children with attention deficit hyperactivity disorder: relating to treatment response to methylphenidate. *Eur Neuropsychopharmacol.* 2005;15:95-101.

175. Stein MA, Waldman ID, Sarampote CS, et al. Dopamine transporter genotype and methylphenidate dose response in children with ADHD. *Neuropsychopharmacology.* 2005;30:1374-1382.

176. Joober R, Grizenko N, Sengupta S, et al. Dopamine transporter 3'-UTR VNTR genotype and ADHD: a pharmaco-behavioral genetic study with methylphenidate. *Neuropsychopharmacology.* 2006;32:1370-1376.

177. Van der Meulen EM, Bakker SC, Pauls DL, et al. High sibling correlation on methylphenidate response but no association with DAT1-10R and DRD4-7 alleles in Dutch sibpairs with ADHD. *J Child Psychol Psychiatry.* 2005;46:1074-1080.

178. McGough JJ, McCracken JT, Swanson J, et al. Pharmacogenetics of methylphenidate response in preschoolers with ADHD. *J Am Acad Child Adolesc Psychiatry.* 2006;45:1314-1322.

179. Mick E, Biederman J, Spencer T, et al. Absence of association with DAT1 polymorphism and response to methylphenidate in a sample of adults with ADHD. *Am J Med Genet.* 2006;141:890-894.

180. Zeni CP, Guimaraes AP, Polanczyk GV, et al. No significant association between response to methylphenidate and genes of the dopaminergic serotonergic systems in a sample of Brazilian children with attention-deficit/hyperactivity disorder. *Am J Med Genet B Neuropsychiatr Genet.* 2007;144:391-394.

181. Purper-Ouakil D, Wohl M, Orejarena S, et al. Pharmacogenetics of methylphenidate response in attention deficit/hyperactivity disorder: association with the dopamine transporter gene (SLC6A3). *Am J Med Genet B: Neuropsych Gene.* 2008;147B:1425-1430.

182. Cheon K, Kim B, Cho S. Association of 4-repeat allele of the dopamine D4 receptor gene III polymorphism and response to methylphenidate treatment in Korean ADHD children. *Neuropsychopharmacology.* 2007;32:1377-1383.

183. Yang L, Wang Y-F, Li J, et al. Association of norepinephrine transporter gene (NET) with methylphenidate response. *J Am Acad Child Adolesc Psychiatry.* 2004;43:1154-1158.

184. Polanczyk G, Zeni C, Gentro JP, et al. Association of the adrenergic alpha-2A receptor gene with methylphenidate improvement of inattentive symptoms in children and adolescents with attention deficit/hyperactivity disorder. *Arch Gen Psych.* 2007;64:218-224.

185. Silva TL, Pianca TG, Roman T, et al. Adrenergic α2A receptor gene and response to methylpheni-date in attention-deficit/hyperactivity disorder-predominantly inattentive type. *J Neural Transm.* 2008;115:341-345.

186. Michelson D, Read HA, Ruff D, et al. CYP2D6 and clinical response to atomoxetine in children and adolescents with ADHD. *J Am Acad Child Adolesc Psychiatry.* 2007;46:242-251.

187. Trapp BD. Pathogenesis of multiple sclerosis: the eyes only see what the mind is prepared to com-prehend. *Ann Neurol.* 2004;55:455-457.

188. Annibali V, Ristori G, Cannoni S, et al. Multiple sclerosis: pharmacogenomics and personalized drug treatment. *Neurol Sci.* 2006;27:347-349.

189. Sriram U, Barcellos LF, Villoslada P, et al. Pharmacogenomic analysis of interferon receptor poly-morphisms in multiple sclerosis.. *Genes Immun.* 2003;4:147-152.

190. Wergeland S, Beiske A, Nyland H, et al. IL-10 promoter haplotype influence on interferon treat-ment response in multiple sclerosis. *Eur J Neurol.* 2005;12:171-175.

191. Sturzebecher S, Wandinger KP, Rosenwald A, et al. Expression profiling identifies responder and non-responder phenotypes to interferon-beta in multiple sclerosis. *Brain.* 2003;126:1419-1429.

192. Piane M, Lulli P, Farinelli I, et al. Genetics of migraine and pharmacogenomics: some consider-ations. *J Headache Pain.* 2007;8:334-339.

193. Wessman M, Kaunisto MA, Kallela M, et al. The molecular genetics of migraine. *Ann Med.* 2004;36:462-473.

194. Haan J , Kors EE, Vanmolkot KR, et al. Migraine genetics: an update. *Curr Pain Headache Rep.* 2005;9:213-220.

195. Russell MB. Tension-type headache in 40-year-olds: a Danish population-based sample of 4000. *J Headache Pain.* 2005;6:441-447.

196. Russell MB. Commentary to comorbidity in Finnish migraine families. *J Headache Pain.* 2006;7:320-321.

197. Russell MB. Genetics in primary headaches. *J Headache Pain.* 2007;8:190-195.

198. Colombo B, Annovazzi PO, Comi G. Therapy of primary headaches: the role of antidepressants. *Neurol Sci.* 2004;3:171-175.

199. Tfelt-Hansen P. Acute pharmacotherapy of migraine, tension-type headache, and cluster headache. *J Headache Pain.* 2007;8:127-134.

200. MaassenVanDenBrink A, Vergouwe MN, Ophoff RA, et al. 5-HT1B receptor polymorphism and clinical response to sumatriptan. *Headache.* 1998;38:288-291.

201. Cacabelos R, Alvarez XA, Lombardi V, et al. Pharmacological treatment of Alzheimer disease: from psychotropic drugs and cholinesterase inhibitors to pharmacogenomics. *Drugs Today.* 2000;36:415-499.

202. Giacobini E. Cholinesterase in human brain: the effect of cholinesterase inhibitors on Alzheimer's disease, related disorders. In: Giacobini E, Pepeu G, eds. *The Brain Cholinergic System in Health and Disease.* Oxon: Informa Healthcare; 235-264.

203. Loveman E, Green C, Kirby J, et al. The clinical and cost-effectiveness of donepezil, rivastigmine, galantamine and memantine for Alzheimer's disease. *Health Technol Assess.* 2006;10:1-176.

204. Kamboh MI. Molecular genetics of late-onset Alzheimer's disease. *Am Hum Genet.* 2004;68:381-404.

205. van Marum RJ. Current and future therapy in Alzheimer's disease. *Fundam Clin Pharmacol.* 2008;22:265-274.

206. Poirier J, Delisle M-C, Quirion R, et al. Apolipoprotein E4 allele as a predictor of cholinergic defi-cits treatment outcome in Alzheimer's disease. *Proc Natl Acad Sci USA.* 1995;92:12260-12264.

207. Almkvist O, Jelic V, Amberla K, et al. Responder characteristics to a single oral dose of cholinest-erase inhibitor: a double-blind placebo-controlled study with tacrine in Alzheimer patients. *Dement Geriatr Cogn Disord.* 2001;12:22-32.

208. Sjorgren M, Hesse C, Basun H, et al. Tacrine and rate of progression in Alzheimer's disease-rela-tion to ApoE allele genotype. *J Neural Transm.* 2001;108:451-458.

209. Borroni B, Colciaghi F, Pastorino L, et al. ApoE genotype influences the biological effects of done-pezil on APP metabolism in Alzheimer disease: evidence from a peripheral model. *Eur Neuropsy-chopharmacol.* 2002;12:195-200.

210. Aerssens J, Raeymaekers P, Lilinefeld S, et al. APOE genotype: no influence on galantamine treatment efficacy or on rate of decline in Alzheimer's disease. *Dement Geriatr Cogn Disord.* 2001;2:69-77.

211. Raskind MA, Peskind ER, Wessel T, et al. Galantamine in AD: a 6-month randomized, placebo-controlled trial with a 6-month extension. The Galantamine USA-1 Study Group. *Neurology.* 2000;54:2261-2268.

212. Risner ME, Saunders AM, Altman JE, et al. Efficacy of rosiglitazone in a genetically defined population with mild-to-moderate Alzheimer's disease. *Pharmacogenomics.* 2006;6:246-254.

213. MacGowan SH, Wilcock GK, Scott M. Effect of gender and apolipoprotein E genotype on response to anticholinesterase therapy in Alzheimer's disease *Int J Geriatr Psychiatry.* 1998;13:625-630.

214. Rigaud AS, Traykov L, Caputo L, et al. The apolipoprotein E epsilon 4 allele and the response to tacrine therapy in Alzheimer's disease. *Eur J Neurol.* 2000;7:255-258.

215. Rigaud AS, Traykov L, Latour R, et al. Presence of absence of lease one epsilon 4 allele and gender are not predictive for the response to donepezil treatment in Alzheimer's disease. *Pharmacogenomics.* 2002;12:415-420.

216. Petersen RC, Thomas RG, Grundman M, et al. Vitamin E and donepezil for the treatment of mild cognitive impairment. *N Engl J Med.* 2005;352:2379-2388.

217. Bizzro A, Marra C, Acciarri A, et al. Apolipoprotein E epsilon-4 allele differentiates the clinical response to donepezil in Alzheimer's disease. *Dement Geriatr Cogn Disord.* 2005;20:254-261.

218. Cacabelos R. Pharmacogenomics in Alzheimer's disease. *Mini Rev Med Chem.* 2002;2:59-84.

219. Cacabelos R. Pharmacogenomics for the treatment of dementia. *Ann Med.* 2002;34:357-379.

220. Cacabelos R. The application of functional genomics to Alzheimer's disease. *Pharmacogenomics.* 2003;4:597-621.

221. Cacabelos R. Pharmacogenomics and therapeutic prospects in Alzheimer's disease. *Exp Opin Pharmacother.* 2005;6:1967-1987.

222. Cacabelos R. Pharmacogenomics, nutrigenomics and therapeutic optimization in Alzheimer's disease. *Aging Health.* 2005;1:303-348.

223. Cacabelos R. Molecular pathology and pharmacogenomics in Alzheimer's disease: polygenic-related effects of multifactorial treatments on cognition, anxiety, and depression. *Methods Find Exp Clin Pharmacol.* 2007;29:1-91.

224. Cacabelos R, Alvarez A, Fernandez-Novoa L, et al. A pharmacogenomic approach to Alzheimer's disease. *Acta Neurol Scand.* 2000;176:12-19.

225. Cacabelos R, Fernandez-Novoa L, Pichel V, et al. Pharmacogenomic studies with a combination therapy in Alzheimer's disease. In: Takeda M, Tanaka T, Cacbelos R, eds. *Molecular Neurobiology of Alzheimer's Disease and Related Disorders.* Basel: Karger; 2004:94-107.

226. Cacabelos R, Takeda M. Pharmacogenomics, nutrigenomics, and future therapeutics in Alzheimer's disease. *Drugs Future.* 2006;31:5-146.

227. Cacabelos R. Pharmacogenomics and therapeutic prospects in dementia. *Eur Arch Psychiatry Clin Neurosci.* 2008;258:28-47.

228. Cacabelos R. Donepezil in Alzheimer's disease: from conventional trials to pharmacogenetics. *Neuropsychiatr Dis Treat.* 2007;3:303-333.

229. Leender KL. Pathophysiology of movement disorders studied using PET. *J Neural Transm Suppl.* 1997;50:39-46.

230. Gilgun-Sherki Y, Djaldetti R, Melamed E, et al. Polymorphism in candidate genes: implications for the risk and treatment of idiopathic Parkinson's disease. *Pharmacogenomics J.* 2004;4:291-306.

231. Wang J, Si YM, Liu ZL, et al. Cholecystokinin, cholecystokinin-A receptor and cholecystokinin-B receptor gene polymorphisms in Parkinson's disease. *Pharmacogenetics.* 2003;13:365-369.

232. Sander JW. The epidemiology of epilepsy revisited. *Curr Opin Neurol.* 2003;16:165-170.

233. Vickrey BG, Hays RD, Rausch R, et al. Quality of life of epilepsy surgery patients as compared with outpatients with hypertension, diabetes, heart disease, and/or depressive symptoms. *Epilepsia.* 1994;35:597-607.

234. Mann MW, Pons G. Various pharmacogenetics aspects of antiepileptic drug therapy. *CNS Drugs.* 2007;21:143-164.

235. Lee Cr, Goldstein JA, Pieper JA. Cytochrome P450 2C9 polymorphisms: a comprehensive review of the in-vitro and human data. *Pharmacogenetics.* 2002;12:251-163.

236. Rettie AE, Wienkers LC, Gonzalez FJ, et al. Impaired S-warfarin metabolism catalyzed by the R144C allelic variant of CYP2C9. *Pharmacogenetics.* 1994;4:39-42.

237. Haining RL, Hunter AP, Veronese ME, et al. Allelic variants of human cytochrome P450 2C9: baculovirus-mediated expression, purification, structural characterization, substrate stereoselectivity, and prochiral selectivity of the wild-type and 1359L mutant forms. *Arch Biochem Biophys.* 1996;353:447-458.

238. Brandolese R, Scordo MG, Spina E, et al. Severe phenytoin intoxication in a subject homozygous for CYP2C9*3. *Clin Pharmacol Ther.* 2001;70:391-394.

239. Kidd RS, Curry TB, Gallagher S, et al. Identification of a null allele of CYP2C9 in an African-American exhibiting toxic phenytoin. *Pharmacogenetics.* 2001;11:803-808.

240. Mamiya K, Ieiri I, Shimamoto J, et al. The effects of genetic polymorphisms of CYP2C9 and CYP2C19 on phenytoin metabolism in Japanese adult patients with epilepsy: studies in stereoselective hydroxylation and population pharmacokinetics. *Epilepsia.* 1998;39:1317-1323.

241. Soga Y, Nishimura F, Ohtsuka Y, et al. CYP2C9 polymorphisms, phenytoin metabolism and gingival overgrowth in epileptic subjects. *Life Sci.* 2004;74:827-834.

242. Schwarz UI. Clinical relevance of genetic polymorphisms in the human CYP2C9 gene. *Eur J Clin Invest.* 2003;33:23-30.

243. Van der Weide J, Steijins LSW, van Weelden JM, et al. The effect of genetic polymorphism of cytochrome P450 CYP2C9 on phenytoin dose requirement. *Pharmacogenetics.* 2001;11:287-291.

244. Xiao ZS, Goldenstein JA, Xie HG, et al. Differences in the incidence of the CYP2C19 polymorphism affecting the S-mephenytoin phenotype in Chinese Han and Bai populations and identification of a new rare CYP2C19 mutant allele. *J Pharmacol Exp Ther.* 1997;281:604-609.

245. Odani A, Hashimoto Y, Otsuki Y, et al. Genetic polymorphism of the CYP2C subfamily and its effect on the pharmacokinetics of phenytoin in Japanese patients with epilepsy. *Clin Pharmacol Ther.* 1997;62:287-282.

246. Kwan P, Brodie MJ. Phenobarbital for the treatment of epilepsy in the 21st century: a critical review. *Epilepsia.* 2004;45:1141-1149.

247. Mamiya K, Hadama A, Yukawa E, et al. CYP2C19 polymorphism effect on phenobarbital. Pharmacokinetics in Japanese patients with epilepsy: analysis by population pharmacokinetics. *Eur J Clin Pharmacol.* 2000;55:821-825.

248. Hadama A, Ieri I, Morita T, et al. P-hydroxylation of phenobarbital: relationship to (S)-mephenytoin hydroxylation (CYP2C19) polymorphism. *Ther Drug Monit.* 2001;23:115-118.

249. Ho PC, Abbott FS, Zanger UM, et al. Influence of CYP2C9 genotypes on the formation of a hepatotoxic metabolite of valproic acid in human liver microsomes. *Pharmacogenomics J.* 2003;3:335-342.

250. Loscher W, Potschka H. Role of multidrug transporter in pharmacoresistance to antiepileptic drugs. *J Pharmacol Exp Ther.* 2002;301:7-14.

251. Sills GJ, Kwan P, Butler E, et al. P-glycoprotein mediated efflux of antiepileptic drugs: preliminary studies in mdr1 knockout mice. *Epilepsy Behav.* 2002;3:427-432.

252. Dean M, Rzhetsky A, Allikmets R. The human ATP-binding cassette (ABC) transporter superfamily. *Genome Res.* 2001;11:1156-1166.

253. HUGO gene Nomenclature Committee (online). Available at: http://www.gene.ucl.ac.uk/nomenclature/ Accessed October 28, 2008.

254. Siddiqui A, Kerb R, Weale ME, et al. Association of multidrug resistance in epilepsy with a polymorphism in the drug-transporter gene ABCB1. *N Engl J Med.* 2003;348:1442-1448.

255. Zimprich F, Sunder-Plassman R, Stogmann E, et al. Association of an ABCB1 gene haplotype with pharmacoresistance in temporal lobe epilepsy. *Neurology.* 2004;63:1087-1089.

256. Hung CC, Tai JJ, Lin CJ, et al. Complex haplotypic effects of the ABCB1 gene on epilepsy treatment response. *Pharmacogenomics.* 2005;6:411-417.

257. Seo T, Ishitsu T, Ueda N, et al. ABCB1 polymorphisms influence the response to antiepileptic drugs in Japanese epilepsy patients. *Pharmacogenomics.* 2006;7:551-561.

258. Tan NCK, Heron SE, Scheffer IE, et al. Failure to confirm association of a polymorphism in ABCB1 with multidrug resistant epilepsy. *Neurology.* 2004;63:1090-1092.

259. Sills GJ, Mohanraj R, Butler E, et al. Lack of association between the C3435T polymorphism in the human multidrug resistance (MDR1) gene and response to antiepileptic drug treatment. *Epilepsia.* 2005;46:643-647.

260. Kim YO, Kim MK, Woo YJ, et al. Single nucleotide polymorphisms in the multidrug resistance 1 gene in Korean epileptics. *Seizure.* 2006;15:67-72.

261. Leschziner G, Jorgensen AI, Andrew T, et al. Clinical factors and ABCB1 polymorphisms in prediction of antiepileptic drug response: a prospective cohort study. *Lancet Neuro.* 2006;5:668-676.

262. Ott J. Association of genetic loci. *Neurology.* 2004;63:955-958.

263. Cardon LR, Bell JI. Association study designs for complex diseases. *Nat Rev Genet.* 2001;2:91-99.

264. Tate SK, Depondt C, Sisodiya SM, et al. Genetic predictors of the maximum doses patients receive during clinical use of the anti-epileptic drugs carbamazepine and phenytoin. *Proc Natl Acad Sci USA.* 2005;102:5507-5512.

265. Gennis MA, Vemuri R, Burns EA, et al. Familial occurrence of hypersensitivity to phenytoin. *Am J Med.* 1991;91:631-634.

266. Fischer PR, Shigeoka AO. Familial occurrence of Stevens-Johnson syndrome. *Am J Dis Child.* 1983;137:914-916.

267. Foujeau J-C, Stern RS. Severe cutaneous adverse reactions to drugs. *N Engl J Med.* 1994;331(19):1272-1285.

268. Wen-Hung C, Shuen-iu H, Hong-Shang E, et al. A marker for Stevens-Johnson syndrome. *Nature.* 2004;428-486.

269. Lonjou C, Thomas L, Borot N, et al. A marker for Stevens-Johnson syndrome: ethnicity matters. *Pharmacogenomics J.* 2006;6:265-268.

270. Somogyi AA, Barratt DT, Coller JK. Pharmacogenetics of Opioids. *Clin Pharmacol Ther.* 2007;81:429-444.

271. Ikeda K, Ide S, Han W, et al. How individual sensitivity to opiates can be predicted by gene analyses. *Trends Pharmacol Sci.* 2005;26:311-317.

272. Lotsch J, Geisslinger G. Are μ-opioid receptor polymorphisms important for clinical opioid therapy? *Trends Mol Med.* 2005;11:82-89.

273. Cararco Y, Maroz Y, Davidson E. Variability in alfentanil analgesia may be attributed to polymorphism in the mu-opioid receptor. *Clin Pharmacol Ther.* 2001;39:63.

274. Klepstad P, Rakvag TT, Kaasa S, et al. The 118A>G polymorphism in the human μ-opioid receptor gene may increase morphine requirements in patients with pain caused by malignant disease. *Acta Anaesthesiol Scand.* 2004;79:316-324.

275. Coulbault L, Beaussier M, Verstuyft C, et al. Environmental and genetic factors associated with morphine response in the postoperative period. *Clin Pharmcol Ther.* 2006;79:316-324.

276. Hirota T, Ieiri I, Takane H, et al. Sequence variability and candidate gene analysis in two cancer patients with complex clinical outcomes during morphine therapy. *Drug Metab Dispos.* 2003;31:677-680.

277. Lotsch J, Zimmerman M, Darimont J, et al. Does the A118G polymorphism at the μ-opioid receptor gene protect against morphine-6-glucuronide toxicity? *Anesthesiology.* 2002;97:814-819.

278. Sindrup SH, Brosen K, Bjerring P, et al. Codeine increases pain thresholds to copper vapor laser stimuli in extensive but not poor metabolizers of sparteine. *Clin Pharmacol Ther.* 1991;48:686-693.

279. Yue QY, Alm C, Svensson JO, et al. Codeine O-desmethylation co-segregates with polymorphic debrisiquine hydroxylation. *Br J Clin Pharmacol.* 1989;28:639-645.

280. Chen ZR, Somogyi AA, Bochner F. Polymorphic-O-demethylation of codeine. *Lancet.* 1988;2:914-915.

281. Chen ZR, Somogyi AA, Reynolds G, et al. Disposition and metabolism of codeine after single and chronic doses in one and seven extensive metabolizers. *Br J Clin Pharmacol.* 1991;31:381-390.

282. Yue QY, Alm C, Svensson JO, et al. Quantification of O- and N-demethylated and the glucoronidated metabolites of codeine relative to the debrisoquine metabolic ratio in urine in ultrarapid, rapid, and poor debrisoquine hydroxylators. *Ther Drug Monit.* 1997;19:539-542.

283. Williams DG, Patel A, Howard RF. Pharmacogenetics of codeine metabolism in an urban population of children and its implications for analgesic reliability. *Br J Anaesth.* 2002;89:839-845.

284. Heiskanen T, Olkkola KT, Kalso E. Effects of blocking CYP2D6 on the pharmacokinetics and pharmacodynamics of oxycodone. *Clin Pharmacol Ther.* 1998;64:603-611.

285. Otton SV, Schadel M, Cheung SW, et al. CYP2D6 phenotype determines the metabolic conversion of hydrocodone to hydromorphone. *Clin Pharmacol Ther.* 1993;4:463-472.

286. Fromm MF, Hofmann U, Griese E.-U., et al. Dihydrocodeine: a new opioid substrate for the polymorphic CYP2D6 in humans. *Clin Pharmacol Ther.* 1995;58:374-382.

287. Poulsen L, Arendt-Nielsen L, Brosen K, et al. The hypoalgesic effect of tramadol in relation to CYP2D6. *Clin Pharmacol Ther.* 1996;60:636-644.

288. Borlak J, Hermann R, Erb K, et al. A rapid and simple CYP2D6 genotyping assay-case study with analgesic tramadol. *Metabolism.* 2003;52:1439-1443.

289. Filegert F, Kurth B, Gohler K. The effects of tramadol on static and dynamic pupillometry in healthy subjects: the relationship between pharmacodynamics, pharmacokinetics and CYP2D6 metabolizer status. *Eur J Pharmacol.* 2005;61:257-266.

290. Slanar O, Nobilis M, Kventina J, et al. Miotic action of tramadol is determined by CYP2D6 genotype. *Physiol Res.* 2007;56:129-136.

291. Slanar O, Nobilis M, Kventina J, et al. CYP2D6 polymorphism, tramadol pharmacokinetics and pupillary response. *Eur J Clin Pharmacol.* 2006;62:75-76.

292. Pedersen RS, Damkier P, Brosen K. Tramadol as a new probe for cytochrome P450 2D6 phenotyping: a population study. *Clin Pharmacol Ther.* 2005;77:458-467.

293. Eap CB, Broly F, Mino A, et al. Cytochrome P450 2D6 genotype and methadone steady-state concentrations. *J Clin Psychopharmacol.* 2001;21:229-234.

294. Coller JK, Joergensen C, Foster DJ, et al. Lack of influence of CYP2D6 genotype on the clearance of (R)-, (S)- and racemic-methadone. *Int J Clin Pharmacol Ther.* 2007;45:410-417.

295. Sindrup SH, Arendt-Nielsen L, Brosen K, et al. The effect of quinidine on the analgesic effect of codeine. *Eur J Pharmacol.* 1992;42:587-591.

296. Desmeules J, Gascon MP, Dayer P, et al. Impact of environmental and genetic factors on codeine analgesia. *Eur J Clin Pharmacol.* 1991;41:23-26.

297. Enggaard TP, Poulsen L, Arendt-Nielson L, et al. The analgesic effect of tramadol after intravenous injection in healthy volunteers in relation to CYP2D6. *Anesth Analg.* 2006;102:146-150.

298. Poulsen L, Brosen K, Arendt-Nielson L, et al. Codeine and morphine in extensive and poor metabolizers of aparteine: pharmacokinetics, analgesic effect and side effects. *Eur J Clin Pharmacol.* 1996;51:289-295.

299. Eckhardt K, Li S, Ammons S, et al. Same incidence of adverse drug events after codeine administration irrespective of the genetically determined differences in morphine formation. *Pain.* 1998;76:27-33.

300. Persson K, Sjostrom S, Sigurdardottir I, et al. Patient-controlled analgesia (PCA) with codeine for postoperative pain relief in ten extensive metabolisers and one poor metaboliser of dextromethorphan. *Br J Clin Pharmacol.* 1995;39:182-186.

301. Poulsen L, Riishede L, Brosen K, et al. Codeine in post-operative pain: study of the influence of sparteine phenotype and serum concentrations of morphine and morphine-6-glucuronide. *Eur J Clin Pharmacol.* 1998;54:451-454.

302. Maddocks I, Somogyi A, Abbott F, et al. Attenuation of morphine-induced delirium in palliative care by substitution with infusion of oxycodone. *J Pain Symptom Manage.* 1996;12:182-189.

303. Stamer UM, Stuber F. Impact of CYP2D6 genotype on postoperative tramadol analgesia. *Pain.* 2003;105:231-238.

304. Caraco Y, Sheller J, Wood AJ. Pharmacogenetic determination of the effects of codeine and prediction of drug interactions. *J Pharmacol Exp Ther.* 1996;278:1165-1174.

305. Mikus G, Trausch B, Rodewald C, et al. Effect of codeine on gastrointestinal motility in relation to CYP2D6 phenotype. *Clin Pharmacol Ther.* 1997;61:459-466.

306. Hasselstrom J, Yue QY, Sawe J. The effect of codeine on gastrointestinal transit in extensive and poor metabolisers of debrisoquine. *Eur J Clin Pharmacol.* 1997;53:145-148.

307. Contopoulos-loannidis DG, Alexious GA, Gouvias TC, et al. An empirical evaluation of multifarious outcomes in pharmacogenetics: a beta-2 adrenoceptor gene polymorphisms in asthma treatment. *Pharmacogenet Genom.* 2006;16:705-711.

Chapter 10

Infectious Diseases

Tawanda Gumbo, MD; John D. Cleary, Pharm.D.

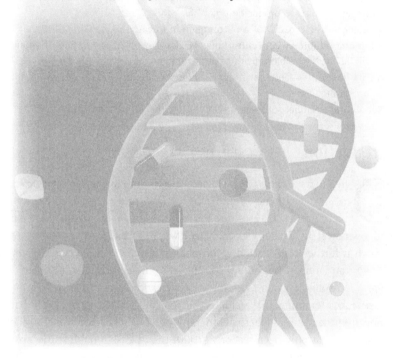

Learning Objectives

After completing this chapter, the reader should be able to

- Define the underlying concepts for application of pharmacogenetic data to therapy of infectious diseases, for anti-infective choice, dose size, and dosing schedule.
- Demonstrate the current use of pharmacogenetics in the derivation of new antimicrobial doses.
- Discuss the current use of pharmacogenetics in infectious diseases clinical practice.

Key Definitions

Antimicrobial pharmacokinetics—A study of absorption, distribution, metabolism, and excretion of antimicrobial drugs.

Antimicrobial pharmacodynamics—The study of how antimicrobial drugs exert their effects on target organisms.

Pharmacokinetic variability—The variability observed in drug absorption, distribution, metabolism, and excretion between different individuals.

Drug dose—The specific quantity of therapeutic agent or drug administered to a patient.

Pathogen—A disease-producing organism.

Virulence—The capacity of a microorganism to cause disease.

Minimum inhibitory concentrations (MIC)—Lowest concentration of an antimicrobial that will inhibit the visible growth of a microorganism.

Innate immunity—The human bodies non-specific, first line of defense against invasion by foreign organisms.

Xenobiotic—Natural substances that are foreign to the body.

Introduction

Our understanding of pharmacogenetics role in the biologic processes of human disease is in its infancy. Pharmacogenetic studies are more complex in infectious diseases than in other diseases due to a second organism's genetic diversity added to the patient's own diversity. This is especially true when the pathogen is a eukaryote (yeast or mould). Research is further complicated when pharmacotherapy has a direct effect on gene transcription and translation of not only the pathogen, but also the host. One can find such a complex scenario for example when assessing invasive candidiasis treated with amphotericin B.

Research attempting to elucidate the role of gene transcription in diagnosis of disease, pathogen virulence, and pharmacotherapy outcomes has been ongoing for many years. Unfortunately, it has only been recently (2000) that the National Institutes of Health "Road Map" for translational medicine and the National Institute of General Medical Sciences (http://www.nigms.nih.gov) has dedicated resources toward genomic or proteomic approaches focused on understanding trauma and inflammatory diseases. Specific initiatives are directed toward Models of Infectious Disease Agent Study (http://www.nigms.nih.gov/Initiatives/MIDAS/), a Pharmacogenetics Research Network (http://www.nigms.nih.gov/Initiatives/PGRN/), and a Pharmacogenetics and Pharmacogenomics Knowledge Base (PharmGKB: www.pharmgkb.org/), to name a few. The NIH Pharmacogenetics Research Network was formed to enable multi-disciplinary research groups to conduct studies in pharmacogenetics and pharmacogenomics and contribute to a knowledge gene base (PharmGKB).

Genetics in the Diagnosis and Monitoring of Infectious Diseases

Numerous studies have evaluated the usefulness of gene transcription as a basis for identification and diagnosis of infectious diseases. This identification can be achieved by assessing changes in host gene transcription in response to an individual pathogen. As an example, David Relman and colleagues have attempted to identify gene-expression patterns associated with the biological processes in Kawasaki disease, Ebola hemorrhagic fever, homopolymeric tracts in *Bordetella pertussis*, acute Dengue hemorrhagic fever, or patients presenting with febrile illnesses.[1-4] They have suggested that gene expression patterns could be used to effectively diagnose a patient. Pharmacists should be aware of these developments, since discoveries in this field of science could be used to monitor pharmacotherapeutic outcomes.

Genetics in Monitoring Virulence of Pathogens and Host Defenses

Changes in the pathogenesis of infecting organisms can be associated with changes in immune response to infection or alterations in organism virulence. Transcriptional changes in pathogen genes are numerous and beyond the scope of this chapter. Investigations into infectious processes associated with alterations in immune response have led to some promising findings. Specifically, the changes in innate immunity that have been identified in humans or other mammals infected by pathogens has been enlightening. For example, genetic alterations in immune responses and clinical outcomes with yeast or mould infections have been identified in humans and animals. The altered gene expression usually results in decreased immune activation associated with pathogen invasion and poor responses to therapy. This has been reported with myeloid differentiation primary response gene (88) (MyD88), interleukin 17, toll-like receptor 4 (TLR-4), and mannose binding lectin.[5-10] Moreover, impressive results have been discovered when evaluating polymorphisms with manganese transport protein MntH gene and susceptibility to mycobacterial pneumonia, specifically, pulmonary tuberculosis along with interleukin12 receptor B1 (IL-12RB1) deficiency with recurrent leishmaniasis or recurrent Salmonella bacteremia.[11-14]

Genetics and Antimicrobial Therapy

Infectious diseases differ from other diseases in that in addition to the usual pharmacokinetic and pharmacodynamic factors associated with the pharmacologic agent, there is behavior of the microbe itself to consider. In other words, what the pathogen does to the antimicrobial drug and what the drug does to the pathogen is also crucial to understand. Antimicrobial pharmacokinetics-pharmacodynamics (PK/PD) is the science that relates antimicrobial drug exposure to microbial effects such as microbial kill and resistance suppression.[15-17] In the same way a patient's genetics play a central role in their pharmacokinetic-pharmacodynamic (PK/PD) response, the pathogen's genes play their own unique role in antimicrobial PK/PD. In addition, since the microbe interacts with the patient, the patient's genetic makeup also influences various aspects of their inflammatory reaction to the pathogen. This unique inflammatory reaction often influences pharmacokinetic variability. On the other hand, influenced by its own genetic makeup, the micro-organism affects the patient (pathology) and sometimes even the patient's PK/PD parameters. These interactions are shown in Figure 10-1, in which arrows indicate direction of effect. The possible pathways modified by the patient's genetic make-up are italicized. This complex interaction is actually still a simplification. In pregnant women for example, the interaction map increases to three organisms (the woman, unborn child, and microbe) each affecting the other. The pharmacogenetic factors implicated in these interactions are only beginning to be investigated and understood. In this chapter, recent use of pharmacogenetics on some of these pathways and its role in the development of new antimicrobial dosing regimens will be discussed. Clinical practices that already employ pharmacogenetics will also be discussed with regards to choice of antimicrobial agent, magnitude of medication dose, dosing schedule, and expected efficacy.

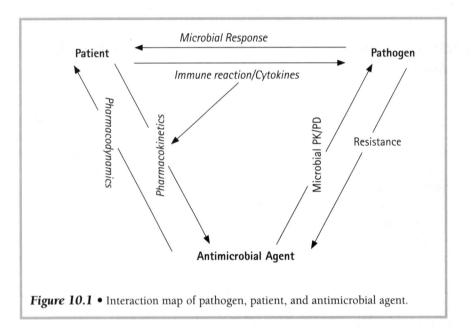

Figure 10.1 • Interaction map of pathogen, patient, and antimicrobial agent.

Principles of Pharmacogenetics in Infectious Disease

Pharmacogenetic data can be used at any of the several decision points represented in Figure 10-1. However, it is important to emphasize that these data are only useful in conjunction with other clinical information (i.e., susceptibility data, microbial PK/PD data, and even anthropometric data such as weight). In other words, pharmacogenetics is only part of several considerations when it comes to infectious diseases pharmacotherapy. First, the diagnosis of an infectious disease should, as much as possible, include the identification of a pathogen by the microbiology laboratory. Even after that, it is to be understood that many infectious diseases are self limiting and may not require chemotherapy. If a decision is made to treat, then the next decision is choice of antimicrobial agent.

When it comes to anti-infective choice, variation in the microbe's genes can play a critical role. The evolutionary history of the pathogen with respect to a specific anti-infective is best determined using a common phenotypic assessment such as, antimicrobial susceptibility tests. However, in some instances such as HIV and *M. tuberculosis*, direct genetic evidence of mutations associated with medication resistance is also commonly used. If the pathogen is resistant to the anti-infective, typically it would be unwise to use the agent as part of a regimen to treat the infection. In fact, the best practice when phenotypic tests are used should be to utilize actual minimum inhibitory concentrations (MIC), rather than just rely on the "resistant" versus "susceptible" dichotomy. A clinically relevant example can be found with Gram positive infections. There is a two-fold difference in clinical outcome when methicillin resistant *Staphylococcus aureus* (MRSA) with an MIC of 0.5 and 1.0 mg/L are treated with the standard dose of vancomycin, even though both are technically susceptible to the vancomycin.[18] There are exceptions to the susceptibility rule. As an example, lamivudine is used together with zidovudine in patients with lamivudine resistant HIV infection due to the M184V mutation. This mutation increases the viral sensitivity to zidovudine 10-fold. Finally, even with low MICs, some pathogens such as *Mycobacterium tuberculosis* are well known to exhibit phenotypic tolerance to some antibiotics.

Once the antibiotic choice has been narrowed down based on susceptibilities, the choices can be narrowed down further based on pharmacogenetic considerations. For some antimicrobial agents, certain patient genotypes predict a high risk of adverse events. In this situation, genotypic tests lead to exclusion of these anti-infectives from the possible regimen, thus minimizing the risk of adverse events. The principle employed here is identification of certain single nucleotide polymorphisms (SNPs) that have an adverse effect on the pharmacodynamics of the anti-infective.

Clinical Pearl

Pharmacogenetic tests can be used to avoid anti-infectives with a high toxicity profile in a group of patients carrying risk associated gene mutations and alleles. This is a pharmacogenomic based decision.

The second important decision point, once an antimicrobial agent has been chosen, is the dose to be employed for the particular patient, disease, and pathogen. This decision is based on population pharmacokinetic variability as well as pharmacodynamics in general, and more specifically, antimicrobial PK/PD exposures associated with optimal kill of pathogen and with resistance suppression. Antimicrobial PK/PD information makes infectious disease pharmacology unique in that specific exposures and exposure patterns can be targeted to achieve optimal efficacy, unlike therapeutics of many other pharmaceuticals. Drug exposures achieved are based on patient specific pharmacokinetics and the variability of these parameters, as well as pathogen factors such as MIC. Pathogens such as *M. tuberculosis* also demonstrate the need to consider the "metabolic" status of the pathogen. In order to better understand how this is used in decision making, one needs to consider the importance of patient pharmacokinetics.

Pharmacokinetic variability is an evolutionary advantage. The human species has been exposed to many plant and fungal chemicals during its evolution. In response to different substances encountered during evolution, genetic variability for the xenobiotic metabolism of these chemicals has developed.[19] As a result, many antimicrobial agents that are metabolized by these enzymes have a wide distribution of systemic clearance. The clinical consequence is that a single fixed dose of antimicrobial agent can achieve different concentrations in different patients. Some individuals will have sub-therapeutic concentrations while others will achieve toxic concentrations. To a certain extent, therapeutic anti-infective monitoring can help monitor this variability, and therefore, guide decisions on the size of the dose used. However, in some instances pharmacogenetic data may be better than using single data points of medication concentrations to adjust dose. Another covariate of pharmacokinetic variability may be the particular pathogen and disease itself. The extensive genetic variability encountered within the immune system means that even if patients were to be infected with the same bacterial isolate, they will have different immune responses. This immune reaction, especially high cytokine concentrations, may be associated with high pharmacokinetic variability in some instances. As an example, one study showed that anidulafungin clearance was significantly higher in patients with invasive candidiasis, compared to other patient groups.[20] There are many such examples, but the main point is that pharmacokinetic variability is not only driven by pharmacogenetic factors, but can also be driven by the disease process caused by the pathogen itself. Thus when taking genetic based variability into consideration in decision making, it should always be remembered that host-pathogen interactions may further alter the effect of genes on pharmacokinetics.

It is possible that as our understanding of the function and regulation of protein transporters (i.e. P-glycoprotein) increases, genetic tests will guide medication selection based on characteristics like distribution into exclusive sites of infection. Practitioners may one day select pharmacotherapy based on the patient's P-glycoprotein genotype and specific transporters of anti-infectives into certain infected sites such as the meninges. Pharmacogenetic correlates of pharmacokinetic variability are increasingly being described, as in the examples of treatment of *H. pylori* related peptic ulcer disease and isoniazid discussed later, and should be used for selection of both dose size and dose schedule.

Clinical Pearl

Pharmacogenetic correlates of pharmacokinetic variability are useful in determination of dose size and dose schedule for some antibiotics.

The usefulness of understanding pharmacokinetic variability for dose size and dose schedule is further maximized when used in conjunction with microbial dynamics. Antimicrobial exposure patterns associated with optimal microbial kill and resistance suppression do not themselves depend on pharmacogenetics, but rather on the interaction of anti-infective and pathogen.[15] In antimicrobial PK/PD science, exposure patterns such as the shape of the concentration-time curve to minimum inhibitory concentration (MIC), peak concentration to MIC (C_{max}/MIC), the 0-24h area under the concentration-time curve to MIC ratio (AUC_{0-24}/MIC), and % of dosing interval that concentration persists above MIC (T_{MIC}), are related to microbial effect.[15-17] Microbial effects (kill or resistance suppression) of antibacterial, anti-viral and anti-fungal drugs tend to be optimized by one of these three parameters, and tend to be generally well preserved across disease systems. Therefore, they can be used for translation from preclinical models to patients. The particular PK/PD parameter associated with the effect dictates the dosing schedule. In the selection of anti-infectives for which C_{max}/MIC optimizes effect, it is advantageous to combine several doses into one to achieve a higher C_{max}. This is the strategy behind once a day aminoglycoside dosing. Selection of anti-infectives for which T_{MIC} optimizes effect, it is advantageous to dose frequently if the agent's half-life is short, as is employed for penicillins. For AUC/MIC driven agents (or AUC/EC_{95} for antivirals), dosing schedule does not matter, as long as the optimal total AUC/MIC is achieved. Examples include fluoroquinolones, triazole antifungal compounds, and nucleoside reverse transcriptase inhibitors.[16,21,22] AUC/MIC driven anti-infectives dosing schedule may also be driven by toxicity issues. This is the case of daptomycin. Once a day daptomycin dosing is associated with less skeletal muscle toxicity and preferred in pharmacotherapy compared to dosing several times a day.[23,24] A second important aspect of antimicrobial PK/PD properties is the optimal exposure (T_{MIC}, AUC/MIC or C_{max}/MIC) associated with optimal kill. This is often the exposure associated with 80-90% of maximal effect, or the exposure associated with resistance suppression. These optimal exposures need to be achieved at the site of infection, if the best microbial effect is to be achieved. To the extent that pharmacogenetics is the foundation for pharmacokinetic variability and leads to a large number of patients failing to achieve these exposures, the interaction of antimicrobial PK/PD and pharmacogenetics becomes paramount. The best dose is that which achieves the optimal antimicrobial PK/PD exposure at site of infection despite pharmacokinetic variability. In other words if an antimicrobial drug dose is administered to patients, genetic based pharmacokinetic variability leads to it achievement of a wide distribution of antimicrobial PK/PD exposure (C_{max}/MIC, or AUC/MIC or T_{MIC}) values at site of infection. The best dose is that which achieves the antimicrobial PK/PD exposure associated with either optimal kill or resistance suppression at site of infection in the majority of patients (often taken as 90% of patients).[25] An example of the use of antimicrobial PK/PD exposure together with pharmacogenetics comes from the arena of isoniazid and pyrazinamide based therapy for tuberculosis, which shall be discussed later.

Clinical Pearl

Antimicrobial pharmacodynamics enable integration of microbial response to pharmacogenetic factors associated with pharmacokinetic variability to optimize anti-infective dose design.

A third important principle in considering pharmacogenetic based antimicrobial dosing is that the patient's genes may also determine both the clinical and microbial response. Despite adequate achievement of anti-infective concentration, a patient's genes may lead to sub-therapeutic responses in some patients. In this case, patient genetic factors may alter the chemical microenvironment at sites of infection in such a way that microbial kill by the antimicrobial agent is compromised. A well recognized example of this scenario is patients with genotypic associated deficiencies in mannose binding lectin. Mannose binding lectin is a pathogen recognition receptor that scavenges foreign bodies that contain mannose. Many pathogenic yeast, bacteria, and some medications contain mannose and can bind to these lectins. Once binding has occurred, complement is usually activated. In other cases, a patient's genes may alter clinical response, so that although the pathogen may be killed. Pharmacogenetic factors may also lead to poor clinical outcomes. A classic example encompasses patients who overexpress inflammatory cytokines (interleukin-1β and tumor necrosis factor α). Even though effective therapy has been administered, the cascade of inflammatory responses leads to cardiovascular collapse and multi-system organ failure.

Clinical Pearl

Despite optimal microbial exposures, some patients may still have anti-microbiological failure, or good microbiologic success but poor clinical outcomes, based on pharmacogenetic factors.

In summary, there are pharmacogenetic decision points for the proper use of antimicrobial agents. Thus, pharmacogenetic data should not be just limited to drug choice, but is important also for drug dose and dosing schedule considerations, as well as determining patient outcomes despite adequate pharmacotherapy. The principles of navigating this thought process are discussed above. As the era of individualized anti-infective therapy dawns, these decisions will take center stage in the clinic. Pharmacists will play a central role in crafting genomic based individualized dosing regimens, both in terms of anti-infective choice, agent dose, and dosing schedule, as well as monitoring serum concentrations to reduce toxicity. To illustrate this, pharmacogenetic data that are being used in the clinic will be discussed. Thereafter, the use of pharmacogenetics in design of optimal drug regimens will also be discussed.

Current Clinical Use of Pharmacogenetics in Antimicrobial Chemotherapy

Glucose-6-Phosphate Dehydrogenase (G6PD) Deficiency

G6PD is essential for protection of red cells against oxidative damage. The gene encoding G6PD is on the X-chromosome. G6PD deficiency is common, and affects close to half a billion people worldwide, making it the most common enzyme deficiency. It is believed that this enzymopathy developed via natural selection as a protection against severe malaria.[26] Hundreds of different mutations have been documented as causing G6PD deficiency, resulting in a spectrum that varies from mild to severe enzyme deficiency. The most common variant is G6PD A-, due to Asn126Asp and Val68Met mutation. While G6PD deficiency may protect against malaria, it nevertheless may lead to severe hemolysis in patients treated with certain oxidant agents, especially the antimicrobials dapsone, primaquine, chloroquine, sulfonamides, nalidixic acid, and nitrofurantoin. Although the most common tests for G6PD deficiency are phenotypic, this in fact is one of the most common pharmacogenetic decisions made in clinical care. As an example, in many clinics that take care of patients with AIDS, practitioners often perform G6PD tests prior to prescription of *Pneumocystis jiroveci* pneumonia prophylaxis with sulfonamides. In a recent study in Rwanda, severe hemolysis was shown to be common in children with malaria treated with chlorproguanil-dapsone and artemusate, leading to the recommendation of G6PD screening prior to treatment of all malaria in children in that area.[27] Even in the USA, pharmacists and physicians should be aware of this in the treatment of malaria.

Clinical Pearl

Prior to start of antimalarials, dapsone, or sulfonamides, G6PD status should be elicited in addition to laboratory tests if available and resources permit.

Treatment of Helicobacter Pylori Infection

Helicobacter pylori infection has prevalence rates of up to 80% in some countries, with higher rates in the elderly, and rates lower than 20% in young people. *H. pylori* is the causative organism of peptic ulcer disease and gastric mucosa associated lymphoid tissue lymphoma (MALT). The former is one of the most common medical conditions, with an estimated life-time prevalence of 10-20% in individuals infected with *H. pylori*. Infection is also a major risk factor for the development of gastric cancer. However, *H. pylori* infection can be treated by a combination of a proton pump inhibitor (PPI), clarithromycin, and amoxicillin.

The site of *H. pylori* infection is the gastric and duodenal mucosa, at an acidic pH. Relatively small pH changes, such as ~1 pH unit decrease, markedly reduce microbial kill by clarithromycin. Thus PPIs play a dual role, one of which is increase in pH at site of infection enabling antimicrobial killing by the macrolide. The *H. pylori* infection itself modulates pH by induction of the pro-inflammatory cytokines interleukin-1β (IL-1β) and tumor necrosis factor, which inhibit acid production. Many PPI are oxidized by CYP2C19, whose polymorphs result in three phenotypes: poor metabolizers, intermediate metabolizers, and extensive metabolizers. The relative proportions of the phenotypes vary considerably by ethnic group, with poor metabolizers accounting for 3% of some populations but up to 70% of others. In one clinical study performed in Japan, the 3 most important risk factors for failure of therapy were *H. pylori* resistance to clarithromycin, the CYP2C19 genotype, and an IL-1β-511 polymorphism.[28,29] In addition to human mutations, *H. pylori* resistance to clarithromycin is associated with a bacterial 23S rRNA genotype. Given these factors, Furuta et al randomized 300 patients to either standard therapy of lansoprazole 30 mg bid, clarithromycin 400 mg bid, and amoxicillin 750 mg bid or an experimental regimen based on pharmacogenetics and bacterial genetics.[30] In the experimental group, patients with the *H. pylori* 23S rRNA genotype associated with resistance were randomized to a group that excluded clarithromycin but had amoxicillin of 500 mg qid. Patients in the experimental arm with *H. pylori* that was susceptible were treated with clarithromycin 200 mg tid. CYP2C19 genotyping was then performed, and extensive metabolozers were treated with lansoprazole 30 mg bid, intermediate metabolizers with 15 mg tid, and poor metabolizers with 15 mg bid; all patients received amoxicillin 500 mg bid. Thus all three agents in the regimen were individualized with respect to dose, dose schedule, and agents used in combination. The eradication rate was significantly superior (96%) in the individualized regimens which utilized pharmacogenetics but only 70% in the standard regimen. When cost of genetic tests was taken into consideration, the experimental regimen cost $669 per successful eradication versus $657 for standard regimen.[30] This study demonstrates several important aspects: the therapeutic regimen selection based on bacterial resistance, doses and dosing schedules based on pharmacogenetics, and pharmacogenetic based regimens can be cost neutral while significantly improving outcomes.

Clinical Pearl

Pharmacogenetic based pharmacotherapy can be superior to standard therapy, and if well designed may have not cost significantly more than standard therapy.

Pharmacogenetic Use in the AIDS Clinic

Many SNPs have been implicated as causes of the pharmacokinetic variability in antiretroviral therapy. However, with a few possible exceptions, most of the findings have not been reproduced in large studies. Two examples, however, demonstrate how pharmacogenetics can be used to make informed decisions in the clinic concerning when to start anti-retroviral therapy (possibly), and to predict anti-infective toxicity.

HIV entry into cells is facilitated by an integral membrane protein on the patient's cells called chemokine receptor 5 (CCR5). Some mutations of genes that control this protein influence susceptibility to HIV infection, and the development of AIDS. The CCR5Δ32 mutation has been well studied in this respect, leading to the development of a new class of antiretrovirals in current clinical use (i.e. Maraviroc). It has also been demonstrated that the gene copy number (gene dose) of its ligand CCL3L1 is associated with altered susceptibility to HIV infection. The CCL3L1-CCR5 genes and gene dose also influence the development of HIV to AIDS, with lower copy numbers predicting a more extensive loss of immunological function. Ahuja et al have further demonstrated that in patients with low CCL3L1 copy numbers and detrimental CCR5 genotypes treated with highly effective antiretroviral therapy, there was poor recovery of CD-4 cells (with a CD-4 nadir less than 350 cells/mL).[31] This observation was true despite complete viral suppression, as opposed to patients with other genotypes who had a robust immune recovery with viral suppression.[31] Recovery of CD-4 cell counts improved stepwise with increase in CCL3L1 copy numbers when individuals were treated with highly active antiretroviral therapy. In this case, pharmacogenetic data would be used as a basis of when to start antimicrobial therapy. Specifically, antiretroviral therapy should be initiated prior to severe immune depletion (CD-4 count < 350 cells/mL) in patients with low CCL3L1 copy numbers for the particular ethnic group and detrimental CCR5 genes. This has not yet been implemented in the clinic, but has great potential.

Once a decision is made to treat the AIDS patient, an optimized highly active anti-retroviral regimen is chosen. Optimized regimens have many configurations, but often consist of a base of nucleoside analogues together with either a protease inhibitor or a non-nucleoside reverse transcriptase inhibitor. The best combinations used are based on numerous prior randomized controlled studies. One popular anti-viral in these regimens is abacavir, a nucleoside reverse transcriptase inhibitor that is part of several once a day regimens. The main limitation of abacavir use, other than viral resistance to the anti-infective in some patients, is the development of a life threatening hypersensitivity reaction. Abacavir hypersensitivity is encountered in ~5% of patients. A definitive immunological diagnosis can be made by use of the abacavir skin patch test. It has been demonstrated that most patients with immunologically proven abacavir hypersensitivity carry the major histocompatibility allele HLA-B*5701.[32,33] Mallal et. al. performed a study in which patients to be started on abacavir were randomized to a pharmacogenetic screen for HLA-B*5701 versus the standard clinical approach.[34] Patients who carried this allele were treated with a non abacavir containing regimen. No patient in the HLA-B*5701 screened arm developed immunologically proven abacavir hypersensitivity compared to 2.7% with the standard approach. Thus the pharmacogenetic test had a 100% negative predictive value, and a positive predictive value of ~50%. This genetic test is currently available for clinical use and has also been used to screen Chinese patients for risk of Stevens Johnson Syndrome and flucloxacillin associated drug-induced liver injury.[35]

Clinical Pearl

In all patients being contemplated for abacavir therapy, tests for HLA-B*5701 should be performed prior to initiation of therapy. In the future, this test may be used to screen for the risk of Stevens Johnson Syndrome with selected drug therapy.

Use of Pharmacogenetics to Develop Optimized Antimicrobial Dose Regimens

Current clinical use of pharmacogenetics has centered on finding genes that predict a higher rate of adverse events, and excluding those anti-infectives from the treatment regimen. Recently, an exciting development has been use of pharmacogenetics to develop doses that may optimize pharmacotherapy. Two such studies have been performed with anti-tubercular compounds; isoniazid and pyrazinamide. These examples will be used to illustrate a process that pharmacists will increasingly be involved with, decision of dose to individualize therapy in the clinic.

While the general notion has been that the treatment of tuberculosis is highly effective, recent data have brought that into question. It had been hoped that short course directly observed therapy (DOT), would ensure improved effectiveness and reduce multidrug resistance. However, an examination of 11 randomized clinical trials has thrown considerable doubt as to weather DOTs is more effective than self administered therapy.[36] Secondly, DOT is only associated with a 62% successful clinical outcome in some countries. Thirdly, when successful DOTs for pulmonary tuberculosis were followed by 2 years of observation in a low HIV setting, mortality was 15% per year, recurrence was 23% of new tuberculosis cases with pan-susceptible tuberculosis and 60% in previously treated patients with MDR-tuberculosis.[37] Long term mortality in patients with tuberculosis meningitis successfully treated with DOTs was close to 60% in one study.[38] Even when patients complete DOTs for pulmonary tuberculosis, it is now clear that more than half of patients develop poor pulmonary function based on pulmonary function tests.[39] It is therefore clear that current therapy needs to be optimized and individualized for all of the three major anti-mycobacterials used to treat tuberculosis: isoniazid, pyrazinamide, and rifampin.

Pharmacogenetic Based Optimization of Isoniazid

Based on two independent studies, isoniazid is best optimized by increasing the AUC/MIC ratio.[40,41] Thus, the Hill-type relationship between exposure and effect is best described by AUC/MIC versus microbial kill. That means, in each patient the determinants of microbial kill will be total AUC/MIC exposure, which are based on dose size and clearance (AUC=dose/clearance) as well as the MIC for each isolate. The metabolism of isoniazid by n-acetyltransferase 2 (NAT-2) has been known for decades to be transcribed and translated by a polymorphic gene.[42] Indeed, 88% of the variability in systemic clearance of isoniazid is due to *nat-2* polymorphisms, with weight and any other factors accounting for the remainder of the variation.[43] Based on this observation, Monte Carlo simulations were performed to determine the rate of microbial kill for 300 mg a day of isoniazid based *nat-2* genotype frequencies in different populations of Hong Kong, China, Japan, India, South Africa, and the United States of America.[41] The kill rates encountered in simulated subjects in Hong Kong, Cape Town, and Chennai, were virtually identical with those encountered in clinical trials, demonstrating that these simulations strongly mirrored clinical outcome. In those countries such as China and Japan where the genotypes associated with fast acetylations are common, the standard 300 mg dose of isoniazid achieved AUC/MIC ratios associated with suboptimal kill, especially in patients with high isoniazid MICs still in the "susceptible" range. Since doses of 600 mg a day have been given in the clinic with little increase in toxicity, such doses should be tested in nat-2 genotype patients with fast acetylation in areas where isoniazid MICs are high.

Gender and Weight Based Optimization of Pyrazinamide Dosing

On the other hand, pyrazinamide has experienced somewhat of an improvement in status of late, and is no longer considered the weakest of the three standard anti-infectives. Traditionally, relapse has been believed to be controlled by both rifampin and pyrazinamide. However, in a recent clinical study by Chideya et al., only pyrazinamide concentrations predicted relapse in patients treated with standard four drug therapy.[44] In addition, a recent analysis demonstrated that weight is the most important determinant of relapse of patients treated with standard DOTs therapy in some parts of the USA.[45] It is known that the three important determinants for pyrazinamide pharmacokinetic variability are weight of the patient, genotype (gender), and oral absorption phenotype (slow versus fast).[46] While gender tends not to be regarded as part of pharmacogenetics, it is nevertheless strictly a pharmacogenetic trait, with women achieving a higher clearance of pyrazinamide than men. In addition, systemic clearance of the drug increases progressively as weight increases above 48 kg. Thus, clearance is high in obese patients. Obesity is often part of the metabolic syndrome, likely polygenic and linked to adipokine, lipoprotein, and ectonucleotide pyrophosphatase genes, among many.[47] Pyrazinamide microbial kill is AUC/MIC linked, with optimal effect at an AUC_{0-24hr}/MIC ratio of 209.[48] That means the three most important determinants of microbial kill are weight, gender, and the dose administered to patients. However, resistance suppression is also linked to T_{MIC}. The clinical effectiveness of pyrazinamide in patients with pulmonary tuberculosis is best predicted by AUC/MIC ratios achieved in the epithelial lining fluid.[48] Monte Carlo simulations of 10,000 patients revealed that standard doses of 15-30 mg/kg resulted in success in only 15-53% of patients. Doses of ≥60 mg/kg performed better.[48] This simulation controlled for gender and weight based pharmacokinetic variability as encountered in the USA where 67% of patients are obese along with the MIC distribution in clinical isolates. While doses greater than 40 mg/kg have been associated with higher hepatotoxicity rates in the past, this was based on studies that treated patients for longer than the current 8 weeks of pyrazinamide therapy, and was based in patients of weights lower than currently encountered in the USA. Thus, these higher doses (> 60 mg/kg) are now ready to be tested in the clinic, based on patient weight and gender. In this case, optimized doses were designed for patients with a common co-morbid condition that is under polygeneic control.

Clinical Pearl

Pharmacogenetic based pharmacokinetic variability such as nat-2 genotypes, as well as variability based on anthropometric factors such as weight (itself under polygenic control), can now be incorporated into dose size design using the tools of Monte Carlo simulations and pharmacodynamics, and represent a rational and scientific approach of integrating pharmacogenetics into dose selection.

Summary

There are several points at which pharmacogenetic data can be used in the therapy of infectious diseases. However, pharmacogenetic data is only useful in conjunction with other pharmacokinetic-pharmacodynamic considerations and microbial PK/PD exposures, as well as genotypes of the microbe itself. Firstly, pharmacogenetic data can be used to exclude use of some anti-infectives which would be associated with a high risk of adverse events. An example of that is abacavir and HLA-B*5707, and G6PD in the treatment of malaria. Secondly, a genotypic data may be used in the future to decide timing of initiation of antiretroviral therapy. Thirdly, the actual anti-infective dose and dosing schedule of antimicrobials can be altered based on pharmacogenetic data, as in the case of treatment of peptic ulcer disease and CYP2C19. Fourthly, pharmacogenetics has begun to be prospectively utilized to develop new dosing regimens in the arena of antituberculosis therapy. Knowledge of these processes will place the pharmacist at the center of designs for individualized anti-infective regimens.

References

1. Gogol EB, Cummings CA, Burns RC, et al. Phase variation and microevolution at homopolymeric tracts in *Bordetella pertussis*. *BMC Genomics*. 2007;8:122.
2. Popper SJ, Shimizu C, Shike H, et al. Gene-expression patterns reveal underlying biological processes in Kawasaki disease. *Genome Biol*. 2007;8:R261.
3. Rubins KH, Hensley LE, Wahl-Jensen V, et al. The temporal program of peripheral blood gene expression in the response of nonhuman primates to Ebola hemorrhagic fever. *Genome Biol*. 2007; 8:R174.
4. Simmons CP, Popper S, Dolocek C, et al. Patterns of host genome-wide gene transcript abundance in the peripheral blood of patients with acute dengue hemorrhagic fever. *J Infect Dis*. 2007;195:1097-1107.

5. Marr KA, Balajee SA, Hawn TR, et al. Differential role of MyD88 in macrophage-mediated responses to opportunistic fungal pathogens. *Infect Immun.* 2003;71:5280-5286.

6. Bochud PY, Chien JW, Marr KA, et al. Toll-like receptor 4 polymorphisms and aspergillosis in stem-cell transplantation. *N Engl J Med.* 2008;359:1766-1777.

7. Hung LY, Velichko S, Huang F, et al. Regulation of airway innate and adaptive immune responses: the IL-17 paradigm. *Crit Rev Immunol.* 2008;28:269-279.

8. Kleinnijenhuis J, Joosten LA, van d V, et al. Transcriptional and inflammasome-mediated pathways for the induction of IL-1beta production by *Mycobacterium tuberculosis. Eur J Immunol.* 2009 Jun 19.

9. Sealy PI, Garner B, Swiatlo E, et al. The interaction of mannose binding lectin (MBL) with mannose containing glycopeptides and the resultant potential impact on invasive fungal infection. *Med Mycol.* 2008;46:531-539.

10. Donders GG, Babula O, Bellen G, et al. Mannose-binding lectin gene polymorphism and resistance to therapy in women with recurrent vulvovaginal candidiasis. *BJOG.* 2008;115:1225-1231.

11. Tanaka G, Shojima J, Matsushita I, et al. Pulmonary *Mycobacterium avium* complex infection: association with NRAMP1 polymorphisms. *Eur Respir J.* 2007;30:90-96.

12. Bellamy R, Ruwende C, Corrah T, et al. Variations in the NRAMP1 gene and susceptibility to tuberculosis in West Africans. *N Engl J Med.* 1998;338:640-644.

13. Sanal O, Turkkani G, Gumruk F, et al. A case of interleukin-12 receptor beta-1 deficiency with recurrent leishmaniasis. *Pediatr Infect Dis J.* 2007;26(4):366-368.

14. Ozen M, Ceyhan M, Sanal O, et al. Recurrent Salmonella bacteremia in interleukin-12 receptor beta1 deficiency. *J Trop Pediatr.* 2006;52:296-298.

15. Drusano GL. Antimicrobial pharmacodynamics: critical interactions of 'bug and drug'. *Nat Rev Microbiol.* 2004;2:289-300.

16. Ambrose PG, Bhavnani SM, Rubino CM, et al. Pharmacokinetics-pharmacodynamics of antimicrobial therapy: it's not just for mice anymore. *Clin Infect Dis.* 2007;44:79-86.

17. Craig WA. Pharmacodynamics of antimicrobials: General concepts and applications. In: Nightangle CH, Ambrose PG, Drusano GL, et al., eds. *Antimicrobial Pharmacodynamics in Theory and Practice.* 2nd ed. New York: Informa Healthcare USA, Inc.; 2007:1-19.

18. Moise-Broder PA, Sakoulas G, Eliopoulos GM, et al. Accessory gene regulator group II polymorphism in methicillin-resistant Staphylococcus aureus is predictive of failure of vancomycin therapy. *Clin Infect Dis.* 2004;38:1700-1705.

19. Gonzalez FJ, Nebert DW. Evolution of the P450 gene superfamily: animal-plant 'warfare', molecular drive and human genetic differences in drug oxidation. *Trends Genet.* 1990;6:182-186.

20. Dowell JA, Knebel W, Ludden T, et al. Population pharmacokinetic analysis of anidulafungin, an echinocandin antifungal. *J Clin Pharmacol.* 2004;44:590-598.

21. Andes D. In vivo pharmacodynamics of antifungal drugs in treatment of candidiasis. *Antimicrob Agents Chemother.* 2003;47:1179-1186.

22. Bilello JA, Bauer G, Dudley MN, et al. Effect of 2',3'-didehydro-3'-deoxythymidine in an in vitro hollow-fiber pharmacodynamic model system correlates with results of dose-ranging clinical studies. *Antimicrob Agents Chemother.* 1994;38:1386-1391.

23. Oleson FB, Jr., Berman CL, Kirkpatrick JB, et al. Once-daily dosing in dogs optimizes daptomycin safety. *Antimicrob Agents Chemother.* 2000;44:2948-2953.

24. Louie A, Kaw P, Liu W, et al. Pharmacodynamics of daptomycin in a murine thigh model of *Staphylococcus aureus* infection. *Antimicrob Agents Chemother.* 2001;45:845-851.

25. Gumbo T. Integrating pharmacokinetics, pharmacodynamics and pharmacogenomics to predict outcomes in antibacterial therapy. *Curr Opin Drug Discov Devel.* 2008;11:32-42.

26. Ruwende C, Khoo SC, Snow RW, et al. Natural selection of hemi- and heterozygotes for G6PD deficiency in Africa by resistance to severe malaria. *Nature.* 1995;376:246-249.

27. Fanello CI, Karema C, Avellino P, et al. High risk of severe anaemia after chlorproguanil-dapsone+artesunate antimalarial treatment in patients with G6PD (A-) deficiency. *PLoS One.* 2008; 3:e4031.

28. Furuta T, Shirai N, Xiao F, et al. Polymorphism of interleukin-1beta affects the eradication rates of *Helicobacter pylori* by triple therapy. *Clin Gastroenterol Hepatol.* 2004;2:22-30.

29. Sugimoto M, Furuta T, Shirai N, et al. Influences of proinflammatory and anti-inflammatory cytokine polymorphisms on eradication rates of clarithromycin-sensitive strains of *Helicobacter pylori* by triple therapy. *Clin Pharmacol Ther.* 2006;80:41-50.

30. Furuta T, Shirai N, Kodaira M, et al. Pharmacogenomics-based tailored versus standard therapeutic regimen for eradication of *H. pylori*. *Clin Pharmacol Ther.* 2007;81:521-528.

31. Ahuja SK, Kulkarni H, Catano G, et al. CCL3L1-CCR5 genotype influences durability of immune recovery during antiretroviral therapy of HIV-1-infected individuals. *Nat Med.* 2008;14:413-420.

32. Mallal S, Nolan D, Witt C, et al. Association between presence of HLA-B*5701, HLA-DR7, and HLA-DQ3 and hypersensitivity to HIV-1 reverse-transcriptase inhibitor abacavir. *Lancet.* 2002;359:727-732.

33. Hetherington S, Hughes AR, Mosteller M, et al. Genetic variations in HLA-B region and hypersensitivity reactions to abacavir. *Lancet.* 2002;359:1121-1122.

34. Mallal S, Phillips E, Carosi G, et al. HLA-B*5701 screening for hypersensitivity to abacavir. *N Engl J Med.* 2008;358(6):568-579.

35. Daly AK, Donaldson PT, Bhatnagar P, et al. HLA-B*5701 genotype is a major determinant of drug-induced liver injury due to flucloxacillin. *Nat Genet.* 2009;41:816-819.

36. Volmink J, Garner P. Directly observed therapy for treating tuberculosis. *Cochrane Database Syst Rev.* 2007;4:CD003343.

37. Cox H, Kebede Y, Allamuratova S, et al. Tuberculosis recurrence and mortality after successful treatment: impact of drug resistance. *PLoS Med.* 2006;3:e384.

38. Shaw JET, Gumbo T. TB meningitis has poor long term outcome despite standard therapy. Paper presented 48th Interscience Conference of Antimicrobial Agents and Chemotherapy and 46th Infectious Diseases Society of America, Oct 25, 2008; Washington, DC.

39. Pasipanodya JG, Miller TL, Vecino M, et al. Pulmonary impairment after tuberculosis. *Chest.* 2007;131:1817-1824.

40. Jayaram R, Shandil RK, Gaonkar S, et al. Isoniazid pharmacokinetics-pharmacodynamics in an aerosol infection model of tuberculosis. *Antimicrob Agents Chemother.* 2004;48:2951-2957.

41. Gumbo T, Louie A, Liu W, et al. Isoniazid bactericidal activity and resistance emergence: integrating pharmacodynamics and pharmacogenomics to predict efficacy in different ethnic populations. *Antimicrob Agents Chemother.* 2007;51:2329-2336.

42. Evans DA, Manley KA, McKusick VA. Genetic control of isoniazid metabolism in man. *BMJ.* 1960;2:485-491.

43. Kinzig-Schippers M, Tomalik-Scharte D, Jetter A, et al. Should we use N-acetyltransferase type 2 genotyping to personalize isoniazid doses? *Antimicrob Agents Chemother.* 2005;49:1733-1738.

44. Chideya S, Winston CA, Peloquin CA, et al. Isoniazid, rifampin, ethambutol, and pyrazinamide pharmacokinetics and treatment outcomes among a predominantly HIV-infected cohort of adults with tuberculosis from Botswana. *Clin Infect Dis.* 2009;48:1685-1694.

45. Pasipanodya JG, Hall G, Weis S, et al. Fat, fractals and failure of antituberculosis therapy. Paper presented 49th Interscience Conference of Antimicrobial Agents and Chemotherapy, Sept 14, 2009; San Francisco.

46. Wilkins JJ, Langdon G, McIlleron H, et al. Variability in the population pharmacokinetics of pyrazinamide in South African tuberculosis patients. *Eur J Clin Pharmacol.* 2006;62:727-735.

47. Joy T, Lahiry P, Pollex RL, et al. Genetics of metabolic syndrome. *Curr Diab Rep.* 2008;8:141-148.

48. Gumbo T, Siyambalapitiyage Dona CS, Meek C, et al. Pharmacokinetics-pharmacodynamics of pyrazinamide in a novel in vitro model of tuberculosis for sterilizing effect: A paradigm for faster assessment of new antituberculosis drugs. *Antimicrob Agents Chemother.* 2009;53:3197-3204.

Chapter 11

Respiratory Diseases

Emily Weidman-Evans, Pharm.D., AE-C, CPE;
W. Greg Leader, Pharm.D.

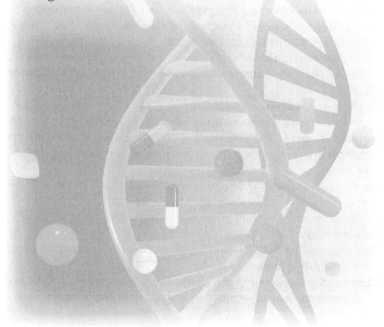

Learning Objectives

After completing this chapter, the reader should be able to

- Describe the interpatient variability in therapeutic efficacy and adverse effects seen in asthmatic patients with β_2-agonists, inhaled corticosteroids, and leukotriene modifiers.
- Explain the genetic variants that can affect the response to treatment with the above drug classes in asthmatic patients.
- Discuss the pros and cons of genetic testing in asthma.
- Describe the role of the cystic fibrosis transmembrane conductance regulator in the pathophysiology of pulmonary disease in cystic fibrosis.
- Discuss the various classes of mutations in the cystic fibrosis transmembrane conductance regulator and their relation to cystic fibrosis phenotype.
- Explain the potential role of "correctors" and "potentiators" in the treatment of cystic fibrosis.

Key Definitions

Allele—One of a pair of genes on a specific location of a chromosome that control the same trait.

Binding motif—A short, highly conserved region in a protein sequence that is involved in binding.

Biofilm—Structural layer of microorganisms adhered to a surface and held together and protected by a polymeric matrix formed from secreted or extracellular substances.

Bronchiectasis—Localized and irreversible dilation of the bronchiole or bronchi due to airway inflammation and obstruction.

Chemoattractant—Inorganic or organic substance that induces or influences cell migration.

Forced expiratory volume in 1 second (FEV1)—The volume of air that can be forced out in the first second after taking a deep breath.

Interpatient variability—Differences in response to drug(s) between patients.

Isoflavone—Naturally occurring organic compounds derived almost exclusively from the bean family.

Nasal potential difference—A measurement of the voltage across the nasal epithelial cell determined by using a high impedance voltmeter between two electrodes, one placed on the inside and one on the outside of the epithelia. The nasal potential difference characterizes the voltage created by the secretion or absorption of chloride ions that are abnormal in cystic fibrosis.

Opsonophagocytosis—The process by which a foreign body (usually microbial) is identified by compliment or antigens to phagocytes resulting in a more efficient energy dependent endocytosis (or engulfment) of the microbe by the phagocytic cell (usually a neutrophil or macrophage).

Peak expiratory flow (PEF)—The maximum airflow during a forced expiration beginning with the lungs fully inflated.

Ubiquitination—Degradation of a protein caused by modification of the protein by covalent attachment of ubiquitin, a regulatory protein, which directs the protein to proteosomes for degradation.

Introduction

Asthma and cystic fibrosis (CF) are two very different conditions that both have major effects on the respiratory system. Asthma is defined by chronic inflammation of the airways and bronchoconstriction, both results of multiple genetic and environmental factors. Cystic fibrosis is a genetic condition that also affects other organ systems, with a mutation in the gene encoding for one single channel identified as causing the condition. The presence of other genetic and environmental factors affect the severity and presentation of both of these diseases. There are a large number of effective medications for the control of asthma symptoms, and well-accepted clinical guidelines to direct treatment. Treatment for CF is symptomatic, and, for the most part, palliative. Deaths resulting from asthma are relatively rare, especially with appropriate treatment. Cystic fibrosis is almost always fatal.

In keeping with these many differences, the pharmacogenomic research that has been applied to the conditions differs, as well. In asthma, a large degree of interpatient variability in response to the available treatments has led to retrospective pharmacogenetic analyses to identify genetic differences that may affect responses to currently accepted therapy. The identification of mutations that can impact the efficacy and safety of treatment might then allow for rational changes in drug therapy before an exacerbation or adverse effect occurs. In CF, on the other hand, genetic mutations that affect the severity of the disease have been identified, and new therapies are being prospectively investigated that will address the physiologic effects of the mutations at the level of the affected protein. The results of this research may result in alterations of the actual disease process, which has not been available to date. In spite of the differences in approach, however, the end result of the pharmacogenomic research in both of these conditions may be improved patient health and clinical outcomes, which is the ultimate goal of all healthcare providers.

Asthma

Introduction

Asthma is a chronic, often progressive, inflammatory disorder of the airways that is characterized by airway hyperresponsiveness, airflow limitation, and respiratory symptoms like wheezing and coughing.[1] It affects over 22 million people in the United States, over ¼ of which are children. The severity and type of presentation, or phenotype, of the disease is highly variable, and classified based upon spirometric markers, as well as reported symptoms and medication use. It is now accepted that the presence of inflammation in asthma is consistent regardless of disease severity and is regulated by a vast number of inflammatory cells and mediators. However, there is even a large degree of interpatient variability in the concentration and types of these cells and mediators.

As shown in Table 11-1, asthma treatment modalities have been designed to target the underlying inflammatory process as well as the resultant bronchospasm and constriction. Inhaled corticosteroids (ICS), the current mainstay of "controller" therapy, as well as leukotriene (LT) modifiers, cromolyn, and the anti-IgE antibody omalizumab all target various steps in the inflammatory process. Long- and short-acting β_2-agonists (LABA and SABA) and theophylline target bronchoconstriction.

Table 11-1
2007 National Asthma Education and Prevention Program Treatment Recommendations[1]

Severity Classification	Preferred Treatment	Alternative Treatment
Step 6	High-dose ICS + LABA + oral corticosteroid	Consider adding omalizumab for those with allergies
Step 5	High-dose ICS plus LABA	Consider adding omalizumab for those with allergies
Step 4	Medium-dose ICS plus LABA	Medium-dose ICS plus either theophylline or LTRA
Step 3	Low-dose ICS plus LABA –or– Medium-dose ICS	Low-dose ICS plus either theophylline or LTRA
Step 2	Low-dose ICS	Cromolyn sodium –or– LTRA –or– Sustained release theophylline
Step 1 (intermittent)	No daily medication needed	
ALL patients	SABA as needed for symptoms	

ICS = inhaled corticosteroid; LABA = long-acting β2-agonist; LTRA = leukotriene receptor antagonist; SABA = short-acting β2-agonist.

Genetics

Asthma perhaps is one of the most studied applications of pharmacogenomics. There are several possible reasons for this. It has long been established that there is a genetic link in asthma, although the etiology is complex, involving interactions of multiple genes and a variety of environmental factors, including allergens and infections.[2] Independent genome-wide screens have found regions of linkage with asthma susceptibility and severity on chromosomes 5, 6, 11, 12, 13, 16, 17 and 19. It is only logical, then, to begin pharmacogenomic research based upon differences in these genetic regions.

In spite of the well-accepted treatment guidelines for this condition, a large degree of interpatient variability in treatment response was noted in drug studies. Fortunately, we do have a relatively good grasp on the precise mechanisms of the drugs that are being used to treat asthma. Therefore, identifying potential genetic targets that involve the receptors or mediators affected by the drugs is easier. To date, specific genes have been identified that affect bronchodilation directly, the production and action of drug receptors, and a number of steps in the inflammatory process (including T-cell proliferation and recruitment, macrophage recruitment, mast cell proliferation, antigen presentation, and inhibition of cytokine activity).[3] The genetic variances that impact three common classes of drugs used in asthma are presented below.

β_2-Agonists

Beta-2 adrenergic receptors (B_2AR) are widely distributed throughout the respiratory tract and when activated, couple with adenylate cyclase and induce airway relaxation.[4] They are also thought to increase airway smooth muscle relaxation by acting directly to increase the flux of potassium out of the muscle cell and thus decrease the membrane potential. Based upon this dual mechanism for airway relaxation, B_2AR agonists (a.k.a. β_2-agonists) are among the most prescribed drugs for asthma. They are used to produce prompt bronchodilation and provide symptomatic relief.[5] As shown in Table 11-1, short-acting β_2-agonists (SABAs) such as albuterol or pirbuterol are recommended as symptomatic "rescue" treatment for ALL patients diagnosed with asthma.[1] Long-acting β_2-agonists (LABAs) such as salmeterol or formoterol are recommended as add-on "controller" therapy when low- or medium-dose inhaled corticosteroids (ICSs) are not adequately controlling asthma symptoms.

Interpatient Variability

While the current clinical guidelines are clear in their recommendations for the appropriate use of β_2-agonists (short- and long-acting), as many as 70% to 80% of patients will have some variability in their response to these drugs, both in terms of symptom relief and adverse effects.[6] There was actually an increase in asthma mortality rates worldwide in the 1960's with the introduction of β_2-agonists to the market.[7] Regularly scheduled SABA use has been shown to increase bronchial hyperreactivity in many patients, and has also been repeatedly associated with tolerance to the drug's effects and thus, a further worsening of symptoms.[7, 8]

There is more recent controversy surrounding the use of LABAs as well. After numerous post-marketing reports to the FDA, the results of the Salmeterol Multi-center Asthma Research Trial (SMART) showed 2 asthma-related deaths per 1000 patient-years of salmeterol use, a four-fold increase over those not receiving the drug.[9] A meta-analysis of nineteen trials (n = 33,826, including the 26,000 from SMART) comparing a LABA to placebo showed similar results, with a 0.06% to 0.07% absolute increase in asthma-related deaths, as well as increases in severe asthma exacerbations and asthma-related hospitalizations.[7] These increases were more pronounced in the black subjects.

Clinical Pearl

It was theorized at the time that the disparity seen in black subjects in the SMART trial was due to either more severe underlying disease and/or the fact that the baseline ICS use in this sub-population was lower.

Genetic Variants Affecting Treatment

The high degree of interpatient variability in response to β_2-agonists, as well as the possible relationship between treatment and race exhibited in SMART, leads to questions regarding a possible genetic cause of the variability. Table 11-2 shows the three coding single nucleotide polymorphisms (SNPs) in the B_2AR gene, which is located on chromosome 5q31-32, that could contribute to some of the demonstrated differences in individual responses to β_2-agonists in asthma and other respiratory diseases.[5,10] These SNPs are substitutions of glycine for arginine at the 16th amino acid (Gly-16), of glutamate for glutamine at the 27th amino acid (Glu-27), and of isoleucine for threonine at the 164th amino acid (Ile-164). While it has been hypothesized that one or more of these polymorphisms predict the susceptibility or severity of disease, all three occur with the same frequency in both asthmatic and non-asthmatic patients, showing that none of them are the cause of asthma, per se.[5,11]

Table 11-2
Clinically Significant SNPs of the B_2AR

SNP	Frequency of (homozygotes)[6,11,12,118,119]	Response to β_2-agonists[5,11]
Gly-16	Overall: 54.8–60.4 White: 60.7 Asian: 46.0 Black: 45.0	Enhanced down-regulation → maximal down-regulation from endogenous catecholamines → decreased tachyphylaxis to regular administration of drug
Glu-27	Overall: 24.7–47.2 White: 36.1 Asian: 13.6 Black: 18.0	Inability to down-regulate → no tachyphylaxis with regular administration of drug
Ile-164	Overall: 5.0	Decreased coupling with adenylate cyclase; decreased binding of drug to receptor → decreased drug activity *(theoretical)*

Gly-16

This relatively common polymorphism might be associated with a more severe asthma phenotype.[12] Several studies have shown that those patients with the wild-type receptor (Arg-16) who were receiving a regularly scheduled SABA experienced decreases in peak expiratory flow readings (PEFR) and forced expiratory volume (FEV_1). This patient population also exhibited a worsening of daily symptoms, increases in the amount of rescue medication required, and an increased number of exacerbations.[13-15] Those who were homozygous for Gly-16 did not experience these negative changes, and some even improved. Furthermore, those patients who were only receiving intermittent (as needed) therapy with a SABA did not exhibit these negative outcomes. As Gly-16 results in enhanced down-regulation of the B_2AR, it is theorized that endogenous catecholamines lead to maximal down-regulation of the receptors in those with this polymorphism. Thus, they cannot be further down-regulated by the SABA, leading to a decrease in the tachyphylaxis seen in the wild-type receptor with regular SABA administration.

Due to the relationship between genotype and response to SABAs, as well as the recent controversy surrounding the use of LABAs, several studies have been conducted to determine the relationship between LABAs and the Gly-16 SNP, unfortunately the results are conflicting. A pharmacogenetic analysis conducted by Bleeker and colleagues of two trials that used either

salmeterol or formoterol showed no difference between genotypes in exacerbations, spirometric measures (PEFR and FEV1), or adverse effects.[16] All of the subjects in this analysis received
ICS in addition to a LABA. Conversely, a similar analysis conducted by Weschler and colleagues
of two large studies utilizing salmeterol showed that those subjects who were homozygous for
the wild-type receptor had lower spirometric measures and increased symptoms and albuterol
use regardless of concurrent ICS use.[17] Those homozygous for Gly-16 all showed an improvements in spirometric and symptomatic measures during the study periods. A retrospective
study in 546 children and young asthmatics showed a two-fold increase in exacerbations in
those with Arg-16. In those who were receiving salmeterol, the risk increased to over three
times that of those with Gly-16.[18]

Glu–27

The Glu-27 polymorphism is actually considered protective since it is associated with decreased airway reactivity.[12] While it does not affect the bronchodilator response to SABAs, studies have shown that patients with this polymorphism do not experience the increase in adverse
events with regularly scheduled albuterol noted with the Arg-16 genotype. This beneficial effect
is likely due to a lack of down-regulation of the receptor, and thus a lack of tachyphylaxis to
the drug's effects.[13,18,19] A study in young asthmatics showed that this polymorphism had no
impact on exacerbations, regardless of salmeterol use.[18]

Ile–164

Since the Ile-164 is a rare polymorphism, very little research has been conducted as to the
clinical implications for those patients with asthma who harbor this SNP. In vitro, however, the
activity of the receptors displaying this polymorphism was about half that of wild-type receptors.[11]
Furthermore, studies in transgenic mice showed a decreased cardiac response to isoproterenol
when compared to mice with the wild-type receptor, leading to the hypothesis that those with this
polymorphism could also have a lower baseline bronchodilator response to inhaled β_2 agonists.

Inhaled Corticosteroids

Inhaled corticosteroids (ICS) are recommended as first-line therapy for nearly all patients with
asthma (Table 11-1).[1] While they may vary in dosage form, administration schedule, potency,
and systemic bioavailability, all of the ICS exert their anti-inflammatory effects primarily by
binding to the glucocorticoid receptor (GR).[20] This in turn activates various anti-inflammatory
genes and represses the expression of pro-inflammatory genes.

Interpatient Variability

Interpatient variability in response to corticosteroids has been demonstrated in a number of
disease states including inflammatory bowel disorder (IBD), psoriasis, nephritic syndrome, and
various cancers. The term "glucocorticoid resistance" has been coined to define this variability.
In asthma, it has been shown that 5% to 10% of patients will have a reduced response to ICS.[10]
This number increases to 35% in those with severe disease, and to as many as 40% of black
patients with asthma. A 12-week study showed that 22% of subjects experienced a decrease in
their FEV1 of 5% or more with inhaled beclomethasone therapy, while 10% improved by more
than 40%.[21] Another study showed 38% of subjects respond minimally to beclomethasone or
fluticasone over 24 weeks of therapy.[22] In both of these studies, the average response was about
a 10% increase in FEV1.

There is less evidence regarding variability in the frequency and severity of adverse effects associated with ICS, most likely because systemic adverse effects are relatively rare. However, one study showed a significant relationship between doses of inhaled triamcinolone, a highly bioavailable ICS, and decreases in bone density. Analysis of individual response showed a large amount of variability in the degree of bone loss experienced between patients that was independent of the number of puffs per day, suggesting factors other than dose contributing to this adverse effect.[23]

Genetic Variants Affecting Treatment

Due to the broad effects of corticosteroids, it is more difficult to pinpoint appropriate genetic targets for focus in pharmacogenomic studies involving ICS. Studies involving genes that code for several key receptors, however, have shown promise in identifying hypo- and hyper responders to ICS.

Corticotropin Releasing Hormone Receptor-1

The gene that encodes for corticotropin releasing hormone receptor-1 (CRHR1) was chosen as a potential target for research because it is the primary receptor mediating the release of adrenocorticotropin hormone (ACTH), a major regulator of glucocorticoid and catecholamine synthesis.[24,25] This gene, located on chromosome 17q21-22, has been implicated in the pathogenesis of inflammatory diseases, and is located in a region linked to asthma in some genome-wide screens. It is hypothesized that alterations in the expression or function of this receptor as a result of genetic variation can lead to decreased ACTH release. This will, in turn, decrease cortisol release in response to inflammation and possibly upregulate corticosteroid receptors. When a patient is given exogenous corticosteroids, then, they will have a more pronounced response.[25]

Variations in CRHR1 have been associated with double to quadruple the response to ICS, when compared to those without the variations.[25] One SNP in particular, rs242941, has been linked to a significant increase in response. This SNP, however, is intronic, so it does not have any effect on the CRHR1 unless it is present in a specific haplotype, designated GAT. This haplotype is present in 27% of whites. A retrospective pharmacogenetic analysis showed that, while all patients on ICS had improved FEV1 after 8 weeks of therapy, GAT homozygotes experienced a two- to three-fold increase in that improvement. Heterozygotes' response fell in between that of homozygotes and those without the GAT haplotype.

T-box Expressed in T Cells (Transcription Factor T-bet)

Transcription factor T-bet plays an important role in the inflammatory process. It influences the development of naïve T-lymphocytes, induces the production of interferon-gamma and represses the production of interleukins 4 and 5.[26] The gene that encodes for T-bet, TBX21, is also located on chromosome 17q21.[27] It has been shown that asthmatic patients have a decreased number of T-cells that express TBX21, and that deletion of this gene in mice results in airway hyperresponsiveness. Furthermore, several mutations of TBX21 have been associated with both asthma susceptibility and severity in humans.[27] The SNP rs2240017, which results in the substitution of glutamine for histidine at the 33rd amino acid (Gln-33), has been linked to a significant increase in response to ICS.[26] A retrospective pharmacogenetic analysis in 701 children showed that those with the SNP had about a three-fold improvement in their PC20 (provocative concentration of histamine causing a 20% fall in FEV1; a measure of airway responsiveness), when compared to those with the wild-type gene. In fact, the mean PC20 for those subjects on ICS with the SNP was 27.7 mg/mL. Anything >25 mg/mL indicates "normal" airway responsiveness. FEV1 increased to a similar extent in all subjects receiving ICS, regardless of the presence of the SNP. The subjects included in this analysis, about 4.5% of the study population, were all heterozygotes for the SNP. The frequency of homozygosity for this beneficial mutation varies greatly based upon race: white 2.7% to 3.0%; black 0.4% to 2%; Hispanic 7.1%; and Korean 11.8%.[27]

Glucocorticoid Receptor Gene (GR/NR3C1)

Another logical genetic target would be the gene that encodes for the glucocorticoid receptor (GR) itself. This receptor has two naturally occurring isoforms: GRα, which is functional and involved in regulating proinflammatory mediators, and GRβ, which has no hormone binding activity and is actually considered an endogenous inhibitor of actions mediated by the GR.[10] An imbalance of either of these isoforms due to a genetic anomaly can lead to glucocorticoid resistance. It is known that 95% of patients with glucocorticoid resistance have type I resistance, which is associated with an increased expression of GRβ.[28,29] The patient will often present with severe systemic side effects, but will have minimal therapeutic effects. Conversely, Type II glucocorticoid resistance is associated with a decrease in GRα, which results in a generalized primary cortisol resistance. These patients typically do not experience either therapeutic or adverse effects when administered ICS. However, the specific mutation(s) that result(s) in this imbalance have not yet been identified.

Leukotriene Modifiers

Leukotrienes (LT) are synthesized from arachidonic acid via the 5-lipoxygenase (ALOX5) pathway.[6] Three of these substances in particular, LTC4, LTD4, and LTE4 (the "cysteinyl leukotrienes," or cys-LT) are known to contribute to many of the abnormalities seen in asthma including airway obstruction, excess mucus secretion, edema, and eosinophil recruitment. Leukotriene modifiers include receptor antagonists (LTRAs), such as montelukast and zafirlukast, and ALOX5 inhibitors, such as zileuton. LTRAs are important as add-on or alternative therapy in patients with all stages of asthma (Table 11-1).

Interpatient Variability

While not as widely studied as the β$_2$-agonists and ICS, one study showed the distribution of responses with montelukast to be similar to that seen with inhaled beclomethasone. Forty-two percent of those receiving montelukast had an increase in FEV1 of more than 10%, while 34% of patients had no improvement or a worsening in FEV1.[21] Since LT appear linked to asthma susceptibility and severity, it is theorized that variations in therapeutic response to this class of drugs are at least partially mediated by the concentration of LT.[6] This suggests that asthma may be mediated by factors other than LT and that LT modifiers will be less effective in those patients with lower concentrations of LT. Conversely, higher concentrations of these mediators could indicate a better response to LT modifiers.

Serious adverse effects with the LTRAs are relatively rare, but zileuton has been linked to hepatotoxicity and even rare causes of hepatic failure. One safety surveillance study showed that 4.4% of subjects receiving zileuton (600 mg four times daily) had elevations in ALT (alanine aminotransferase) to greater than three times the upper limit of normal; 1.3% had elevations greater than 8 times the upper limit.[30] Women were more likely than men to experience these significant elevations, as were the elderly. No genetic studies have been performed, but it is possible that the genetic mutations discussed below, or others, could contribute to this adverse effect.

Clinical Pearl

Zileuton was removed from the U.S. market, but re-released in 2005, at the urging of health-care professionals. In July 2008, the four times daily immediate release drug was replaced by a once-daily formulation.

Genetic Variants Affecting Treatment

Based upon the hypothesis presented above, genes encoding for three key enzymes involved in LT production have been identified as possible targets.

5-Lipoxygenase Promoter Gene

The enzyme 5-lipoxygenase (ALOX5) is involved very early in the LT synthesis process, converting arachidonic acid to 5-hydroperoxyeicosatetraenoic acid (5-HPETE), and then converting 5-HPETE to LTA4.[31] The promoter gene for this enzyme, located on chromosome 10q11, contains a regulatory region with five tandem repeats of the binding motif.[32,33] Table 11-3 shows the frequencies of the variants of this and other enzyme promoter genes in the LT synthesis pathway, and highlights the racial differences that exist.[34]

Table 11-3
Frequency and Effects of Variant Promoter Genes in the LT Synthesis Pathway

Variant Promoter Gene	Homozygotes (%)[34]	Heterozygotes (%)[34]	Effect on FEV1[6,34,35,38]	Effect on Exacerbations[34]
ALOX5	Overall: <1 White: 3.6 Black: 24.6	Overall: 36 White: 33 Black: 57	+/−	−
LTC4 synthase	Overall: 11	Overall: 38	+	−
LTA4 hydrolase	Overall: 8	Overall: 44	NE	+

LT = leukotriene; FEV1 = forced expiratory volume in 1 second; ALOX5 = 5-lipoxygenase.
+ = Increased.
− = Decreased.
+/− = Conflicting evidence.
NE = Not evaluated.

It has been theorized that certain variant alleles result in a decrease in LT production; therefore, it is likely that the airway obstruction experienced in patients with these altered promoter genes is caused by mechanisms other than LT. Patients with these variants will be less responsive to LT modifiers.[6] This theory is supported by two studies that showed significant increases in FEV1 (9.1% to 18.8%) in subjects homozygous for the wild-type gene, compared to a small decrease (1.1% to 2.3%) in those with mutations of the gene.[6,35] Another study showed that those homozygous for the polymorphism had no change in FEV1, β_2-agonist use, or number of asthma exacerbations after 12 weeks of montelukast treatment, while those homo- and heterozygous for the wild-type gene had significant improvements in each of these parameters.[36] Other research, however, has shown opposite outcomes. One study that compared percent change in FEV1 and exacerbations with montelukast showed that homozygotes for the variant gene had a fifteen-fold greater increase in FEV1 when compared to homozygotes for the wild-type gene.[34] In addition, those with at least one mutant allele had a 73% reduction in exacerbations (at least one during the 6-month study period). Obviously, further studies are necessary to clarify this apparent discrepancy.

Leukotriene C4 Synthase Promoter Gene

Leukotriene C4 (LTC4) synthase is a late-stage enzyme in the LT production process that is responsible for converting LTA4 to LTC4.[37] One specific variant in the promoter gene for this enzyme, located on chromosome 5q35, is the SNP A(-444)C (rs730012), has been identified in 32% of non-asthmatic patients, 56% of those with severe asthma, and 76% of those with aspirin intolerant asthma (AIA).[38] This variant enhances the expression of LTC4 synthase, thus increasing LTC4 production. It is hypothesized that since LTC4 and its products contribute so significantly to asthma physiology, those with this SNP would be good responders to LT modifiers. This theory is supported by a small study that involved administering zafirlukast for 2 weeks to 23 subjects with severe asthma and 31 non-asthmatic subjects. Those subjects with at least one variant allele for the promoter gene had a 9% increase in FEV1, compared to a 12% decrease in those with the wild-type gene. Furthermore, subjects homo- or heterozygous for the mutant gene had an 80% reduction in exacerbations while taking montelukast.[34] Interestingly, those with at least one variant allele receiving placebo also had a significant decrease in exacerbations (69%), when compared to those homozygous for the wild-type gene.

Leukotriene A4 Hydrolase Promoter Gene

The Leukotriene A4 (LTA4) hydrolase enzyme is responsible for converting LTA4 to LTB4. The presence of one SNP (rs2660845) in its promoter gene, located on chromosome 12q22, has been linked with up to a four-fold increase in the risk of patients having at least one exacerbation when taking montelukast.[34] This difference was not observed between genotypes in those receiving placebo. The effect on LTA4 hydrolase activity as a result of this SNP is unknown. It is possible that the increase in exacerbations results from a decrease in the activity of LTA4 hydrolase, which leads to more LTA4 being converted to LTC4 and increased asthma symptoms. Conversely, the variant could increase the activity of LTA4 hydrolase, thus decreasing the production of the cys-LT. This would result in a decreased therapeutic response to LT modifiers.

Case Study

RP is an 8-year-old African American male admitted for the third time this year as a result of an asthma exacerbation. His current medications include fluticasone/salmeterol (dry powder inhaler) 500 mcg/50 mcg twice daily, montelukast 5 mg daily, and albuterol (metered-dose inhaler) 1–2 puffs as needed. At his last admission, he was sent home with a 10-day course of prednisone, started on montelukast, and his dose of fluticasone/salmeterol was increased from 250 mcg/50 mcg. In the 24 hours prior to this admission, RP's mother states that he probably used his albuterol ten times, and that it "just didn't seem to work." Furthermore, you note that his FEV1 is currently only 50% of expected, and that it is not reversing with the administration of albuterol via nebulizer. Since he is on an appropriate therapeutic regimen, the clinical team decides that RP is a good candidate for genetic testing.

1. How would you explain to RP's mother the specific benefits and risks of genetic testing to her son?
2. For what variants would you test in RP? Why?
3. How would you adjust RP's therapy, based upon the possible results of those tests?

Clinical Implications

The data for each of the genetic variants discussed above strongly suggest that clinical measures are being affected by the presence or absence of certain polymorphisms. It can be proposed that knowledge of specific genetic variants could help healthcare providers individualize therapy, and make adjustments before a patient has an exacerbation or adverse effect. There are assays currently available for identifying the mutations discussed above, but they are not commonly used in practice due to their high cost. The debate continues regarding the clinical, legal, and ethical implications surrounding widespread genetic testing. The impact of pharmacogenomic testing on clinical decision making, patient privacy, and costs of healthcare is discussed throughout this book. For example, there are proven racial differences in the frequencies of many of the mutations covered here. African Americans are less likely than whites to have the beneficial variants in B2AR and CRHR1, but more likely to have the potentially positive mutation in ALOX5. Could this finding lead to racial profiling in the application of genetic testing, prior to initiating or altering therapy, or in obtaining healthcare insurance?

There is some overlap in genetic polymorphisms with regards to the pathophysiology and susceptibility of asthma with that of both chronic obstructive pulmonary disease (COPD) and allergic rhinitis/atopic dermatitis.[39-41] This genetic overlap is important since there are many similarities in the treatments of these conditions. As per the 2007 Global Initiative for Chronic Obstructive Lung Disease guidelines, β_2-agonists and corticosteroids are indicated for a large proportion of patients with COPD. Similarly, the 2008 update of the World Health Organization's Allergic Rhinitis and its Impact on Asthma guidelines state intranasal corticosteroids are the most effective treatment for allergic rhinitis, and the LT modifier montelukast should be considered in all patients over the age of six.[42,43] While no definitive studies have been done, given these similarities in etiology and treatment, the question must be asked if the genetic variants identified as having a potential effect on asthma therapy will have similar effects in COPD and allergic rhinitis.

To Test or Not to Test?

In the case of asthma, the possibility of widespread genetic testing is not simply a far-off dream. There is presently an at-home test for the Gly-16 polymorphism. This test kit is commercially available from a number of sources for patients to order independent of a healthcare provider (in most states).[44] The test involves a self-performed cheek swab that is mailed to the testing company. The cost to the patient is approximately $300. The patient will then receive a report to discuss with his or her healthcare provider. The ready availability of this test leads to a number of questions, which could be applied to any class of medication for which testing is made available, regarding its utility, implications for therapeutic decision making, and cost-effectiveness.

The test claims 99% sensitivity, and is simple to perform, but results in a report fairly heavy with medical jargon that might be difficult for many patients to understand.[44,45] If the report is not discussed with a healthcare provider there is the concern that a patient may discontinue therapy on his or her own, which could result in further negative outcomes. Likewise, the amount of knowledge and training that the interpreting healthcare provider has will also impact the action that is taken, and whether it is appropriate or not.

Each of the drug classes discussed above play a very large role in the treatment and management of asthma. Therefore, it is important to consider the alternatives in patients for whom these drugs might not be optimal. There is a likelihood that a large proportion of the asthmatic population with the polymorphisms discussed in this chapter may possess more than one at a time. The usefulness of testing for only one variant involving one drug class must be questioned. The overall genetic make-up of the patient must be considered since addressing only one polymorphism could actually be detrimental. If a patient is tested and has the Arg-16 B_2AR, the alternatives for the β_2-agonists (SABA and LABA) are limited. The current options for short-acting bronchodilation are limited to anticholinergics like ipratropium, which has a longer onset and duration of action than albuterol. Higher doses of ICS might be necessary to obtain adequate long-term control, in lieu of adding a LABA. If the patient also has an increased therapeutic response to ICS through variants in the CRHR1 or TBX21 genes, or has Type I glucocorticoid resistance, they could be more at risk for systemic adverse effects from the higher-dose ICS. Alternatively, a LT modifier could be added to a patient's regimen, but the efficacy and safety of these drugs as the sole "controller" medications have been questioned, especially if the patient is a non-responder who possesses the LTC4 synthase promoter gene SNP A(-444)C.

The commercially available test for the B2AR mutation is fairly expensive to the patient, and is likely not to be covered by third-party payers at this time. Arguments for universal testing could be made from a cost-effectiveness standpoint, however. In 2008 dollars, the average direct cost of an asthma-related emergency department visit is $315, which is only slightly more than the cost of the test itself.[46] An asthma-related hospitalization costs about $4,150, but ranges anywhere from $2,700 to more than $20,000. Currently there is no data linking the frequency of negative asthma outcomes with genetic makeup, but these figures suggest that it might be cost-effective to test as many as thirteen patients, if one asthma-related hospitalization could be prevented through changes in the approach to therapy. Considering the complex relationships between outcomes, genetics, and environment, no recommendation could be made based upon these numbers alone, however.

A lack of long-term outcomes studies make it unclear whether there is a role for universal genetic screening of asthmatic patients, due to therapeutic limitations and cost-effectiveness concerns. However, the pharmacogenomic data related to β_2-agonists, ICS, and LT modifiers suggest the need for consideration of genetic factors in patients who are not responding optimally to therapy sooner rather than later.

Cystic Fibrosis

Introduction

Cystic fibrosis (CF), the most common lethal genetic disease in the Caucasian population, is an autosomal recessive disorder that results from a mutation at a single gene location on chromosome 7 resulting in mutations in the CF transmembrane conductance regulator (CFTR) protein. In 1989 the gene was identified by positional cloning,[47] and today over 1600 mutations of the CFTR have been reported.[48] This defect affects exocrine glands in epithelial cells lining the lungs, intestinal tract, pancreatic ducts, sweat glands, biliary tree and vas deferens resulting in a complex disease state with symptoms being seen in the pulmonary, gastrointestinal, and reproductive tracts.[49]

The diagnosis of CF is based on clinical symptoms or a sibling history of CF that is confirmed through documentation of CFTR dysfunction (Table 11-4). Newborn screening for CF via the identification of elevated blood immunoreactive trypsinogen is currently being used more frequently in the United States to identify potential CF patients. CF occurs more commonly in the Caucasian population, but the disease affects all races. Approximately 30,000 people in the United States have CF, and one out of every 31 Americans is a heterogeneous carrier for the disease.[50] CF occurs in approximately 1 out of every 3,200 live births in the Caucasian population, and although the disease is not limited to the Caucasian population, incidence rates in the African American (1 per 15,000), Asian American (1 per 31,000), native American (1 per 10,900), and Hispanic populations (1 per 9,200) are quite low.[51] In 2006, there were approximately 24,500 patients in the Cystic Fibrosis Foundation Registry with a racial make-up of 94.6% Caucasians and 3.9% African-Americans. In 2006, 6.8% of patients in the registry listed ethnicity as Hispanic.[52]

Table 11-4
Diagnosis of Cystic Fibrosis[114]

One or more clinical features characteristic of CF[a], or history of CF in a sibling, or positive newborn screening test (elevated immunoreactive trypsinogen)
AND
Laboratory evidence of an abnormality in the CFTR gene or protein (positive sweat chloride or nasal potential tests) or identification of CF causing CFTR mutations on both copies of the CFTR gene

[a]Chronic sinopulmonary disease manifested by colonization/infection with typical CF pathogens, chronic cough and sputum production, persistent abnormalities on chest radiograph such as atelectasis, bronchiectasis, infiltrates, and hyperinflation, airway obstruction with wheezing and air trapping, nasal polyps in conjunction with radiographic or tomographic abnormalities of the paranasal sinuses; gastric and nutritional abnormalities including meconium ileus, distal intestinal obstruction syndrome, rectal prolapse, pancreatic insufficiency, recurrent acute pancreatitis, chronic pancreatitis, prolonged neonatal jaundice, chronic hepatic disease manifested by clinical or histological evidence of focal biliary cirrhosis or multilobar cirrhosis obstructive, and nutritional deficiencies resulting in failure to thrive, protein malnutrition with edema or complications secondary to fat soluble vitamin deficiency; salt-wasting syndromes such as acute salt depletion or chronic metabolic alkalosis, or genetic abnormalities causing obstructive azoospermia.

When CF was initially described, survival past childhood was uncommon. Advances in the diagnosis of CF and the treatment of complications related to CF have dramatically increased the lifespan of CF patients; however, effective methods to correct the genetic defect, and thus affect a cure, remain elusive. Despite the fact that CF has been commonly referred to as a pediatric disorder, more and more practitioners who normally deal with adult populations are now caring for patients with CF. In 1970 the median predicted survival for a CF patient was 16 years; however, in 2006, the median predicted survival had increased to 36.9 years.[52] Adult CF patients are more common today, and in 2006, 44.6% of the patients in the Cystic Fibrosis Foundation Registry were 18 years of age or older.[52]

In 2006, 362 CF deaths were recorded in the CF database sponsored by the Cystic Fibrosis Foundation.[50] Over 90% of all CF deaths are related to pulmonary complications of the disease.[53]

Pathophysiology

CF is caused by a genetic defect in the production of the CFTR protein, which is a member of the adenosine triphosphate (ATP)-binding cassette transporter ATPases. CFTR is a 1480 amino acid glycoprotein that functions as a cyclic adenosine monophosphate (cAMP)-regulated chloride channel. The protein consists of two transmembrane domains, which contribute to the ion pore with two cytoplasmic nucleotide binding domains (NBD) linked by a cytosolic regulatory domain. Chloride transport is controlled by cAMP dependent protein kinase A (PKA) phosphorylation of the R-domain with ATP binding and hydrolysis at the NBDs.[47,54]

CFTR is expressed on the apical plasma membrane of the epithelial cell where it is a part of a multiprotein assembly in close proximity to a number of other ion channels and membrane receptors.[54] In addition to acting as gated-chloride channel, CFTR appears to play a role in the regulation of other apical ion transport processes including the epithelial sodium channel (ENaC) whose activity is inhibited by CFTR in the normal airway.[55,56] In addition to CFTR, luminal chloride secretion in airway epithelial cells can also occur through alternative chloride channels such as those activated by P2Y2 receptors or intracellular calcium. These fluid and ion secretion and absorption processes are responsible for maintaining appropriate airway surface liquid (ASL) hydration.

In the airways, the most important factor in mucus clearance is hydration of the airway surface. The primary physiologic defect in the airways in CF is a thick tenacious mucus that is poorly cleared due to dehydration of the ASL. The ASL consists of fluid in the mucus layer and the periciliary liquid (PCL). The mucus layer of the airway lies over the PCL, which is a low viscosity polyanionic fluid or gel layer that facilitates ciliary movement.[53] Thus, the PCL serves as a lubricant between the mucus layer and the airway allowing ciliary movement of the mucus layer. ASL volume regulation is not completely understood; however, it appears that, in the normal lung, chloride secretion by the CFTR and alternative chloride channels, and sodium absorption via ENaC work in conjunction to maintain ASL. The balance between sodium absorption and chloride secretion maintains the proper hydration and tonicity of secretions. In CF, the CFTR is either missing or non-functional; thus, this balance is disrupted. In addition to the loss of CFTR chloride secretion, ENaC related sodium absorption appears to be increased leading to dehydration of the ASL, collapse of the PCL, and the inability of airway cilia to clear mucus.[53,56] Epithelial cells in CF retain their ability to secrete chloride via non-CFTR chloride channels; however, this function is not sufficient to maintain ASL homeostasis.

The dehydration of the mucus and the loss of the PCL results in adhesion of mucus to the airway surface and the formation of mucus plaques. Adhesive secretions obstruct submucosal glands and the distal airways.[54] Mucus stasis and airway obstruction occur. Because of the mucus stasis, inhaled bacteria are not efficiently cleared, and bacterial colonization develops resulting in a neutrophilic inflammation. Mucus stasis may prevent neutrophil migration and the diffusion of antimicrobial substances produced in the lungs, decreasing the efficiency of the immune reaction. In addition, neutrophil elastase and other related proteases damage structural proteins in the lungs leading to bronchiectasis and decrease opsonophagocytosis, thus perpetuating chronic infection.[57] Furthermore, DNA and other breakdown products released upon neutrophil death contribute to decreased mucus viscoelasticity. This mucus may create a hypoxic environment that is favorable for bacterial growth and biofilm development. In addition, evidence exists demonstrating impaired production or trafficking of CFTR may cause activation of nuclear factor-kappa B resulting in increased interlukin-8, the principal neutrophil chemoattractant in the lung; thus, airway inflammation may exist independent of infection in the CF lung.[57,58]

The genetic defect in CF results in a chronic neutrophilic inflammatory disease of the airways with poor mucus clearing and bacterial colonization. Clinically, this translates into episodic exacerbations of acute viral and bacterial pulmonary infections leading to further airway structural damage resulting in bronchiectasis, air trapping, and hyperinflation of the lungs. Increased airway obstruction and a progressive decline in lung function lead to chronic hypoxia.

Genetic Defects

The expression and activation of CFTR is complex. Briefly, mRNA transcribed from DNA in the nucleus migrates to cytoplasmic ribosomes where amino acid translation occurs. Protein synthesis then occurs at the membrane of the endoplasmic reticulum followed by glycosylation and folding of the protein in the Golgi body. In normal cells, appropriately folded CFTR is then trafficked to the cell surface. Truncated, unstable, or misfolded protein is degraded by the endoplasmic reticulum.[59]

Mutations of the CFTR can be classified based on how they disrupt CFTR function (Table 11-5). Class I mutations are splicing or nonsense mutations and are caused by a premature stop codon, which results in an unstable mRNA or a shortened or unstable protein that is degraded in the cell. Class I mutations result in the CFTR not being expressed at the cell membrane. Molecules that suppress premature stop codons and allow translation to continue may be used to increase apical membrane protein expression in this class of mutations. This type of mutation is associated with 5% to 10% of CFTR mutations and results in a severe phenotype exhibiting both pulmonary disease and pancreatic insufficiency.[60] The W1282X mutation is the most common mutation among Israeli CF patients of Ashkenazi Jewish descent where it is seen in up to 60% of alleles; however, it is rare in other populations.[61]

Table 11-5
Classification of Cystic Fibrosis Transmembrane Regulator Dysfunction

	Class I	Class II	Class III	Class IV	Class V
Functional defect	Premature stop codon	Amino acid deletion	Amino acid substitution	Amino acid substitution	Promoter or splicing errors
Results on CFTR expression and/or function	Shortened dysfunctional CFTR protein that is degraded in the ER	Misfolding of the CFTR protein that is degraded in the ER	Dysregulation of CFTR protein at the cellular membrane	Altered channel architecture leading to decreased conductance or channel gating	Decreased CFTR expression at the apical membrane with differing levels of activity
Representative genotypes	G542X, R553X, W1282X	ΔF508, N1303K, G85E	G551D, G1349D	R117H, R334W, R234P, D1152H	D565G, IVS85T, G576A, 3849 + 10kb C→T
Typical phenotypes	Severe disease; pancreatic insufficiency	Severe disease; pancreatic insufficiency	Severe disease; pancreatic insufficiency	Milder disease; pancreatic sufficiency	Varied severity dependent on expression of functional CFTR protein
Potential protein repair therapy	Gentamicin, Ataluren	Sodium phenylbutyrate	Genistein, Sildenafil Vardenafil, VX770	Genistein, milrinone, VX-770	Genistein, Sodium butyrate

ER = endoplasmic reticulum.

Class II mutations are mutations caused by impaired processing of the CFTR protein which results in degradation of CFTR by the endoplasmic reticulum degradation processes, and a lack of functional CFTR expression at the cell membrane. Class II mutations are similar to Class I mutations; however, they result in a more severe form of CF that includes respiratory disease and pancreatic insufficiency. The most common Class II mutation, ΔF508, is caused by the deletion of a phenylalanine at the 508 amino acid position. This mutation is seen in 70% of defective alleles and 90% of CF patients in the United States.[54] Because of its frequency, most research has been directed at understanding and correcting this defect. It is thought that calnexin and the heat shock protein HSC70 are involved in the trafficking of the protein as it matures. They may associate with the protein and assist it in the folding process before releasing it to the Golgi body for glycosylation. Because the ΔF508 mutation impedes proper folding, there is prolonged association with calnexin and HSC70 resulting in ubiquitination and degradation in the endoplasmic reticulum.[59,62] It is estimated that greater than 99% of ΔF508 protein is degraded by this mechanism.[59] When expressed at the membrane, the ΔF508 mutation retains chloride-channel activity, but it does not function as well as the wild type channel.[54] This decrease in relative function may be related to a decreased open time for the channel.[63]

Class III mutations are caused by full-length proteins that are properly processed and trafficked to the membrane but have significantly decreased chloride ion transport capabilities. The lack of channel activity appears to be caused by the protein's resistance to phosphorylation, ATP binding, or hydrolysis. The most common Class III mutation is a glycine to aspartic acid interchange at amino acid position 551 (G551D), which is present among 3.1% of CF chromosomes.[59,64] Patients with class III mutations usually present with severe disease that includes both pancreatic insufficiency and respiratory disease.

Class IV mutations, like Class III mutations, are properly processed and expressed at the apical membrane. The protein is appropriately regulated by PKA and cAMP; however, amino acid substitutions result in changes in channel architecture that alter chloride conductance or channel gating.[65] These mutations are relatively rare. When expressed on the apical membrane, the ΔF508 mutant CFTR retains some chloride conductance and may exhibit class IV mutant properties. Because the CFTR protein is appropriately expressed on the apical membrane and maintains some function, the mutation is associated with pancreatic sufficiency and milder disease.[66]

Class V mutations result from promoter or splicing errors leading to decreased expression of the functional protein at the apical membrane. This may be due to decreased numbers of the CFTR protein or adequate numbers with decreased function. Class V mutations account for approximately 12% to 13% of mutations worldwide.[7] Presentation of CF in patients with class V mutations is quite variable, and disease severity has been shown to be inversely related to the number of correctly spliced transcripts.[65] Mutations that generate both correctly and aberrantly spliced transcripts (3849 + 10kb C→T) confer a milder phenotype with more variable disease, whereas mutations that completely abolish exon recognition (621 + 1 G→T) result in an absence of correctly spliced transcripts and a relatively severe phenotype.[67] Additional classification categories have been used to describe mutations that result in increased protein turnover at the membrane or proteins presenting with altered regulatory properties.[54]

Clinical Pearl

Although the most common mutation in Caucasians in the United States is the ΔF508 mutation, the prevalence of mutation in other races and ethnicities is not as predictable. Population mixing may alter the prevalence of mutation in different racial and ethnic groups over time.

Genetic Modifiers of Phenotype

Significant variability in disease severity occurs, even in patients with the same genotype.[68] In addition to environmental factors, genetic factors that affect ion transport through non-CFTR mechanisms and the inflammatory response may play a role in phenotypical differences. Alterations in genes for alpha$_1$-antitrypsin, angiotensin converting enzyme I, beta$_2$-adrenergic receptors, mannose binding lectin, major histocompatibility class II alleles, secretory leukocyte protease inhibitor, transforming growth factor beta$_1$ (TGFβ1), tumor necrosis factor alpha, as well as others have been associated with CF.[69,70] However, a study of these factors in 808 patients homozygous for the ΔF508 mutation found that genetic and allelic association with phenotype was only identified for the gene encoding for TGFβ1 with the TGFβ1 codon 10CC genotype being associated with more severe lung disease.[71] More recently, a study evaluating the mannose-binding lectin (MBL2) and TGFβ1 genes as modifiers of CF lung pathophysiology in 1,019 pediatric CF patients found that MBL2 deficiency was associated with a decrease in FEV_1 as well as an earlier onset of infection with *Pseudomonas aeruginosa* (PA). These effects were more significant in patients carrying a high producing TGFβ1 genotype demonstrating a significant gene-gene interaction.[72] TGFβ1 genotype alone was associated with pulmonary function decline but not age of first infection with PA. The potential importance of these findings in choosing drug therapy is not clear.

Pharmacotherapy

Current therapies available for the treatment of CF are outlined in Table 11-6. Treatment consists of replacing pancreatic enzymes, correcting nutritional deficiencies, and preventing pulmonary deterioration through preventing and treating infectious exacerbations. These measures are supportive/palliative, and at best slow pulmonary progression. Current research is focused on development of further therapies to slow pulmonary progression, insert a corrected copy of the CFTR gene into airway epithelial cells, or to enhance expression or function the CFTR protein. The latter may be accomplished by correcting transcription, processing and trafficking of the protein, or potentiating the activity of the protein.[60]

Table 11-6
Pharmacotherapy of Cystic Fibrosis[120-122]

Therapy	Comments
Microencapsulated pancreatic enzymes	Pancreatic insufficiency leads to malnutrition and fat-soluble vitamin deficiency due to decreased digestion and absorption of dietary fat and protein and fat-soluble vitamins.
Multivitamin	Used for supplementation of fat soluble vitamins.
Percussion and postural drainage	Increases clearance of airway mucus.
Recombinant Human DNAse	Decreases viscosity of airway mucus, increases clearance of airway mucus, improves pulmonary function, and decreases frequency of pulmonary exacerbations.
Hypertonic saline (7%)	May improve hydration of airway surface liquid, improves lung function and quality of life, and decreases exacerbations.
β-agonists/theophylline	Improves pulmonary function in patients with reactive airway disease. Responsiveness to bronchodilators should be identified prior to initiating chronic therapy.
Corticosteroids	Oral corticosteroids (1–2 mg/kg) decrease inflammation associated with disease, but have undesirable effects. The efficacy of inhaled corticosteroids is not proven.

Continued on next page

Table 11-6 *(Continued)*

Ibuprofen	High dose ibuprofen decreases CF associated inflammation; however, there is an increased risk of gastrointestinal adverse effects.
Aerosolized tobramycin	Improves lung function and quality of life. Decreases pulmonary exacerbations and intravenous antibiotic use.
Azithromycin	Recommended for use in patients 6 years of age or older with *Pseudomonas aeruginosa*. Treatment improves lung function and reduces exacerbations.

Gene Therapy

The correction of the genetic defect of CF through gene transfer has not been successful to date. Despite the fact that more than 140 CF patients have been treated with recombinant adeno-associated virus vectors of gene therapy, no significant progress has been made in this area or in the development of vectors that successfully deliver the transgene to the cell.[73] Based on current therapeutic trials, lung gene therapy does not appear to be a viable therapeutic alternative in the near future.

Protein Repair Therapy

Protein repair therapy is directed at correcting the underlying defect in CF by targeting the processing, trafficking, and activity of the CFTR and could theoretically target patients with specific CFTR mutations.[74] Agents aimed at improving the expression of CFTR on the apical membrane through enhanced gene transcription, protein processing, or trafficking of the protein are termed "correctors." Agents in this class could be targeted for treatment of patients with Class I, II, and V mutations. Molecules aimed at improving the function of the CFTR protein by increasing chloride conductance are termed potentiators, and agents in this class would be directed toward patients with Class III and IV mutations. Because in some cases mutations may take the characteristics of more than one mutation (e.g., ΔF508), combination therapy may be required for certain patients.

Correctors

Several compounds have been identified that affect CFTR processing and trafficking. The aminoglycoside antibiotic gentamicin is known to interfere with the proof reading process of transfer mRNA by inducing read throughs of premature stop codons and disturbing the codon-anticodon matching process. This activity allows for random amino acid insertion resulting in continued translation and the production of full-length CFTR proteins. While these proteins retain chloride channel activity, they may contain missense mutations that result in decreased expression or activity of the protein.[65]

Class I Mutations. Gentamicin increases CFTR expression in CFTR nonsense mutation transfected cells and in a bronchial epithelial cell line expressing a nonsense mutation.[75,76] Gentamicin nasal drops (given three times a day for 14 days) caused a significant decrease in nasal potential difference (NPD), a measurement of chloride secretion and sodium absorption across the epithelia, in response to a chloride-free isoproterenol solution in patients homozygous for the W1282X stop mutation (n = 4) or heterozygous for the W1282X and G542X (n = 3), ΔF508 (n = 1), or 3849 + 10kb C→T (n = 1) mutation.[77] No differences were seen in basal

NPD. In a follow-up double-blind, placebo controlled crossover trial, nasally administered gentamicin was evaluated in 19 CF patients homozygous for the W1282X mutation (n = 11) or heterozygous for the W1282X and ΔF508 mutations (n = 8) and 5 patients homozygous for the ΔF508 mutation.[78] In patients carrying the W1282X mutation (homozygous or heterozygous), a significant decrease in basal and isoproterenol-treated NPD was associated with gentamicin administration; however, the response was not seen in all patients. When homozygous and heterozygous W1282X patients were evaluated separately, NPD was significantly decreased in the homozygous population but not the heterozygous population. No changes in basal NPD or response to chloride free isoproterenol solution were seen in patients homozygous for ΔF508. *Ex vivo* analysis of full-length CFTR protein in nasal epithelial cells before and after gentamicin treatment in two heterozygous patients who had a response to therapy demonstrated increased cellular membrane localization of CFTR. A more recent study evaluating intranasal gentamicin and tobramycin in CF patients heterozygous for a premature stop mutation (n = 11) or CF patients without a stop mutation (n = 18) found no differences in basal or isoproterenol stimulated NPD over 28 days.[79] *Ex vivo* evaluation of nasal epithelial cells likewise demonstrated no increases in membrane localization of CFTR. The effect of systemically administered gentamicin was evaluated in five CF subjects heterozygous for one premature stop mutation and five CF subjects without premature stop mutations.[80] Subjects were administered gentamicin for 7 days with doses adjusted to achieve peak serum concentrations of 8–10 mg/L and trough concentrations <2 mg/L. Chloride sweat test, basal NPD and response to chloride-free isoproterenol administration were measured at baseline, during (days 3, 4, 5 and 6) and after gentamicin administration and again one to four weeks after treatment. No difference between the two groups was seen in the chloride sweat test or basal NPD; however, patients with the stop mutation had a significant increase in the number of NPD readings indicating increased chloride transport. As with the other studies, not all patients responded.

Differences in these trials may be related to population differences since it has been recently demonstrated that response to gentamicin may be related to initial levels of CFTR expression, enhanced nonsense mediated mRNA decay, or be stop mutation specific.[81,82] Furthermore, early studies demonstrating success with gentamicin have been conducted in populations of patients having at least one mutation containing W1282X. It has been demonstrated that W1282X CFTR retains partial chloride channel function that is enhanced after suppression of the stop codon.[83] Finally, although none of the trials reported significant adverse effects, long-term systemic administration of gentamicin would raise safety concerns because of its well-documented toxicities.

Because of the early success with gentamicin and the recognized toxicity and administration issues, considerable interest exists in the development of compounds that can safely suppress premature stop codons. Ataluren is an orally available oxadiazole identified via high through-put screening of low molecular weight compounds that may have the potential to treat disease caused by nonsense mutations. At low concentrations, ataluren has been shown to promote dose-dependent read through in nonsense mutations and is a more potent nonsense suppressor than gentamicin.[84] Phase I trials of ataluren indicated the drug was safe for further clinical study.[85] A phase II trial in adult CF patients with at least one nonsense mutation in the CFTR gene evaluated the effectiveness of ataluren given in two 28-day cycles.[86] The first cycle (n = 23) consisted of 16 mg/kg per day of ataluren given in three divided doses for 14 days followed by 14 days without drug. In cycle two, 21 of the cycle one patients received ataluren 40 mg/kg/ day in three divided doses for 14 days followed by 14 drug-free days. Significant increases were seen in total chloride transport in both treatment cycles, and total chloride transport entered the normal range for 57% of patients in cycle 1 and 43% of the patients in cycle 2. Adverse effects were mild. This study demonstrated the short-term efficacy and safety of ataluren. Phase II trials for ataluren with treatment durations up to 84 days have been completed in adult and pediatric patients with CF, and a 48-week Phase III trial is planned for early 2010.[87]

Clinical Pearl

Tobramycin 600 mg per day has become standard maintenance therapy for prevention of pulmonary exacerbations of CF; however, it does not appear to have the same efficacy as gentamicin in inducing read through of premature termination codons.

Class II Mutations. Class II mutations, particularly ΔF508, are responsible for the majority of mutations seen in CF. It is postulated that the defective CFTR protein can be "rescued" from the endoplasmic reticulum and intracellular trafficking improved, thus enhancing expression of functional protein.[88] One agent, sodium butyrate, has been shown to prevent breakdown of mutated proteins at the cellular level; however, poor bioavailability and toxicities preclude its clinical use.[62] Sodium 4-phenylbutyrate (4-PBA), a derivative of butyrate used for treatment increased blood ammonia in urea cycle disorders, has also been shown to increase trafficking of ΔF508.[89] It is thought that 4-PBA reduces the expression of heat shock protein HSC-70 resulting in decreased HSC-70 association with ΔF508 leading to decreased ΔF508 degradation in the endoplasmic reticulum.[60] The effect of 4-PBA on NPD and sweat chloride response was evaluated in CF patients homozygous for the ΔF508 mutation in a randomized, double-blind, placebo-controlled trial.[90] Subjects were given placebo or 19 grams of 4-PBA in divided doses three times a day. Patients in the pilot trial treated with 4-PBA (n=9) showed significant improvement in NPD after infusion of a chloride-free isoproterenol solution when compared to placebo treated patients. No differences were seen in amiloride sensitive NPD or sweat chloride concentrations. A phase I/II trial of 4-PBA in 19 adult CF patients homozygous for ΔF508-CFTR demonstrated a significant increase in isoproterenol stimulated chloride transport in nasal epithelia. The maximal response was seen with a daily dose of 20 grams for 1 week.[91] Peak response occurred between days three and four with a decrease in response seen at day 7. It is possible that this decrease in response could be related to increased ENaC activity since a recent *in vitro* study showed that 4-PBA induces a time-dependent increase in ENaC protein in the apical membrane in conjunction with increased apical amiloride-sensitive sodium current.[92] Therefore, increased CFTR expression may be offset by increased ENaC related sodium absorption.

It was postulated that curcumin, a sarcoplasmic/endoplasmic reticulum calcium pump inhibitor and a major constituent of the spice turmeric, could increase ΔF508 expression by interfering with calcium dependent protein chaperones like calnexin. In an early study with homozygous ΔF508-CFTR mice, treatment with curcumin corrected both basal and isoproterenol stimulated NPD.[93] However, subsequent studies of curcumin in cell culture or whole animals could not reproduce these results.[94-96] A phase I study of curcuminoid compounds in adult CF patients homozygous for ΔF508 has been completed, but no results have been reported.[97]

Class V Mutations. Class V mutations are caused by aberrantly spliced transcripts. The severity of the disease depends on the number of correctly spliced transcripts. One method for increasing the numbers of correctly spliced transcripts, and thus the expression of CFTR at the apical membrane, is to overexpress splicing factors which increases the amount of correctly spliced RNA.[98] Sodium butyrate has been previously shown to modify the alternative splicing pattern of exon 7 in the survival motor neuron-2 (SMN2) gene thus increasing the number of full-length SMN mRNA transcripts and exon 7 containing SMN protein in spinal muscular atrophy lymphoid cells.[99] Based on these results, the effect of sodium butyrate function and expression of CFTR in an epithelial cell line from a nasal polyp of a patient with the 3849 + 10kb C→T mutation was evaluated.[67] Sodium butyrate significantly decreased the amount of aberrantly spliced transcripts and activated CFTR. The utility of these findings is unknown as sodium butyrate is not well suited for clinical use; however, other agents such as valproic acid have also demonstrated the ability to increase SMN2 transcripts and proteins and may have application in this area.

Potentiators

A second approach to improving CFTR function is to increase the proportion of CFTR chloride channels that are open either by directly inducing channel opening or by lengthening the time that the channel remains open. This approach to therapy requires that a full-length CFTR protein be localized to the apical membrane and would be directed at Class III and IV mutations. Genistein, a soybean derived isoflavone, has been shown to increase CFTR chloride transport in both wild type and mutant CFTR. In patients with at least one G551D mutation, perfusion of the nasal mucosa with genistein was shown to hyperpolarize NPD in both healthy and CF patients indicating it stimulates chloride conductance in the nasal epithelia.[100] It appears that genistein enhances CFTR activity by decreasing the closing rate of the channel at low concentrations, but may inhibit channel activity at high doses by binding to a low affinity site that decreases the opening rate of the channel.[101,102] Genistein's clinical usefulness may be limited by its low potency and rapid metabolism.

The compound 8-cyclopentyl-1,3-dipropylxanthine (CPX) also activates CFTR, probably through direct binding to the protein and may have some selectivity for ΔF508-CFTR.[59,103,104] A phase I trial of in 37 adult patients homozygous for ΔF508-CFTR demonstrated the drug to be safe in humans; however, a single dose of CPX had no effect on NPD or sweat chloride measurements.[105] In nasal epithelial cells expressing G551D-CFTR, genistein, but not CPX, increased chloride conductance.[106]

Phosphodiesterase inhibitors have likewise been shown to activate CFTR chloride conductance *in vitro*, however, an *in vivo* study with milrinone in mice and humans could not reproduce this response.[107] At supraphysiologic doses (300 x doses used for erectile dysfunction), the phosphodiesterase V specific inhibitor, sildenafil, corrects trafficking of ΔF508-CFTR and localization to the apical plasma membrane in nasal epithelial cells from CF patients homozygous or heterozygous for ΔF508.[108,109] More recently, an in vivo study of pharmacologic doses of sildenafil and vardenafil demonstrated that both agents stimulated chloride conductance in ΔF508del mice, a mouse model with decreased expression of ΔF508-CFTR; however, the drugs had no effect on sodium transport.[108] Currently, no clinical data concerning the effect of these drugs in human CF patients are available.

VX-770, an orally active small molecule identified via high throughput screening, has the ability to increase chloride secretion in cells expressing ΔF508- and G551D-CFTR. The molecule is currently in phase II trials in patients with the G551D mutation.

Combination Therapy

Because some CFTR mutations like ΔF508 may exhibit characteristics of more than one mutation type, combination therapy with a corrector and potentiator may be a feasible option. *In vitro* studies demonstrated that pretreatment of cells expressing ΔF508-CFTR with the corrector, 4-PBA, enhances the response to the potentiator, genistein; however, the response to CPX in 4-PBA pretreated cells is not enhanced.[110,111] Currently, the combination of 4-PBA and isoflavone extracts containing genistein is being evaluated in two Phase II trials for the treatment of patients homozygous or heterozygous for ΔF508-CFTR.[112,113]

Case Study

ARL is a 15-year-old white female with cystic fibrosis who is being discharged from the hospital after her second exacerbation in the last 18 months. Her home medications include Vitamax® 2 tablets daily, Pancrease MT20® 2 capsules with meals and one capsule with snacks, aerosolized tobramycin 300 mg nebulized twice a day, Pulmozyme® 2.5 mg nebulized daily, albuterol 2.5 mg nebulized three times a day, hypertonic saline 7% 4 mL nebulized twice a day, Flovent® HF® 220 mg inhaled twice a day, and Azithromycin 500 mg three times a week. She is very adherent to her medication regimen and takes very good care of herself. Her FEV1 was 75% of predicted at her clinic visit one month ago. She keeps up with innovations in cystic fibrosis therapy and is concerned about the impact of the disease on the quality and length of her life. As a child, she underwent genetic testing and is known to be homozygous for ΔF508-CTR. ARL is curious about drugs in the pipeline and would like to know what agents may be available to treat her type of cystic fibrosis in the next 10 years.

1. What information could you provide ARL concerning agents that may be available to improve therapy in her specific phenotype?
2. ARL is interested in enrolling in a clinical trial at the hospital for a new investigational drug that has been shown to have positive effects in cells and animals with Class III and Class IV mutations. What information can you provide ARL concerning the potential benefits she may have if she receives the study drug?

Clinical Implications

Despite ongoing research efforts, correction of CFTR activity through gene transfer therapy continues to face significant challenges in delivering the transgene effectively. High throughput screening of small molecules has identified a number of agents that may be effective for protein repair therapy. Some agents such as ataluren and VX-770 have shown clinical promise and have progressed into phase II trials. Identification of specific mutant alleles in CF is common, and current genetic screening panels can identify approximately 90% of CF mutations.[114] Therefore, identification of specific medications that correct or potentiate specific CF mutations or classes of mutations would allow for individualized therapy for that genotype. Furthermore, it has been suggested that significant pulmonary morbidity may be decreased by restoration of as little as 10% to 35% of normal CFTR activity.[115] Thus, relatively small improvements in protein expression and activity could have a significant impact on the disease.

Genetically targeted therapies have the potential to significantly enhance quality of life and increase life expectancy in CF patients; however, none of these products has currently made it past phase II clinical trials. Because these molecules work at the cellular level and interfere with basic cellular processes, potential long-term adverse effects are unknown. Additionally, ASL homeostasis is a complex process and CFTR may play a role in regulating other ion channels that contribute to ASL homeostasis. Restoration of the CFTR protein or enhancement of its chloride channel function may not restore its regulatory activity.[116] The future progress of these agents and others through the discovery and regulatory process can be monitored at the cystic fibrosis foundation web site (http://www.cff.org/research/drugdevelopmentpipeline/).[117]

Summary

In spite of the many differences in the pathophysiology, epidemiology, severity, and current treatments of asthma and CF, they are two conditions affecting the respiratory system for which ongoing pharmacogenomic research could result in improved treatment. With regards to asthma, the application of ongoing and future research could allow practitioners to optimize therapy based upon genotype, and reduce negative outcomes. In CF patients, enhanced understanding of the basic genetic defect and its variations have led to the development of a number of investigational drugs that may actually modify the disease process based upon the specific mutations in the gene encoding for the CFTR the patient possesses. Research into the genetic basis and modifiers of both asthma and CF and their influence on the response to therapy has created opportunities for individualized therapy. However, this knowledge must be translated into clinical practice through rigorous pursuit of genetic-based drug development and outcome measures for these disease states.

References

1. National Asthma Education and Prevention Program. Expert Panel Report 3: Guidelines for the diagnosis and management of asthma.: U.S. Department of Health and Human Services, Public Health Services, National Institutes of Health, National Heart, Lung, and Blood Institute; 2007.
2. Noguchi E, Arinami T. Candidate genes for atopic asthma: Current results from genome screens. *Am J Pharmacogenomics.* 2001;1:251-261.
3. Howard T, Meyers D, Bleecker E. Mapping susceptibility genes for asthma and allergy. *J Allergy Clin Immunol.* 2000;105(suppl):S477-481.
4. Johnson M. The beta -Adrenoceptor. *Am J Respir Crit Care Med.* 1998;158:146S-153.
5. Ortega VE, Hawkins GA, Peters SP, et al. Pharmacogenetics of the [beta]2-adrenergic receptor gene. *Immunol Allergy Clin North Am.* 2007;27:665-684.
6. Drazen JM, Silverman EK, Lee TH. Heterogeneity of therapeutic responses in asthma. *Br Med Bull.* 2000;56:1054-1070.
7. Salpeter SR, Buckley NS, Ormiston TM, et al. Meta-analysis: effect of long-acting beta-agonists on severe asthma exacerbations and asthma-related deaths. *Ann Intern Med.* 2006;144:904-912.
8. Salpeter SR, Ormiston TM, Salpeter EE. Meta-analysis: respiratory tolerance to regular {beta}2-agonist use in patients with asthma. *Ann Intern Med.* 2004;140:802-813.
9. Nelson HS, Weiss ST, Bleecker ER, et al, the SSG. The salmeterol multicenter asthma research trial: A comparison of usual pharmacotherapy for asthma or usual pharmacotherapy plus salmeterol. *Chest.* 2006;129:15-26.

10. Morrow T. Implications of pharmacogenomics in the current and future treatment of asthma. *J Manag Care Pharm.* 2007;13:497-505.

11. Liggett SB. The pharmacogenetics of B2-adrenergic receptors: Relevance to asthma. *J Allergy Clin Immunol.* 2000; 105(suppl):S487-492.

12. Contopoulos-Ioannidis DG, Manoli EN, Ioannidis JP. Meta-analysis of the association of beta2-adrenergic receptor polymorphisms with asthma phenotypes. *J Allergy Clin Immunol.* 2005;115:963-972.

13. Israel E, Chinchilli VM, Ford JG, et al. Use of regularly scheduled albuterol treatment in asthma: genotype-stratified, randomised, placebo-controlled cross-over trial. *The Lancet.* 2004;364:1505-1512.

14. Israel E, Drazen JM, Liggett SB, et al. The effect of polymorphisms of the beta(2)-adrenergic receptor on the response to regular use of albuterol in asthma. *Am J Respir Crit Care Med.* 2000;162:75-80.

15. Taylor DR, Drazen JM, Herbison GP, et al. Asthma exacerbations during long term beta agonist use: influence of beta 2 adrenoceptor polymorphism. *Thorax.* 2000;55:762-767.

16. Bleecker ER, Postma DS, Lawrance RM, et al. Effect of ADRB2 polymorphisms on response to long-acting beta2-agonist therapy: a pharmacogenetic analysis of two randomised studies. *Lancet.* 2007;370:2118-2125.

17. Wechsler ME, Lehman E, Lazarus SC, et al. beta-Adrenergic receptor polymorphisms and response to salmeterol. *Am J Respir Crit Care Med.* 2006;173:519-526.

18. Palmer C, Lipworth B, Lee S, et al. Arginine-16 B2 adrenoceptor genotype predisposes to exacerbations in young asthmatics taking regular salmeterol. *Thorax.* 2006;61:940-944.

19. Israel E, Drazen JM, Liggett SB, et al. Effect of polymorphism of the beta(2)-adrenergic receptor on response to regular use of albuterol in asthma. *Int Arch Allergy Immunol.* 2001;124:183-186.

20. Weiss ST, Lake SL, Silverman ES, et al. Asthma steroid pharmacogenetics: a study strategy to identify replicated treatment responses. *Proc Am Thorac Soc.* 2004;1:364-367.

21. Malmstrom K, Rodriguez-Gomez G, Guerra J, et al. Oral montelukast, inhaled beclomethasone, and placebo for chronic asthma: A randomized, controlled trial. *Ann Intern Med.* 1999;130:487-495.

22. Szefler SJ, Martin RJ, King TS, et al. Significant variability in response to inhaled corticosteroids for persistent asthma. *J Allergy Clin Immunol.* 2002;109:410-418.

23. Israel E. Genetics and the variability of treatment response in asthma. *J Allergy Clin Immunol.* 2005;115(suppl):S532-S538.

24. Weiss S, Litonjua A, Lange C, et al. Overview of the pharmacogenetics of asthma treatment. *Pharmacogenomics J.* 2006;6:311-326.

25. Tantisira K, Lake S, Silverman E, et al. Corticosteroid pharmacogenetics: Association of sequence variants in CRHR1 with improved lung function in asthmatics treated with inhaled corticosteroids. *Hum Molec Gen.* 2004;13:1353-1359.

26. Tantisira KG, Hwang ES, Raby BA, et al. TBX21: A functional variant predicts improvement in asthma with the use of inhaled corticosteroids. *Proc Nat Acad Sci USA.* 2004;101:18099-18104.

27. Raby BA, Hwang E-S, Steen KV, et al. T-Bet Polymorphisms are associated with asthma and airway hyperresponsiveness. *Am J Respir Crit Care Med.* 2006;173:64-70.

28. Leung D, Spahn J, Szefler S. Steroid-unresponsive asthma. *Semin Respir Crit Care Med.* 2002;23:387-398.

29. Bray P, Cotton R. Variations of the human glucocorticoid receptor gene (NR3C1): pathological and in vitro mutations and polymorphisms. *Hum Mutat.* 2003;21:557-568.

30. Watkins PB, Dube LM, Walton-Bowen K, et al. Clinical pattern of zileuton-associated liver injury: results of a 12-month study in patients with chronic asthma. *Drug Saf.* 2007;30:805-815.

31. Weschler M, Israel E. Pharmacogenetics of treatment with leukotriene modifiers. *Curr Opin Allerg Clin Immunol.* 2002;2:395-401.

32. Hoshiko S, RÃ¥dmark O, Samuelsson B. Characterization of the human 5-lipoxygenase gene promoter. *Proc Nat Acad Sci USA.* 1990;87:9073-9077.

33. Drazen JM, Yandava CN, Dube L, et al. Pharmacogenetic association between ALOX5 promoter genotype and the response to anti-asthma treatment. *Nat Genet.* 1999;22:168-170.

34. Lima JJ, Zhang S, Grant A, et al. Influence of leukotriene pathway polymorphisms on response to montelukast in asthma. *Am J Respir Crit Care Med.* 2006;173:379-385.

35. Anderson W, Kalberg C, Edwards L, et al. Effects of polymorphisms in the promoter region of 5-lipoxygenase and LTC4 synthase on the clinical response to zafirlukast and fluticasone. *Eur Respir J.* 2000;16(suppl):183S.

36. Telleria J, Blanco-Quiros A, Varillas D, et al. ALOX5 promoter genotype and response to montelukast in moderate persistent asthma. *Resp Med.* 2008;102:857-861.

37. Wechsler M, Israel E. Pharmacogenetics of treatment with leukotriene modifiers. *Curr Opin Allerg Clin Immunol.* 2002;2:395-401.

38. Sampson AP, Siddiqui S, Buchanan D, et al. Variant LTC4 synthase allele modifies cysteinyl leukotriene synthesis in eosinophils and predicts clinical response to zafirlukast. *Thorax.* 2000;55(suppl):S28-31.

39. Chien Y-H, Hwu W-L, Chiang B-L. The genetics of atopic dermatitis. *Clinical Reviews in Allergy and Immunology.* 2007;33:178-190.

40. Molfino N. Current thinking on genetics of chronic obstructive pulmonary disease. *Curr Opin Pulm Med.* 2007;13:107-113.

41. Wood A, Stockley R. The genetics of chronic obstructive pulmonary disease. *Resp Res.* 2006;7: 130-43.

42. Global Strategy for the Diagnosis, Management and Prevention of COPD, Global Initiative for Chronic Obstructive Lung Disease (GOLD). www.goldcopd.org. Accessed October 1, 2008.

43. Allergic rhinitis and its impact on asthma. World Health Organization. http://www.whiar.org/. Accessed October 1, 2008.

44. Asthma Drug Response Test: B16AsthmaGEN(TM). http://www.consumergenetics.com/DNA-Tests/Asthma-Drug-Response.php. Accessed October 8, 2008.

45. Sample B16AsthmaGEN(TM) Drug Response Test Report. http://www.consumergenetics.com/pdfs/AsthmaGenResultSample.pdf. Accessed October 8, 2008.

46. Weiss KB, Sullivan SD. The health economics of asthma and rhinitis. I. Assessing the economic impact. *J Allergy Clin Immunol.* 2001;107:3-8.

47. Gadsby DC, Vergani P, Csanády L. The ABC protein turned chloride channel whose failure causes cystic fibrosis. *Nature.* 2006;440:477-483.

48. Cystic Fibrosis Mutation Database. CFMDB statistics. http://www.genet.sickkids.on.ca/cftr/StatisticsPage.html. Accessed 3 November, 2008.

49. Strausbaugh SD, Davis PB. Cystic Fibrosis: a review of epidemiology and pathobiology. *Clin Chest Med.* 2007;28:279-288.

50. Cystic Fibrosis Foundation. Frequently Asked Questions. Available at: http://www.cff.org/AboutCF/Faqs/. Accessed 28 October, 2008.

51. Hamosh A, FitzSimmons SC, Macek M, Jr., et al. Comparison of the clinical manifestations of cystic fibrosis in black and white patients. *J Pediatr.* 1998;132:255-259.

52. Cystic Fibrosis Foundation. *Patient Registry 2006 Annual Data Report.* Bethesda, MD: Cystic Fibrosis Foundation; 2008.

53. Boucher RC. Airway surface dehydration in cystic fibrosis: pathogenesis and therapy. *Ann Rev Med.* 2007;58:157-170.

54. Rowe SM, Miller S, Sorscher EJ. Cystic fibrosis. *N Engl J Med.* 2005;352:192-2001.

55. Mehta A. CFTR: more than just a chloride channel. *Pediatric Pulmonol.* 2005;39:292-298.

56. Donaldson SH, Boucher RC. Sodium channels and cystic fibrosis. *Chest.* 2007;132:1631-1636.

57. Elizur A, Cannon CL, Ferkol TW. Airway inflammation in cystic fibrosis. *Chest.* 2008;133:489-495.

58. Weber AJ, Soong G, Bryan R, et al. Activation of NF-κB in airway epithelial cells is dependent on CFTR trafficking and Cl⁻ channel function. *Am J Physiol Lung Cell Mol Physiol.* 2001;281:L71-L78.

59. Kerem E. Pharmacological induction of CFTR function in patients with cystic fibrosis: mutation specific therapy. *Pediatric Pulmonol.* 2005;40:183-196.

60. Kerem E. Mutation specific therapy in CF. *Peadiatr Resp Rev.* 2006;7(suppl):S166-S169.

61. Shoshani T, Augartan A, Gazit E, et al. Association of a nonsense mutation (W1128X), the most common mutation in the Ashkenazi Jewish cystic fibrosis patients in Israel, with presentation of severe disease. *Am J Hum Genet.* 1992;50:222-228.

62. Roomans GM. Pharmacological approaches to correcting the ion transport defect in cystic fibrosis. *Am J Respir Med.* 2003;2:413-431.

63. Zeitlin P. Novel pharmacologic therapies for cystic fibrosis. *J Clin Investig.* 1999;103:447-452.

64. Becq F. On the discovery and development of CFTR chloride channel activators. *Curr Pharm Design.* 2006;12:471-484.

65. MacDonald KD, McKenzie KR, Zeitlin PL. Cystic fibrosis transmembrane regulator protein mutations. 'Class' opportunity for novel drug innovation. *Pediatr Drugs.* 2007;9:1-10.

66. Rubenstein RC. Targeted therapy for cystic fibrosis. Cystic fibrosis transmembrane conductance regulator mutation-specific pharmacologic strategies. *Mol Drug Ther.* 2006;10:293-301.

67. Nissim-Rafinia M, Aviram M, Randell SH, et al. Restoration of the cystic fibrosis transmembrane conductance regulator function by splicing modulation. *EMBO Rep.* Nov 2004;5:1071-1077.

68. The Cystic Fibrosis Genotype-Phenotype Consortium. Correlation between genotype and phenotype in patients with cystic fibrosis. *N Engl J Med.* 1993;329:1308-1313.

69. Soferman R. Immunophysiologic mechanisms of cystic fibrosis lung disease. *IMAJ.* 2006;8:44-48.

70. Büscher R, Grasmann H. Disease modifying genes in cystic fibrosis: therapeutic option or one-way road? *Naunyn-Schmiedeberg's Arch Pharmacol.* 2006;374:65-77.

71. Drumm ML, Konstan MW, Schluchter MD, et al. Genetic modifiers of lung disease in cystic fibrosis. *N Engl J Med.* 2005;353:1443-1453.

72. Dorfman R, Sandford A, Taylor C, et al. Complex two-gene modulation of lung disease severity in children with cystic fibrosis. *J Clin Investig.* 2008;118:1040-1049.

73. Saeed Z, Wojewodka G, Marion D, et al. Novel pharmaceutical approaches for treating patients with cystic fibrosis. *Curr Pharm Des.* 2007;13:3252-3263.

74. Ratjen F. New pulmonary therapies for cystic fibrosis. *Curr Opin Pulm Med.* 2007;13:541-546.

75. Howard M, Frizzell RA, Bedwell DM. Aminoglycoside antibiotics restore CFTR function by overcoming premature stop mutations. *Nat Med.* 1996;2:467-469.

76. Bedwell DM, Kaenjk A, Benos DJ, et al. Suppression of a CFTR premature stop mutation in a bronchial epithelial cell line. *Nat Med.* 1997;3:1280-1284.

77. Wilschanski M, Famini C, Blau H, et al. A pilot study of the effect of gentamicin on nasal potential difference measurements in cystic fibrosis patients carrying stop mutations. *Am J Respir Crit Care Med.* 2000;161:860-865.

78. Wilschanski M, Yahav Y, Yaacov Y, et al. Gentamicin-induced correction of CFTR function in patients with cystic fibrosis and CFTR stop mutations. *N Engl J Med.* 2003;349:1433-1441.

79. Clancy JP, Rowe SM, Bebok Z, et al. No detectable improvements in cystic fibrosis transmembrane conductance regulator by nasal aminoglycosides in patients with cystic fibrosis with stop mutations. *Am J Resp Cell Mol Biol.* 2007;37:57-66.

80. Clancy JP, Bebok Z, Ruiz F, et al. Evidence that systemic gentamicin suppresses premature stop mutations in patients with cystic fibrosis. *Am J Respir Crit Care Med.* 2001;163:1683-1692.

81. Linde L, Boelz S, Nissim-Rafinia M, et al. Nonsense-mediated mRNA decay affects nonsense transcript levels and governs response of cystic fibrosis patients to gentamicin. *J Clin Investig.* 2007;117:683-692.

82. Sermet-Gaudelus I, Renouil M, Fajac A, et al. *In vitro* prediction of stop-codon suppression by intravenous gentamicin in patients with cystic fibrosis: a pilot study. *BMC Medicine.* 2007;5:5.

83. Rowe SM, Varga K, Rab A, et al. Restoration of W1282X CFTR activity by enhanced expression. *Am J Resp Cell Mol Biol.* 2007;37:347-356.

84. Welch EM, Barton ER, Zhuo J, et al. PTC124 targets genetic disorders caused by nonsense mutations. *Nature.* 2007;447:87-91.

85. Hirawat S, Welch EM, Elfring GL, et al. Safety, tolerability, and pharmacokinetics of PTC124, a nonaminoglycoside nonsense mutation suppressor, following single- and multiple-dose administration to healthy male and female adult volunteers. *J Clin Pharmacol.* 2007;47:430-444.

86. Kerem E, Hirawat S, Armoni S, et al. Effectiveness of PTC124 treatment of cystic fibrosis caused by nonsense mutations: a prospective phase II trial. *Lancet.* 2008;372:719-727.

87. ClinicalTrials.gov [Internet]. Bethesda (MD): National Library of Medicine (US). 2000 Feb 29. [Cited 2009 June 22.] Available at: http://clinicaltrials.gov/.

88. Rubenstein RC. Novel, mechanism-based therapies for cystic fibrosis. *Curr Opin Pediatr.* 2005;17:385-392.

89. Rubenstein RC, Egan ME, Zeitlin PL. In vitro pharmacologic restoration of CFTR-mediated chloride transport with sodium 4-phenylbutyrate in cystic fibrosis epithelial cells containing ΔF508-CFTR. *J Clin Investig.* 1997;100:2457-2465.

90. Rubenstein RC, Zeitlin PL. A pilot clinical trial of oral sodium 4-phenylbutyrate (Buphenyl) in ΔF508-homozygous cystic fibrosis patients: partial restoration of nasal epithelial CFTR function. *Am J Resp Crit Care Med*. 1998;157:484-490.

91. Zeitlin PL, Diener-West M, Rubenstein RC, et al. Evidence of CFTR function in cystic fibrosis after systemic administration of 4-phenylbutyrate. *Mol Ther*. 2002;6:119-126.

92. Pruliere-Escabasse V, Planes C, Escudier E, et al. Modulation of epithelial sodium channel trafficking and function by sodium 4-phenylbutyrate in human nasal epithelial cells. *J. Biol. Chem.* 2007;282:34048-34057.

93. Egan ME, Pearson M, Weiner SA, et al. Curcumin, a major constituent of turmeric, corrects cystic fibrosis defects. *Science*. 2004;304:600-602.

94. Dragomir A, Björstad J, Hjelte L, et al. Curcumin does not stimulate cAMP-mediated chloride transport in cystic fibrosis airway epithelial cells. *Biochem Biophys Res Commun*. 2004;322:447-451.

95. Song Y, Sonawane ND, Salinas D, et al. Evidence against the rescue of defective ΔF508-CFTR cellular processing by curcumin in cell culture and mouse models. *J Biol Chem*. 2004;279:40629-40633.

96. Grubb BR, Gabriel SE, Mengos A, et al. SERCA pump inhibitors do not correct biosynthetic arrest of ΔF508 CFTR in cystic fibrosis. *Am J Resp Cell Mol Biol*. 2006;34:355-363.

97. Ramsey B, Seer Pharmaceuticals, CF Therapeutics Development Network Coordinating Center, Cystic Fibrosis Foundation. Safety study of orally administered curcuminoids in adult subjects with cystic fibrosis (SEER) Available at: http://clinicaltrials.gov/show/NCT00219882 NLM Identifier: NCT00219882.

98. Nissim-Rafinia M, Kerem B. Splicing modulation as a modifier of the CFTR function. *Prog Mol Subcell Biol*. 2006;44:233-254.

99. Chang JG, Hsieh-Li HM, Jong YJ, et al. Treatment of spinal muscular atrophy by sodium butyrate. *Proc Natl Acad Sci USA*. 2001;98(17):9808-9813.

100. Illek B, Zhang L, Lewis NC, et al. Defective function of the cystic fibrosis-causing missense mutation G551D is recovered by genistein. *Am J Physiol*. 1999;277(4 Pt 1):C833-C839.

101. Wang F, Zeltwanger S, Yang IC-H, et al. Actions of genistein on cystic fibrosis transmembrane conductance regulator channel gating. Evidence for two binding sites with opposite effects. *J Gen Physiol*. 1998;111:477-490.

102. Moran O, Zegarra-Moran O. A quantitative description of the activation and inhibition of CFTR by potentiators: genistein. *FEBS Letters*. 2005;579:3979-3983.

103. Eidelman O, Guay-Broder C, Van Galen PJM, et al. A₁ adenosine-receptor antagonists activate chloride efflux from cystic fibrosis cells. *Proc Natl Acad Sci USA*. 1992;89:5562-5566.

104. Arispe N, Ma J, Jacobson KA, et al. Direct activation of cystic fibrosis transmembrane conductance regulator channels by 8-cyclopentyl-1,3-dipropylxanthine (CPX) and 1,3-diallyl-8-cyclohexylxanthine (DAX). *J Biol Chem*. 1998;273:5727-5734.

105. McCarty NA, Standaert TA, Teresi M, et al. A phase I randomized, multicenter trial of CPX in adult subjects with mild cystic fibrosis. *Pediatr Pulmonol*. 2002;33:90-98.

106. Zegarra-Moran O, Romio L, Folli C, et al. Correction of G551D-CFTR transport defect in epithelial monolayers by genistein but not by CPX or MPB-07. *Br J Pharmacol*. 2002;137:504-512.

107. Smith SN, Middleton PG, Chadwick S, et al. The in vivo effects of milrinone on the airways of cystic fibrosis mice and human subjects. *Am J Resp Cell Mol Biol*. 1999;20:129-134.

108. Lubamba B, Lecourt H, Lebacq J, et al. Preclinical evidence that sildenafil and vardenafil activate chloride transport in cystic fibrosis. *Am J Resp Crit Care Med*. 2008;177:506-515.

109. Dormer RL, Harris CM, Clark Z, et al. Sildenafil (Viagra) corrects ΔF508-CFTR location in nasal epithelial cells from patients with cystic fibrosis. *Thorax*. 2005;60:55-59.

110. Andersson C, Roomans GM. Activation of ΔF508 CFTR in a cystic fibrosis respiratory epithelial cell line by 4-phenylbutyrate, genistein and CPX. *Eur Resp J*. 2000;15:937-941.

111. Lim M, McKenzie KR, Floyd AD, et al. Modulation of ΔF508 cystic fibrosis transmembrane regulator trafficking and function with 4-phenylbutyrate and flavonoids. *Am J Resp Cell Mol Biol*. 2004;31:351-357.

112. Children's Hospital of Philadelphia, Cystic Fibrosis Foundation, National Centers for Research Resources (NCRR). Phenylbutyrate/genistein duotherapy in delta F508-homozygous (for cystic fibrosis). Available at: http://clinicaltrials.gov/show/NCT00016744 NLM Identifier: NCT00016744.

113. Children's Hospital of Philadelphia, Cystic Fibrosis Foundation. Phenylbutyrate/genistein duo-therapy in delta F508-heterozygotes (for cystic fibrosis). Available at: http://clinicaltrials.gov/show/NCT00590538 NLM Identifier: NCT00590538.

114. Farrell PM, Rosenstein BJ, White TB, et al. Guidelines for diagnosis of cystic fibrosis in newborns through older adults: Cystic Fibrosis Foundation consensus report. *J Pediatr.* 2008;153(suppl):S4-S14.

115. Kerem E. Pharmacologic therapy for stop mutations: how much CFTR activity is enough? *Curr Opin Pulm Med.* 2004;10:547-552.

116. Clarke LL. Phosphodiesterase 5 inhibitors and cystic fibrosis. Correcting channel dysfunction. *Am J Resp Crit Care Med.* 2008;177:469-472.

117. Cystic Fibrosis Foundation. Drug Development Pipeline. Available at: http://www.cff.org/research/drugdevelopmentpipeline/. Accessed March 19, 2009.

118. Reihsaus E, Innis M, MacIntyre N, et al. Mutations in the gene encoding for the beta 2-adrenergic receptor in normal and asthmatic subjects. *Am J Respir Cell Mol Biol.* 1993;8:334-339.

119. Sabato MF, Irani A-M, Bukaveckas BL, et al. A simple and rapid genotyping assay for simultaneous detection of two ADRB2 allelic variants using fluorescence resonance energy transfer probes and melting curve analysis. *J Mol Diagn.* 2008;10:258-264.

120. Flume PA, O'Sullivan BP, Robinson KA, et al. Cystic fibrosis pulmonary guidelines: chronic medications for maintenance of lung health. *Am J Respir Crit Care Med.* 2007;176:957-969.

121. Dalcin P deTR, Abreu e Silva FA de. Cystic fibrosis in adults: diagnostic and therapeutic aspects. *J Bras Pneumol.* 2008;34:107-117.

122. Milavetz G. Cystic fibrosis. In: Dipiro JT, Talbert RL, Yee GC, et al., eds. *Pharmacotherapy: A Pathophysiologic Approach.* 7th ed. New York: McGraw-Hill, Inc.; 2007:535-546.

Chapter 12

Toxicogenomics

Helen E. Smith, MS, Ph.D., R.Ph.

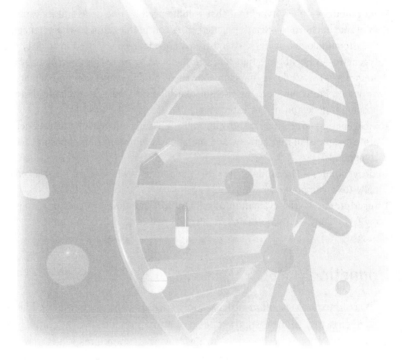

Learning Objectives

After completing this chapter, the reader should be able to
- Define key terminology used in the field of toxicogenomics.
- Discuss the tools used in toxicogenomics and toxicogenetics.
- Discuss how toxicogenomics is utilized in drug development.
- Discuss the potential and current clinical use of toxicogenomics and toxicogenetics to personalize the use of medicines.

Key Definitions

Biomarker—A biological characteristic that can be measured to indicate the presence of a biologic or pathogenic process, predict a pharmacological response to a therapeutic intervention, indicate an exposure, or predict the risk of disease or adverse effect due to an exposure.

Metabolomics—The study of the relative production of metabolites in animals, cells, or tissues. Metabolomics may be used in toxicological studies to evaluate the effects of an exposure on protein expression and activity.

Monogenetic—A phenotypic trait that is influenced by one gene and its variants.

Phenotypic anchoring—Relating gene expression profiles to well-characterized endpoints such as histopathology or clinical chemistry parameters typically used in toxicity studies.

Polygenetic—A phenotypic trait that is influenced by more than one gene and their variants.

Proteomics—The study of the relative levels of protein expression and activity in animals, cells, or tissues. Proteomics may be used in toxicological studies to evaluate the effects of an exposure on gene and mRNA expression.

Toxicogenetics—The study of how an individual's genetic makeup affects gene expression, protein expression and activity, and metabolism in response to exposures to potentially toxic compounds.

Toxicogenomics—The study of how the genome as a whole responds to exposures to potentially toxic compounds.

Transcriptomics—The evaluation of mRNA expression levels in cells or tissues using microarray technology. Transcriptomics are also referred to as expression profiles.

Introduction

Classic toxicology often utilizes tools such as clinical chemistry, histology, and electron microscopy to measure the effects of a toxin on a tissue. In contrast, toxicogenomics is an emerging discipline that studies how the genome responds to toxic exposures. Gene transcription, protein expression and activity, and metabolic activity may all be evaluated to measure the genome response to exposures. Toxicogenetics is the study of how an individual organisms' genetic makeup affects its response to environmental stressors or toxins. The terms toxicogenomics and toxicogenetics (as well as pharmacogenomics and pharmacogenetics) are often used synonymously, but there is a distinction. Toxicogenomics focuses on the genome as a whole, while toxicogenetics focuses on variants of individual genes. Toxicogenetics investigations usually evaluate the influence of the variants of one or just a handful of genes, rather than the whole genome. The distinction between these two terms is apparent in their applications.

The discipline of toxicogenomics grew out of pharmacogenomics in the 1990s as tools of pharmacogenomics began to be applied to toxicology questions. The development of microarray technologies at that time enabled high throughput investigations of the affects of exposures on gene expression. This allowed toxicogenomics development and progress to move forward rapidly.[1] Toxicogenetics has been a part of clinical medicine for some time, although it was not until recently that it has been given that title. One of the first examples of the application of toxicogenetic concepts to medicine was the discovery during the Korean War that soldiers of certain ethnic backgrounds developed severe haemolysis when given the antimalarial primaquine.[2] Deficiencies in the activity of the glucose 6-phosphate dehydrogenase (G6PD) enzyme caused this susceptibility to haemolysis. Originally, G6PD activity in patient red blood cells was measured to predict the amount of risk for this adverse response to primaquine, whereas now genotyping can be done to determine this risk. This is an example of how an individual's phenotype affected the individual's response to a drug.

Toxicogenomics is used with the goal of understanding the deleterious effects of environmental exposures as well as the underlying causes of adverse effects of medications. Toxicogenomics is therefore very pertinent to the field of pharmacy. It is emerging as a tool in both drug development and in medicine. In drug development, toxicogenomics methods are used to both investigate the mechanisms of and to predict the toxicities of medications. Toxicogenetics is applied in clinical medicine to identify patients at risk for developing adverse drug reactions based on their genotypes.

In the following sections of this chapter, the tools utilized in toxicogenomics and toxicogenetics, the use of toxicogenomics in drug development, and examples of current and potential applications of toxicogenetics in clinical pharmacy practice are presented.

Case Study—Toxicogenomics of Abacavir

A.B. is a 45-year-old Caucasian male that is HIV+. Clinicians wish to prescribe abacavir to A.B. for a second time. A.B. has no other underlying disease states other than being HIV+. The patient tolerated abacavir in the past, showing no signs of hypersensitivity. Although this is one of the medications caregivers feel is best to use in treating this patient, A.B. is quite anxious about taking this medication again. He has read it is possible to develop a severe hypersensitivity reaction to this drug even though it was previously well tolerated. As a pharmacist involved in this patient's care, what recommendations would you make in an effort to help A.B. decide whether or not to take abacavir again?

Questions:

1. You discuss with A.B. the information regarding the current understanding of the toxicogenomic aspects of hypersensitivity to abacavir. Based on A.B.'s ethnicity, which gene variant do you suggest he be genotyped for in an effort to determine his risk for developing abacavir-induced hypersensitivity?

   Answer: HLA-B*5701

2. Does the FDA mandate that patients be screened for this genetic polymorphism before administration of abacavir?

   Answer: No, the FDA does not require that patients be screened for their HLA-B status, but the agency does recommend that such screening be done.

3. What is the rationale for screening patients for this polymorphism before the administration of abacavir?

   Answer: Screening patients for this polymorphism will identify patients very likely to develop abacavir hypersensitivity. Given the knowledge that a patient carries an HLA-B*5701 allele, clinicians should be extremely cautious if they choose to administer this drug to such patients, as the presence of that allele puts the patients at significant risk of suffering a serious adverse drug effect.

4. If the patient is homozygous for the wild-type allele, may it be assumed with certainty he will not develop hypersensitivity to abacavir?

   Answer: No. Patients that carry this polymorphism have a significantly greater risk of developing abacavir hypersensitivity compared to patients that have at least one allele for HLA-B*5701. However, patients that are homozygous wild type should be monitored for signs of abacavir hypersensitivity even though they do not have a known genetic risk factor predisposing them to developing abacavir hypersensitivity. Some patients without the HLA-B*5701 genotype may have as yet undiscovered risk factors for abacavir hypersensitivity.

Tools of Toxicogenomics and Toxicogenetics

The development and implementation of tools used in toxicogenomics and toxicogenetics investigations have changed rapidly over time, and will probably continue to do so as technologies evolve. Their use has sometimes been challenging as scientists struggle with the best technological ways to approach the questions they wish to address and how best to analyze the results produced using these tools. In general, these tools evaluate changes in gene expression, protein production, or metabolite production as a result of an exposure to a toxic substance. Two general approaches are taken. The first approach involves comparing simultaneous changes in gene expression, protein production, or metabolite production as a result of an exposure. The second approach involves evaluation of sequential changes in gene expression, protein production, or metabolite formation as a result of an exposure and allows for an investigation into biological pathways of response. Both approaches provide a means of describing the response and a means of investigating the mechanism of a toxicological response.[3,4] The data produced may be used to classify unknown compounds and predict the toxicity of new compounds, investigate mechanisms of toxicity, and predict the risk of patients developing adverse effects as a result of exposures. Toxicogenomics is being utilized in the environmental and occupational health fields, in various chemical industries, in the pharmaceutical and biopharmaceutical industries, and in medicine.

Probably the most significant tool in toxicogenomics to date is the microarray. There are several kinds of array technologies, with DNA arrays the first to become available. DNA arrays include gene expression arrays, genotyping arrays, and identifying arrays. These arrays each have different applications in toxicogenomics. Gene expression arrays measure the relative changes in gene expression as a result of an exposure in cultured cells or the tissues of an exposed organism compared with the gene expression patterns of cells or tissues prior to exposure. These changes in gene expression, when measured as changes in mRNA expression, are called transcript profiles. Studies using transcript profiles may be designed to evaluate gene expression changes across different doses, across exposures at different times in growth or development, for different lengths of time, or across different species. With the development of arrays that are able to measure the response of thousands of genes and in some cases the entire genome of various organisms, the potential to investigate at the genome level the toxic responses of a huge number of genes and across a variety of animals has evolved. Genotyping arrays are another DNA array technology commonly used in toxicogenomics. Genotyping detecting single nucleotide polymorphisms (SNPs), alternative splice variants, or chromosome copy number may be done using SNP arrays, alternative splice arrays, or comparative genomic hybridization arrays, respectively. Assays used to identify contaminating organisms in foods, feeds, or water are a third type of DNA array commonly used in toxicogenomics. Contaminants may be identified by their unique genetic fingerprint that can be detected using these arrays. GeneID is a commercial array used for this purpose that is available at this time. More information on these various types of DNA arrays may be found at the National Center for Biotechnology Information (NCBI) website (http://www.ncbi.nlm.nih.gov/About/primer/microarrays.html).

Data from DNA microarray toxicogenomics studies may be complemented by proteomics and metabolomics studies. Technologies for evaluating protein and metabolic activity and production have been rapidly evolving. Currently, changes in protein expression following exposure to a potential toxin may be analyzed using two-dimensional polyacrylamide gel electrophoresis, protein arrays, antibody arrays, and mass spectrometry.[5] Analysis of altered metabolite formation in biological samples following toxin exposure is currently evaluated using mass spectrometry and NMR spectroscopy.[6] For a detailed discussion of proteomics and metabolomics methodologies, see reviews by Boguski and McIntosh and Kaddurah-Daouk et al.[5,6]

The tools of toxicogenetics are those used to indirectly or directly determine an individual's genetic makeup. Indirect determinations of a patient's genotype involve using a surrogate marker of the genotype of interest such as determining the kinetics of an exogenously administered probe drug in a patient or measuring enzyme activity in accessible tissues such as blood. These techniques identify a patient's phenotype that is known to correlate with a genotype, thus identifying the genotype indirectly. Direct genotyping of patient DNA may be done using a number of techniques such as restriction fragment length polymorphism (RFLP) assays, genotyping utilizing Sanger biochemistry in semi-automated capillary-based assays, or the high-throughput hybridization genotyping microarray presented above. The use of microarrays for genotyping allows for a large number of alleles to be identified at one time for one patient or for many patients to be genotyped at the same time. However, the use of microarrays for genotyping is limited at this time due to their expense and accessibility. New DNA sequencing technologies, often referred to as "next-generation DNA sequencing" methods, are being developed and may eventually replace microarrays for high-throughput genotyping. These next-generation DNA sequencing techniques such as cyclic-array sequencing methods may prove to be less costly and perhaps more accurate compared to microarray genotyping methods. A comprehensive discussion of these techniques is beyond the scope of this chapter, but information about them may be found in recent reviews.[7,8]

Application of Toxicogenomics to Drug Development

Toxicogenomics is opening the door to advancing our knowledge of mechanisms of toxicity and may provide tools to more quickly identify potentially hazardous compounds. This is important for compounds used in industry, those that are environmental contaminants, and for the development of new medications. In drug development, traditional toxicology studies are conducted on potential new medications as part of the drug development process. A variety of toxicity assessments are conducted on these new drug entities depending on their anticipated toxicity. These assessments include the use of in vitro assays as well as testing compounds for toxicity in animals (animal bioassays). These studies provide data for predicting toxicities and early identification of general mechanisms of toxicity. These studies are typically done early in the drug development process. Animal bioassays are also used late in the drug development process to investigate in more depth the mechanisms of the toxicities observed in the earlier assays and to predict long-term effects such as the potential for carcinogenicity. The process of identifying and understanding the potential toxicities of a new drug takes time, is very expensive, may require relatively large amounts of the new compound, and often requires large numbers of animals. For these reasons, alternative methods for evaluating the toxicities of a new drug are being proposed. The tools of toxicogenomics, such as microarray technologies, may help reduce costs of toxicity testing in the drug development process.

Gene expression microarray technologies are being used to predict the toxicity of drugs and to assist in the identification of mechanisms of toxicity. Toxicity prediction using gene expression microarrays makes the assumption that structurally similar drugs or drugs with the same mechanisms of toxicity will have similar effects on gene expression profiles. The transcript profiles of unknown compounds can be compared to the transcript profiles generated for known compounds. The databases of transcript profiles of known compounds must be well-characterized with regard to the toxicological and pathological responses they cause in biological systems for this comparison to be valid and useful. This approach to the classification of unknown compounds, the prediction of compound toxicity, and the investigation of mechanisms of toxicity has been validated. Waring et al. were able to show that compounds with similar mechanisms of toxicity produced similar gene expression profiles in transcription microarrays in rat hepatocytes treated for 24 hours with known hepatotoxins.[9] Waring et al. also demonstrated that the gene expression in livers of rats treated with known hepatocytes correlated with the histopathology and clinical chemistry parameters measured in those treated rats.[10] This second study by Waring is quite important in that it showed that changes in gene expression as a result of exposures and measured by microarrays are valid when compared to traditional measures of toxicity such as histopathology and clinical chemistry. Hamadeh et al. showed that animals treated with agents in the same pharmacological class (for example, all animals were treated with peroxisome proliferators) had very similar gene expression profiles. They also demonstrated that animals treated with drugs of differing chemical classes (some animals were treated with peroxisome proliferators while some were treated with enzyme inducers) have very different gene expression profiles.[11] Table 12-1 lists the compounds tested in the studies by Waring and Hamadeh mentioned above.

Table 12-1
Compounds Used in Microarray Validity Testing

Compounds Tested		Reference
Known Hepatotoxins:		9, 10
Allyl alcohol	Diquat	
Amiodarone	Etoposide	
Aroclor 1254	Indomethacin	
Arsenic	Methapyrilene	
Carbamazepine	Methotrexate	
Carbon tetrachloride	3-Methylcholanthrene	
Diethylnitrosamine	Monocrotaline	
Dimethyl-formamide		
Peroxizome proliferators:	**Enzyme inducer:**	11, 12
Clofibrate	Phenobarbital	
Wyeth 14,643		
Gemfibrozil		

For microarrays to be useful in predicting mechanisms of toxicity or classification of unknown compounds into toxic categories, the transcript profiles of the test compounds need
to be compared to the transcript profiles of model compounds whose profiles have been
well-defined. Hamadeh et al. illustrated that unidentified compounds could be identified using comparisons of cDNA microarrays.[12] In this study, the investigators created a database of
transcription profiles generated by exposing rats to compounds that are either enzyme inducers
or peroxizome proliferators. The expression profiles from these known compounds were then
compared to the expression profiles generated from the livers of rats exposed to unidentified
compounds. The investigators were blinded to the identity of the unknown compounds the
rats were exposed to as they compared the gene expression profiles. The unknown compounds
were able to be correctly identified using the transcription database of the known compounds.[12]
The compounds investigated in this study are also listed in Table 12-1.

Several public and commercial databases of transcript profiles of model compounds have
been developed.[13] Primary databases are those that publish in-house expression data; secondary databases are those that publish in-house and collaborator data. Tertiary databases are those
that house data from unrelated parties that meet submission criteria.[14] Table 12-2 lists the three
currently existing public transcript profile databases. Investigators may submit their expression
array data to these public databases for the benefit of the scientific community. Data submitted to theses databases must meet the quality criteria listed in the Minimal Information About
Microarray Experiments (MI-AME) standards.[13,16]

Table 12-2
Public Transcript Profile Databases

Public Databases

Database Name	Publisher	Website	Reference
Gene Expression Omnibus (NCBI GEO)	National Center for Bio-technology Information (NCBI)	http://www.ncbi.nlm.nih.gov/geo	13, 14
ArrayExpress	European Molecular Biol-ogy Laboratory—Euro-pean Bioinformatics Institute (EMBL-EBI)	http://www.ebi.ac.uk/arrayexpress	13, 15
Center for Informa-tion Biology gene EXpression Data-base (CIBEX)	DNA Databank of Japan (DDBJ)	http://cibex.nig.ac.jp/index.jsp	16, 17

It is hoped that microarray technologies, specifically the use of expression arrays, will be
significantly useful to the field of toxicology in several ways. It is anticipated that microarrays
will improve the ability to predict drug toxicity by speeding up the drug development process.
The data from expression arrays illustrating the effects of a drug exposure on genomic expression may identify early in the drug developmental process medications likely to fail in the
development pipeline due to toxicity. Such early failures would preclude the need to continue
with more toxicity studies. Microarray expression data may also be very useful in contributing

to the early understanding of mechanisms of toxicity and may help direct further, more traditional, toxicity testing to investigate mechanisms of toxicity or may reduce the need for these studies. In a review of the usefulness of toxicogenomics in the pharmaceutical industry, Lühe et al. suggest that toxicogenomics is already able to predict the toxicities of compounds, especially those that are hepatotoxins or nephrotoxins.[13] Another application of pharmacogenomics in drug development is the potential to limit drug toxicity in volunteers during clinical trials. Using proven biomarkers of toxicity generated from transcript profiles to identify subjects likely at risk for known and significant adverse reactions would allow investigators to prevent such subjects from participating in these studies that might be dangerous to them. Some of these anticipated advantages of microarrays are being seen in the pharmaceutical industry during drug development. These advantages, however, are modulated by several caveats. The cost-effectiveness of toxicogenomics in predicting toxic events may be limited to those toxicities that are usually seen after long term exposures, such as the development of cancer. Furthermore, the current difficulties in interpreting the large amounts of data generated from these microarray studies limits being able to understand the results of multiple exposure expression studies, or for comparisons of toxic effects across species.[13]

Proteomics and metabolomics techniques will also be useful in the drug development process by providing data that complements that generated from microarray and traditional toxicology studies. These techniques will contribute to investigations of mechanisms of drug toxicity and drug toxicity prediction. These techniques are not used yet to a great extent due to limitations caused by the massive amounts of data generated from these methodologies. Techniques for analyzing this data are still being developed. If this challenge of data analysis is overcome, the integration of genomics, proteomics, and metabolomics is anticipated to lead to a better understanding of adverse drug responses. Another benefit anticipated from understanding the complete sequence of events caused by an exposure, from gene expression to the influence on metabolism, is a better understanding of the phenomenon that the adverse effects of a medication likely affect multiple genes in addition to being influenced by multiple environmental factors.

Current and Potential Applications of Toxicogenetics to Clinical Practice

Pharmacogenomics is proving useful in drug development and toxicity screening as discussed above. Pharmacogenetics, since it is the evaluation of the influence of variants of individual genes on the response to a drug, leads to its use in the individualization of medicine. There are several examples where advances in the knowledge of genetic variants have identified relationships between polymorphisms and the risk for drug toxicity. Genetic polymorphisms may increase the adverse effects of drugs either by increasing the potential for side effects of a drug used alone or by increasing the likelihood of drug-drug interactions when drugs are used simultaneously. Genes that influence drug toxicity have been generally grouped into one of three categories: those that code for drug metabolizing enzymes, those that code for transporters, and those that code for Human Leukocyte Antigens (HLAs).[18] The pharmacokinetics of various drugs may be affected by variants of drug metabolizing enzymes. When polymorphisms decrease the activity of metabolizing enzymes, biologically active parent drugs or metabolites may accumulate and thus reach toxic levels. Two such examples are the polymorphisms found in cytochrome P450s (CYPs) and in glutathione S-transferase (GST) isoforms. Several of the known polymorphisms in these genes are well characterized regarding their influence of drug pharmacokinetics. Specifically, low activity variants of the important drug metabolizing enzyme CYP2D6 have been found to be related to increased toxicity from narrow therapeutic index drugs such as antidepressants and antipsychotics. Davies et al. identified a relationship between levels of glutathione S-transferase (GST) T1 expression and the risk for developing toxicity to antileukemic medications, especially in children being treated for acute myeloid leukemia. Children that do not express GSTT1 had increased toxicity and decreased survival compared to children that expressed at least one GSTT1 allele.[19]

Attempts to discover correlations between genotypes and the risk of developing drug toxicities are pursued with the hope that the information found may be clinically useful. Understanding the relationship between genotype and risk for toxicity may aid in identifying patient populations whose polymorphisms put them at relatively higher risk for drug toxicities compared to populations without those polymorphisms. This information may help at-risk patients avoid using drugs that could prove to be harmful to them. This information may also be useful in determining appropriate doses for patients with varying drug toxicity risks if their genotype allows for limited use of the drug. However, not all correlations between genotype and risk of drug toxicity identified thus far clinically utilized at this time. The clinical usefulness of known correlations between genotypes and drug response may be quite complicated and confounded by other variables. For example, identification of a genotype known to increase the risk for developing drug toxicity in one population may not cause as significant an increase in the risk of developing toxicity in another population. This discrepancy across populations may be caused by a monogenetic risk for drug toxicity in the first population and an unidentified polygenetic or other multifactorial risk of drug toxicity in the second population. In other words, the drug toxicity seen in the first population is due to a gene variant while the drug toxicity seen in the second population could have been caused by variants of several genes or the variant found in the first population and other factors such as disease state or environmental exposures. A second reason why known genotype/phenotype correlations may not be used is that these genetic biomarkers that have potential as predictive risk factors of adverse drug effects need extensive validation before they may be clinically useful. Attempts are currently being made to develop guidelines for drug dosing that incorporate polygenic traits.[20]

In reality, scientists have probably uncovered little of the potential of genomics and genetics in the individualization of medicine. There are several medications, however, for which the known relationships between genotype and risk of toxicity is being utilized clinically in an attempt to reduce the incidence of severe adverse effects. The U.S. Food and Drug Administration (FDA) published several documents focused on pharmacogenomics and toxicogenomics of which clinicians need to be aware. One such document is the FDA's Table of Valid Genomic Biomarkers in the Context of Approved Drug Labels.[21] This document lists drugs whose labeling includes information on genomic biomarkers and ranks these medications with a designation of whether genotyping before administration of the medication is required or suggested by the FDA. A 1designation in the table denotes the FDA requires genotyping before the drug may be administered. A 2 designation indicates the FDA strongly recommends genotyping before the patient be given the drug. A designation of 3 reflects the Agency's opinion that genotyping would provide useful information in guiding the use of the medication but is not necessary. Of course, patients for whom a drug may be prescribed are the usual subject of the genotyping, especially when testing is being done to avoid drug toxicities. In some instances, however, genotyping may be done on an infectious agent such as the HIV virus or cells of a tumor being treated to determine the virus' or the tumor cells' susceptibility to a medication. At this time, all drugs listed in the FDA table as a category 1 medication require genotyping to determine whether or not the medication will be efficacious rather than identifying patients at risk of developing adverse reactions to a drug. For many of the drugs in the table listed as category 2 or 3 medications, the FDA is recommending patient genotyping to identify those that may be at increased risk of developing drug toxicity. A wide variety of medications have toxicities that are associated with genetic variants, including anticoagulants, chemotherapeutics, antimicrobials, and anticonvulsants. Below is a discussion of several medications for which patient genotyping may be done to decrease the incidence of adverse effects, as indicated in current FDA labeling.

Warfarin is a narrow therapeutic index drug used as an anticoagulant. The most common adverse reaction to this medication is an increased risk for bleeding events. It is often difficult to determine the starting dose in some patients and then to maintain their anticoagulant levels appropriately. At this time, it is known that variants of the warfarin metabolizing enzymes CYP2D9 and Vitamin K epoxide reductase complex 1 (VKORC1) contribute to the variability in required starting and maintenance doses for patients. Several studies have found that patients with lower activity variants of CYP2C9, the primary hepatic P450 responsible for the metabolism and subsequent elimination of warfarin, are at higher risk for over-anticoagulation or bleeding complications while on this medication compared to patients with normal activity CYP29 activity (22, 23, and 24). VKORC1 also has several polymorphic alleles, and the 1173C/T variant has been found to be significantly associated with dose variability and to contribute to the risk of patients experiencing over-anticoagulation or bleeding events.[25] Interestingly, not all the variability of warfarin dosing is accounted for by these known variants of CYP2C9 and VKORC1. Efforts are being made to validate the significance of these variants, and dosing guidelines incorporating variations of both these genes are being developed.[20] The fact that not all the dose variability is accounted for by CYP2C9 and VKORC1 variants implies there are other factors affecting warfarin dose.

Clinical Pearl

Most adverse drug effects will be polygenetic rather than monogenetic in nature, complicating our understanding and use of this information.

A deficiency in the enzyme glucose-6-phophsate dehydrogenase (G6PD) puts patients at risk for developing severe, life-threatening oxidative hemolytic anemia when exposed to certain medications. A patient may have a G6PD deficiency because the gene coding for that enzyme has variants that decrease or eliminate the enzyme's activity. There are many known variants of G6PD that result in lowered or no activity of the enzyme. The most significant variants have the highest prevalence in people of African, Mediterranean, or Asian ancestry. Patients with these backgrounds should be evaluated for G6PD-deficiency before they are administered certain drugs. It was during the Korean War that the G6PD-deficiency was found to be responsible for the severe hemolytic anemia suffered by some soldiers. Other medications that can cause hemolytic anemia in the presence of g6PD deficiency include the antimicrobial dapsone used to treat leprosy and rasburicase used to treat Hyperuricemia in cancer patients. The FDA currently recommends that patients be evaluated for their G6PD status before they are given Rasburicase and Dapsone.[26,27]

Carbamazepine is a medication used primarily as an anticonvulsant. Very serious dermatological reactions that include Stevens-Johnson Syndrome (SJS) and toxic epidermal necrolysis (TEN) can occur in some patients taking this medication. An association has been found between the risk of developing SJS and TEN and the presence of a variant of the human leukocyte antigen HLA-B*1502.[28-30] This association appears to be most prevalent in patients of Asian ancestry.[31] The FDA has included information in the labeling of carbamazepine regarding the significance of this association to prompt clinicians to genotype patients for their HLA-B status to help prevent the life-threatening adverse effects this drug can cause. The FDA does caution, however, that the usefulness of genotyping patients based on ethnicity before the administration of carbamazepine is limited due to the variability in the rates of HLA-B*1502 prevalence in ethnic groups.[32] The HLA-B*1502 variant has not been found to be associated with the occurrence of carbamazepine-associated SJS in patients that did not claim Asian descent.[31,33] Those patients that do not carry the HLA-B*1502 allele may still develop carbamazepine-associated severe cutaneous adverse effects. Therefore, HLA-B*1502 is not a universal genetic biomarker for this occurrence of these adverse effects. Efforts to find other genetic biomarkers linked to the development of carbamazepine-induced SJS and TEN are continuing.

Clinical Pearl

One cannot assume that a polymorphism that is associated with an adverse drug effect in one population will also be associated with that adverse drug effect in another population.

Another variant of the HLA-B gene, HLA-B*5701, has been found to be associated with a severe, immunologically mediated hypersensitivity reaction to abacavir. This hypersensitivity reaction is not the SJS or TEN seen with carbamazepine that is linked to the HLA-B*1502 variant, but it is very dangerous to patients. Abacavir is an antiretroviral agent that is a reverse transcriptase inhibitor used to treat HIV. Mallal et al. found that prospectively screening HIV patients for HLA-B*5701 reduced the incidence of hypersensitivity reactions to abacavir.[34] The FDA recommends in the abacavir labeling that patients be screened for their HLA-B*5701 status before using abacavir for the first time, and in patients who have taken and tolerated the medication before but who's HLA-B*5701 status is not known.[35] A negative finding for the presence of HLA-B*5701 does not mean that a patient will not develop sensitivity to the drug, but the chances are much smaller compared to patients who carry a HLA-B*5701 allele.

Clinical Pearl

One should not assume that the absence of an allele known to be associated with an adverse drug effect in a patient guarantees that the adverse effect will not occur.

6-Mercaptopurine (6-MP) is an antimetabolic antineoplastic agent used mostly to treat various leukemias, especially acute lymphatic leukemia. It is an active metabolite of the prodrug azathioprine, which is an antimetabolite used primarily to prevent transplant rejection, and to treat rheumatoid arthritis and inflammatory gastrointestinal diseases. 6-MP is metabolized to cytotoxic metabolites that cause the adverse effects of the medication. 6-MP is inactivated in part by thiol methylation catalyzed by the polymorphic thiopurine S-methyltransferase (TPMT) enzyme. Low activity variants of TPMT have been identified. Patients that are heterozygotes for the low-activity variant of TPMT have intermediate levels of TPMT activity, while those that are homozygotes for the low activity allele have low or no TPMT activity. Decreased TPMT activity puts patients at risk for developing myelotoxicity with azathioprine and 6-MP administration since high levels of 6-MP are then available for metabolism to the cytotoxic metabolite accumulate. TPMT deficient homozygotes have a serious risk of developing life-threatening myelotoxicity on conventional doses of azathioprine.[36] TPMT genotyping has been found to improve the prediction of hematologic side effects of azathioprine.[37,38] Therefore, the FDA recommends that patient TPMT genotype or phenotype status be determined before administered azathioprine and 6-MP to prevent this life-threatening side effect.[39,40]

Irinotecan is an antineoplastic agent whose mechanism of action is due to its inhibition of topoisomerase I. It is metabolized to its active metabolite SN-38 primarily via hepatic carboxylesterase activity. Both the parent drug and SN-38 bind to topoisomerase I after it complexes with DNA, preventing repair of the single-strand breaks caused by topoisomerase I. This complex of irinotecan or SN-38 with the topoisomerase and DNA is cytotoxic, which is both its therapeutic mechanism of action and the mechanism of action for its toxicity. SN-38 is glucuronidated by the polymorphic enzyme UDP-glucuronosyl transferase 1A1 (UGT1A1), allowing it to be eventually eliminated from the body. Low activity variants of UGT1A1 have been identified and have been found to be associated with an increased risk of cancer patients developing severe neutropenia while being treated with irinotecan.[41,42] These variants are associated with increased levels of SN-38, which have been associated with an increased risk for neutropenia at the initiation of irinotecan therapy. The FDA recommends genotyping patients for their UGT1A1 status and reducing the irinotecan starting dose for patients homozygous for the low activity alleles.[43]

The above are examples of the current clinical applications of toxicogenetics to prevent adverse drug responses. Identifying patients at risk for developing severe adverse effects to some medications based on their genotype is very useful when the association between the genotype and adverse effect has been well characterized. There are many associations between genotype and drug response that are not yet fully characterized, but may in the future be useful. For example, many antidepressants, including tricyclics and some selective serotonin reuptake inhibitors (SSRIs) are metabolized by the polymorphic enzyme CYP2D6. Large variations in the pharmacokinetics for these medications across patients have been noted, putting some at risk for drug toxicity. In addition, variants of CYP2C9 may significantly alter the pharmacokinetics of several medications used to treat cardiovascular disease, nonsteroidal anti-inflammatory drugs, and hypoglycemic agents, as well as warfarin as discussed above. The utility of genotyping patients receiving these medications for their CYP2D6 and CYP2C9 status to prevent adverse effects has not been unequivocally proven. Perhaps with more characterization of the associations between these genotypes and the adverse effects caused by these drugs, genotyping will be proven useful in preventing adverse effects of these particular drugs.[44] Besides the significance of polymorphisms in drug metabolizing enzymes, polymorphisms in genes coding for drug transporter enzymes such as the multi-drug resistance transporter 1 (MDR1) may also prove to be clinically significant in the development of adverse drug reactions. Again, genotyping patients for known MDR1 variants is not yet validated to the extent to be clinically useful, but may be in the near future.[45] Another very interesting potential use of pharmacogenomics in the clinical setting that is being evaluated are biomarkers for identifying idiosyncratic adverse reactions. The International Serious Adverse Events Consortium (SAEC) led by the FDA was formed in 2007 to further this application of pharmacogenomics. Efforts are being made to identify genetic variants that may be predictive of these rare, nondose-related but potentially serious adverse reactions to medications. The SAEC is currently working to identify variants that may have a role in the idiopathic development of serious hepatic and dermal adverse drug responses.[46]

Summary

The scientific and regulatory communities are putting great efforts into making toxicogenomics and toxicogenetics useful and valid. Regulatory agencies, academic institutions, and industry groups have joined forces in the form of various consortiums, centers, or funding agencies to promote the use, validation, and effectiveness of toxicogenomic and toxicogenetic technologies and their applications. One agency working on this is the The National Institute of Health (NIEHS), who created the National Center for Toxicogenomics (NCT) in September of 2000. The mission of the center was "to promote the evolution and coordinated use of gene expression technologies and to apply them to the assessment of toxicological effects in humans."[47] Its primary goal was to create a reference system of human gene expression data and develop a database of chemical effects in biological systems. Its second goal was to gain more understanding of mechanisms of toxicity.[47] This Center is no longer in existence in its original form, but has been redistributed within the NIEHS and is now a component of the Environmental Genetics Group, the Environmental Stress and Cancer Group, and the Chemical Effects in Biological Systems (CEBS) database. Links to these groups within NIESH may be found at the NIEHS website http://www.niehs.nih.gov/research/atneihs.nct.cfm.

While the NCT was in its original form, to meet its stated goals, the NCT formed the Toxicogenomics Research Consortium (TRC) in 2000. This consortium was formed and funded by the NIEHS Division of Extramural Research and Training (DERT) with the solicitation of applications for extramural researcher participation. Selected participants coordinated their research efforts in toxicogenomics investigations and had the support of the NIEHS extramural staff, the NIEHS NCT, and access to NCT-supported Resource Contractors. The majority of the researchers involved in the consortium focused their toxicogenomics efforts in the field of environmental health. The investigators involved included the NIEHS Microarray Center and leading scientists at the University of North Carolina (UNC) at Chapel Hill, Duke University in Durham, the Fred Hutchinson Cancer Research Center/University of Washington (UW) in Seattle, the Massachusetts Institute of Technology (MIT) in Cambridge, and the Oregon Health Science University (OHSU) in Portland.[48] Projects undertaken as part of the efforts of the consortium are in various stages of completion. The NIEHS website lists current consortium members and the projects they are working on (http://www.niehs.nih.gov/research/supported/centers/trc/). As listed on the website, the goals for the TRC include the "enhancement of research in the broad area of environmental stress responses using microarray gene expression profiling; development of standards and practices which will allow analysis of gene expression data across platforms and provide an understanding of intra- and inter-laboratory variation; contribute to the development of a robust relational database which combines toxicological endpoints with changes in gene expression profiles; improve public health through better risk detection, and earlier intervention in disease processes." Parallel to the efforts of the TRC is a consortium of pharmaceutical companies under the coordinating guidance of The Health and Environmental Sciences Institute (HESI) of the International Life Sciences Institute (ILSI). Members of this group are evaluating the world-wide harmonization efforts of gene expression data and analysis.[49]

In addition to developing consortiums to further progress in this field, the NIEHS has developed databases as tools for storing, accessing, and comparing data generated by pharmacogenomics studies. NIEHS has developed the toxicogenomics data repository that was the original mission of the NCT. This is the Chemical Effects in Biological Systems (CEBS).[50] This repository is accessible by the public and includes information on study design, clinical chemistry, and histopathology data associated with the study subjects as well as microarray and proteomics data generated in the submitted studies.[50] A second database, the Biomedical Investigation Database (BID), was created as another component of the CEBS. The BID is used to aid in submitting and archiving data to CEBS, as well as archiving additional data not already stored in CEBS. Access to CEBS can be gained by going to http://cebs.niehs.nih.gov, while BID may be accessed at https://dir-apps.niehs.nih.gov/arc/.[50] A second data repository has also been developed by the NIEHS in the Mount Desert Island Biological Laboratory (MDIBL), a Marine and Freshwater Biomedical Science (MFBS) Center of the NIEHS. This data repository, called the Comparative Toxicogenomics Database (CTD), allows scientists to investigate the interactions between chemicals, genes, proteins, and diseases thought to be influenced by environmental exposures. These databases, although focusing on the adverse effects of environmental exposures, are still of interest to healthcare providers as most diseases, either their etiology or the effectiveness or risks of their pharmacological treatment, will be influenced by patient environment.

Another key government agency that is coordinating efforts to develop toxicogenomics and toxicogenetics is the U.S Food and Drug Administration (FDA). The FDA created the National Center for Toxicological Research (NCTR) to conduct research and provide technical advice and training to FDA scientists. These services are provided to assist the FDA in making science-based regulatory decisions with the goal of improving the health of the American public. NCTR research focuses on understanding mechanisms of toxicity and to further the development of new technologies for assessing human exposure, susceptibility to disease, and risk. The NCTR has developed several centers focused on different issues related to toxicogenomics, including the Center for Toxicoinformatics, the Center for Functional Genomics, the Center for Metabolomics, and the Center for Proteomics. The Center for Functional Genomics was established in 2001 to provide NCTR scientists and their collaborators access to microarray technology of high quality, facilitate toxicogenomics research by assisting collaborative efforts between scientists conducting toxicogenomics studies and statisticians, bioinformaticians, and Center scientists. The Center for Functional Genomics was also established to help the FDA integrate genomics into their mission. The Centers for Metabolomics and Proteomics provide scientists access to high tech analytical methods used in those investigational areas, while the Center for Bioinformatics conducts research in bioinformatics and assists scientists in using these capabilities. The Center for Bioinformatics also offers several software packages for genomics data management, mining, analysis, and interpretation. Links providing more information regarding these FDA Centers for Excellence related to toxicogenomics may be found at the FDA NCTR website http://www.fda.gov/nctr/index.html.

Besides providing leadership in the development of toxicogenomics and toxicogenetics, the

FDA is encouraging the pharmaceutical and biopharmaceutical industry to submit pharma-cogenomics data with Investigational New Drug (IND) applications, New Drug Applications (NDAs), and Biologic License Applications (BLAs). Their guidance documents *Guidance for Industry: Pharmacogenomic Data Submissions* delineates when pharmacogenomics and pharmacogenetics data must be submitted to the agency and when it may be voluntarily submitted.[51,52] At this time, there is concern in the pharmaceutical and biopharmaceutical industry regarding how toxicogenomics data will be interpreted and used in the drug development process. Efforts are being made by both the FDA and companies developing drugs and biologicals to come to an understanding of the use of toxicogenomics in the drug development process.[53]

As evidenced by the many efforts of scientists, clinicians, and government agencies to discover, validate, and use toxicogenomics and toxicogenetics in drug discovery, toxicity prediction and understanding, and in the personalization of medicine, this field has become very important. Although there are still limitations to the ability to use the information generated by toxicogenomics investigations, there is great promise in its eventual more complete utility. On the flip side, as more is learned about the influence of genetic variants on drug toxicity and response, it will likely be found that the application of this information is more difficult. This is because most adverse responses to medications, when influenced by genomics, will rarely be monogenetic. These types of examples will likely be limited compared to the numbers of adverse drug reactions that will prove to be polygenic. The adverse effects of medications will also likely be found to be influenced by the effects of the medications themselves on multiple genes, as well as by other environmental factors that influence the expression of those same genes. This moves toxicogenomics into the realm of another new discipline called systems biology. This science is attempting to look at how gene-gene interactions and gene-environment interactions influence an organism's responses to exposures to either environmental factors or medications.[54]

It is important that pharmacists keep up to date with the evolution of toxicogenomics and toxicogenetics as professionals in the field of pharmacy are involved in drug development, investigations of adverse effects, and in ensuring the safe use of medications in clinical practice. Familiarity and frequent perusal of medical literature focusing on toxicogenomics and toxicogenetics investigations and new clinical applications is necessary for the practitioner that wishes to keep abreast of this rapidly evolving field.

References

1. Weber WW. Toxicogenomics: history and current applications. *ASM News.* 2004;70:364-370.
2. Cappellini MD, Fiorelli G. Glucose-6-phosphate dehydrogenase deficiency. *Lancet.* 2008;371:64-74.
3. Schmidt CW. Toxicogenomics. *Environ Health Perspect.* 2002;110:A750-A755.
4. Hayes KR, Bradfield CA. Advances in toxicogenomics. *Chem Res Toxicol.* 2005;18:403-414.
5. Boguski MS, McIntosh MW. Biomedical informatics for proteomics. *Nature.* 2003;422:233-237.
6. Kaddurah-Daouk R, Kristal BS, Weinshilboum RM. Metabolomics: a global biochemical approach to drug response and disease. *Ann Rev Pharmacol Toxicol.* 2008;48:653-683.
7. Shendure J, Mitra RD, Varma C, et al. Advanced sequencing technologies: methods and goals. *Nature Reviews Genetics.* 2004;5:335-344.
8. Shendure J, Hanlee J. Next-generation DNA sequencing. *Nature Biotechnology.* 2008;26:1135-1145.
9. Waring JF, Ciurlionis R, Jolly RA, et al. Microarray analysis of hepatotoxins in vitro reveals a correlation between gene expression profiles and mechanisms of toxicity. *Toxicol Lett.* 2001;120:359-368.
10. Waring JF, Jolly RA, Ciurlionis R, et al. Clustering of hepatotoxins based on mechanism of toxicity

using gene expression profiles. *Toxicol Appl Pharmacol*. 2001;175:28-42.

11. Hamadeh HK, Bushel PR, Jayadev S, et al. Gene expression analysis reveals chemical-specific profiles. *Toxico Sci*. 2002;67:219-231.

12. Hamadeh HK, Bushel PR, Jayadev S, et al. Prediction of compound signature using high density gene expression profiling. *Toxico Sci*. 2002;67:232-240.

13. Lühe A, Suter L, Ruepp S, et al. Toxicogenomics in the pharmaceutical industry: Hollow promises or real benefit? *Mutation Research*. 2005; 75:02-115.

14. Edgar R, Domrachev M, Lash AE. Gene expression omnibus: NCBI gene expression and hybridization array data repository. *Nucleic Acids Research*. 2002;30:207-210.

15. Brazma A, Parkinson H, Sarkans U, et al. ArrayExpress-a public repository for microarray gene expression data at the EBI. *Nucleic Acids Research*. 2003;31:68-71.

16. Brazma A, Hingamp P, Quackenbush J, et al. Minimum information about a microarray experiment (MIAME)-toward standards for microarray data. *Nature Genetics*. 2001;29:365-371.

17. Ikeo K, Ishi-i J, Tamura T, et al. CIBEX: Center for Information Biology gene expression database. *CR Biologies*. 2003;326:1079-1082.

18. Wilke RA, Lin DW, Roden DM, et al. Identifying genetic risk factors for serious adverse drug reactions: current progress and challenges. *Nat Rev Drug Discovery*. 2007;6:904-916.

19. Davies SM, Robison LL, Buckley JD, et al. Glutathione S-transferase polymorphisms and outcome of chemotherapy in childhood acute myeloid leukemia. *J Clin Onc*. 2001;19:1279-1287.

20. Anderson JL, Horne BD, Stevens SM, et al. Randomized trial of genotype-guided versus standard warfarin dosing in patients initiating oral anticoagulation. *Circulation*. 2007;116:2563-2570.

21. US Food and Drug Administration. Table of valid genomic biomarkers in the context of approved drug labels. Available at: http://www.fda.gov/cder/genomics/genomic_biomarkers_table.htm. Accessed March 23, 2009.

22. Coumadin [package insert]. Princeton, NJ: Bristol-Myers Squibb Company; August 2007.

23. Momary KM, Shapiro NL, Viana MA, et al. Factors influencing warfarin dose requirements in African Americans. *Pharmacogenomics*. 2007;8:1535-1544.

24. Lima MV, Ribeiro GS, Mesquita ET, et al. CYP2C9 genotypes and the quality of anticoagulation control with warfarin therapy among Brazilian patients. *Eur J Clin Pharmacol*. 2008;64:9-15.

25. Limdi NA, Veenstra DL. Warfarin pharmacogenetics. *Pharmacotherapy*. 2008;28:1084-1097.

26. ElitekTM [package insert]. New York, NY: Sanofi-Synthelabo Inc; November 2004.

27. AczoneTM [package insert]. Fort Collins, CO: QLT USA; 2005.

28. Chung WH, Hung SI, Hong HS, et al. Medical genetics: a marker for Stevens-Johnson syndrome. *Nature*. 2004;428-486.

29. Hung SI, Chung WH, Jee SH, et al. Genetic susceptibility to carbamazepine-induced cutaneous adverse drug reactions. *Pharmacogenet Genomics*. 2006;16:297-306.

30. Man CB, Kwan P, Baum L, et al. Association between HLA-B*1502 allele and antiepileptic drug-induced cutaneous reactions in Han Chinese. *Epilepsia*. 2007;48:1015-1018.

31. Lonjou C, Thomas L, Borot N, et al. A marker for Stevens-Johnson syndrome: ethnicity matters. *Pharmacogenomics J*. 2006;6:265-268.

32. Tegretol [package insert]. East Hanover, NJ: Novartis Pharmaceuticals Corporation; December 2007.

33. Kaniwa N, Saito Y, Aihara M, et al. HLA-B locus in Japanese patients with anti-epileptics and allopurinol-related Stevens-Johnson syndrome and toxic epidermal necrolysis. *Pharmacogenomics*. 2008;9:1617-1622.

34. Mallal S, Phillips E, Carosi G, et al. HLA-B*5701 screening for hypersensitivity to abacavir. *N Engl J Med*. 2008;358:569-579.

35. Ziagen® [package insert]. ResearchTrianglePark, NC: GlaxoSmithKine, July 2008.

36. Eichelbaum M, Ingelman-Sundberg M, Evans WE. Pharmacogenomics and individualized drug therapy. *Ann Rev Med*. 2006;57:119-137.

37. Relling MV, Hancock ML, Rivera GK, et al. Mercaptopurine therapy intolerance and heterozygosity at the thiopurine S-methyltransferase gene locus. *J Natl Cancer Inst*. 1999;91:2001-2008.

38. Heckmann JM, Lambson EM, Little F, et al. Thiopurine methyltransferase (TPMT) heterozygosity and enzyme activity as predictive tests for the development of azathioprine-related adverse events. *J Neurol Sci*. 2005;231:71-80.

39. Imuran [package insert]. San Diego, CA: Prometheus Laboratories Inc; May 2008.

40. Purinethol® [package insert]. Sellersville, PA: DSM Pharmaceuticals Inc; August 2003.
41. Innocenti F, Undevia SD, Iyer L, et al. Genetic variants in the UDP-glucuronosyltransferase 1A1 gene predict the risk of severe neutropenia of irinotecan. *J Clin Oncol.* 2004;22:1382-1388.
42. Marcuello E, Altés A, Menoyo A, et al. UGT1A1 gene variations and irinotecan treatment in patients with metastatic colorectal cancer. *Br J Cancer.* 2004;91:678-682.
43. Camptosar® [package insert]. New York, NY: Pfizer; July 2005.
44. Kirchheiner J, Seeringer A. Clinical implications of pharmacogenetics of cytochrome P450 drug metabolizing enzymes. *Biochimica et Biophyicas Acta.* 2007; 1770:489-494.
45. Zhou S, Di YM, Chan E, et al. Clinical pharmacogenetics and potential application in personalized medicine. *Curr Drug Metab.* 2008;9:738-784.
46. Holden A. The innovative use of large-scale industry biomedical consortium to research the genetic basis of drug induced serious adverse events. *Drug Discover Today: Technologies.* 2007;4:5-87.
47. Tennant RW. The National Center for Toxicogenomics: using new technologies to inform mechanistic toxicology. *Environ Health Perspect.* 2002;110:A8-A10.
48. Medlin J. Toxicogenomics research consortium sails into uncharted waters. *Environ Health Perspect.* 2002;110:A744-A746.
49. Pennie W, Pettit SD, Lord PG. Toxicogenomics in risk assessment: an overview of an HESI collaborative research program. *Environ Health Perspect.* 2004;112:417-419.
50. Waters M, Stasiewicz S, Merrick BA, et al. CEBS—chemical effects in biological systems: a public data repository integrating study design and toxicity data with microarray and proteomics data. *Nucleic Acids Res.* 2008;36:D892-D900.
51. US Department of Health and Human Services; Food and Drug Administration; Center for Drug Evaluation and Research (CDER); Center for Biologics Evaluation and Research (CBER); and Center for Devices and Radiological Health (CDRH). Guidance for Industry: Pharmacogenomic Data Submissions. Rockville, MD: Food and Drug Administration; March 2005.
52. US Department of Health and Human Services, Food and Drug Administration, Center for Drug Evaluation and Research (CDER), Center for Biologics Evaluation and Research (CBER), and Center for Devices and Radiological Health (CDRH). Attachment to Guidance on Pharmacogenomic Data Submissions: Examples of Voluntary Submissions or Submissions Required Under 21 CFR 312, 314, or 601. Rockville, MD: Food and Drug Administration; March 2005.
53. Freeman K. Toxicogenomics data: the road to acceptance. *Environ Health Perspect.* 2004;112:A678-A685.
54. Olden K. Toxicogenomics—a new systems toxicology approach to understanding of gene-environment interactions. *Ann NY Acad Sci.* 2006;1076:703-706.

Part III

Important Issues in Pharmacogenomics

Chapter 13

The Role of Pharmacists in Pharmacogenomics

Ajoy Koomer, Ph.D., MS, E.M.B.A.; Miriam A. Ansong, Pharm.D.

Learning Objectives

After completing this chapter, the reader should be able to

- Recognize the role of the pharmacist in pharmacogenomics education.
- Explain the impact pharmacists may have on educating healthcare professionals. on the use of pharmacogenomics information in clinical practice.
- Recognize the pharmacist's role in pharmacogenomics research.

Key Definitions

Formulary management—The use of various techniques to match the drugs stored in a formulary system for individuals enrolled in a prescription drug plan. As per ASHP guidelines, formulary system refers to the methods for evaluation and selection of suitable drug products that are to be stored in the formulary of organized healthcare settings.

Postmarketing surveillance—Refers to the regular monitoring of pharmaceutical drug products and devices after they are released into the market. Because most drug products are approved based on clinical trials on a small controlled sample tailored for the experiment, post marketing surveillance can further refine, confirm or deny the safety of a drug after it has been used by the global population who might be exposed to a wide array of diseases and other medical complications, not experienced in the sample population group.

Managed care programs—A term used to describe a variety of techniques intended for mitigating the unnecessary healthcare costs and improve the quality of care organizations that use these techniques or render them as services to other organizations. Sometimes the definition also encompasses systems that finance and render healthcare benefits to enrollees organized around managed care concepts.

Benefit management programs—In the context of pharmacy, it refers to a true client based solution that provides for the appropriate medication usage with least amount of administration at an optimal price.

Prior authorization programs—Refers to a program or process that mandates the prescriber or physician to consult with the company's contractor who might have suggested the use of a particular medication under a medical assistance program to ensure that the patient meets the predetermined criteria for coverage under that specified program.

Drug utilization review—Refers to evaluation of clinical information of a particular patient according predetermined criteria and conveying the results of findings to a clinician.

Phenotype—Refers to the outward manifestation of an individual's genotype.

Genotype—Refers to the complete set of genes carried by an individual.

High through screening—Coupled with combinatorial chemistry and bioinformatics, it is an automated method for rapidly screening the activity of thousands of potential drug candidates to further the investigation of those compounds that show promise in the initial screening methods.

Introduction

Pharmacogenomics relates to multiple genetic variations in determining drug response.[1-5] An offshoot of this concept is pharmacogenetics, which studies the effect of inter-individual genetic variations on pharmacokinetic and pharmacodynamic profiles of drugs administered to patients. Notably, pharmacogenetics is likely to be one of the greatest developments of the post genomic era and one which will refute the concept that "one medication fits all size" and lead "to the concept of customized or tailor made medicines." All healthcare professionals can play pivotal roles in ensuring that pharmacogenetic information is disseminated properly and effectively in healthcare settings.[1] Pharmacists as educators, clinical consultants, and providers of healthcare can affect the way that the concept of personalized medications based on genetic profiling is handled in practice.[1-5] One goal of pharmacogenomics is to improve on the current data that indicates that therapeutic responses to drug therapy only averages about 50% and increase it to 75% or more.[6] Though not clearly defined in the literature, pharmacists will play unique and dynamic roles in pharmacogenetics that may include participation in patient and health provider education, including genetic counseling, medication safety management, formulary management, developing research methodologies in collaboration with scientists and implementing bench work pharmacogenetics tests in clinical settings. Some of the potential roles for pharmacists in pharmacogenomics are summarized in Table 1-1.

Table 1-1
Possible Roles for Pharmacists' in Pharmacogenomics

Roles	Anticipated Functions
Educators	• Serve as a conduit for educating other healthcare providers about TDM and adverse drug reactions that may have direct correlation with a patient's drug-gene interaction pattern. • Provide continuous education programs for fellow pharmacists. • Offer genetic counseling of patients and possible interpretation of genetic test results.[1]
Clinical pharmacists/specialists	• Facilitate use of genotyping information for patients by physicians and pharmacy benefit sponsoring programs that may result in mitigation of adverse drug reactions and less healthcare expenditure from suboptimal therapy. • Pharmacist's knowledge of pharmacogenetics may guide drug selection, drug dose, and duration of usage, which are very important considerations in determining prescription coverage. • Pharmacists should be able to inform physicians whether drug targets generated by a rare genotype could affect formulary or nonformulary drugs, and this decision might affect formulary management. • Knowledge of genetics should help pharmacists in providing a robust drug utilization review.[4]
Clinicians/research scientists	• Develop research methodologies and aid implementation of pharmacogenetics in clinical practice through development of proof of principle, proof of efficacy, and proof of cost effectiveness.[1]

Case Study—The Potential Role of Pharmacists in Anticoagulation Clinics

With the scope of pharmacogenetic testing rapidly escalating it is quite possible that pharmacists managing warfarin patients in anticoagulation clinics might be entrusted with the additional responsibility of warfarin genotyping followed by genetic counseling.

Questions:

1. Are there any ethical concerns using the results of warfarin genotyping for making health-care decisions?
2. Are there limitations to be considered for confidential reporting of pharmacogenetic tests?
3. How might genotyping reduce healthcare costs associated with congenital diseases?
4. What criteria must be met in order to make a pharmacogenetic test like CYP 2C9 genotyping clinically relevant?
5. Are there any examples available that one can benchmark as models for application of genetic testing in clinical settings?

Pharmacists as Educators for Patients and Healthcare Providers

With advances in genomics, the FDA will likely become more involved in reviewing and approving pharmacogenetic tests related to the clinical use of medications that are seen in community pharmacist settings. According to ACCP, in the near future, about 25% of FDA approved drugs will have pharmacogenetic information in the package inserts.[1-5] A number of medical centers and major laboratories are offering pharmacogenetic tests related to warfarin and tamoxifen therapy. The FDA has likewise approved AmpliChip (Roche) and UGT1A1-Invader (Third Wave Technologies) for clinical use.[1-5] For physicians TPMT genotyping is recommended as a useful adjunct to a regimen that includes 6-MP (6-mercaptopurine) or azathioprine. Physicians can also recommend CYP 2C9 and VKOR-C1, CYP 2D6 and UGTA1 genotyping before prescribing warfarin, tamoxifen, Strattera, or Camptosar (high intensity irinotecan). [13] Patients might ask pharmacists questions about these tests after discussion with their prescribers or pharmacists may be called in to counsel the patients and interpret their results. Physicians may ask pharmacists how pharmacogenomic test results impact a patient's present or prospective drug regimens. Pharmacists by virtue of their knowledge in pharmaco-dynamic and pharmacokinetic profiles and drug interactions can be the "go-to" persons so far as education of physicians and patients are concerned, and may one day be asked to provide genetic counseling services.[1-5]

In light of the rapid advancement of pharmacogenomics research, the American Association for Colleges of Pharmacy (AACP) academic affairs committee in 2001/2002 laid down the competencies in pharmacogenomics expected from a pharmacist. In 2005, the International Society for Pharmacogenomics (ISP) published their recommendations to the deans of the schools of medicine, pharmacy, and nursing schools, which suggested global guidelines regarding pharmacogenomics education for health professionals. As detailed in Chapter 15, surveys have shown that schools of pharmacy across continental America and Western Europe have been the frontrunners in modifying their professional pharmacy curriculum to embrace pharmacogenomics.[7] In fact today genomics is offered in many different courses of the didactic curriculum starting from toxicology and pharmacology to pharmacotherapeutics.[7] Anecdotal evidence suggests that pharmacogenomics is being incorporated into pharmacy practice experiences as well. In response to the needs of practicing pharmacists, various professional pharmacy organizations (see Chapter 15) have started offering 3–5 credit hour continuing education programs in genomics.[3,8]

Although the role of pharmacogenomic testing in healthcare settings is not fully established, it is evident that due to advances in technologies, genetic testing for variations in drug metabolizing enzymes have been increasing.[1] The FDA is also mandating genomics inserts for different drug categories, which may be relevant not only for hospital pharmacists but for retail also. Being the drug experts pharmacists can serve as conduits for educating other healthcare providers about therapeutic drug monitoring (TDM) and adverse drug reactions (ADR) that may have direct correlation with a patient's drug-gene interaction pattern.[1] Anecdotal evidence suggests that many pharmacists are performing that role in selective situations today. It is encouraging to find that pharmacy educational institutes and professional organizations are taking a lead role in enlightening pharmacists to this new field.

Pharmacists' Role in Formulary Management, Medication Safety, and Drug Expenditure

A number of factors that can influence decisions regarding formulary systems include cost, Pharmacy and Therapeutics committees' reviews, and third-party payers or managed care systems. Each of these factors is discussed in detail below.

Drug Expenditure

Healthcare cost is on the rise. Part of this increase is attributed to drug expenditure, which will likely continue to increase. While it is easy to blame this on pharmaceutical companies, the overall drug development process needs to first be examined. It may take years to develop and market a drug at a cost of many millions of dollars. Often times, even a promising drug does not make it to the market. Postmarketing surveillance can lead to withdrawal of some drugs approved by the FDA and marketed. In either case, the government does not control drug cost in the U.S. as it does in some other countries.[9] Although the FDA does not currently require pharmacogenomic testing in clinical trials, curent evidence continues to support the importance of such tests in clinical practice.[9] Therapeutic failure, adverse drug reactions, and complications of drug therapy that increase healthcare cost may be offset by the availability of pharmacogenomic information. Pharmacists and other clinicians can then make effective drug therapy decisions for patients utilizing such information. The availability of genetic information will permit individualized treatment to be devised, facilitate concrete decisions about formulary drug selections, and many patients will be accommodated for their therapy. This may offer the most cost effective way of treatment, improve patients' quality of life, and reduce healthcare cost.[9,10]

Pharmacists and Therapeutics (P&T) Committees

Drug formulary management is a responsibility of pharmacists. Pharmacists conduct objective assessment of drug or drug classes based on scientific information, critical treatment pathways, and clinical experiences. This assessment is used to make decisions with respect to formulary establishment and maintenance in their various institutions. The drug formulary is approved by the P&T committees in various institutions. Pharmacy and Therapeutics committees are present in institutions and organizations such as managed care, pharmacy benefit management, State Medicaid Boards, State Department Public institutions, and many others. The P&T committee consists of physicians, nurses, other health professionals, and a designated pharmacist.

The pharmacist implements policies for drug formulary selection, addition, and management. Before a formulary addition is made, drug monographs are prepared by the pharmacist and submitted to the P&T committee for review and approval. Other relevant information such as pharmacokinetics and pharmacology are also included in the formulary. Pharmacogenomics, quality of life, and clinical outcomes are expected to be included in the future for evaluating drug monographs. Cost effective analysis studies are crucial for making selection based on efficacy and safety.[10] However, data may often be limited and clinicians might depend solely on cost analysis for such decisions. The effectiveness of drug response due to genetic variability can be attributed to differences in drug metabolism, target organ, and drug distribution or transport.[4] Many drugs undergo metabolism through several metabolic pathways that utilize enzyme systems. Examples of these enzyme systems that exhibit genetic variability and have been studied include cytochrome P-450 (CYP450) enzymes, N-acetyltransferase (NAT), thiopurine S methyltransferase (TPMT), and uridine diphosphate glucuronosyltransferase (UGT). The isoenzyme CYP2D6, alone, accounts for metabolism of about 30% of all drugs currently available in the market.[4] Selected examples of drugs that exhibit genetic variability include anticoagulants, immunosuppressants, antidepressants, antipsychotics, antiseizure agents, beta-blockers, and antiarrthythmics.[4] Drug distribution or transport is promoted by several proteins that are found in certain organs such as the kidney, liver, intestines, and blood brain barrier.[4] These proteins show genetic differences among people based on the different genes that may code for a particular protein.[4] This transport system may eventually affect the distribution of drugs at their functional target organs. As a result drugs may fail to reach their target cells or organs, which may eventually lead to drug resistance or toxicity elsewhere.[4] Drugs that have been noted for such transport mechanisms include digoxin, antiretroviral agents, and certain antineoplastics. The above highlights the necessity of incorporating genetic variability information when making formulary decisions.[4,11,12]

Drugs often interact with tissues and organs through receptors. Genetic variability in these receptors or their effector mechanisms can result in different responses to drug effectiveness or toxicities among individuals depending on their receptor related activities.[4] Certain individuals may be more or less responsive to certain drugs or a class of drugs based on such variability. The pharmacist can make an impact on patients by making recommendations to the formulary to help accommodate such individuals.[4]

Appropriate drug dosing and cost analysis can affect formulary drug selection. Dose of a drug such as warfarin can be affected by the individual genetic make up. Cost of therapy may be higher or lower based on the strength, quantity, and duration of therapy that a patient may need. Medication misadventures resulting from wrong drug or inappropriate duration of therapy can then be prevented with the availability of genetic information. Pharmacogenomic data will be paramount in clinical decisions, medication safety, and formulary management. Reducing the occurrences of therapeutic failures and increasing the chances of successful therapy will eventually reduce overall healthcare costs.[9,12,13]

Pharmacists and Managed Care Systems

Third-party payers or managed care organizations have different prescription benefit programs. The significance of pharmacogenomics information will impact drug policies such that individuals with genetic differences may be allowed a nonformulary drug in a specific plan. Prior authorization programs help to control drug cost. Rules and regulations are implemented by these organizations to control the unnecessary use of certain drugs. This process can be very tedious for plan holders, physicians, and especially pharmacists. The availability of individual pharmacogenomics information will eliminate some steps and ultimately improve the efficiency of the prior authorization process. Additionally, managed care organizations will be better informed, pharmacists can perform effective drug use reviews and create expanded formulary, prescription drug coverage policies will significantly improve, and hopefully drug expenditure may decrease.[4,11,12]

Clinical Pearl

Pharmacists can use pharmacogenetics to provide safe and cost-effective TDM (therapeutic drug monitoring).

The FDA has mandated TDM of narrow therapeutic index (NTI) drugs. TDM is required for these drugs since a very small change in dosage levels could result in either sub therapeutic and toxic levels with the consequences for adverse drug reactions that may result in pain, frequent visits to emergency rooms, hospitalization, and even death.[15] As reported by physicians the significant candidates are digoxin, warfarin, and phenytoin. But how does TDM fit into pharmacogenetics and what role should clinical pharmacists play it? In hospitals TDM is usually conducted by the clinical laboratory in consultation with clinical pharmacists. The clinical pharmacist generally works with general medicine teams, surgery units, subspecialty services, and intensive care specialists to evaluate the appropriate of drug therapy and interpreting serum concentration levels.[15] Because pharmacists are expert in gene-drug interactions apart from drug-drug interactions, they can play a pivotal role in mitigating ADRs by educating physicians and other healthcare providers about the clinically relevant genetic variants which NTI drugs usually possess, and the ramifications of drug responses in patients who might carry these allelic variations.[15] For example, P-glycoprotein of MDR1 gene decreases the bioavailability of digoxin in the intestine by localizing the drug in intestinal lumen. In the kidney the same glycoprotein increases the secretion of the drug in urine. Genetic variants of P-glycoproteins that express clinically relevant polymorphisms at amino acids 2677 and 3435 result in proteins with low transport activity. These polymorphisms reverse the normal functions (increased drug bioavailability in intestine and decreased secretion in the urine) of the efflux protein. A prior knowledge of genetic variations in drug transporter proteins for NTI drugs through consultation with the clinical pharmacist may help the physician to optimize drug levels for patients without running the risk of ADRs.[15]

Pharmacists' Role in Pharmacogenomics Research

Though it is anticipated that pharmacists' contribution to research in pharmacogenomics will be patient centered, limited to disease management and "quality of life" outcomes improvement, some researchers have differing views.[1-5] It can be argued that pharmacists by virtue of their knowledge of pharmacokinetic/pharmacodynamic profile of drugs could spearhead research methodologies development in different stages of genomics investigation in industry and academic settings. In fact many of them are currently gearing up to this role. One example was cited El-lbriary et al. of a pharmacist in UCSF, who as a part of interdisciplinary epileptic management team, had developed detailed reaction and metabolism pathways for the antiseizure drug phenytoin and was successful in constructing a phenotyping instrument for pharmacoresponse.[1] The main criterion for selection of the pharmacist in the research team was the complex pharmacokinetic variations for antiepileptic drugs.[1] If one dissects the entire genomics research scheme, starting from developing robust methodologies and culminating in its implementation in clinical practice, it consists of four stages: proof of principle, proof of efficacy, proof of cost-effectiveness and proper implementation.[3] It should be emphasized that biomedical and analytical industries play a crucial role in developing robust and reliable assays for pharmacogenomics testing. This testing requires the development of new methodologies, an area where pharmacists can contribute.[3] However, a major challenge in this stage is the lack of impetus for pharmaceutical industries to participate in this investigation, "because of market segmentation and an end to an era of blockbuster drugs," even though findings in 2004 suggest that applications of genomics in drug research can reduce cost by $300 million and the lag time by 2 years.[3] It is encouraging to note that regulatory agencies like FDA are attempting to rectify the situation by mandating genomics label for certain drugs like 6-mercaptopurine and irinotecin.[3] In addition, pharmacists can collaborate with scientists and other healthcare providers to develop diagnostic criteria for genomics testing.[3] A crucial challenge in implementing the findings of pharmacogenomics research from bedside to clinics is lack of ability to predict "accurate outcomes for drug treatment." In order to correlate positive association studies with drug response variation, it is imperative to codify drug response phenotypes.[1] This is difficult to attain for most studies since phenotypic research is out of tune with advances in genotypic research, thus necessitating more studies.[1] Pharmacists' input into the process can help realize the full potential of genomic research in high through put screening. Pharmacists too have roles in selecting clinically relevant pharmacogenomic studies and developing guidelines and protocols for their implementation in clinics.[1] They can help mould the physicians' opinions favorably towards genomics tests and drugs thus indirectly helping in its acceptance in medication. First hand knowledge about the clinical and economic factors that guide healthcare decisions can help the pharmacists in attaining this goal.[3]

The role of PG in drug development can work several ways. First drugs can be designed for specific responders based on their genetic profile. However, will it be cost effective for companies to develop and market drugs to such a limited population? Also, patients with certain genetic susceptibilities to the drug toxicity may be selective excluded from clinical trials and thus make the results of the clinical trial more robust. Pharmacists can help refine the criteria used to codify drug response phenotypes and play a pivotal role in advancing pharmacogenomics from bench side to clinics.

Even though present knowledge of pharmacogenomics justifies the integration of this concept into clinical practice, a major impediment prevents the realization of its full potential in the field of modern medicine. Many genotype-phenotype relationships are unknown and the cause-effect phenomenon that leads to identification of such associations are hindered by the lack of statistical power for clinical trials and prospective studies.[16] Scientists agree that advances in "drug response phenomics" have lagged behind the progress in genomics leading to difficulties in quantification or specification of drug response phenotypes.[1] As noted by El-lbiary et al., ambiguity still exists in defining a successful drug response outcome.[1] Pharmacists who by virtue of their profession monitor clinical outcomes of drug treatments for success and failure can play a crucial role in defining standardized criteria for clinical drug responses and help set up pharmacogenetic models that can be used as benchmarks for future studies. For example, pharmacists working in anticoagulation clinics can cite a number of clinically relevant outcomes that could be of potential interests for scientists conducting pharmacogenetic studies in establishing an association between genotypes and the clinical outcomes of warfarin therapy as evaluated by minor/major bleeding events, INR ratio, and time for stable warfarin dosage.[1]

Summary

Because variations in drug responses in some cases is related to genetic variability, pharmacogenomics or pharmacogenetics show promise in generating positive pharmacotherapy outcomes by mitigating adverse drug reactions. With companies developing quick tests to evaluate drug metabolizing enzymes, many large medical centers are conducting *direct-to-consumer* or *direct-to-physician* marketing of selected pharmacogenetic tests.[5] Anecdotal evidence in North Carolina suggests that many patients are coming to pharmacists for interpretation of these tests.[5] Thus it is imperative that pharmacists who are experts in analyzing drug-drug interactions on patients are well equipped to integrate this genetic variability component into their clinical practice skills so that they can better serve the patients. It is also imperative that pharmacists collaborate with other healthcare providers in pharmacogenomics research, discovery and clinical applications.[1] With the rapid strides in this field, it is possible that in the near future pharmacists in all settings (clinical, institutional, or community) will be mandated to interpret a patient's genetic profile, counsel them, or be involved in genetic screening to ensure a safe and efficacious dosing regimen for the patient.[1] Being the natural drug experts, pharmacists have a greater depth in comprehension of absorption, distribution, action, elimination, and excretion of drugs, which can play a pivotal role in defining their roles in pharmacotherapy disease management process.[1]

References

1. El-lbriary YS, Cheng C, Alldredge B. Potential roles for pharmacists in pharmacogenetics. *JAPhA.* 2008;48:e21-e31.
2. Bishop JR. Clinical applications of pharmacogenomics in retail pharmacy. Drug Store News. 2007;March/April:C31, C36.
3. Swen JJ, Huizinga TW, Gelderblom H, et al. Translating pharmacogenomics: challenges on the road to the clinic. PLoS Med. 2007;4:e209.
4. Teagarden JR. Pharmacogenomics and its potential uses in managed care pharmacy. *Hospital Pharmacy.* 2006;41:477-482.
5. Foxhall K. Pharmacogenetics: pharmacists should own it, not fear it. *US Drug Topics.* 2006;April:C4, C5.
6. Hines RN, McCarver DG. Pharmacogenomics and the future of drug therapy. *Pediatr Clin N Am.* 2006;53:591-619.
7. Zdanowicz MM, Huston SA, Weston GS. Pharmacogenomics in the professional pharmacy curriculum: content, presentation and importance. *IJPE.* 2006;2:1-12.

8. Brock TP, Faulkner CM, Williams DM, et al. Continuing-education programs in pharmacogenomics for pharmacists. *Am J Health Syst Pharm.* 2002;59:722-725.

9. Haga SB, Burke W. Using pharmacogenetics to improve drug safety and efficacy. *JAMA.* 2004;291:2869-2871.

10. Case LA. Does pharmacogenomics provide an ethical challenge to the utilization of cost-effectiveness analysis by public health-systems? *Pharmacoeconomics.* 2005;23:445-447.

11. Malone PM, Mark AM, Nelson PJ, et al. Pharmacy and therapeutic committee. In: Malone PM, Mosbell KW, Kier L, et al., eds. *Drug Information: A Guide for the Pharmacists.* 3rd ed. New York: McGraw Hill; 2006:483-532.

12. Malone PM, Mark AM, Nelson PJ, et al. Drug evaluation monographs. In: Malone PM, Mosbell KW, Kier L, et a., eds. *Drug Information: A Guide for the Pharmacists.* 3rd ed. New York: McGraw Hill; 2006:533-589.

13. Evans WE, Relling MV. Moving towards individualized medicine with pharmacogenomics. *Nature.* 2004;429:464-468.

14. Temple-Smolkins R. The year in pharmacogenomics. Available at: http://www.mostgene.org/2008_conference. Accessed March 20, 2009.

15. Bukaveckas BL. Adding pharmacogenetics to the clinical laboratory. *Arch Pathol Lab Med.* 2004;128:1330-1333.

16. Frueh FW, Gurwitz D. From pharmacogenetics to personalized medicine: a vital need for educating health professionals and the community. *Pharmacogenomics.* 2004;5:571-579.

Chapter 14

Pharmacogenomics and Clinical Testing

James W. Fetterman, Jr., Pharm.D.; Pamela F. Hite, Pharm.D.

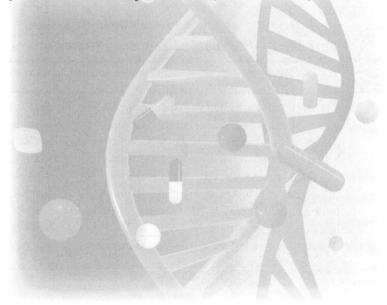

Learning Objectives

After completing this chapter, the reader should be able to

- Define the clinical implications of pharmacogenomics in daily practice.
- Describe the difference between the various genetic markers used for determining patient's response to therapy.
- Identify which valid biomarkers are approved by the FDA for use in the treatment of patients with various disease states.
- Describe the factors that are involved in evaluation of the cost versus the benefit of pharmacogenomic testing.

Key Definitions

Valid biomarkers—A biomarker that is measured in an analytical test system with well-established performance characteristics and for which there is an established scientific framework or body of evidence that elucidates the physiologic, toxicologic, pharmacologic, or clinical significance of the test results.

Genetic variants—An alteration in a gene distinct from the normal, wild-type allele.

Pharmacogenomics—The branch of pharmacology that deals with the influence of genetic variation on drug response in patients by correlating gene expression or single-nucleotide polymorphisms with a drug's efficacy or toxicity.

Clinical validity—The accuracy with which a test identifies or predicts a patient's clinical status.

Case Study—Psychiatric Disorders: Extreme Anxiety

B.J., a 25-year-old female, presents with a recent history of extreme anxiety. She has been on fluoxetine 20 mg daily for about 2 months. She has a history of Type II Diabetes and is treated with metformin 500 mg bid. She is otherwise healthy. B. J. was doing better after about 2 weeks, but then she began the following signs and symptoms: the inability to sit still and recently she has noticed a persistent tremor as well as excessive sweating. She has been on two other medications to treat her anxiety prior to fluoxetine and has had to stop them because of severe side effects. Her labs were as follows: CMP within normal limits, blood glucose 175, A1C 7, fluoxetine levels were 2 ½ times normal limits. Pharmacogenomic testing for CYP2D6 and CYP2C9 were ordered and the results were no mutations on CYP2C9 but multiple mutations on CYP2D6*3,*4,*5 *6 *12, which are nonfunctional alleles and *9 *10 *17, which represent decreased function.

Questions:

1. Given the information above, what additional pharmacogenomic testing would you recommend?
2. Which variants of the alleles could cause this problem?
3. Is B.J. a fast or poor metabolizer?

Introduction

Because the successful mapping of the human genome, the possibilities of being able to successfully determine the specific gene variant(s) that will help determine what drug to use for which patient has been vigorously studied and reported. Many alleles have been identified to affect several different diseases and the susceptibility of the disease to the medication to be used. It is the purpose of this chapter to assist the practitioner in determining which clinical tests are available for use in practice and which disease that particular test will be most valuable for. Such knowledge will enable the practitioner to better care for the patient and ensure optimum response to the drug or dosage chosen. In this chapter, we will look at several disease states cardiovascular, hematology/oncology, CNS/psychiatric, and infectious disease states and discuss the practicality of pharmacogenomic testing within each area as it relates to clinical practice.

Clinical Implications

Starting with pharmacokinetics, medicinal chemistry and pharmacology, students of pharmacy are told that each drug may work differently in different patients or each patient may respond differently to the same drug given to another patient. There are known variabilities of drug response due to genetic variations or genetic mutations caused by environmental exposure to various toxins.[1] According to Zineh, while there is a large amount of research being conducted on the top 200 most prescribed drugs, there is a much smaller amount of research being conducted in the area of pharmacogenomics-based prescribing for these drugs.[2] As a result, such information is not widely found in the manufacturer's product insert (PI). Although more extensive research on the vast majority of drugs needs to be conducted to establish the efficacious use of pharmacogenomics (PG), there are those drugs with a narrow therapeutic index, such as warfarin, that have been studied and shown to be candidates for the clinical application of PG.

There are so many polymorphisms that have been identified thus far that it can be difficult to determine which polymorphism(s) have clinical impact and thus should be tested for. The Food and Drug Administration (FDA) has approved several PG-related clinical tests and are now requiring manufacturers to include that information within their PIs. Approximately 10% of the drugs approved by the FDA currently contain PG information in their PIs.[3] This information is based on valid genomic biomarkers, which can help the practitioner to identify those patients who may be responders or nonresponders to various drugs with the goal of decreasing adverse drug reactions (ADR) or identifying those patients who will respond better to certain drugs. According to the FDA definition, a valid biomarker is "one for which an established and validated assay exists for which an established body of evidence exists that supports its pharmacological and/or clinical significance."[4]

Clinical Pearl

Approximately 10% of all prescription medications within the U.S. have genetic testing options available.

The genomic biomarkers listed on the labels of certain drugs are classified according to their effect on clinical response and the indication of risk to the patient. These genomic biomarkers are used to assist in determining the dose, as well as to identify the susceptibility, resistance, differential diagnosis, and polymorphic targets. Not all of the FDA-approved labels make recommendations for required pretesting or dosing guidelines based on PG. Some are provided only for informational purposes, thereby alerting the practitioner to the possible effects of the biomarker or any polymorphisms that might be present for that drug.

The following sections will review selected biomarkers and their potential effects on the treatment of cardiovascular diseases, hematology/oncology, CNS/psychiatric disorders, infectious diseases, respiratory disease, and drug toxicity. Table 14-1 provides a list of valid biomarkers that are associated with the FDA Approved Drug Labels along with the appropriate recommendations for genomic testing.[3,5,6] As of Fall 2008, the FDA modified the need to test or not list in the Table of Valid Biomarkers; however, they are no longer included because the level of evidence is constantly evolving and may not necessarily reflect the current clinical standard of practice.[7]

Table 14-1
List of Valid Biomarkers Associated with FDA-approved Drug Labels and Recommendation of Genomic Testing Requirements[3,5,6]

Clinical Presentation	Pharmacogenomics Biomarker	Drug	FDA Test Classification[a]
Cardiovascular	CYP2C9 variants	Warfarin	TR
	Protein C deficiencies	Warfarin	TR
	VKORC1	Warfarin	TR
	CYP2D6 PM and EM	Metoprolol	I
		Propranolol	I
		Carvedilol	I
		Propafenone	I
	CYP2D6	Timolol Maleate (Ophth. Solution)	I
	NAT variants	Isosorbide and Hydralazine HCL	I
	Familial Hypercholester-olemia	Atorvastatin	TR
	CYP2C19 (*1,*2,*3)	Clopidogrel	NRG

Continued on next page

Cardiovascular Disease

One of the most commonly used drugs in the treatment of various cardiovascular diseases is warfarin. As a vitamin K antagonist, it is clinically indicated in the treatment of patients presenting with a variety of diseases requiring anticoagulation such as deep vein thrombosis (DVT), atrial fibrillation, myocardial infarction, pulmonary embolism, and patients with certain types of artificial heart valves. Warfarin is primarily metabolized by cytochrome P-450 isoenzymes 2C9 (CYP2C9), which is responsible for the metabolism of approximately 60% to 70% of the S-warfarin isomer.[8,9] Variations in this enzyme, more specifically the single nucleotide polymorphisms (SNPs) CYP2C9*2 and CYP2C9*3, are responsible for affecting warfarin clearance.[4,10,11] Those patients who carry either one or both of these variants tend to metabolize warfarin more slowly and therefore have a greater risk of increased bleeding secondary to elevated levels of warfarin. In cases such as this, the dose of warfarin would need to be reduced to prevent an ADR.

As equally important to the potential of ADRs is the effect that vitamin K epoxide reductase (VKORC1) variants (especially -1639G>A) can have in the sensitivity of warfarin and its effects on the international normalized ratio (INR).[8] These variants will also have an effect on the anticoagulant proteins C, S, and Z, but especially C. The effects on a patient who presents with either CYP2C9*2, CYP2C9*3, or the VKORC1 variants or a combination of any of the three, could prove to be life-threatening if the patient is not dosed appropriately and closely monitored.

Table 14-1 (*Continued*)

Clinical Presentation	Pharmacogenomics Biomarker	Drug	FDA Test Classification[a]
Hematology/oncology	c-KIT expression	Imatinib mesylate	I
	DPD deficiency	Capecitabine	I
		Fluorouracil topical	I
	EGFR expression	Erlotinib	I
	CYP2D6 variants	Tamoxifen	I
	EGFR expression	Cetuximab (head and neck cancer)	I
		Gefitinib	I
		Cetuximab (colorectal cancer)	I
		Panitumab	R
	G6PD deficiency	Gefitinib	R
	Her2/neu over-expression	Rasburicase	TR
		Trastuzumab	R
		Lapatinib	R
	Philadelphia Chromo-some-positive responders	Busulfan	I
	Philadelphia Chromo-some-positive responders	Dasatinib	R
	PML/RAR alpha gene expression	Tretinoin	I
		Arsenic oxide	I
	UGT1A1 variants	Nilotinib	I
	Del(5q)	Lenalidomide	I
	UGT1A1 variants	Irinotecan	TR
	TPMT variants	Thioguanine	TR
		Mercaptopurine	TR

Continued on next page

When dosing a patient with warfarin, one should strongly consider all aspects that could have an effect on the metabolism of the drug and the clinical outcome of the patient. Sconce et al. have developed a dosing regimen taking into consideration the patient's age as well as CYP2C9 and VKORC1 genotype and height.[11] They showed that when all of the variables were taken into consideration, the incidence of ADRs were greatly decreased, and that when

Table 14-1 *(Continued)*

Clinical Presentation	Pharmacogenomics Biomarker	Drug	FDA Test Classification[a]
CNS/psychiatric disorders	CYP2C19	Diazepam	I
	CYP2D6	Fluoxetine	I
		Olanzapine	I
		Cevimeline	I
		Tolterodine	I
		Clozapine	I
		Aripiprazole	I
		Tramadol and acetomorphine	I
		Thioridazine	I
		Protriptyline	I
	UCD deficiency	Valproic acid	TR
		Na phenylacetate and Na benzoate; Na phenyl butyrate	TR
	HLA-B*1502 allele presence	Carbamazepine	TR (for at risk patients)
	CYP2D6 variants	Atomoxetine	I
		Venlafaxine	I
		Risperidone	I
	CYP2C19 variants (PM or EM)	Omeprazole	I
		Pantoprazole	I
		Esomeprazole	I
		Rabeprazole	I
Infectious diseases	CCR5-Chemokine C-C motif receptor	Maraviroc	R
	CYP2C19 variants	Voriconazole	I
		Nelfinavir	I
	CYP2D6 (PM and EM)	Terbinafine	I
	G6PD	Dapsone	TR
	G6PD	Primaquine	I
		Chloroquine	I
	HLA-B*5701 allele presence	Abacavir	TR
	NAT variants	Rifampin, isoniazid, and pyrazinamide	I
	TPMT variants	Azathioprine	TR

Continued on next page

Table 14-1 *(Continued)*

Clinical Presentation	Pharmacogenomics Biomarker	Drug	FDA Test Classification[a]
Respiratory	CYP2D6 variants	Tiotropium bromide inhalation	I
Other	CYP2C9 variants	Celecoxib	I

R = required testing; TR = testing recommended; I = for information only; NRG = no recommendation given.

[a]These designations were assigned as of Fall 2008; however, they are no longer included on the website because the level of evidence is constantly evolving and may not necessarily reflect the current clinical standard of practice.[7]

comparing the dose of warfarin to a 90-year-old patient with that of a 30-year-old (both having the same genotypes), the dose for the older patient was over 6 times lower than the dose for the younger patient.[11] The International Warfarin Pharmacogenetics Consortium, which is composed of more than 25 medical centers from around the world (21 research groups, 9 countries, and 4 contents), developed an algorithm for dosing warfarin based on 5,700 patients.[12] Of the 5,700 patients, the study focused on the 5,052 patients who had a targeted INR of 2–3. The consortium of investigators collected many specific clinical factors to determine the efficacy of using a PG-based warfarin dosing algorithm. Data collected included demographic characteristics, primary indications for warfarin therapy, mean INR, target INR, current medication history (grouped into those drugs that would either increase or decrease the INR), and the presence of genotype variants of CYP2C9 (including all three variants *1, *2, and *3) and VKORC1. The study showed that the use of the pharmacogenomic algorithm worked best in those patients requiring ≤21 mg/week or ≥49 mg/week of warfarin when compared to the use of a standard dosing algorithm. Those patients who required >21 mg/week and <49 mg/week were not as accurate in achieving required stable therapeutic doses as when the pharmacogenomic algorithm was used. Even though patients who were dosed based on the pharmacogenomic algorithm showed a better response to the dose than if they were dosed by the standard method, this is only the beginning. PG-based dosing is an ever evolving science; therefore, the results of the International Warfarin Pharmacogenetics Consortium's study on PG-based warfarin dosing algorithm may or may not be the same in the future as we find out more about the various interactions of warfarin and other variants that have yet to be discovered.

Clopidogrel, an inhibitor of platelet aggregation, is used routinely in patients with recent myocardial infarction (MI), stroke, peripheral arterial disease (PAD), or acute coronary syndrome (ACS), and is also metabolized by CYP450. Specifically, CYP2C19 is involved in the formation of both the active metabolite as well as those metabolites with less function. The CYP2C19*1 allele correlates to fully functional metabolism of the drug, whereas the *2 and *3 alleles show reduced metabolism. Mega et al. and Simon et al. in two separate studies have shown that those patients being treated with clopidogrel who have one or more reduced-function allele (typically >30% of patients) have a higher rate of cardiovascular events than those patients that are considered ultra or fast metabolizers of the drug. The studies showed that depending on the expression of the variant alleles both the pharmacokinetic and pharmacodynamics of the drug were affected.[13,14] Even though the FDA Table of Valid Biomarkers no longer recommends whether to test or not to test, the manufacturer in their package insert states that "pharmacogenomic testing can identify genotypes associated with variability in CYP2C19 activity."[15]

Clinical Pearl

Saliva testing may prove to be as efficacious as blood testing, as seen with the recently released clopidogrel saliva test.

Other cardiovascular drugs are also affected by variants in the genome. Beta-blockers are also affected by several variants of the CYP2D6 gene polymorphisms.[16] A possible interaction with timolol and inhibitors of the CYP2D6, such as quinidine and SSRIs, may cause potentiating effects of systemic beta-blockade.[17] Metoprolol, propranolol, and carvedilol are also affected by CYP2D6 polymorphisms. The extent to which these agents are affected is dependent on the variability of the polymorphism found in each patient. Of the beta-blockers mentioned above, metoprolol is affected most due to having the greatest dependency on the CYP2D6 pathway. As shown in Table 14-1, the CYP2D6 variants indicates that it can be expressed in the population as either a poor metabolizer (PM) or an extensive metabolizer (EM). Because 70% to 80% of metoprolol is metabolized via this route, those patients who are classified as PM (either genetically or by drug induced changes) can have an increase in blood levels by several-fold or a decreased cardioselectivity of the drug.[16,17] Because propranolol and carvedilol do not rely as heavily on the CYP2D6 metabolic pathway, they are affected by polymorphic variabilities within this pathway to a lesser extent and therefore patient response to these medications is not as sensitive to a patient's metabolic classification (i.e., PM or EM).

Theoretically, those patients who are PMs would require a lower dose and those who are EMs would require higher doses; however, there does not appear to be any significant differences in efficacy or adverse effects between these two groups when treated with similar doses.[16,17] According to the FDA, due to the lack of clinical applicability of PG testing in beta-blocker therapy, the use of pharmacogenomic testing in these patients would be for informational purposes only.

Other areas of interest in the treatment or prevention of cardiovascular disease includes drugs used to treat familial hypercholesterolemia. Although there are several drugs in this class, the one that has been addressed by the FDA is atorvastatin. Atorvastatin is metabolized by CYP3A4 and it has been shown that when atorvastatin is given concomitantly with drugs that inhibit CYP3A4 (i.e., clarithromycin) there is a significant increase in plasma levels of atorvastatin which can potentially lead to uncomplicated myalgia, myopathy, or rarely, rhabdomyolysis with acute renal failure secondary to myoglobinuria. Concomitant administration of those drugs that induce CYP3A4 (i.e., efavirenz and rifampin) may cause a decrease in plasma concentrations of atorvastatin. The effect this change in plasma concentrations has on low density lipoprotein-cholesterol (LDL-C) levels, the main target of familial hypercholesterolemia therapy, is currently unknown.[18] As seen in Table 14-1, the FDA recommends testing for homozygous familial hypercholesterolemia and to adjust dosing according to the individual patient, with doses of between 10–80 mg/day. Heterozygous patients aged 10–17 years have been studied and results showed that plasma levels of total cholesterol, LDL-C, triglycerides, and apolipoprotein-B were significantly decreased with atorvastatin 10–20 mg/day.[18]

For patients with hypertension, the combination drug, BiDil® (isosorbide and hydralazine HCl) has been included in the list of valid biomarkers for informational purposes. Hydralazine is metabolized by N-acetyltransferase (NAT), and there are patients who may present with an NAT variant (slow acetylators and fast acetylators). Those patients who are slow acetylators have a tendency to exhibit toxic effects of the drug secondary to higher plasma levels as opposed to the fast acetylators who will have a tendency to metabolize and excrete the drug faster; either way, the dose should be adjusted according to the clinical manifestations presented.

Clinical Pearl

Pharmacogenomics can be used in daily practice to facilitate appropriate therapy in various disease states, including cardiovascular, hematology/oncology, CNS and psychiatric, and infectious disease states.

Hematology/Oncology

Choosing the right drug treatment for the initial management of a disease or condition is always important; however, due to the high morbidity and mortality associated with the wide range of disease states within the hematology/oncology arena it is of extreme importance. Using PG tests to aid in the appropriate selection of chemotherapeutic agents has been shown to be of significant therapeutic benefit. Several PG tests are recommended or even required during treatment for certain cancers and with certain chemotherapy agents, while many are done for informational purposes (Table 14-1).

Current chemotherapeutic regimens are considered to be patient specific, but how is this specificity achieved? Evidence based guidelines show what agents have been effective in clinical trials so that is where treatment often begins. After that, it is based on patient response and adverse effects to the medication(s) selected. Some examples of how PG testing can take treatment guidelines to the next level and make treatment patient specific on the genetic level include testing for variations in c-KIT expression when using imatinib, dihydropyrimidine dehydrogenase deficiencies (DPD) with the use of capecitabine, variants of CYP2D6 metabolic pathways when using tamoxifen, ability to respond to the Philadelphia chromosome when using dasatinib or busulfan, as well as Her2/neu overexpression when using trastuzumab or lapatinib (Table 14-1).

CNS/Psychiatric Disorders

Central nervous system (CNS) and psychiatric disorders are particularly difficult to treat due to the subjective nature of these disorders. PG testing has the potential to be extremely useful within this area of medicine. At this point in time testing is either recommended or for informational purposes, rather than required (Table 14-1).

Patients with variations within the CYP2C19 metabolic pathway who are receiving diazepam may be affected by variations within this pathway. Diazepam is metabolized into an active metabolite, which contributes to the prolonged activity that some patients may experience. Knowing how a patient would specifically metabolize diazepam could help determine the dosing frequency necessary to appropriately treat signs and symptoms. However, there has not been conclusive evidence to support enough clinical benefit that testing be required or even recommended by the FDA. Testing is currently for informational purposes only (Table 14-1).

Certain antidepressants (fluoxetine, venlafaxine) and antipsychotics (risperidone) have tests available to detect variants within the CYP2D6 metabolic pathway. According to the FDA, these tests are currently only for informational purposes. These classes of medications can be difficult to dose appropriately. This difficulty can be due to either having to wait several weeks for the patient to experience the full effect of an antidepressant or having to balance efficacy with adverse effects of an antipsychotic. For the patient, the trial and error period that occurs when titrating a dose can be especially difficult. Therefore, it is of utmost importance to pharmacogenomically test a patient to determine optimal dosing, due to the complex nature of the CNS, variations in genetic abilities to control various neurotransmitters, as well as variations within medication metabolic pathways (Table 14-1).

Infectious Disease

With the increase in multidrug resistant organisms and a decrease in the development of novel antimicrobial agents, selecting an appropriate antibiotic when treating infectious diseases is highly important. PG testing in this area of medicine is mostly informational at this point; however, there are a few tests that are recommended, and one that is required (Table 14-1).

When treating patients with voriconazole or nelfinavir, checking for variants within the CYP2C19 metabolic pathway could help direct therapy. Approximately 3% to 8% of patients receiving abacavir may develop hypersensitivity reactions (HSR). The PREDICT-1 study showed that only about 6% of whites carry the HLA-B*5701 allele, which has been shown to increase the chance of HSR. Therefore, screening for the HLA-B*5701 allele has been recommended for those patients where abacavir in indicated.[19] For patients with tuberculosis, the presence of NAT variants (discussed previously in the cardiovascular section of this chapter) could provide useful information regarding the use of rifampin, isoniazid, and pyrazinamide. HIV patients who are to receive the new drug maraviroc to block the entry of HIV into the cell, must first receive PG testing to determine if the drug will be efficacious or not. Because there is more than one receptor that HIV can use to enter a cell, it is essential to determine if the patient's HIV is using the CCR5 receptor that maraviroc inhibits or the CXCR4 receptor that maraviroc does not inhibit to gain entry (Table 14-1).[20]

Economic Impact of Pharmacogenomic Testing

As with any new and innovative procedure or test, one must always consider the cost of the test and whether some portion of the cost to the patient will be covered by the insurance or other third-party carrier. Before such PG testing occurs, one must determine whether the cost (i.e., up to $1600 per test) is justified by clinical benefit.[21] For those drugs in Table 14-1 that have the recommendation of genetic testing for informational purposes only, the patient and the practitioner should evaluate whether the benefit to the patient will be worth the expense, especially if the patient either is not covered by a third party payer or the third-party payer will not cover the test. One argument that can be made for such testing is that based on the results of the test, the patient's medication would be more accurately monitored and the possibility of costly adverse effects is greatly decreased. For those drugs with the designation of "testing recommended," there could be a much stronger argument made for testing based on the fact that potentially life-threatening toxicities could be avoided by testing for genetic variants (i.e., increased risk of bleeding with warfarin and a patient carrying the CYP2C9*2 or *3 alleles). Likewise, for those drugs identified by the FDA that require testing in order to determine whether the patient will respond to the therapy or not (i.e., HER2/over expression and trastuzumab), the argument can be made that valuable time, money and resources can be saved by choosing the correct medication or treatment modalities to the patient the first time.

In a retrospective study, Stallings et al. developed simulated models using data from a health claims database for patients presenting with asthma to estimate the difference, if any, between testing patients for a nonresponse genotype before initiating therapy and not testing at all. The cost per test chosen was $200 (range $0 to $1600) and was based on reported costs for currently available commercial tests. They concluded from their simulated asthma model that there was an offset in costs between the up-front pharmacogenomics tests when compared to the costs that were avoided with the patients not tested and thus treated with the more traditional method of trying first line therapy then second line, etc. The authors also concluded that their model can be used to predict the economic impact of genetic pretesting patients presenting with other diseases.[21]

Summary

Although there are many unanswered questions, it appears that the way of treating certain disease states will be to perform pretesting to determine a patient's genetic predisposition to respond to medications. Examples of this are shown in Table 14-1 and have been discussed throughout this chapter. Making sure the patient receives appropriate treatment is the primary concern; however, cost should always be taken into consideration. Care can be maximized for the patient by ensuring the patient is receiving the correct drug at the correct dose. This will also greatly decrease the risk of inappropriate dosing and adverse events, which has the potential to be much more costly in the long run. After all we are here to offer the best possible care for our patients, because ultimately they are why we are here and why we chose to do what we do.

References

1. Zhang W, Ratain MJ, Dolan ME. The HapMap resource is providing new insights into ourselves and its application to pharmacogenomics. *Bioinform Biol Insights*. 2006;2:15-23.
2. Zinch I, Pebamco GD, Aquianto CL, et al. Discordance between availability of pharmacogenetics studies and pharmacogenetics-based prescribing information for the top 200 drugs. *Ann Pharmacother*. 2006;40:639-644.
3. US Food and Drug Administration, Center for Drug Evaluation and Research. Table of valid genomic biomarkers in context of the approved drug labels. Available at: http://www.fda.gov/cder/genomics/genomic_biomarkers_table.htm. Accessed April 28, 2009.
4. Shin J, Kayser SR, Langaee TY. Pharmacogenetics: from discovery to patient care. *Am J Health Syst Pharm*. 2009;66:625-637.
5. Weinshilboum R, Wang L. Pharmacogenomics: bench to bedside. *FOCUS*. 2006;IV:431-441.
6. Veteran's Administration Technology Assessment Program, Office of Patient Care Services (11T). Available at: http://www.va.gov/vatap. Accessed August 18, 2009.
7. Zineh I [e-mail]. Silver Spring, MD: US Food and Drug Administration, Office of Clinical Pharmacology; October 19, 2009.
8. Gulseth MP, Grice GR, Dager WE. Pharmacogenomics of warfarin: uncovering a piece of the warfarin mystery. *Am J Health Syst Pharm*. 2009;66:123-133.
9. Ndegwa S. Pharmacogenomics and warfarin therapy In: *Issues in Emerging Health Technologies*. Issue 104. Ottawa, Canada: Canadian Agency for Drugs and Technologies in Health; 2007.
10. Phillips KA, Veenstra DL, Ramsey SD, et al. Genetic testing and pharmacogenomics: issues for determining the impact to healthcare delivery and costs. *Am J Managed Care*. 2004;10:425-432.

11. Sconce EA, Khan TI, Wynne HA, et al. The impact of CYP2C9 and VKORC1 genetic polymorphism and patient characteristics upon warfarin dose requirements: proposal for a new dosing regimen. *Blood*. 2005;106:2329-2333.

12. The International Warfarin Pharmacogenomics Consortium. Estimation of the warfarin dose with clinical and pharmacogenetic data. *NEJM*. 2009;360:753-764. Retrieved April 15, 2009, from Research Library Core database. (Document ID: 1655927791).

13. Simon T, Verstuyft C, Mary-Krause M, et al. Genetic determinants of response to clopidogrel and cardiovascular events. *N Engl J Med*. 2009;360:363-375.

14. Mega JL, Close SL, Wiviott SD, et al. Cytochrome P-450 polymorphisms and response to clopidogrel. *N Engl J Med*. 2009;360:354-362.

15. Plavix (Clopidogrel) [package insert]. Bridgewater, NJ: Bristol-Myers Squibb/Sanofi Pharmaceutical Partners; 2009.

16. Shin J, Johnson JA. Pharmacogenetics of beta-blockers. *Pharmacotherapy*. 2007;27:874-887.

17. US Food and Drug Administration, Center for Drug Evaluation and Research. Table of valid genomic biomarkers in context of the approved drug labels. Available at: http://www.fda.gov/cder/genomics/genomic_biomarkers_notes.htm. Accessed April 28, 2009.

18. Lipitor [package insert]. Dublin, Ireland: Pfizer Ireland Pharmaceuticals; September 2007.

19. Mallal S, Phillips E, Carosi G, et al. HLA-B*5701 screening for hypersensitivity to abacavir. *N Engl J Med*. 2008;358:568-578.

20. Selzentry [package insert]. New York, NY: Pfizer Inc; 2007.

21. Stallings SC, Huse D, Finkelstein SN, et al. A framework to evaluate the economic impact of pharmacogenomics. *Pharmacogenomics*. 2006;7:853-862.

Chapter 15

Pharmacogenomics in Pharmacy Education

Ajoy Koomer, Ph.D., MS, E.M.B.A.

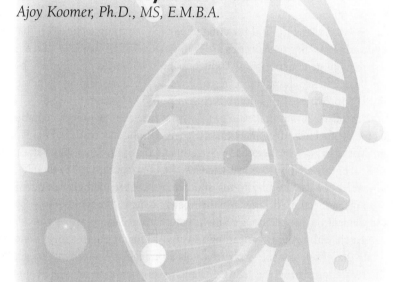

Learning Objectives

After completing this chapter, the reader should be able to

- Comprehend the present state of pharmacogenomics education in schools of pharmacy in U.S. and Canada.
- Interpret the clinical pearl associated in this chapter.
- Recall the modes of pharmacogenomics content delivery and teaching methodologies used in present professional pharmacy curriculum.
- Summarize faculty perceptions of the importance of pharmacogenomics in profession pharmacy curriculum.
- Understand the importance of continuing education programs in pharmacogenomics for pharmacists.

Key Definitions

NCHPEG—National Coalition for Health Professional Education in Genetics
ISP—International Society of Pharmacogenomics
NHGRI—National Human Genome Research Institute

Introduction

The vision of personalized medication is becoming a reality with recent advances in pharmacogenomics/genetics (PGx).[1] Owing to technological advances in genotyping as the well as the ground breaking haplotype mapping technology that catalogues human genetic variations, new discoveries are being made which correlate differential drug responses to variations in gene expression. Though at present genetic testing may be applicable to only 2% of the estimated population, researchers at National Human Genome Research Institute (NHGRI) approximates this number to go up to 60% within a decade.[1] Thus it is imperative that pharmacists should be aware of new gene-drug interactions to complement their knowledge of identified new drug interactions when offering medication therapy management to patients.[1] This view is corroborated by Streetman who opines that without a clear cut knowledge about PGx and related biomedical sciences, the pharmacists will be unable to match with other health professionals like physicians and nurses in convincingly laying claims for any direct roles (in drug selection, dosing, and therapeutic drug monitoring) with respect to utilization of PGx in clinical practice.[2] Though individual pharmacists are actively involved in cutting-edge PGx research with some even leading research teams in pharmacogenomics (PGRN), it is unfortunate that if one considers pharmacy as a profession then there is a general disconnection in effectively translating the fruits of bench work genomics research into clinical practice.[2] Because of this apparent confusion, minimal attention is paid to the educational aspects of PGx for prospective pharmacists (both community and hospital settings) and society at large.[3] To circumvent this perception and in order to better prepare future pharmacy graduates for this new and challenging concept, the academic affairs committee of the American Association for Colleges of Pharmacy (AACP) in their 2001/2002 background paper identified the core competencies in pharmacogenomics and pharmacogenetics expected from a competent pharmacist.[3] These competencies were partially developed from Core Competencies in Genetics Essential for All Health-Care Professionals originally developed by National Coalition for Health Professional Education in Genetics (NCHPEG) in 2001.[4] This report was followed by a background paper and recommendations and actions for the deans of colleges of pharmacy, medicine, and nursing by International Society of Pharmacogenomics (ISP) in 2005, regarding implementation of genetics in professional curriculum. Its suggestions were much more concrete than those laid down by AACP.

ISP Recommendations and Directives Regarding Implementation of a Genetics Curriculum

1. We call upon Deans of Education at Medical, Pharmaceutical, and Health Schools worldwide to incorporate the teaching of pharmacogenomics as an integral part of their core pharmacology curricula, as soon as possible.

2. We call upon policymakers and government agencies involved with medical education, and education sections of National Pharmacology Societies, and the European and International Pharmacology Organizations to recommend the incorporation of the teaching of pharmacogenomics globally in the basic education of physicians, pharmacists, and nurses.

3. Basic MD pharmacogenomics education should ideally encompass at least 4 hour and ideally about 8 hours of teaching, as part of the basic pharmacology curricula for MD /pharmacy students. It should include background information on the large scope of human genome variation and on the scientific methods employed to utilize this variation for the benefit of medical practice. It should emphasize the potential of pharmacogenomics applications for improving the quality and safety of pharmacotherapy for chronic diseases in several organ systems. Finally, it should present in detail common genetic polymorphisms in drug-metabolizing enzymes affecting drug pharmacokinetics and hence drug safety, such as the CYP450 enzyme family and the TPMT. Examples of polymorphisms that seem to affect drug pharmacodynamics, such as the beta-2 adrenergic receptor and apolipoprotein E, should also be taught. This might be incorporated as a case-based learning module in pharmacology/toxicology or pathology courses.

4. More extensive teaching in pharmacogenomics should be offered to graduate students in Pharmaceutical, Life Sciences, and Health Schools.

5. Pharmacogenomics is a rather new field that has not been part of the curricula of practicing clinicians today. Efforts for continuing medical education (CE) on pharmacogenomics should be initiated in major academic hospitals worldwide.

6. Oncology teaching and continuous education (CE) programs, in particular, must include a focused emphasis on pharmacogenomics, since personalized, genotype-based treatments have effectively entered the clinic for several types of malignancies.

7. The content of pharmacogenomics educational material should be updated regularly, keeping up-to-date with the latest developments and technical innovations.

8. We call upon publishers of basic and clinical pharmacology textbooks to dedicate a separate chapter to pharmacogenomics in their upcoming editions. Meanwhile, review articles, web resources, and case studies should be employed as teaching materials.

Source: Reprinted with permission from Gurwitz D, Lunshof JE, Dedoussis G, et al. Pharmacogenomics education: International Society of Pharmacogenomics recommendations for medical, pharmaceutical, and health schools deans of education. Pharmacogenomics J. 2005;5:221-225.

This chapter will discuss the extent and depth PGx education (in the present state) globally in the schools and colleges of pharmacy, with special emphasis on U.S. educational institutes in compliance with AACP and ISP recommendations. In addition, a brief review on the state of CE programs in pharmacogenomics/genetics for the practicing pharmacists is offered by different pharmacy professional organizations. Like AACP, the American Society of Health-System Pharmacists (ASHP), American Pharmacists Association (APhA), and American College of Clinical Pharmacy (ACCP), and others will complement the chapter. The chapter will be partly based on the published surveys conducted by Latif and Zdanowicz in 2005 and 2006 with the U.S. and Canadian colleges of pharmacy. The data from the authors' unpublished survey regarding the extent of pharmacogenomics/genetics education in the U.S., Canadian, and UK colleges of pharmacy in 2008 (presented at AACP conference in Chicago, IL) will also be included in this chapter.[1,3-6]

The Present State of Pharmacogenomics/Genetics Education in Professional Pharmacy Curriculum

Pioneering works by Latif and Zdanowicz published in *The American Journal of Pharmaceutical Education (AJPE)* and the International Journal of Pharmacy Education (IJPE) in 2005 and 2006, throws light on the current state of PGx education in U.S. and Canadian schools of pharmacy.[5,6] Latif's survey conducted in 2005 reported that 78% of the respondent schools of pharmacy had incorporated PGx as a part of their professional curriculum.[5] This percentage escalated to 95% in Zdanowicz's survey conducted a year later, showing the appreciation of the importance of genomics training in pharmacy education keeping in tract with the changing profession of pharmacy with advances in genetics.[6] In our unpublished survey, conducted in 2008, we reported that 96% of the respondent schools (Table 15-1) have embraced PGx in their curriculum which is in accordance with the current trend.[7] Our current survey data reported in Table 15-1 also revealed that out of 39 schools in U.S. and Canada, 36 in the U.S. and three in Canada have incorporated PGx in education; 73% offered it integrating it with other courses; while 12% and 9% offered it as stand alone required or electives, with 6% offering a combination of the above.[7] Thus, in 3 years, the percentage of schools offering PGx as an integrated curriculum increased roughly 1.5-fold.[5,7] Also our current follow-up survey conducted in 2008 demonstrated that the majority of institutions offered between 4 and 72 contact hours of PGx study with the mean content being 12.6 hours with a S.E ± 2.54 (refer to Table 15-1), compared to 10.1 ± 1.16 contact hours in Zdanowicz's survey conducted 2 years earlier.[6,7]

Table 15-1
PGx Content in the Professional Curriculum in U.S. and Canadian Schools of Pharmacy

Survey Questions	Yes	No
Have you incorporated pharmacogenomics/pharmacogenetics (PGx) information as an integral part of professional pharmacy curriculum?	95% N = 39	5% N = 2
What is the status of (PGx) information in the professional curriculum?	Stand alone, Required 12% N = 5 Stand alone, Elective 9% N = 4 Of Other Courses 73% N = 28 All of the above 6% N = 2	NA
How many contact hours of PGx are included in professional curriculum?	Mean = 12.6 Std. Error = 2.54	NA
PGx is being taught in what year of the professional pharmacy curriculum? (Check out all that apply to you.)	PY1 60% N = 24 PY2 52.5% N = 21 PY3 40% N = 16 PY4 5% N = 2	NA

The data in Table 15-1 (our unpublished survey) reveals that schools mainly taught PGx content spread across the first 3 years of the professional curriculum with the majority of schools (60%) stressing this content in the first professional year.[7] Out of the schools that had embraced PGx content, only 5.0% taught it during the fourth professional year.[7] Figure 15-1 lists the specific courses in which PGx content is integrated. While PGx content was distributed in a wide array of disciplines, the most common courses include pharmacology and toxicology (PT) (35%), pharmacokinetics (PK)/integrated sequence (IT) (32% each), and cellular and molecular biology (CMB)/pharmacotherapeutics (PT) (29% each) followed by biochemistry (Biochem) and medicinal chemistry (med chem and genetics (gen). "Other" included 21% of schools that offered PGx content in a course not corresponding with those listed on the survey. Some examples of "other" courses that included PGx content were human response to diseases, foundation of diseases, principles of drug design, fundamentals of biotechnology, total patient care, and biomedical sciences modules.[7]

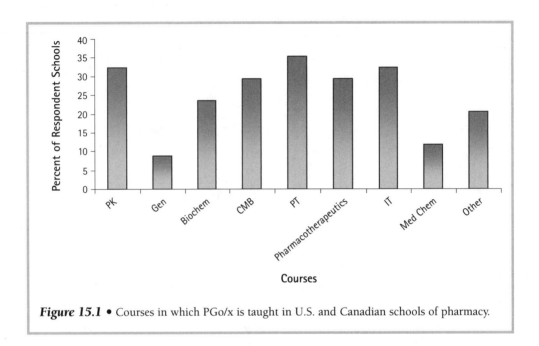

Figure 15.1 • Courses in which PGo/x is taught in U.S. and Canadian schools of pharmacy.

Table 15-2 presents a breakdown of specific PGx content areas that respondent schools included in their curriculum.[7] The majority of the PGx content areas listed on the survey were common to the curriculum of at least 63% of the schools of pharmacy who included PGx. Approximately 85% of respondents stressed topics such as gene polymorphisms, the role of pharmacogenomics in drug metabolism, and clinical applications of pharmacogenomics in diseased states, while 71% focused on the role of genomics in drug transport. Approximately 54% of schools concentrated on genotyping, while 34% of the schools also focused on bioethics in genetics. These findings are partially validated by a study designed as continuing education (CE) for practicing pharmacists. Pittenger et al. used semistructural interviews conducted with a selected group of faculty members (interested in genomics) from University of Minnesota College of Pharmacy to design a CE course in PGx. The topics that were considered relevant included genetic variations with drug response, pharmacists' role in application of PGx, and importance of legal, ethical, and societal considerations in genetic screening.[12] Our survey also indicated that in 37% of the schools that had incorporated PGx, a single faculty member was responsible for teaching the discipline, 40% of the schools had two or three faculty teaching the course, and in the remaining schools the discipline was team-taught by several faculty members coordinating the course.[7] Most of the schools we surveyed (72%) reported that they had no intention to hire any additional faculty for this discipline in the next 4 years, while the remaining schools plan to hire more.[7] This represented a deviation from Latif's survey conducted in 2005, when 63% of respondent schools indicated their intention to hire more faculties in the next 2 years.[5,7] The plateau effect observed was due to the fact that most schools already filled in the vacant faculty positions for genomics.

Table 15-2
PGx Course Content in U.S. and Canadian Schools of Pharmacy[a]

PGx Course Content	Percent of Respondents
Fundamentals of genetics and human genome project	63(26)
Role of PGx in drug discovery and development	66(27)
Gene polymorphisms, including single nucleotide polymorphisms	85(35)
Genotyping methods in PGx	54(22)
PGx of phase I and phase II drug metabolizing enzymes	85(35)
PGx of drug transporter proteins	71(29)
Clinical applications of PGx in diseased states	85(35)
Bioethics	34(14)
Other	2(1)

[a]Numbers in ( ) refer to the actual number of respondents who focus on the respective topics.

Clinical Pearl—Integrating Pharmacogenomics in Pharm.D. Curriculum[8]

PGx is offered as a three-credit-hour course to professional pharmacy students at Ohio State University in the third professional year. Designed by Jeffrey Johnson and Daren Knoell, this course consists of the modules ranging from applied molecular and cellular biology and principles of genetic medicine to pharmacogenomics of cancer, pulmonary disease, neurological disorders, and cardiovascular disease.[8] Initially there was reluctance among the students to accept this discipline as a mandatory requirement for this curriculum, as there was a disconnection between theory and its perceived applications in day-to-day pharmacy activities. To circumvent this, course faculty focused on clinically relevant examples of HER 2, TPMT, and CYP2D6 polymorphisms.[8] In addition they implemented a novel, longitudinal classroom genotyping exercise that connected across multiple lectures from day one to the end of the year in a sequence specific manner. This activity was designed to give the students a first-hand experience of data collection and acquisition and interpretation of genetic data and application to patient care. Student feedback revealed that it was well-appreciated and aroused significant interest in this challenging discipline.[8]

The Mode of Content Delivery

As shown in Table 15-3, our survey indicated that the schools mainly use lectures for delivering PGx content (98%) followed by individual projects (34%) and tutorials (17%).[7] Around 12% of respondents used both case presentations with groups and integrated virtual learning environment (IVLE) while 7% employed continuous assessments. "Others" accounting for 10% included workshops, laboratory exercises, interpretation and comparison of lay media, and peer-reviewed journal articles.[7] The decline in the schools using case presentations as a means for content delivery in 2008, compared to Zdanowicz's survey conducted in 2006 (64%), is intriguing.[6,7] As shown in Figure 15-2, in 2008 74% and 78% of faculty used a specific textbook or journal, respectively, as their main teaching resources. These percentages are almost up by twofold, since the last comprehensive survey conducted by Zdanowicz in 2006.[6] These results are not surprising given rapid advances in PGx research in the past 2 years. It should be noted that keeping with this trend, 66% of the instructors use website resources for PGx teaching, compared to 46% in Zdanowicz's publication.

Table 15-3
Methods of PGx Content Delivery in Professional Pharmacy Programs

PGx Content Delivery Methods	Percent of Respondents
Lectures	98(40)
Tutorials	17(7)
Individual projects	34(14)
IVLE	12(5)
Group (case) presentations	12(5)
Continuous assessments	7(3)
Others	10(4)

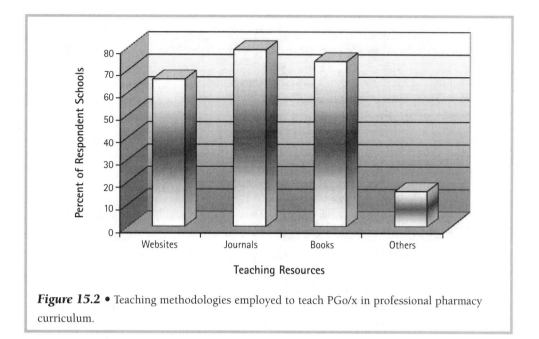

Figure 15.2 • Teaching methodologies employed to teach PGo/x in professional pharmacy curriculum.

Faculty Perception of Pharmacogenomics

It is evident from Figure 15-3 that 49% of surveyed faculty felt that the current level of PGx content in their curriculum was sufficient, and 47% felt it was insufficient while 4% felt it was more than adequate.[7] Compared to Zdanowicz's survey in 2006, it is encouraging to find that more faculties are feeling confident that appropriate attention is being given to PGx in professional pharmacy curriculum.[6,7] Also 97% of the faculties appreciated the importance of PGx education in curriculum regardless of whether their schools are presently offering it or not. Even faculty members from two schools who are not offering any PGx courses strongly felt that they would be incorporating the discipline in their curriculum in the near future. It is encouraging to find that 100% faculties in schools of pharmacy across U.S. and Canada consider knowledge of genomics to be vital for both current students and community and health system pharmacists at large to perform medication therapy management (MTM), which includes genetic counseling of patients.[7]

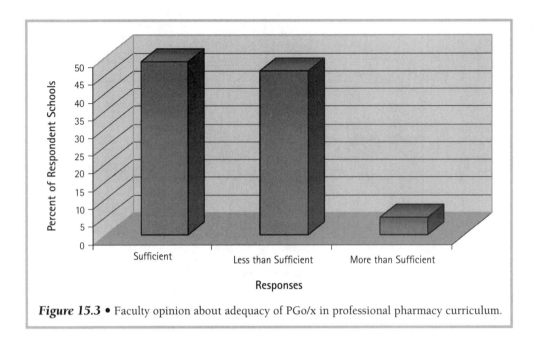

Figure 15.3 • Faculty opinion about adequacy of PGo/x in professional pharmacy curriculum.

State of Continuing Education (CE) Programs in Pharmacogenomics

Pioneering work by Sansgiry in 2003 demonstrated that community pharmacists' overall confidence in knowledge in human genome project, genetic testing, and pharmacogenomics was moderate.[9] Our unpublished survey in 2008, regarding pharmacists' perception of PGx in their profession, revealed that for the selected group of pharmacists in hospital settings and community and managed care facilities in metro Louisville, KY, the confidence level in all the disciplines (mentioned above) ranged from low to moderate.[10] Despite the fact that our population was small and catered to a specific area, the survey highlights the point that even 5 years following Sansgiry's studies, knowledge of practicing pharmacists in this field has not kept pace with the advancement in this field.[10] Thus it appears there is greater need for continuing education programs for present pharmacists who may be out of tune with recent advances in genomics. Researchers in 2002 looked at the educational program agendas for the three national pharmacy organizations' (namely ACCP, APhA, and ASHP) previous annual or midyear meetings.[11] Their objective was to quantitate the amount of continuing education credits awarded to genomics, genetics, and gene therapy in these conferences. Research revealed that on average, pharmacists could spend up to 50% of the total continuing education contact hours in genomics-related disciplines.[11] In spite of these endeavors, more efforts are clearly needed to increase the frequency of genomics continuing education credits. Our survey in 2008 revealed that 5% of the pharmacy schools in U.S. and Canada that have embraced PGx in their curriculum offer five credits of continuing education in PGx to pharmacists.[10] These efforts supplemented by national organizations like American Association for Colleges of Pharmacy (AACP) and American Pharmaceutical Scientists (AAPS) have started offering continuing education credits in PGx. In fact in 2007 ACCP inaugurated an online course in PGx for pharmacists. Completion of this module ensures continuing education credits to pharmacists. Recently the Skaggs School of Pharmacy and Pharmaceutical Sciences at UC San Diego (in partnership with APhA, ASHP, and AACP) has announced its intention to launch a nation-wide pharmacogenomics educational program known as "PharmGenEd" to target more than 100,000 pharmacy practitioners and students. This program has the dual intent of educating pharmacists and other healthcare providers about sequence differences in the human genome and its effects on therapeutic outcomes. It will also focus on increasing the participants' awareness to pharmacogenetic testings and its potential applications.[13]

Summary

More schools of pharmacy are incorporating PGx content in their curriculum following the AACP and ISP guidelines. However, there is huge dispersion so far as PGx content is concerned and different topics receive differential attraction across pharmacy curricula. The majority of the schools were of the opinion that the amount of PGx content in their current curriculum was sufficient. Nowadays pharmacy instructors presenting PGx content readily use texts, reference journals, or websites, which are widely available. Content knowledge in PGx was considered vital for prospective as well as present pharmacists working in different settings, ranging from hospital settings to managed care facilities as they offer MTM to patients. It is encouraging that in order to facilitate the pharmacists increasing depth of genomics education, many pharmacy organizations and schools of pharmacy have implemented or are in the process of implementing continuing education credits for the pharmacists.

Acknowledgment: We would like to acknowledge Dr. Latif and Dr. Zdanowicz for kindly letting us use their survey contents for conducting our follow-up survey in 2008.

References

1. Foxhall K. Pharmacogenetics: pharmacists should own it, not fear it. *Drug Topics.* 4 2008.
2. Streetman DS. Emergence and evolution of pharmacogenetics and pharmacogenomics in clinical pharmacy over the past 40 years. Available at: http://www.theannals.com. Accessed May 14, 2009.
3. Gurwitz D, Lunshof JE, Dedoussis G, et al. Pharmacogenomics education: International Society of Pharmacogenomics recommendations for medical, pharmaceutical, and health schools deans of education. *Pharmacogenomics J.* 2005;5:221-225.
4. Johnson JA, Bootman JL, Evans WE, et al. *Pharmacogenomics: A Scientific Revolution in Pharmaceutical Sciences and Pharmacy Practice Report of the 2001/02 Academic Affairs Committee.* Alexandria, VA: American Association for Colleges of Pharmacy; 2001.
5. Latif DA. Pharmacogenetics and pharmacogenomics instruction in schools of pharmacy in the USA: is it adequate? *Pharmacogenomics.* 2005;6:317-319.
6. Zdanowicz MM, Huston SA, Weston GS. Pharmacogenomics in the professional pharmacy curriculum: content, presentation and importance. *Int J Pharm Edu.* 2006;2:1-12.
7. Koomer A, Dutta AP, Tran HT. Current state of pharmacogenomics/pharmacogenetics information in the schools and colleges of US, Canada and UK. Paper presented at: Annual Meeting of the American Association for Colleges of Pharmacy; July 19-23, 2008; Chicago, IL.
8. Johnson J, Knoell D. Integrating pharmacogenomics into the Pharm.D. curriculum. Paper presented at: Annual Meeting of the American Association for Colleges of Pharmacy; July 19-23, 2008; Chicago, IL.
9. Sansgiry SS, Kulkarni AS. The Human Genome Project: assessing confidence in knowledge and training requirements for community pharmacists. *Am J Health-Syst Pharm.* 2003;67:1-10.

10. Koomer A, Dutta AP, Sansgiry SS. Pharmacists' perception of pharmacogenomics/genetics in their profession. Paper presented at: Annual Meeting of the American Association for Colleges of Pharmacy; July 19-23, 2008; Chicago, IL.

11. Brock TP, Faulkner CM, Williams DM, et al. Continuing-education programs in pharmacogenomics for pharmacists. *Am J Health-Syst Pharm.* 2002;59:722-725.

12. Pittenger A, Janke K, Ejim I. Needs assessment for pharmacist education in pharmacogenomics. Paper presented at: Annual Meeting of the American Association of Colleges of Pharmacy; July 14, 2007; Florida.

13. Pharmacogenomics: UC San Diego to lead nationwide program to educate pharmacists. Available at: http://www.rxpnews.com/UC. Accessed May 14, 2009.

Chapter 16

Ethical Considerations in Pharmacogenomics

Sally A. Huston, Ph.D.

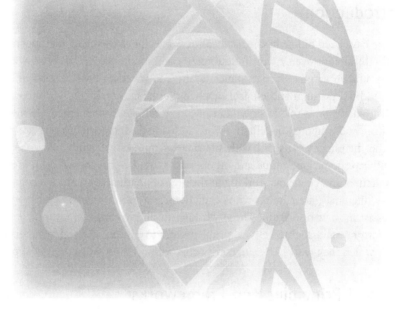

Learning Objectives

After completing this chapter, the reader should be able to

- Describe the ethical principles most frequently applied to medical ethics.
- Explain Veatch's ethical framework for considering ethical problems.
- Recognize ethical issues that can arise in pharmacogenomics at the individual and societal level.
- Summarize legal protections and regulations related to genetic information.
- Explain clinician's and researcher's roles and responsibilities related to the ethics of pharmacogenomics.

> ### Key Definitions
>
> **Autonomy**—Autonomy involves the right of individuals to do as they wish or to choose their own path.
>
> **Beneficence**—Beneficence is to do good for or to prevent harm to an individual.
>
> **Ethics**—Ethics is the process of thoughtfully considering and evaluating choices that individuals make.
>
> **Justice**—Justice involves rights that individuals have, as well as fair and equitable treatment.
>
> **Non-malfeasance**—Non-malfeasance means to avoid doing harm or evil to another individual.

Introduction

There have been biomedical ethical controversies since the time of Hippocrates, if not earlier,[1,2] and ethical controversy will undoubtedly continue in the relatively new area of scientific inquiry known as pharmacogenomics. Many controversies have already arisen in regard to its use, in both research and clinical practice. Public concerns will undoubtedly influence future policies and play a role in how pharmacogenomics is implemented.[3] While there are exciting existing and potential benefits for both individuals and society, there are risks as well. Many of the dilemmas associated with pharmacogenomics are similar to those in other areas of healthcare, some are unique and others may as yet be unrecognized.[4] It is important that both researchers and clinicians working in the area of pharmacogenomics recognize and understand these dilemmas, are familiar with regulations and protections, and have an ethical framework to assist in their resolution. Those working in pharmacogenomics must know how to reduce and/or prevent associated ethical problems and to educate affected members of the populations with which they work. This chapter begins with a review of basic ethical principles.

Ethical Principles and Frameworks

Although guidelines and regulations are being established in regard to pharmacogenomics, many ethical issues are not covered by these policies and laws. Persons involved in pharmacogenomics should understand and be able to apply ethical principles and moral rules to help determine moral actions. Ethical decisions must be made more often than is realized. One situation that frequently arises is the need for researchers and clinicians to determine what information truly constitutes informed consent. Determining an ethical course of action is not always easy: it is not unusual in medical situations for rules and principles to conflict. As one example, an individual may prefer to keep the results of a genetic test private, consistent with the principle of autonomy. Yet beneficence suggests the knowledge should be shared with family members who could use this information to reduce their risks of harm. Should the patient share this information? If the patient does not, should the clinician?

Moral principles, moral rules, and ethical theories are important. But just what are they? At its core, ethics deals with the meaning and value of human life.[2] There is held to be a common morality, which is a set of rules that guide correct actions.[5] These actions can be positive or negative, meaning that there are obligations as well as proscriptions. It is commonly held that one should not kill a fellow human being, or cause them pain and suffering. Proactively, one should tell the truth, take care of the helpless, and prevent harm or suffering when possible.[5]

Medical morality goes beyond the common morality, however. In medical situations, clients are especially vulnerable, and medical professionals are held to have a social contract, with a duty to hold the welfare and benefit of their clients higher than their own under normal circumstances.[6]

Moral principles discussed in medical ethics generally include: respect for autonomy, non-malfeasance, beneficence, and justice, and moral rules include veracity, privacy, confidentiality, and fidelity.[5]

Autonomy

Autonomy involves the ability of an individual to do as they wish, and has strongly been associated with Kantian ethics.[7] In practical terms, this means that the individual is free from others interfering control, understands relevant situations sufficiently that they can make meaningful choices, and are able to act according to their own desire or plan.[5] Autonomy is a concept; the moral principle is respect for autonomy.[5] Autonomy exists on a continuum; few of us enjoy perfect autonomy. Indeed, substantial autonomy may be sufficient in some circumstances.

Moral rules are generally derived from moral principles such as respect for autonomy. Moral rules can be supported by more than one principle at a time however. Moral rules derived primarily from the principle of autonomy are[5]:

- Veracity (truth-telling)
- Respect for privacy
- Confidentiality
- Informed consent for interventions
- When asked, help others make important decisions.

Some individuals have inherently diminished autonomy, while others may face diminished autonomy in specific situations. Prisoners, children, cognitively impaired, and severely ill or unconscious individuals are generally held to have diminished autonomy. Inadequate information can result in situationally diminished autonomy as well.

Case Study

During a routine office visit, Dr. McGinnis finds that Mary Campbell, a 48-year-old Caucasian woman, has total cholesterol of 250 mg/dL, with an LDL value of 160 mg/dL and an HDL of 30 mg/dL. Dr. McGinnis prescribes simvastatin 20 mg daily. Her triglyceride value is 150 mg/dL. After 3 months, Mary's cholesterol has improved only slightly, so the Dr. increases the dose to 40 mg daily. Three months later there is still no improvement. Dr. McGinnis asks Mrs. Campbell if she would be willing to undergo pharmacogenetic testing (for the E4 variant of the APOE gene), because it would help determine if she is a non-responder to statins. She hands Mrs. Campbell an informed consent, but does not read it to her. Mrs. Campbell signs, but does not read the form. Mrs. Campbell is not informed that this E4 variant of the APOE gene is associated with an increased risk of Alzheimer disease.

Questions:
1. Does Mrs. Campbell have substantial understanding about the genetic test?
2. Is Mrs. Campbell acting autonomously when she consents to the test?
3. Is the physician acting in a paternal manner, meaning the physician assumes authority without the patient actually delegating it?

Beneficence and Non-malfeasance

Beneficence and non-malfeasance are complementary, but there is a difference between the two. Both are expressed in the Hippocratic oath, "I will use treatment to help the sick according to my ability and judgment, but I will never use it to injure or wrong them." Non-malfeasance focuses on doing no evil or harm to someone, or causing someone to be at risk of evil or harm.[5] Non-malfeasance can be considered passive. In contrast, beneficence is an active obligation, centering on preventing or removing evil or harm, and doing or promoting good.[5] Beneficence is the core principle of utilitarianism.[7] Individuals are expected to act without malfeasance, but beneficence is somewhat more optional. One would not be expected to put his or her own life at risk to rescue someone, but if it could do done without causing significant harm to oneself, most people would expect the effort.[5]

Moral rules deriving primarily from the principle of beneficence are[5]:

- Protect and defend the rights of others
- Prevent harm from occurring to others
- Remove conditions that will cause harm to others
- Help persons with disabilities
- Rescue persons in danger

Moral rules deriving from non-malfeasance are[5]:
- Do not kill
- Do not cause pain or suffering
- Do not incapacitate
- Do not cause offense
- Do not deprive others of the goods of life

Non-malfeasance and beneficence can be at odds with each other, as illustrated by the case study of Mrs. Campbell. A test to determine if she is a genetic non-responder to statins may be helpful in determining which therapy to try next. But, if Mrs. Campbell would choose not to know if she was at increased risk for Alzheimer disease and she received this information with her lab results or discovered the information in a magazine article, she has been put at increased risk for harm from the test. Non-malfeasance usually takes priority over beneficence, although this can vary depending on the particulars of the case.[5] Consider what could happen if Mrs. Campbell's employer gains access to her medical records. Her employer could decide to terminate her employment to keep insurance premiums for the remaining employees down. While this would certainly be beneficial for the remaining employees, most members of society would not consider the harm caused to Mrs. Campbell acceptable.

Justice

Justice involves "fair, equitable, and appropriate treatment," and involves having a right to something.[5] Distributive justice involves distributing both benefits and harms equitably and with fairness. In research, a major focus of justice has been protection from harm. During the 1990s, with the advent of HIV/AIDS activism, considerations of justice in research have also included its benefits.[5] If something is considered unjust, it is often viewed as denying someone a thing they are entitled to. The formal principle of justice suggests that equals must be treated equally.[5]

Determining precisely what is just or who is equal can be difficult, however; it often depends on perspective. To each person an equal share of healthcare seems quite reasonable until you consider that every person may not need an equal share. To each according to his or her need? But then, are acne treatments or Botox injections really needed? Who makes that decision? Society finds it difficult to make these types of choices. One potential solution is to provide for "fundamental needs,"[5] but this too has proven difficult. Oregon attempted to expand Medicare healthcare coverage by rationing according to need, as well as effectiveness and public values. A list of healthcare services was created and ranked. Since its 1994 implementation, amid much controversy, the list has been revised and the range of services provided under Medicaid has actually expanded.[8]

Another consideration is age. Should the same effort should be put forth to save the life of a 70-year-old compared to a 7-year-old? On what is the decision based; the intrinsic value of a human life or potential productive years gained and the resulting value to society? This is not an improbable question. A notorious study conducted for Philip Morris suggested it would be cost-effective for the Czech Republic to allow people to smoke and die at relatively younger ages, rather than to encourage smoking cessation and incur housing and healthcare costs for citizens who were no longer working.[9] A tradeoff like this contravenes the Kantian viewpoint that life itself is sacred.

One set of potential distributive principles is[10]:

1. To each person an equal share
2. To each person according to need
3. To each person according to effort
4. To each person according to contribution
5. To each person according to merit
6. To each person according to free-market exchanges

Different groups may reject some of these principles, while others may accept all but elevate some of these principles over others.[5] Smoking cessation programs probably will not be implemented based on future contributions to society, but on need. Case specifics, context, societal perspectives, and/ or additional ethical principles must be considered in most situations.

An ethical framework popular in pharmacy has been provided by philosopher and medical ethicist Robert M. Veatch, Ph.D.[11,12] This framework provides four general steps that should be taken to resolve an ethical dilemma. The first step is to ensure that all facts of the case are known. If all of the facts are known, it may turn out that no ethical dilemma actually exists. If all the facts are known, and an ethical dilemma remains, move to the second step. Step two involves applying moral rules, such as confidentiality, informed consent or do not cause someone to suffer. Moral rules may not provide appropriate guidance, or perhaps they conflict. Perhaps confidentiality says information should not be revealed, while the rule of preventing harm says the information should be disclosed. If the conflict cannot be resolved using moral rules, move to step three. In step three ethical principles such as respect for autonomy or non-malfeasance are invoked. If these are not useful, step four involves the use of ethical theories.

Principle-based ethical theories are most often applied to resolving healthcare dilemmas, as opposed to virtue based theories which is the other major domain of traditional Western morality.[7] Principle-based ethical theories that have strongly influenced Western medical ethics include Kant's rule-based "deontological" theories, and Bentham and Mill's teleological theory of utilitarianism.[7] Kant sees persons as being important in and of themselves, rather than the means to some other end.[5] Deontological theories such as Kant's focus on "constraints," where as teleological theories such as utilitarianism are more proactive.[5] Utilitarian theories center on outcomes, advocating courses of action that result in maximal utility, meaning the most good for the most people.[7] Two other theories used in medical ethics are "rights theory" and "communitarianism." Rights are "justified claims" based on "liberal individualism."[5] Rights language is embedded in the U.S. Constitution, and is often used to protect individuals from societal imposition.[5] Communitarians value the common good and cooperation, with families being seen as small communities within the larger community.[5] People should act in accordance with the rights and values of the community and for the benefit of the community.[5]

All of these theoretical stances have been useful in thinking critically about medical dilemmas. Each dilemma must be considered carefully, according to both the specifics of the case and the context. An appreciation of the multiple potential perspectives should contribute to one's understanding of the ongoing discussion.

Potential Benefits of Pharmacogenomics

In thinking about the ethical implications of pharmacogenomics it is important to understand both the potential benefits and the potential risks since both benefits and risks will accrue to individuals and society. Although some effects may be described as affecting society as a whole, various societal groups such as clinicians, the pharmaceutical industry, and insurance companies, will be differentially affected.

Individual Benefits

There are two major categories of potential pharmacogenomics benefits, improved drug safety and the ability to optimize individual therapy, although these two categories can be intertwined. Many patients currently experience adverse drug reactions (ADRs), and this is an international problem. A meta-analysis of U.S. hospitals showed a 2.1% (95% CI 1.9% to 2.5%) incidence of serious ADRs in already hospitalized patients, while the incidence on admission was 4.7% (95% CI 3.1% to 6.2%).[13] A recent review involving reports from five continents (Europe, Asia, Australia, and North and South America) found the median prevalence rate of ADRs requiring hospitalization was 5.3% of admissions.[14] These ADRs ranged from mild to severe, and involved all ages.[14] The problem is bigger than that, however, as not all ADRs require hospital admission. Often an adverse reaction can result in a patient not taking the medication, or adhering poorly to his or her therapy.[15] Side-effects were associated with SSRI discontinuation rates of approximately 10% to 13%.[16] Many adverse drug reactions appear to be a result of genetic polymorphisms.[15,17] CYP2D6 and CYP2D9 polymorphisms are widely recognized as influencing drug enzyme activity, with various alleles resulting in decreased, intermediate, or extensive drug metabolism.[18] For example, CYP2D6 polymorphisms are clinically important considerations in the use of antipsychotics (tardive dyskinesia), antiarrhythmics (proarrhythmia and other toxic effects), and β-adrenoreceptor antagonists (increased β-blockade).[17] In addition to reducing ADRs, another benefit of personalizing medicine is to optimize therapy by identifying the most effective drugs for patients. Patients will benefit from not only from the best drug, but by avoiding time wasted with ineffective or less than optimal drug therapies.[17] Antidepressants are a good example: it can takes weeks of therapy to determine if a particular antidepressant will work in a patient, and between 30% to 40% of patients prescribed antidepressants do not respond to the first drug they are prescribed.[19] This condition is known as treatment resistance.[15] Much of this non-response is likely due to genetic polymorphisms.[20] Optimal initial drug selection should result in fewer adverse effects, quicker resolution of problems, and reduced costs. Individual genetic testing could also be used to identify disease early, allowing early intervention,[21] or perhaps even prevention.

Besides selecting the appropriate drug, selecting the appropriate dose is another potential way to optimize individual therapies. In addition to selecting the appropriate antidepressant, some dosing recommendations based on CYP450 polymorphisms have also been made.[20] Another example would be to test patients for genetic variability in CYP2C9, which is involved in warfarin metabolism, or VKORC1, which is a warfarin target, to help determine the appropriate warfarin dose.[22] Optimal dosing is particularly important for drugs such as warfarin which have a narrow therapeutic window. Testing for CYP2C9 or VKORC1 could also help identify a need for increased venous thrombosis monitoring.[22] Characterizing a patient as a slow or fast cytochrome P450 2D6 metabolizer can help determine the optimal dose for patients complaining of inadequate pain relief from taking opioids.[21] This can be done using a non-invasive and accurate test by measuring O-demethylated metabolite excretion in the urine.[21] Such testing could also help clinicians determine if a patient is seeking drugs for some other purpose.

While the current and potential uses of personalized medicine are exciting, there are definitely limitations. Although the potential for pharmacogenomics is great, its use in clinical practice is still limited.[18] One reason pharmacogenetic testing is rarely used in clinical practice is because tests are not widely available. Additionally, it seems likely that several genes or genetic polymorphisms may influence metabolic pathways and thus responses to particular drugs.[20] Therefore, information about only one gene may be only suggestive.[23] Many non-genetic factors also influence drug metabolism, side-effects and effects.[15] In addition, randomized clinical trials have not yet been conducted to determine if genetic testing truly results in improved outcomes for patients.[15]

Societal Benefits

Society as a whole, as well as individuals, stands to benefit from pharmacogenomics. One area of benefit is the cost savings resulting from a reduction in the number of adverse drug reactions and more optimized therapy. Better knowledge could improve screening programs as well.[24] An additional potential area in which society could benefit from pharmacogenomic information is policy-making. For example, when exposed to environmental contaminants, Portuguese populations may be at greater risk of developing bladder cancer than are other European populations.[25] Portuguese health officials could choose to mount campaigns for reducing environmental toxins, and the Portuguese might benefit from increase bladder cancer screenings as a result of this information.

An additional benefit is more efficient and improved drug development. Systematic methods of drug discovery could lead to discovery of a variety of receptors and enzymes that could be modified, related to genes associated with a disease, or to disease susceptibility,[4] resulting in more and better therapies. For example, a recent study suggests UGT1A1 as a potential drug target because of its strong influence on bilirubin metabolism and associated risk of cardiovascular disease.[26] It is estimated that eventually somewhere between 5,000 to 10,000 novel protein targets may be identified.[27] Gene therapy itself could be used to treat diseases like hemophilia B, Duchenne muscular dystrophy, Parkinson's or familial hypercholesterolemia.[9] Older drugs could be re-purposed that, while unsafe or ineffective for general use, could be beneficial to more limited populations.[28]

The testing process can also be streamlined. More drugs should make it through the pipeline. Drugs that may have been stopped because of adverse affects could still move forward if there are identifiable groups that do not experience these adverse effects. Smaller, more targeted Phase III clinical trials could include only those likely, based on phenotype, to benefit from the drug[23] This should result in drugs becoming available more quickly and with greater safety to the public. Drug trials could be targeted to those who would not be expected to suffer severe adverse events, or could target only those for whom it is anticipated the drug will work.[4] Another potential benefit could derive from genotyping patients who experience adverse effects during post-marketing surveillance.[29] Restricting use in patients with genotypes associated with adverse effects could improve safety.

At this point, the benefits described above are not certain. It may be that there is so much variability in genotype and drug response that it would not be worthwhile to conduct genetic tests.[29] It is also possible that the number and complexity of genes influencing a particular drug reaction makes genetic testing impractical.[29] And finally, multiple factors influence drug response, and genetic differences may not have the largest impact.[29] Only over time will we discover if pharmacogenomics can significantly benefit drug research and development.

Risks and Ethical Issues

The ethical principles that apply to pharmacogenomics are the same that apply to healthcare and medical research in general: respect for autonomy, beneficence, non-malfeasance, and justice, and rights derived from these principles such as the right to privacy and informed consent, and increasingly, a right to health.[30] As in any clinical or research situation, the benefits must be balanced against the risks. Many of the risks to patients or study participants associated with pharmacogenomics will be familiar to clinicians and medical researchers: loss of privacy, discrimination, emotional harm, and economic harm. While not entirely unique to pharmacogenomics, the loss of an open future is a risk that must be considered when genetic testing is performed. Reserving an open future means to hold autonomy in trust for children.[31] Once autonomy is attained they can then determine for themselves if they wish to have this knowledge. Pharmacogenomic information can also have an impact on families and communities.[24] There are potential negative social consequences and/or political harms as well.[32] An additional ethical principle that should be considered is "respect for communities." [24,33]

Ancillary Information

A major source of the risks associated with pharmacogenomics is ancillary information, the revelation of more information than originally sought.[22] Ancillary information can arise from either an acquired variant or an inherited variant, due to pleiotropy or polygenics.[22,24] Pleiotropy occurs when a single gene controls more than one phenotypic trait, while polygenics is when more than one gene influences a phenotypic characteristic. The prospect of harmful ancillary information is greatest with inherited variants.[22] Some have argued that "abbreviated SNP linkage disequilibrium profiles" could provide very limited information such as a response to medication, but not much more than that.[34] More recent research indicates that SNPs could provide a significant amount of information if they can be associated with a haplotype.[35] At least twenty-two gene variants already have disease risk associated with them, and information unrelated to the disease under investigation is often revealed.[36] An example is provided by G308A, which is associated with sensitivity to carbamazepine, and has been associated with "risk for rheumatoid arthritis, tuberculosis, celiac disease, and ulcerative colitis."[36] A second example is provided by the MTHFR gene. The C667T variant has been associated with methotrexate therapy toxicity, while other variants have been associated with "several types of cancer, migraine, neural tube defects, and stroke."[36] As the field progresses it is likely that the potential for ancillary information will increase. While there may be future benefits from ancillary information, these are not certain.[22] Harm could strike immediately, or far into the future, due to increased knowledge or if unauthorized parties obtain the information.[22]

Not all ancillary information will be harmful. The potential for harm depends on several factors, such as the type of information, the attitude of the patient, and who else becomes aware of it. Some patients may wish to know if they are at increased risk of a disease, especially if preventive steps could be taken. For others however, knowledge of future disease risk could be unwelcome. If others become aware of it, ancillary risk information could also result in stigma, discrimination, and both economic and emotional harms. For instance, an individual having a test for the E4 variant in the APOE gene, which may be associated with warfarin therapy,[37] could also discover she was at greater risk for Alzheimer's disease.[22] This patient could experience great distress and worry over this possibility, even though she might never develop the condition. She could also experience stigma, discrimination, and economic harm with their corresponding emotional consequences if her genetic information fell into the hands of the wrong parties.[38]

An instructive example is provided by patients testing positive for Huntington's disease, who had negative experiences when revealing their test results to employers.[39] A total of 8 out of the 9 patients who revealed their genetic information stated they would not reveal the results to future employers. Even patients in the study who did not reveal the information felt "stuck" in their jobs, worried about performance evaluations and career advancement.[39] This type of worry is not unfounded. More than 200 cases of genetic discrimination by employers, insurance companies and others were reported in a 1996 survey.[40] In one egregious situation the Burlington Northern Santa Fe Rail Company performed genetic testing on employees without consent, to see if they had a predisposition for carpal tunnel syndrome, even though such tests are probabilistic at best.[41] Another major concern of the patients with Huntington's disease was social consequence; all of the patients noticed differential treatment within their families when the genetic information was revealed.[39] Most reported at least one relationship for which the news had a negative impact. Study participants were also afraid to reveal their genetic status to insurance companies.[39]

Legal Protections and Regulations

If the benefits of pharmacogenomics are to be realized, protections must be in place and be perceived as adequate. In a 1997 study, 85% thought employers should not have access to genetic information, and 63% said they would refuse genetic testing if insurers or employers would have access to the results.[42] In the U.S., some protections are in place, most notably the Americans with Disabilities Act (ADA), the Health Insurance Portability and Accountability Act (HIPAA) and the genetic information non-discrimination Act (GINA).[43] In addition, more than half of US states have ratified legislation prohibiting genetically based employment discrimination.[44] However, these protections are not complete.[22]

The ADA provides some protection, although it does not specifically mention genetic discrimination.[42] Protection appears to be extended only to those already exhibiting symptoms of the condition.[42] For instance, a lawsuit was brought when one employee who filed for carpal tunnel syndrome based compensation refused to provide a blood sample and was threatened with dismissal. Only after the federal Equal Employment Opportunity Commission became involved, arguing that basing employment decisions on the basis of a genetic test was a violation of the Americans with Disabilities Act, was the case was settled. The Burlington Company agreed to discontinue the practice.[41]

With regards to insurance, HIPAA bars the use of genetic information to establish a pre-existing condition if there has not yet been a diagnosis, although family histories can be exchanged between insurers and have been used to deny coverage in the past.[32] GINA was passed in April of 2008, and focuses on making the use of genetic information for setting health insurance payments or premiums or determining coverage illegal. It does not apply to life insurance or to long-term care insurance.[15] GINA also prohibits genetically based employment discrimination, although employers can gain access to information through benefit records, which are not considered medical information.[32] Even when legal protections are in place it is not always possible to prove an abuse or seek redress. For instance, one of the Huntington's Disease patients mentioned above was denied employment after reaching a third round interview in which he or she finally revealed their disease status; "nobody said anything about the Huntington's but they said other things about why they didn't hire me."[39]

Firewalls between healthcare personnel and insurance/employers may be desirable. One option for firewalls is to release only the "medicine response result," but withhold gene-specific and ancillary information.[29] The test result itself could provide a clue to the actual genetic and ancillary information however, and knowing that a patient is unlikely to benefit from "the only drug available for a serious condition" could be sufficient to result in discrimination.[29] Another method of utilizing a firewall could be to have a neutral and trusted third party hold the sample and related information, but this poses risks as well.[29] There have been numerous situations in which large data repositories holding personal information have been breached, including supposedly secure repositories such as those held by banks and the government.

Age is another consideration when thinking about ancillary information, especially in regard to children. The dangers faced by adults are also faced by children, and could be even more far-reaching, since the affected time span could be longer and include crucial developmental periods. Children must be able to comprehend medical information in order to truly give informed consent. Elements that can be understood by children around the age of 9 include the purpose of a test, what a procedure will involve, and the risks and benefits of clinical treatment options.[45] Generally the type of information that can be understood increases with developmental maturity.[46] It may be difficult for children to understand the implications of heredity and probability, necessary for understanding the meaning of ancillary information. In one recent qualitative study, a 10-year-old child did exhibit understanding of the probability concept.[46] While children in this age range may be able to understand the information, it may take more time, explanation and effort, with an opportunity for the children to personalize the implications of the test.[46] There is an important distinction between testing when beneficial action is possible vs. testing when nothing can be done to prevent or ameliorate the condition.[46] Diseases for which little or nothing can be done, such as sickle cell trait or alpha-1-antitrypsin deficiency have had negative psychosocial impacts on both children and their parents.[47] Several organizations, including the American Society of Human Genetics, discourage childhood genetic testing for diseases for which nothing can be done.[32]

Ancillary information also has potential relevance for family members.[4,32] As with the individual patient, stigma, discrimination and other harms are potential problems for family members of patients at genetic risk of disease.[32,38] Genetic information could have a long-term family impact if descendants face future job discrimination, reduced insurability,[24] or higher insurance premiums.[48] If family members are put at risk because of genetic information, do they have a right to know? What if they could benefit from it? Direct genetic testing is not the only potential source of this type of harm to family members however. Results of other disease tests can be sensitive, and disclosure is an important consideration.[48] In addition, health history information has long been used in determining insurance risk.[32] Patients will undoubtedly be concerned about this issue if it is brought to their attention, and healthcare professionals and researchers should be prepared to discuss the potential impact of ancillary pharmacogenetic information on patients' families.

The risks posed by ancillary information should be considered when genetic testing is offered. Clinical and research personnel have a duty to educate their clients: it is unlikely that lay persons will be familiar with the potential risks and they have a right to truly informed consent.

Implementation and Evidence

Another ethical issue concerns determining when the pharmacogenomic evidence is adequate and under which circumstances findings should be utilized in clinical practice. Much evidence thus far has been retrospective,[49] with small numbers of participants,[49] and from pharmacokinetic or observational studies.[15] Results have not been consistent nor were underlying mechanisms well understood.[15] While retrospective studies can be very useful, they cannot distinguish between cause and effect, nor can they distinguish between common causes.[50] The problem is further exacerbated when study numbers are small. Observational studies suffer from similar weaknesses. Many non-genetic factors influence drug metabolism and outcomes, including age, gender, ethnicity, diet, method of drug administration, drug-drug and drug-diet interactions.[15] Randomized controlled trials (RCT) comparing standard treatments with genetic testing and personally tailored treatment would be helpful in determining their clinical applicability.[15] RCTs would allow greater numbers of participants, increasing the generalizability of results as well, but they are also time-consuming and expensive to implement.

While RCT would be useful, they are not necessarily needed before incorporating all pharmacogenomic testing into clinical practice. Where reasonable alternative therapies are available, routine testing could be recommended, despite the weak evidence.[49] A case in point involves tamoxifen and CYP2D6 genotyping.[49] Relatively small retrospective studies have shown that certain slow CYP2D6 metabolizers do not produce the most active tamoxifen metabolite, endoxifen, apparently resulting in a greater chance of relapse and poorer survival rates.[51,52] Other drugs that impact CYP2D6 pathways, such as selective serotonin reuptake inhibitors (SSRIs), could also result in poor clinical outcomes by reducing tamoxifen metabolism.[51] These data were retrospective and did not involve more than a few hundred patients.[49] Despite the fact that the evidence is weak, there are alternatives to SSRIs for women using tamoxifen, and for women with hormone-positive breast cancer who are post-menopausal.[49] Routine testing for these women could be considered acceptable. These test results could provide additional information to use, in conjunction with other clinical factors, to inform therapy decisions. Existing alternatives involve ovarian suppression and are not necessarily reasonable for pre- and peri-menopausal women because they could have undesirable side-effects or suppress fertility. While there is little or no benefit to genetic testing in this case, harm to the patient could occur; if not now, at some future point as knowledge continues to advance. Routine use of pharmacogenomic information for situations in which there is neither an effective nor an alternative treatment is not ethical because the benefits do not outweigh the risks.

A final implementation issue is the limited number of FDA approved pharmacogenomic tests.[29] Many testing labs currently offer genetic testing using their own procedures and reagents.[29] The FDA recently issued the *Guidance for Industry and FDA Staff: Pharmacogenetic Tests and Genetic Tests for Heritable Markers* on June 19, 2007.[53] Recent approvals include the first genetic test for warfarin sensitivity, approved September 17, 2007,[54] a test for HER2, approved July 8, 2008, which is used to help determine if Herceptin is an appropriate treatment for breast cancer,[55] and a test for UGT1A1 variations, approved August 22, 2005, used to determine variations in the enzyme UDP-glucuronosyltransferase, which is active in irinotecan metabolism.[56] Dosage adjustments for irinotecan based on UGT1A1*28 allele status are recommended in the package insert, although the insert does not specifically require genetic testing.[57] New approved tests may hit the market in conjunction with new drugs, especially for new drugs approved only for certain genotypes.[29] Gaining FDA approval for a pharmacogenomic test is both time consuming and expensive, so the number of approved tests may be slow to increase, especially for existing or off-patent medications.

Implementation and Access

There are several access issues. One is whether third party payers will include pharmacogenomic tests in their coverage, and the second is whether drug access will be restricted based on test results.[29] Buchanan et al. suggest the tests will be covered if they are perceived as cost-effective, but could result in restricted access. Even if the chance of a response is low, or of adverse effects are high, situations could arise in which these drugs would be rational choices for a patient.[29] This is the distributive justice question raised earlier; how are the rights of the individual balanced against those of society?

Another issue could result from the use of closed, partially open, or negative formularies by third-party payers. In a closed formulary, only approved medications are included on the list, although there may be exceptions under certain circumstances.[58] Partially open formularies include certain drug classes, while negative formularies exclude certain drugs classes or drugs.[58] If an optimal drug, as determined through pharmacogenetic testing, is not included within a formulary, seeking coverage for it as an exception may force the revelation of test results.

Informed Consent in Clinical Practice

Should informed consent be sought before administering a pharmacogenetic test in clinical practice? There remains some controversy about this. Although the potential risks can be great, as illustrated above there is a great deal of variation in cases. The Nuffield Council on Bioethics has suggested that this issue will need to be determined for each situation on an individual basis.[59] A 1999 report to the U.S. House of Representatives Science Committee "strongly" advocated for written informed consent in clinical practice, stating that potential consequences should be included within the consent.[60]

In practice clinicians may not be obtaining informed consent from their patients before pharmacogenetic testing. Whether or not it is obtained appears to depend on the situation, and whether the test is considered as similar to other medical tests, or bundled in with them as part of a larger work-up.[61] If the test is for something that is not heritable, such as HER2 overexpression, clinicians may not feel it is a real genetic test and therefore does not require informed consent.[61] Some clinicians believe they don't have time to discuss it with their patient.[61] Paternalism may play a role as well. For newly diagnosed patients, especially those with a significant disease like breast cancer, information overload can be a real problem.[61] Other clinicians want to avoid disappointing patients by giving them false hope that doesn't bear out.[61]

One recommendation has been to obtain consent for higher risk pharmacogenomic tests,[22,62] but it may be difficult to classify the risk of these tests, especially as information and knowledge continues to advance.[63] Tests for inherited variants would likely pose greater risks than tests for acquired variants because of the greater potential for ancillary information and familial implications.[22] While in some situations genetic counseling may be needed, it is probably not practical in many clinical situations.[22,63] At the least, patients should be informed that they are receiving a genetically-based test, that ancillary information may be revealed now or in the future as knowledge progresses, how the data and/or tissues are being stored and handled, potential future uses of the material, and if employers or insurers will have access to the results. Administering a potentially risky genetic test to someone who is unaware of the potential risks would be a failure to respect their autonomy, especially within the context of a trust-based professional relationship.

Research

Pharmacogenomics in research involves several concerns in addition to those described above. While genetic material may be collected for a specific project and then destroyed, some is being collected with long-term use, data-mining, and commercial profit anticipated.[32] When these are the goals, community representation and benefit-sharing become issues.[32] At the individual and family level, research poses several unique issues that should be considered for inclusion in the informed consent. Many of these issues are connected to the preservation of confidentiality and privacy. Pharmacogenomic research also involves societal level issues, revolving around justice, access and non-malfeasance. These include setting research priorities and genetic colonialism, in which research by Westerners is seen as exploiting developing populations,[32] or as regarding them as "experimental animals."[64]

Risk levels will depend to some degree on the level of genome penetrance in the population, the types and level of identifiable data required, and disease association. There is greater risk for those with genes having low penetrance or those associated with serious diseases.[65] When research considerations permit, risks should be minimized by the choice of genetic markers that reveal minimal ancillary information, and firewalls should be considered to reduce the chance of accidental confidentiality breaches.[29] One method of protecting information but maintaining its usefulness is "pseudonomyzation," which involves replacing patient identifiers with new identifiers, and perhaps even the use of triple coding as is done in the GENOmatch system.[66] Even when "frank identifiers such as names, addresses, or patient identification numbers are removed from the data, the remaining data may uniquely identify an individual."[41] Vaszar et al. suggest protecting pharmacogenomic data by keeping identifiable subsets of cases larger than 5.[41] This means that if multiple characteristics are entered into the data base, the smallest group of cases meeting those criteria should be larger than five. If the number of cases identified via a particular search is 5 or smaller, then some data may need to be removed or modified before the information is released to a researcher. An example would be to remove the birth date and substitute the birth year.[41]

The U.S. National Bioethics Advisory Commission has suggested that research on unidentifiable material not be considered research on a human subject, and therefore no longer subject to the protections of the Common Rule.[67] To be classified as unidentifiable, any personal identifiers must not be retrievable if they were collected, or must never been collected. If information is unlinked, it is still considered human subjects research, although it could be considered eligible for IRB exemption under 45 CFR 46.101(b)(4). If information is coded, and that code could be linked to identifying information, it is considered research on human subjects and is regulated by the Common Rule, although it could be considered for expedited review if the risk is minimal. Coded or identified samples that are publicly available could be eligible for exemption.[67]

Informed Consent in Research

Informed consent is important when considering pharmacogenomic research; study participants are exposed to even more risk than clinical patients. Similar potential risks include emotional harm from genetic knowledge or ancillary information and/or harms resulting from the loss of privacy. There are also potential risks from long-term storage and access, and unanticipated future uses of their genetic material.

Prospective participants may not be aware of these potential risks and will need to be informed and educated about them.[68] Consent documents will need to include information about how the genetic sample will be handled, including storage, access, identifiable information, and length of retention.[24] Participants should know if their sample could be used in future research,[24] and researchers should spell out if they will obtain consent each time, or if they are asking for a blanket consent.[29] See Table 16-1 for a list of elements and samples of suggested language to be used in an informed consent for research. An informed consent template has been developed by a multidisciplinary group from the Centers for Disease Control and Prevention, and is available at http://www.cdc.gov/genomics/population/publications/consent.htm.

Table 16-1
Summary of Suggested Informed Consent Language*

Template Element	Excerpts of Sample Language
Introduction Identify the organizations conducting the research and the object of the study. Explain how prospective participants have been chosen.	The Centers for Disease Control and Prevention (CDC) and the Heart Alliance are doing a research study to find out more about how genes affect a person's risk of getting heart disease.
Why is this study being done? Summarize the problem and explain the research question(s) to be addressed.	Scientists have also found many genes that may be linked with heart disease and we expect they will find more in the future. The purpose of our study is to find out which genes are the most important for heart disease. This may help us begin to learn why some people get heart disease and others do not.
What is involved in the study? Describe how the biological sample will be obtained, any questionnaire or interviews, and whether participants will be asked to grant access to their medical records.	If you decide to provide a sample for this study, we will draw about 2 tbsp of blood from a vein in your arm. We will also ask you to fill out a survey about your health, diet, and exercise and your use of tobacco, alcohol, and medicines. There will be no medicines to take and no experimental treatments to undergo in this study.
How will information about me be kept private? Describe security measures and describe the extent to which confidentiality of records identifying the participant will be maintained.	Once we take your blood sample, we will assign it a code number. We will separate your name and any other information that points to you from your sample. We will keep files that link your name to the code number in a locked cabinet. Only the study staff will be allowed to look at these files. We will only release study information if it is ordered by a court of law.
What are the risks of the study? Describe relevant physical risks, informational risks, and potential group harms.	Although your name will not be with the sample, it will have other facts about you such as your race, ethnicity, and sex. These facts are important because they will help us learn if the factors that cause heart disease to occur or get worse are the same or different in men and women and in people of different racial or ethnic backgrounds. Thus, it is possible that study findings could one day help peple of the same race, ethnicity, or sex as you. However, it is also possible through these kinds of studies that genetic traits might come to be associated with your group. In some cases, this could reinforce harmful stereotypes.
Are there benefits to taking part in the study? Reiterate the object of the study.	You will not get any direct benefit for providing a blood sample for this study, but you will help us learn more about genes and other factors that may lead to heart disease.

Continued on next page

Table 16-1 *(Continued)*

Template Element	Excerpts of Sample Language
Are any costs or payments involved? Explain whether participants will be reimbursed for time or travel and what compensation or treatment is available if injury occurs. Explain arrangements regarding the development of products with commercial application.	The aim of our research is to improve the public health. Sometimes such research may result in findings or inventions that have value if they are made or sold. We may get a patent on these. We may also license these, which could give a company the sole right to make and sell products or offer testing based on the discovery. Some of the profits from this may be paid back to the researchers and the organizations doing this study, but you would not receive any financial benefits.
How will I find out about the results of the study? Include description of any general communication (eg, newsletters) about the study.	The studies we do are to add to our knowledge of how genes and other factors affect health and heart disease. We are gathering this knowledge by studying groups of people, and the study is not meant to test your personal medical status. For these reasons, we will not give you the results of our research on your sample. However, you can choose to get a newsletter that will tell you in general about the research studies we are doing. If you have questions about whether any genetic tests would be useful to you, you should ask your doctor.
What will happen to my sample after the study is over? Describe how the samples will be stored, where, and for how long. Clarify plans for future research to the extent possible.	After our study is over, we would like to keep any unused blood left over for future research. We don't have specific research plans at this time, but we would like to use the sample for future studies of heart disease. An institutional review board, like the one that helps protect you during this research project, will review and approve all future projects.
What are my rights as a participant? Include provisions for withdrawal following storage for future research.	You may choose not to have your sample stored for future research and still be part of this study. Also, you may agree to have your sample stored and later decide that you want to withdraw it from storage. If so, you should call the study person and tell him or her to discard your sample. He or she will discard your sample, but any data from testing your sample until that point will remain part of the research.
Whom do I call if I have questions or problems? Provide contact information for questions, rights, and injury.	If you have any questions about how this study works, contact _____. If you have any concerns about your rights in the study, contact _____. If you think that being in this study injured you, contact _____.

Continued on next page

Table 16-1 *(Continued)*

Template Element	Excerpts of Sample Language
Consents and signature Include separate section for consent to storage for future research. Offer option to receive general study communications.	My choice about having my sample stored and used for future research under the conditions described is (please check ONE box): ☐ I refuse to have my blood sample stored or used for studies of heart disease. ☐ It is OK to store my blood sample with a code number and to use it for studies of heart disease. I would like to receive a newsletter that will tell me about the research study and what researchers are learning in the future studies about genes and disease. Please circle ONE: Yes/No

*The examples used throught the templates are fictitious and were not drawn from any actual research project. The risk column contains only excerpts of sample language and does not necessarily include all of the elements listed in the left column. See http://jama.ama-assn.org/Issues/v286n18/ abs/jlm10008.html for complete template and sample language.

An important consideration is whether genetic information derived from the research should be disclosed to the participants. These decisions could be influenced by the type of genetic test being used, differing between FDA approved tests and non-approved laboratory gene tests.[29] The Nuffield Council on Bioethics recommended that study participants should be offered a choice to receive the information during the informed consent process if the information could be expected to be useful.[59] If feedback is planned the information cannot be anonymized, and other steps such as pseudonomyzation must be used. Researchers will need to determine and spell out how the information will be delivered to the participant, how the participants and researchers will remain in contact, how far into the future the patient would want to be contacted, and if they want to be contacted for as yet undetermined future tests.[29] One potential solution would be to contact the patient when a discovery is made, and allow them to access the information if he or she chooses to utilizing a password provided by the researcher.[66] Depending on the situation, it may be desirable to offer genetic counseling[29] or medical help.[67] A decision may also have to be made as to whether information should be included in the participants' medical records.[29]

From the researchers point of view there may be concern that a lengthy consent process and the issues brought up will discourage research participation. Evidence suggests that is not the case, however. Approximately 85% of participants in the National Health and Nutrition Examination Survey for 1999 and 2000 agreed to have a blood sample stored in a national repository for future research.[69]

Family and Children

While genetic research has implications for individual participants, family members also have a stake in the information revealed. Family members often play a role in genetic research by disclosing health information and loss of privacy and potential discrimination are serious risks for the entire family. In addition, traditional healthcare relationships with providers may be altered.[24] For example, privacy and beneficence are key principles underlying patient-provider relationships, but when the entire family is involved, the welfare of the group also factors in.[24] This is one place where "respect for communities" comes into play.[24] Although most research is conducted on the basis of personal consents, recently there has been interest in family consent procedures.[38] This does not refer to a family member giving consent for another family member, but involves consent by each member of the family. It is acknowledged however that reaching consensus could be difficult in practice.[38]

Children's participation in research may raise special concerns. Research in young people will be needed because gene expression can change considerably as children develop and mature.[70] Many maturational changes occur in receptor systems, neural networks and the production of drug metabolizing enzymes, and some diseases affecting children have no adult correlates.[71] For example, cytochrome P450 (CYP) 1A2 is not really active until after 4 months, although some of the other CYPs do perform some of its activities before then.[70] There may be a great deal of interaction between nutrition and the environment and gene expression as well. For example, breast fed children metabolize caffeine differently than non-breast fed children.[70] Potential therapeutic targets may exist for only a period of time as children mature, and it will be important to know not only where to look, but when.[71]

Despite advances in non-invasive techniques, tissue samples from organs like the intestine, liver or kidney remain necessary to understand gene expression.[70] This means that progress will be slow. Fetal research will undoubtedly remain controversial, and it will be difficult to obtain transplant tissues since they are (and should be) usually used to save the lives of sick children.[71] Although research should not be started unless it can reasonably be anticipated that the study will include a sufficient number of participants to answer the question, this may not happen in studies with children.[70] IRBs will need to determine if "some data is better than none," since the alternative is to do no research and continue dosing children without adequate research data.[70]

It is generally agreed upon that genetic testing should be done in children only if they can expect a direct and timely benefit, and when the parent's consent is obtained.[71] Children older than 7 should also give their assent.[71] Testing should be delayed for conditions that do not appear until adulthood, unless something could be done to treat or prevent it earlier.[71] While both children and parents appear willing to participate in research studies for altruistic reasons, expected benefits appear to play a role.[46] For example, parents of children in families with heart disease were more interested in participating in genetic studies than those in families with breast cancer, and this was linked to the potential for positive behavior changes.[46]

Research Agendas

One of the potential benefits of pharmacogenomics is the ability to streamline clinical trials by including only those who appear likely to benefit or unlikely to experience severe side-effects. The flip side to this is that these drugs would not be tested in the general population. To ensure safe use, genetic tests would be needed, and potential consumers will need to be informed that they are needed. These tests would increase the cost of using the drug. One manufacturer has already been sued for failing to warn consumers that people with HLA-DR4+ genotype would be more susceptible to developing arthritis if they used the Lyme disease vaccine.[72] Assuming the information is included in package inserts, people with unapproved phenotypes would have to use at their own risk. Off-label use of medications is common, with estimates ranging from 7.5% to 40% in adults, and even higher rates in children.[73]

Drug companies will have to decide which diseases and drugs they are going to pursue. One choice will be to go for as broad a market as possible, developing drugs useful for multiple genotypes, or they can choose to concentrate on particular subgroups.[4] Certain groups may appear more desirable, especially those who can pay for the therapy. Sub-groups that are too small or not affluent enough may not provide a viable market, and drugs could end up costing more for smaller markets.[4] These kind of decisions may result in an increase in "orphan phenotypes" or "orphan genotypes,"[23] or perhaps even orphan countries.

The discovery of phenotypes or genotypes associated with ethnic group, racial identity or continent of origin could result in "oppression" or discrimination against these groups.[32] If vulnerabilities are identified, there is also the potential risk of genocidal weapons.[30] It would be desirable to include community representatives in decisions about genetic research for these groups, but this could prove difficult.[32] Potential roadblocks include identifying the appropriate community, preventing coercion of individuals within a community, and preserving neutrality in the face of a conflicted community.[32]

Most drugs are developed in the U.S. or in Europe, and drugs are approved on the basis of safety and effectiveness in at least a portion of those populations.[74] It is unclear if these drugs will be safe and effective in other areas of the world, like Africa or Asia, although they are sold and used there.[74] If drugs are targeted for specific genotypes it will probably not be possible to develop the cheaper generics needed for developing countries.[4] Advances in understanding haplotypes may help with this situation, but will probably not be sufficient. Regional SNP-genotyping in developing areas has begun, and needs to be expanded.[74] This information will help determine if drugs developed in the U.S. or Europe can be safely and effectively used in these populations.

Summary and Recommendations

Clearly there are numerous ethical issues for pharmacogenomic researchers and clinicians to consider within the context of their work. Many of these issues can be resolved in advance by ensuring that patients and participants give truly informed consent for pharmacogenomic testing. At a societal level, family and community input should be considered. In addition, all materials and information should be safe-guarded, by the individuals entrusted with them, and legislatively. GINA is a good start, but it has loopholes. Additional legislation and regulations addressing issues such as long term care insurance and life insurance is needed.

Randomized clinical trials, pharmacoeconomic studies, and cost-benefit analyses are needed to determine which pharmacogenomic tests are truly worth incorporating into clinical practice. The development of clinical guidelines and increased education of clinicians and researchers would be beneficial.

It may not always be easy to determine the correct course of action, but a consideration of the facts, moral rules, principles and theories should provide insight. Risks and benefits must be balanced depending on the context and particulars of each case and multiple viewpoints must be acknowledged. The strength of evidence and availability of alternatives should be taken into consideration as well.[15] If there is serious doubt about a situation, try to err on the side of caution.[15] While pharmacogenomics will play an increasingly important role in healthcare, it is important to avoid "geneticisation," the tendency to ascribe everything to a genetic influence, and downplaying the influence of the environment, lifestyle, and behavior.[75]

References

1. Jonsen AR. *The Birth of Bioethics*. New York: Oxford University Press; 1998.
2. Veatch RM. *Medical Ethics*. Sudbury, MA: Jones & Bartlett Publishers, Inc.; 1997.
3. Nielsen LF, Moldrup C. Lay perspective on pharmacogenomics: a literature review. *Per Med.* 2006;3:311-316.
4. van Delden J, Bolt I, Kalis A, Derijks J, Leufkens H. Tailor-made pharmacotherapy: future developments and ethical challenges in the field of pharmacogenomics. *Bioethics.* 2004;18(4):303-321.
5. Beauchamp TL, Childress JF. *Principles of Biomedical Ethics*. 6th ed. New York, Oxford: Oxford University Press; 2009.
6. Wilensky HL. The professionalization of everyone? *Am J Sociol.* 1964;70(2):137-158.
7. King NMP. Health care ethics and the provider's role. In: Henderson GE, King NMP, Strauss RP, Estroff SE, Churchill LR, eds. *The Social Medicine Reader*. Durham & London: Duke University Press; 1997:304-308.
8. Ham CJ. Retracing the Oregon trail: the experience of rationing and the Oregon health plan. *Br Med J.* 1998;316(7149):1965-1969.
9. BBC News. Smoking is cost-effective, says report. *World: Americas* [Tuesday, 17 July 2001; Available at: http://news.bbc.co.uk/1/hi/world/americas/1442555.stm.
10. Rescher N. *Distributive Justice*. Indianapolis, IN: Bobs-Merrill; 1966.
11. Veatch RM. Hospital pharmacy: what is ethical? *Am J Hosp Pharm.* 1989;46:109-115.
12. McCarthy RL, Schafermeyer KW, eds. *Introduction to Health Care Delivery. A Primer for Pharmacists*. 3rd ed. Sudbury, MA: Jones and Bartlett; 2004.
13. Lazarou J, Pomeranz B, Corey P. Incidence of adverse drug reactions in hospitalized patients: a meta-analysis of prospective studies. *JAMA.* 1998;279(15):1200-1205.
14. Kongkaew C, Noyce PR, Ashcroft DM. Hospital admissions associated with adverse drug reactions: a systematic review of prospective observational studies. *Ann Pharmacother.* 2008;42:1017-1025.
15. Rasmussen-Torvik LJ, McAlpine DD. Genetic screening for SSRI drug response among those with major depression: great promise and unseen perils. *Depress Anxiety.* 2007;24(5):350-357.
16. MacGillivray S, Arroll B, Hatcher S, et al. Efficacy and tolerability of selective serotonin reuptake inhibitors compared with tricyclic antidepressants in depression treated in primary care. Systematic review and meta-analysis. *Br Med J.* 2003;326c:1014-1019.
17. Meyer UA. Pharmacogenetics and adverse drug reactions. *Lancet.* 2000;356(9242):1667-1671.
18. Manolopoulos VG. Pharmacogenomics and adverse drug reactions in diagnostic and clinical practice. *Clin Chem Lab Med.* 2007;45(7):801-814.
19. Anonymous. Mayo Clinic offers new genetic test to screen for side effects of antidepressant treatment. *Pharmacogenomics.* 2006;7(6):811.
20. Morley KI, Hall WD. Using pharmacogenetics and pharmacogenomics in the treatment of psychiatric disorders: some ethical and economic considerations. *J Mol Med.* 2004;82(1):21-30.
21. Emilien G, Ponchon M, Caldas C, Isacson O, Maloteaux JM. Impact of genomics on drug discovery and clinical medicine. *Q J Med.* 2000;93(7):391-423.

22. Haga SB, Burke W. Pharmacogenetic testing: not as simple as it seems. *Genet Med.* 2008;10(6):391-395.

23. Rai AK. Pharmacogenetic interventions, orphan drugs, and distributive justice: The role of cost-benefit analysis. *Soc Philos Policy.* 2002;19(2):246-270.

24. Issa AM. Ethical considerations in clinical pharmacogenomics research. *Trends Pharmacol Sci.* 2000;21(7):247-249.

25. Oliveira E, Marsh S, Van Booven DJ, Amorim A, Prata MJ, McLeod HL. Pharmacogenetically relevant polymorphisms in Portugal. *Pharmacogenomics.* 2007;8(7):703-712.

26. Lin JP, Schwaiger JP, Cupples LA, et al. Conditional linkage and genome-wide association studies identify UGT1A1 as a major gene for antiatherogenic serum bilirubin levels—The Framingham Heart Study. *Atherosclerosis.* 2009.

27. Peet NP, Bey P. Pharmacogenomics: challenges and opportunities. *Drug Discovery Today.* 2001;6:495-498.

28. Peterson-Iyer K. Pharmacogenomics, ethics, and public policy. *Kennedy Institute of Ethics Journal.* 2008;18(1):35-56.

29. Buchanan A, Califano A, Kahn J, McPherson E, Robertson J, Brody B. Pharmacogenetics: Ethical issues and policy options. *Kennedy Inst Ethics J.* 2002;12(1):1-15.

30. Bartfai T. Pharmacogenomics in drug development: societal and technical aspects. *Pharmacogenomics J.* 2004;4(4):226-232.

31. Feinberg J. Chapter 5. The child's right to an open future. In: Howie J, ed. *Ethical Principles for Social Policy.* Carbondale and Edwardsville: Southern Illinois University Press; 1983:97-122.

32. Anderlik MR, Rothstein MA. Privacy and confidentiality of genetic information: What rules for the new science? *Ann Rev Genom Hum Genet.* 2001;2:401-433.

33. Weijer C, Miller PB. Protecting communities in pharmacogenetic and pharmacogenomic research. *Pharmacogenomics J.* 2004;4(1):9-16.

34. Roses AD. Pharmacogenetics and the practice of medicine. *Nature.* 2000;405:857-865.

35. Phillips MS, Lawrence R, Sachidanandam R, et al. Chromosome-wide distribution of happlotype blocks and the role of recombination hot spots. *Nat Genet.* 2003;33:382-387.

36. Henrikson NB, Burke W, Veenstra DL. Ancillary risk information and pharmacogenetic tests: social and policy implications. *Pharmacogenomics J.* 2008;8(2):85-89.

37. Wadelius M, Chen LY, Eriksson N, et al. Association of warfarin dose with genes involved in its action and metabolism. *Hum Genet.* 2007;121:23-34.

38. Van der Vorm A, Rikkert MO, Vernooij-Dassen M, Dekkers W, on behalf of the EDCON panel. Genetic research into Alzheimer's Disease: a European focus group study on ethical issues. *Int J Geriatr Psych.* 2008;23:11-15.

39. Penziner E, Williams JK, Erwin C, et al. Perceptions of discrimination among persons who have undergone predictive testing for Huntington's Disease. *Am J Med Genet Part B (Neuropsych Genet).* 2008;147B(3):320-325.

40. Geller LN, Alper JS, Billings PR, Barash CI, Beckwith J, Natowicz MR. Individual, family and societal dimensions of genetic discrimination: a case study analysis. *Sci Eng Ethics.* 1996;2-1:71-88.

41. Vaszar LT, Cho MK, Raffin TA. Privacy issues in personalized medicine. *Pharmacogenomics.* 2003;4(2):107-112.

42. Cornell University ILR School. Genetic information and the workplace—full report. In: US Dept of Labor UDoHaHS, US Equal Employment Opportunity Commission, ed; 1998.

43. H.R. 493—110th Congress. GovTrack.us (database of federal legislation); 2007. Available at: http://www.govtrack.us/congress/bill.xpd?tab=summary&bill=h110-493. Accessed May 18, 2009.

44. Nelson RR. State labor legislation enacted in 2002. *Monthly Labor Review Online.* January, 2003 2003;126(1).

45. Weithorn LA, Campbell SB. The comptency of children and adolescents to make informed treatment decisions. *Child Dev.* 1982;53:1589-1598.

46. Bernhardt BA, Tambor ES, Fraser G, Wissow LS, Geller G. Parents' and children's attitudes toward the enrollment of minors in genetic susceptibility research: Implications for informed consent. *Am J Med Genet A.* 2003;116A:315-323.

47. Newman TB, Browner WS, Hulley SB. The case against childhood cholesterol screening. *JAMA.* 1990;264:3039-3043.

48. Smart A, Martin P, Parker M. Tailored medicine: Whom will it fit? The ethics of patient and disease stratification. *Bioethics.* 2004;18(4):322-343.

49. Hartman AR, Helft P. The ethics of CYP2D6 testing for patients considering tamoxifen. *Breast Cancer Res.* 2007;9(2).

50. Mantel N, Haenszel W. Statistical aspects of the analysis of data from retrospective studies of disease. In: Buck C, Llopis A, Najera E, Terris M, eds. *The Challenge of Epidemiology: Issues and Selected Readings.* Washington, DC: Pan American Health Organization; 1988:533-553.

51. Knox SK, Ingle JN, Suman VJ, et al. The impact of cytochrome P450 2D6 metabolism in women receiving adjuvant tamoxifen. *Breast Cancer Res Treat.* 2007;101:113-121.

52. Grabinski JL, Smith LS, Chrisholm GB, et al. Relationship between CYP2D6 and estrogen receptor alpha polymorphisms on tamoxifen metabolism in adjuvant breast cancer treatment. *J Clin Oncol (Meeting Abstracts).* 2006;24:506.

53. Food and Drug Administration. Guidance for Industry and FDA Staff. Pharmacogenetic tests and genetic tests for heritable markers. Available at: http://www.fda.gov/cdrh/oivd/guidance/1549.pdf. Accessed October 24, 2008.

54. Food and Drug Administration. FDA clears genetic lab test for warfarin sensitivity. Available at: http://www.fda.gov/bbs/topics/NEWS/2007/NEW01701.html. Accessed October 24, 2008.

55. Food and Drug Administration. FDA approves new genetic test for patients with breast cancer. Available at: http://www.fda.gov/bbs/topics/NEWS/2008/NEW01857.html. Accessed October 24, 2008.

56. Food and Drug Administration. FDA clears genetic test that advances personalized medicine. Test helps determine safety of drug therapy. Available at: http://www.fda.gov/bbs/topics/NEWS/2005/NEW01220.html. Accessed May 19, 2009.

57. Pfizer. NDA 20-571 Camptosar® (irinotecan HCl) Final Label; 2005.

58. Pizzi LT, Lofland JH. *Economic Evaluation in U.S. Health Care. Principles and Applications.* Sudbury, MA: Jones and Barlett; 2006.

59. Nuffield Council on Bioethics. *Pharmacogenetics: Ethical Issues: Report of Working Party.* London: Nuffield Council on Bioethics; 2003.

60. Morella CA, ed. Genetics testing in the new millennium: advances, standards, and implications. Hearing before the subcommittee on technology of the Committee on Science. U.S. House of Representatives. One hundred sixth congress; 2001; No. 106-7.

61. Hedgecoe A. 'At the point at which you can do something about it, then it becomes more relevant': Informed consent in the pharmacogenetic clinic. *Soc Sci Med.* 2005;61(6):1201-1210.

62. Robertson JA, Brody B, Buchanan A, Kahn J, McPherson E. Pharmacogenetic challenges for the health care system. *Health Affairs.* 2002;21(4):155-167.

63. Netzer C, Biller-Andorno N. Pharmacogenetic testing, informed consent and the problem of secondary information. *Bioethics.* 2004;18(4):344-360.

64. Kahn P. Genetic diversity project tries again. *Science.* 1994;266:720-722.

65. Beskow LM, Burke W, Merz JF, et al. Informed consent for population-based research involving genetics. *JAMA.* 2001;286(18):2315-2321.

66. Reischl J, Schroder M, Luttenberger N, et al. Pharmacogenetic research and data protection - challenges and solutions. *Pharmacogenomics J.* 2006;6(4):225-233.

67. National Bioethics Advisory Commission. *Research Involving Human Biological Materials: Ethical Issues and Policy Guidance: Executive Summary.* Rockville, MD: U.S. National Bioethics Advisory Committee; 1999.

68. Alcalde MG, Rothstein MA. Pharmacogenomics: Ethical concerns for research and pharmacy practice. *Am J Health-Syst Pharm.* 2002;59(22):2239-2240.

69. McQuillan GM, Porter KS, Agelli M, Kington R. Consent for genetic research in a general population: the NHANES experience. *Genet Med.* 2003;5(1):35-42.

70. Freund CL, Clayton EW. Pharmacogenomics and children. *Bioethics.* 2003;8(6):399-404.

71. Leeder JS, Kearns GL. The challenges of delivering pharmacogenomics into clinical pediatrics. *Pharmacogenomics J.* 2002;2(3):141-143.

72. Rothstein MA. Pharmacogenomics: Ethics, policy, and public perceptions. *Drug Metabolism Reviews.* 2002;34:3-3.

73. Gazarian M, Kelly M, McPhee JR, Graudins LV, Ward RL, Campbell TJ. Off-label use of medicines: consensus recommendations for evaluating appropriateness. *Med. J. Aust.* 2006;185:544-548.

74. Daar AS, Singer PA. Pharmacogenetics and geographical ancestry: implications for drug development and global health. *Nat Rev Genet.* 2005;6(3):241-246.
75. Lippman A. Led (Astray) by genetic maps: the cartography of the human genome and health care. *Soc Sci Med.* 1992;35:1469-1476.

Chapter 17

Future Promise of Pharmacogenomics in Clinical Practice

Jeffery D. Evans, Pharm.D.

Learning Objectives

After completing this chapter, the reader should be able to

- Identify potential areas of pharmacogenomic practice.
- Associate applications of pharmacogenomics with the different practice sites of pharmacists.
- Predict the roles of pharmacists in the future using pharmacogenomics.
- Recognize resources found online and in print that can assist in furthering the reader's understanding of pharmacogenomics.

Key Definitions

Hippocratic oath—An oath taken by physicians and other healthcare professionals that is mainly known for the "first do no harm" statement, though the statement does not appear in the modern Hippocratic oath.

HMG-COA reductase inhibitors—Also known as the "statins." A class of medications used to treat high LDL-cholesterol. They are linked to rare but life-threatening adverse effects.

Point-of-care tests—These laboratory tests provide results to the patient and clinician at the time the test is completed. Most laboratory tests must be sent to the lab; however, these are completed usually in the room where the patient is. They are usually very quick.

Introduction

Before a discussion on the future impact of pharmacogenomics (PG) can occur, it is important to see how the science of pharmacogenomics has evolved. Even though pharmacogenetics was first defined in the 1950s, it is not taught universally, even in schools of pharmacy. However, this is likely to change as old and new medications alike are including pharmacogenetic information in their package labeling.

The previous chapters of this text have discussed what is currently available and possibly what will be available in the near future with regards to pharmacogenomics. This chapter will highlight some of the information found in the previous chapters. Additionally, it will discuss the impact of PG on the practice of pharmacy, including how it will affect the various sites of practice of pharmacists.

In addition to the many disease states in which this book has shown the promise of pharmacogenomics, there are many that still hold promise and should be investigated. For example, pharmacogenomic differences have been associated with varying responses to opioids and HMG-CoA reductase inhibitors (statins), but these relationships have not been fully investigated.[1,2] A specific example of a disease state that has not yet been adequately studied, in relation to pharmacogenomics, is hypertension. In this condition, there are known racial disparities among the effectiveness of different classes of antihypertensive agents.[3] Currently, it has been shown clinically that African Americans with hypertension respond better to calcium channel blockers and diuretics than other populations. After reading this text and reviewing the many areas in which pharmacogenomics have already provided an answer to a question, it is easy to see how this racial variation might be related to pharmacogenomics. Additionally, one might look at the side effects that are both uncommon and common with angiotensin-I converting enzyme inhibitors (ACEIs). Cough is a common adverse event with each ACEI and is thought to be caused by an excess accumulation of bradykinin. Because this reaction occurs in about 3% of the U.S. population, one might wonder if it could be a possible pharmacogenomic reaction?[4] Could the patients developing a cough secondary to using an ACEI actually have a SNP that causes the accumulation of excess bradykinin when they are exposed to an ACEI?

The potential impact of pharmacogenomics on the effectiveness of medications is great. Currently a one-size-fits-all mentality impacts the way that healthcare providers treat patients with medications. When a pharmacist works in a clinic and needs to make a recommendation to another provider, he or she must consult current clinical guidelines and consider the complete list of medications that are available to treat the condition. Unfortunately, many of the medications may not be as effective for the patient as those that could be recommended if they were based on the patient's genetic make-up. As more patients have genetic profiles performed and more information is available about medications and their interactions with different genetic profiles, the pharmacist will be able to tailor a regimen with specific medications and doses for the patient based on the patient's genetic make-up. This customization will be in addition to the other commonly accepted variables used today (age, weight, sex). The pharmacists responsible for the dispensing of the medication also may benefit from the additional information from the patient's profile. It will help them know that the patient is receiving the correct drug and that the dose for the medication is appropriate.

Beyond effectiveness, and perhaps foremost in many pharmacists' minds, is safety. The Hippocratic Oath states that first the physician should do no harm. Pharmacists adopt this mentality, yet are sometimes responsible for causing a patient harm without knowing it. With genetic testing, many of the worst side effects from medications maybe more predictable. HMG-COA reductase inhibitors are an example of a class of medications where genetic testing may have prevented patient deaths from occurring.[4] Additionally, cerivastatin, a medication that was both effective and cheaper than other members of its class, could have been left on the market if its target population had been genetically screened. However, because genetic testing was not completed, the medication was blamed for the deaths of the patients instead of a possible fault in their genetic makeup. As a result the medication was removed from the market, and numerous lawsuits ensued.

Case Study—Hyperlipidemia

R.E. is a 47-year-old female who was recently diagnosed with hyperlipidemia. R.E. is found to have a mutation of the gene that codes for HMG-COA reductase, which alters the ability for HMG-COA reductase inhibitors to bind appropriately to the enzyme.

Questions:
1. What impact would this mutation have on the care of the patient?
2. What cholesterol reducing agents would still be appropriate for this patient?
3. Would a higher dose of HMG-COA reductase inhibitors be recommended for this patient? Would you expect the same level of side effects?

This patient would most likely not respond to HMG-COA reductase medications (statins) thus she would need to find alternatives to those medications. Other agents that lower LDL would still be good choices for this patient. If desired, higher doses of the statin medications could be tried to ensure that maximal binding to the mutated site would occur; however, it is likely that the statins would still bind normally to other sites which could lead to increased site effects.

Obstacles to Applying Pharmacogenomics to Practice

As outlined in the preceding chapters, there are numerous opportunities related to pharmacogenomics that can be utilized, but also roadblocks that must be overcome. The opportunities are clear: improved effectiveness of medications in patients that need them, avoidance of medications that will be ineffective, and a reduction in adverse effects. The roadblocks though are somewhat more difficult to ascertain, but must still be overcome. Each party involved in the patient's care has unique obstacles that must be overcome before they might fully realize the benefits of PG.

The first obstacle is common among all of the people involved in the patient's care—knowledge. Education regarding pharmacogenomics is an issue for schools of medicine where less than half include PG education in the required didactic portion of their curriculums.[5] Surveys of pharmacy schools showed that greater than half of the schools of pharmacy included PG education as a requirement for graduation.[6,7] If the healthcare providers do not understand the role that pharmacogenomics play in patient care, then it is unlikely that they will request the genetic testing needed to determine the effect the patient's genes may have on the medication. Additionally, if the healthcare providers do not have adequate levels of knowledge regarding pharmacogenomics, they can not educate their patients on the importance of genetic testing.

Pharmacists are well trained in how to make recommendations based on medication levels in the blood and diseases that are being treated. The practice of making recommendations based on PG data must also become an integrated portion of the curriculum of schools to ensure that pharmacists in all settings will be able to interpret the results of PG testing and make educated recommendations from these results.

The second obstacle is privacy. Unlike hypertension or hyperlipidemia, there is no treatment for variations in one's genetic makeup. Thus, if the patient is told he or she has a mutation that may put him or her more at risk for developing tachyphylaxis to inhaled beta-2 agonists, what can be done? Should the patient be forced to tell the healthcare providers about his or her genetic condition? Should this information also be considered in the provision of health insurance or be part of the patient's life-insurance premium determination?

Furthermore, if a patient is found to have a genetic mutation, does that not compromise the privacy of his or her parents and their offspring? Most likely the patient inherited the gene from his or her parents and passed it on to their children. Thus, by completing the genetic test, the healthcare provider has not only identified a possible issue with the patient, but also other members of the family that may not be under the care of the healthcare provider.

Additional obstacles are cost, utilization, and usefulness. As mentioned elsewhere, the current cost of genetic testing is considerable. In theory though, if PG becomes more accepted the number of tests will increase and the cost of each test should decrease. However, the initial burden of an entity paying for the tests may be too much, and significant costs may be passed on to the patient. To increase the number of tests performed, the utilization must be increased. There are no data currently available that demonstrate the percentage of patients being screened for PG related issues prior to the initiation of medication; however, it is likely very low. Finally the usefulness of PG testing is an important issue that must be addressed. Until significant time or money savings can be demonstrated with PG testing and utilization, the usefulness of the testing will also be questionable. Healthcare providers can always continue with the trial and error method of prescribing medications, which has been the standard of care for decades.

Clinical Pearl

Some patients with and without insurance do not wish to have a diagnosis such as hypertension or diabetes mellitus added to their history as this may impact the availability of insurance and/or the cost of insurance in the future.

The final roadblock is cost. Currently many of the commercially available genetic tests range from less than $100 to several thousand dollars depending on the nature and quantity of the mutations the test is looking for. Given the limited applicability of many of the genetic tests to current treatment, insurance companies are unwilling to cover them from a cost standpoint. Thus, the cost is shifted back onto the patient who may not be willing to pay for the test and thus cost becomes a limiting issue.

Impact of Pharmacogenomics on Pharmacy Practice

Though the promise of pharmacogenomics will impact the overall practice of pharmacy, each of the individual fields of pharmacy practice may be affected differently.

Community pharmacists may be the first to experience the series of questions and applications of pharmacogenomics. Being the most accessible healthcare professional and one of the most trusted, community pharmacists will have the opportunity and the responsibility to address the questions and concerns of the public.[6] One of the first changes in practice that the field of pharmacogenomics might make to community practice is the potential collection of genetic information. Along with all of the other information that a pharmacist must collect (age, address, allergies), the pharmacist could soon be asked to collect whether or not the patient has any genetic abnormalities he or she wishes to report. This will be important for the pharmacists as the medication dispensing process occurs. Much like the pharmacist must know if a drug–drug interaction is relevant or not, the pharmacist must also have a good understanding of pharmacogenomics to determine if he or she should contact the medication prescriber to warn them of the potential interaction, or just educate the patient.

Community pharmacists also may be at the forefront of genetic testing, willing or not. One of the proposed mechanisms to ensure patient confidentiality is to have the tests available over-the-counter where patients may pick up the test and collect a small blood sample and then send the test off to be analyzed. On completion of the test, the company will mail the results back to the patient. Once the patient has the results in hand, he or she can choose with whom to share the results. This system is already in place for one of the genomic tests important to asthma treatment. Additionally, some genetic screenings may become point-of-care (POC) tests similar to lipid and glucose testing is today. If POC machines do become available for genomic testing, this would be an excellent arena for community pharmacists to develop a service that would provide the exam and then also provide limited information regarding what the results mean. This could become another part of the cognitive services that some pharmacies offer today.

For pharmacists working in hospitals, the promise of pharmacogenomics is slightly different in that required duties, such as discharge counseling and medication histories, will be impacted. One special area of interest may be in the emergency room where certain treatment decisions must be made quickly, yet pharmacogenomic information may not be collected in a timely fashion.

Case Study—Asthma

A 12-year-old African-American male presents to the emergency room with worsening shortness of breath and wheezing. His mother says that he was at home this morning when he started wheezing. She has given him three albuterol treatments via nebulizer, and he initially improved but has not been feeling well since then. His mother states that he had some genomic testing, and it showed he had an asthma variant. She is not sure which. During the interview, the patient starts to become unstable and his O_2 saturation drops to 85%.

Questions:

1. What information is needed to evaluate the patient?
2. In this case, does the pharmacogenomic information help or hurt the care of this patient?
3. With the information presented, how does this change your recommendation for the management of this patient?

This case shows a serious concern that is already occurring with genetic testing that will continue to worsen as more tests are available. What to do with the patient who has had testing, but does not know the results? Some patients do not know what previous therapies they have tried or even what reactions they have had to medications other than they are allergic to them. In the above case, it should be ascertained if the results of the genomic testing recommended using (or not using) a certain medication over another. However, currently the results of the testing are not helping this patient's therapy selection as no information is provided. Thus, even though this patient has completed genomic testing, no benefit is derived from it and the patient will receive the standardized, one size fits all, therapy.

The role of the pharmacist in discharge counseling may also need to be adjusted with wider implementation of genetic testing. The pharmacist is responsible for ensuring that patients understand the medication therapy they will be taking before they leave the hospital in many institutions. What role will pharmacogenomics play in this setting? The pharmacist may be asked and will need to document why the medications were prescribed in the place of other medications. Additionally, the pharmacist may be asked to explain what the different genomic exam results mean and what should be done about them. Additionally, even in the traditional roles of dispensing and distribution in hospital pharmacies, the pharmacist will need to be proficient in what the different pharmacogenomic results mean and be able to input them correctly into the pharmacy system to ensure that the patients do not receive medications or doses that are not recommended for their pharmacogenomic profiles.

Pharmacists working in clinical settings have the most control over the implementation of pharmacogenomics in their practice setting. Pharmacists working in a specific setting, such as an anticoagulation clinic, will be able to handle the large amount of pharmacogenomic information being released in the coming years. In this setting maintaining an adequate and up-to-day database of knowledge regarding pharmacogenomics may be easier, as it will be focused to specific disease states. Pharmacists working in general ambulatory care practices or rounding with medical teams may be overwhelmed by the amount of pharmacogenomic information being released yearly. However, if the pharmacist is able to master this information, he or she will become an even more valued member of the healthcare team and will most likely be the most knowledgeable person regarding pharmacogenomics. The outpatient clinic setting is also where pharmacists will be able to implement the use of pharmacogenomics most thoroughly. With easy access to the patient, healthcare provider, and laboratories, the pharmacist located in a clinic will be able to address many of the areas of concern that pharmacists in other areas of pharmacy can not address. Additionally, the clinic-based pharmacist will have full access to the chart which may include valuable information regarding the patient's genetic makeup and other indicators, such as prolonged QTc, of genetic abnormalities.

Impact of Pharmacogenomics on Drug Development

The use of PG will extend beyond the clinical practice setting. Early adoption of PG by the pharmaceutical industry has already occurred.[8] The pharmaceutical industry intends to utilize PG to "rescue" old drugs, as described below, and to target specific PG profiles that would benefit more from the medication, or experience fewer adverse effects.

One prospective application for pharmaceutical companies is by recovering and re-branding medications that have been pulled off of the market or could possibly be pulled off of the market for safety reasons. If a PG reason can be found to explain why the adverse events occurred, then screening could be completed that would identify patients at risk and avoid the use of the medication in this patients. This does provide some market shrinkage for the company as fewer patients would be eligible to use the medication; however, it may reduce the company's legal risks. An example of this is abacavir, a medication used to treat HIV infection.[8] Though uncommon, a potentially life-threatening hypersensitivity reaction (HSR) was found to be associated with the medication. After broad spectrum testing, patients with the HLA-B57 mutation were found to have a higher incidence of HSR to abacavir. Now labeling for abacavir recommends the use of the genetic test to screen patients for the potential interaction.

Pharmacogenomics can also be used earlier in the drug development process. Tranilast is an allergy medication that had been linked to hyperbilirubinemia in about 10% of patients who took the medication.[8] Potential enzymes were identified, and from these enzymes the genes that code for them were analyzed and a genetic variant was identified. This occurred during phase III trials of the medication; however, the protocol was still able to be updated to exclude patients with this mutation.

A goal of the pharmaceutical industry is to identify potential problems as early as possible. In both of the examples provided above, the PG issue occurred either late in the research process or after the medication was released. Since the Human Genome Project has been completed, it is easier for industry officials to identify potential problems based on PG differences. However, even if a PG problem is identified, the potential market loss by excluding a large number of patients may impact research in the area, leading to decreased numbers of studies on drugs that may be limited by PG variances.

Impact of Pharmacogenomics on the Cost of Healthcare

Before a new medication is readily accepted as standard therapy, it must be shown to be safe, effective, and cost-effective. PG has been shown in previous chapters to impact the way medications interact differently in individual patients. However, cost effectiveness or perceived cost effectiveness may limit its widespread acceptance into standard-of-care therapies. Cost effectiveness just reviewing the effectiveness of medications will probably not be significant.

However, when cost avoidance is considered, through the reduction of adverse events with specific medications and the reduction of time to adequate treatment, PG testing could provide significant cost savings.

In theory, PG testing and implementation will be cost-effective since once a variant is found in a patient, it may positively impact his or her future therapy and thus money may be saved over the lifetime of the patient.[9] Two issues factor into the true cost of the exam and impede the implementation of wide spread genetic testing: cost of the test and prevalence of the mutation. The cost tests vary from less than $100 to significantly more than $1000. As the number of genetic tests increase, the economy of scale should help lower the individual test cost. The frequency of the variant, though, will most likely not change. If the frequency of the variant is very low, this means a significant number of patients must be screened prior to finding a patient who has the mutation.

For maximal cost-effectiveness, the cost of the test must be low and the prevalence of the mutation should be high. The final component considered in cost-effectiveness is how much money is saved from "saving" the patient from medications that may harm them due to genetic variations. This number is hard to obtain due to expression of the PG mutation occurring over the life of the patient with undiscovered therapies whose side effects are unknown along with their interaction with the mutation.[9] In the end, the amount of savings must be higher than the cost of the test divided by the prevalence of the mutation. If this is not true, then the genetic test is not cost-effective and should not be adopted as a standard of care.

Resources for Pharmacists

No textbook can claim to be the most up-to-date reference for pharmacogenomics as the field is changing rapidly and new information is being released monthly that changes practices and reinforces the enormous amount of information that still needs to be discussed. However, there are some sources where pharmacists interested in pharmacogenomics may find valuable information regarding new data or even summaries of recent date.

Journals

- *The Pharmacogenomics Journal,* published by Nature, Inc., is one of the journals focusing only on pharmacogenomics and the clinical applications of pharmacogenomics. Many of the articles published in the journal involve the determination of genomic mutations and their impact on disease progression and the epidemiology of various genomic mutations. This journal is an excellent resource for pharmacists who already have an understanding of pharmacogenomics and how it could be used in the future. Readers should have an understanding of the disease states discussed prior to reading the journal article. The journal is available by subscription at http://www.nature.com/tpj/.
- The journal of *Clinical Pharmacology & Therapeutics* provides basic science research, clinical practice research, and in depth review articles that cover pharmacogenomics. The research presented in the journal is current and provides practice-related insights. As the above journal, some baseline knowledge of PG and the various disease states is needed to obtain the maximum benefit from the journal. The journal is available by subscription at http://www.nature.com/clpt.

- *Future Medicine—Pharmacogenomics* is a journal available online with a subscription that posts both primary research and substantial review articles that could bring a reader with a low comprehension of a pharmacogenomic up to speed. Additionally they often focus on one medication's pharmacogenomic properties, thus allowing the pharmacist to have a complete understanding of how different genomic properties impact that specific drug or even class. The journal is available in print and at http://www.futuremedicine.com/loi/pgs.
- Other journals, such as *Pharmacotherapy* and the *American Journal of Health-System Pharmacy,* which already include pharmacogenomic studies and review articles will increase the frequency of each in the coming years as the need for pharmacists to have this information increases.

Websites

Any time information is gathered from the internet, some fact checking should occur. Additionally if the website is selling something related to the information you should be very suspicious until your feelings are proved wrong. However, there are some well-known and respectable websites that can provide pharmacists with information that is relevant to their practice and accurate.

- http://www.pharmgkb.org/—The Pharmacogenetics and Pharmacogenomics Knowledge Base (PPKB) provides an easy-to-use search function to find information that is very relevant. The website allows the viewer to look at specific diseases, medications, and pathways. Additionally, easy links to primary literature and a brief summary of relevant information is available for each of the sections.
- http://hapmap.org—This site, a database of known genetic variances, and research are funded by both private and public entities. They allow for electronic downloads of their database to spur further research. The site is very scientific and would not be recommended for the general public.
- http://www.genetests.org/— Genetests is a National Institutes of Health funded website that provides database searches similar to the PPKB. They invite authors to provide summaries of current data and provide information to healthcare providers on which tests are available for each of the genetic conditions covered in the database.
- http://www.cdc.gov/genomics/—The National Office of Public Health Genomics provides a wealth of information both for pharmacists and the public. The website provides information for patients on what their family medical histories may mean along with fact sheets detailing what pharmacogenomics is and why it is important. For pharmacists, the site provides a weekly update of pharmacogenomic information along with several references and links to primary literature.
- http://www.fda.gov/cder/genomics/default.htm—The Food and Drug Administration provides updates regarding PG. Patients, industry members, and healthcare providers can find relevant information regarding the FDA's requirements for PG testing in medications and forms to be completed if problems arise.

Summary

The promise of pharmacogenomics on the practice of pharmacy is both exciting and confusing. As the previous chapters have documented, the amount of information already present is large, with new information being released every month. The pharmacist will be responsible for this information in the same way the pharmacist is responsible for knowing drug–drug interactions currently. Other healthcare providers will be turning to the "drug experts" for advice on how to handle the many genomic mutations that will be determined to be clinically relevant. As mentioned in this chapter, all fields of pharmacy practice will likely be impacted, thus more education is needed to ensure that both practicing pharmacists and pharmacy students are prepared to meet the demand for information that will be occurring in the coming years.

Based on their training, pharmacists are ideally suited to interpret PG patient results and make recommendation for specific drugs to their other healthcare providers. Additionally, pharmacists are the most trained healthcare provider when it comes to drug counseling. Pharmacists are in a unique position to take the lead on PG counseling and what it means to patients.

References

1. Somogyi AA, Barratt DT, Coller JK. Pharmacogenetics of opioids. *Clin Pharmacol Ther.* 2007;81:429-444.
2. Group TSC. SLCO1B1 variants and statin-induced myopathy—a genomewide study. *N Engl J Med.* 2008;359:789-799.
3. Johnson JA. Ethnic differences in cardiovascular drug response: potential contribution of pharmacogenetics. *Circulation.* 2008;118:1383-1393.
4. Dicpinigaitis PV. Angiotensin-converting enzyme inhibitor-induced cough: ACCP evidence-based clinical practice guidelines. *Chest.* 2006;129(1_suppl):169S-173S.
5. Gurwitz D, Wetzman A, Rehavi M. Education: teaching pharmacogenomics to prepare future physicians and researchers for personalized medicine. *Pharm Sci.* 2003;24:122-125.
6. Zdanowicz MM, Huston SA, Weston GW. Pharmacogenomics in the professional pharmacy curriculum: content, presentation and importance. Available at: http://www.samford.edu/schools/pharmacy/ijpe/206/206.html. Accessed June 15, 2009.
7. Latif DA. Pharmacogenetics and pharmacogenomics instruction in schools of pharmacy in the USA: is it adequate? *Pharmacogenomics.* 2005;6:317-319.
8. Roses AD. Genome-based pharmacogenetics and the pharmaceutical industry. *Nat Rev Drug Discov.* 2002;1:541-549.
9. Wedlund PJ, de Leon J. Pharmacogenomic testing: the cost factor. *Pharmacogenomics J.* 2001;1:171-174.

Index